Management and Leadership for Nurse Managers

———The Jones and Bartlett Series in Nursing———

Management and Leadership for Nurse Managers

RUSSELL C. SWANSBURG, PH.D., R.N., C.N.A.A.

Professor of Nursing Administration
School of Nursing
Medical College of Georgia

JONES AND BARTLETT PUBLISHERS
Boston

To my wife,
Laurel C. Swansburg, R.N.

Editorial, Sales, and Customer Service Offices

Jones and Bartlett Publishers
20 Park Plaza
Boston, MA 02116

Printed in the United States of America
10 9 8 7 6 5 4 3

Library of Congress Cataloging-in-Publication Data

Swansburg, Russell C.
    Management and leadership for nurse managers / by Russell C.
  Swansburg
      p. cm.
    Includes bibliographical references.
    ISBN 0-86720-439-7
    1. Nursing services—Administration. 2. Leadership. I. Title.
    [DNLM: 1. Administrative Personnel. 2. Nursing, Supervisory. WY
  105 S972m]
  RT89.S89 1990
  362.1′73′068—dc20
  DNLM/DLC
  for Library of Congress   89-71678
                                       CIP

ISBN: 0-86720-439-7

Production Services Coordinator: Judy Salvucci
Production: Editing, Design, & Production, Inc.
Cover design: Rafael Millán

Foreword

Alice looked around her in great surprise. "Why, I do believe we've been under this tree the whole time! Everything's just as it was!"

"Of course it is," said the Queen. "What would you have it?"

"Well, in our country," said Alice, still panting a little, "you'd generally have gotten somewhere else if you ran very fast for a long time as we've been doing."

"A slow sort of country!" said the Queen. "Now, here, you see, it takes all the running you can do, to keep in the same place. If you want to get somewhere else, you must run at least twice as fast as that!"

In the contemporary world of the health-care environment, the nursing manager is often left with the feeling that Alice expresses—a feeling of running exceedingly fast and finding yourself merely "staying even." The words of the Queen seem to be as reflective of our time as they were of 1872, when Lewis Carroll committed them to paper in *Through the Looking Glass.*

I feel deeply honored to have been invited by Russell Swansburg to write the foreword for his book. For the pace that is required of us today as nursing managers, a contemporary guide to our science is necessary. This volume provides the elements of the essential "tool kit" for today's nurse manager.

In his book, Dr. Swansburg has approached nursing management in the same way one might approach any other specialty in nursing today. I truly believe that nursing management is a specialty with its own unique body of complex knowledge and skills. As with texts regarding other nursing specialties, Dr. Swansburg's work describes both the art and the science of contemporary nursing management.

As the art and science of nursing management change, so changes the role of the nurse manager. This book provides those who assume the roles of nursing leadership in today's health-care institutions with both the theoretical and practical knowledge to deal with the shifting demands. As Alice found, as soon as the rules are defined and you think you know what they are, they change. Dr. Swansburg describes the theoretical underpinnings of the historical and current concepts of management. He then gives examples of the application of those concepts from the Institutional to the patient care unit level. By using this approach, the nurse manager is prepared to successfully negotiate the ambiguities of the environment.

To borrow once again from Alice's description of the health-care environment (in *Alice's Adventures in Wonderland* 1865):

"This is very curious!" Alice thought. "But everything is curious today."

Dr. Swansburg's very timely book and approach have provided us with keys.

By taking the little golden key, and unlocking the door, Alice said to herself, "Now, I'll manage better this time."

Jenny R. James, M.S., R.N.
Vice President for Nursing
Brigham and Women's Hospital
Boston, Massachusetts

Preface

This book provides theoretical and practical knowledge that will aid each nurse manager to meet the demands of constantly changing patient-care services. The extreme shortage of nurses is closely related to the management process. Financial considerations have dominated the health-care industry in recent years, making the job of managing scarce and costly human and material resources even more important. As health care has moved out of hospitals, more nurse management positions have evolved in skilled nursing facilities, ambulatory care centers, hospices, home health care agencies, and staffing agencies. New nurse management positions are developing.

This book will focus on management abilities needed by nurse managers, including knowing how to manage nursing activities so that professional nurses will be able to practice the primary functions of clinical nursing: assessment, diagnosis, prescription, and evaluation. It provides essential theoretical and practical knowledge in several areas: first, planning and managing the budget, since those who control budgets thereby control activities paid for by those budgets; second, developing and implementing personnel policies that assist staff to work effectively toward individual goals as well as those of the unit, department, division, and organization; third, learning about leadership skills and employee motivation; and fourth, learning to make sound decisions that contribute to progress.

Managers oversee many tasks involving many people with specialized knowledge and skills. The management role may be played by charge nurses of shifts and head nurses or supervisors of units, wards, departments, clinics, and agencies. This book is intended as an aid to improving communication, enhancing assignment planning and priority setting, and developing training and education programs that lead to staff satisfaction. Through the evaluation process, nurse managers determine whether they are satisfied with the results, from both their viewpoints and that of their constituents.

This book is organized around the four major management functions of planning, organizing, directing (leading), and controlling (evaluating). It is designed for management development of professional nurses. It can be used in all nursing programs as well as staff development programs in health care agencies.

To the Instructor

Extensive student/teaching supplements are available to accompany this text, including:

- *Student Workbook and Study Guide for Management and Leadership for Nurse Managers,* Swansburg
- *Instructor's Resource Manual with Transparency Masters for Management and Leadership for Nurse Managers,* Swansburg
- *Nursing Management/Leadership Video Library*

Russell C. Swansburg

vii

Introduction

Nursing plays an integral part in the complex, dynamic process of providing health care for patients, families, and communities. Nurses utilize their own professional standards and body of knowledge and work in cooperation with other disciplines to maximize potential for the achievement of positive health status. However, this is not easily accomplished. Nursing leadership is needed to plan and implement necessary patient-care services. Acquisition of sufficient resources is necessary to provide those services, and the quality of programs and services must be monitored to maintain a high level of care delivery. Because health care involves many disciplines, interdisciplinary coordination and cooperation must be encouraged. Technology is changing rapidly, and nurses must keep aware of the technological and sociopolitical milieu that affects the ability to offer programs and services.

Nurse managers can provide the needed leadership and support nurses in their professional role. Nurse managers can act as boundary spanners in working with other disciplines to interpret the goals of nursing and develop coordinated and comprehensive patient-care services. Nurse managers can keep aware of the changing environment and work with their staff to respond to those changes in a positive manner.

Knowledge of management science and a repertoire of administrative skills are required by nurse managers to achieve effective performance. This is in addition to the clinical knowledge base and skills in patient care management that the study of nursing provides. This book provides an avenue for nurses to increase their knowledge of management theories, strategies, and techniques and to relate that knowledge to the practice of nursing management. The use of nursing examples throughout the book demonstrates that relationship.

Chapter 1 discusses theories of management and relates those theories to the principles of nursing management and the development of nursing management theory. Chapters 2 through 10 revolve around the planning function of management.

Dynamics and skills necessary for effective planning are presented. Mission statements, philosophy, objectives, and written operational plans are important pieces of the planning process. Development of a staffing plan is essential to the acquisition of resources required to facilitate the provision of services. People are the cornerstone of any organization, and the development of a personnel management system provides a framework for the creation of positive management-employee relationships. In such a climate employees can feel valued for their efforts, supported to facilitate productivity, and motivated to provide the desired level of service. Financial resources are essential to the well-being of an organization and to the ability to provide services. The budget is an operational plan translated into dollars. Effective budgeting skills and the ability to develop potential fund sources and compete for limited resources are presented in Chapter 6.

Planning for the delivery of nursing care services involves an understanding of nursing theory, modalities of care delivery, utilization of the nursing process, and the impact of ethical and legal issues. Policies and procedures facilitate the delivery of nursing services. Regulatory constraints can be adhered to and communicated to the staff through the development and effective use of those policies and procedures. Effective planning depends on the ability to make decisions in complex situations. In Chapter 9, Dr. Claudette Coleman provides models and strategies of decision making that can be utilized in developing and strengthening problem solving skills. Change is inherent in the planning process. The theory and strategies for understanding and working with the ramifications and impact of change are presented in Chapter 10.

Chapters 11 through 13 encompass the organizational functions of management. Organization theory is related to the health care setting and development of a supportive organizational climate for the provision of nursing care. The complexity of health care organizations generates the need to organize the manner in which work can be accomplished, so that work can proceed in a timely and effective fashion. Work organization frequently calls for the use of committees. In many instances the use of selected groups or committees can enhance the productivity of the individual. Techniques that may be utilized to keep committees producing effective results are discussed in Chapter 12. Arguments are then presented for the effective use of participatory management as a means to encourage a healthy work environment and make maximum use of employees' abilities.

The management function of leading and/or directing is discussed in Chapters 14 through 21. Leaders provide the vision and ability to facilitate staff response to the ever changing world of work. Within health care organizations, nursing managers are key players in producing effective patient care systems and directing patient care activities to maintain high levels of care. Nurses are expected to be professional care providers and, as such, have the knowledge, resources, and commitment to take responsibility for their actions. Nurse managers can tap those resources and commitment through common goal setting and effective delegation. Effective use of delegation can reduce the managerial workload to reasonable levels, avoiding work overload for the manager and, at the same time, encouraging a positive sense of responsibility and self-esteem for the employee. In Chapter 15, Dr. Sharon Farley presents a discussion of leadership theory and styles in relation to leadership for nursing and the acquisition of appropriate power to support the leadership role.

Motivation theories and applications to nursing management are presented in Chapter 16. Motivated employees are effective producers, but effective communication is also essential to employee understanding and acceptance of direction. Effective communication is a two-way process, flowing between employees and managers and clarifying and validating individual perceptions. Techniques to recognize barriers and develop effective communication are discussed. Richard Swansburg continues the emphasis on communication with a discussion of technologies available to enhance communication. Computerized management information systems can provide the nursing manager with an array of tools that can be used to enhance managerial decision making. Nurse managers must be aware of system capabilities and how they can be maximized to present information in usable form without producing a data overload. Nurse managers also must be aware of the limitations of the systems.

In Chapter 19, Louvenia Ward presents the principles of supervision and the relationship of leadership style, communication, and motivation to the work of nursing supervision and the goal of quality patient care. In addition to their role as supervisors, effective nurse managers also function as teachers, encouraging the professional growth of their staff. Dr. Sharon Farley discusses principles of adult learning and staff development. Concluding the discussion of leading and/or directing is the recognition of the potential for conflict wherever people interact. Conflict in health care settings occurs among members of professional disciplines, among patients, families, and staff, and among members within a single discipline. Conflict can be constructive as well as destructive. The management of conflict is an essential skill for nursing managers.

The controlling function, or evaluation, is the emphasis for Chapters 22 through 25. Control is identified as being used to determine whether goals are being achieved, and includes coordination, decision-making related to planning and organizing, and information from directing and worker performance evaluation. Quality assurance is identified as a major component of a master evaluation or controlling plan. Standards and management processes involved in quality assurance are discussed. Controlling and evaluation programs are not complete without the recognition of the importance of clarification of job responsibilities as demonstrated in job descriptions and employee performance appraisals. Performance appraisals provide the opportunity for feedback for both employee and manager and can be used constructively to promote growth and reward appropriate performance. The effective use of performance standards and appraisal within a reward system based on merit is the concluding chapter.

Throughout the book, examples relate to real situations and tool formats that have been shown to be effective. Nurse managers in the clinical setting can adapt the practical techniques presented for use in their own setting. Both nurse managers and students should take advantage of the organized presentation of the material and references that can be utilized for further learning.

Arlene J. Lowenstein, Ph.D., RN
Chair, Department of Nursing Administration
Medical College of Georgia
Augusta, Georgia

Contents

Theory of Nursing Management

1

WHAT IS MANAGEMENT?

Modern management theory evolved from the work of Henri Fayol, who identified the administrator's activities or functions as planning, organizing, coordinating, and controlling.[1] Fayol defined management in these words:

> To manage is to forecast and plan, to organize, to command, to coordinate, and to control. To foresee and provide means examining the future and drawing up the plan of action. To organize means building up the dual structure, material and human, of the undertaking. To command means binding together, unifying and harmonizing all activity and effort. To control means seeing that everything occurs in conformity with established rule and expressed demand.[2]

While some persons believed these were technical functions to be learned only on the job, Fayol believed that they could be taught in an educational setting if a theory of administration could be formulated.[3] He also stated that the need for managerial ability increased in relative importance as an individual advanced in the chain of command.[4]

Fayol listed the principles of management as follows:

1. Division of work
2. Authority
3. Discipline
4. Unity of command
5. Unity of direction
6. Subordination of individual interests to the general interest
7. Remuneration
8. Centralization
9. Scalar chain (line of authority)
10. Order
11. Equity

12. Stability or tenure of personnel
13. Initiative
14. Esprit de corps.[5]

Another theorist in the development of the science and art of management was L. Urwick. He indicated that administrative skill is a practical art that improves with practice and requires hard study and thinking. The administrator has to master intellectual principles, the process being reinforced by general reflection about actual problems. From his work Urwick concluded that there are three principles of administration. He described the first principle as that of *investigation* and stated that all scientific procedure is based on investigation of the facts. Investigation takes effect in *planning*. The second principle is *appropriateness*, which underlines *forecasting*, entering into process with *organization* and taking effect in *coordination*. Exercising the third principle, the administrator looks ahead and organizes *resources* to meet future needs. Planning enters into process with *command* and is effected in *control*.[6]

Throughout management literature, the original functions of planning, organizing, directing (command and coordination), and controlling as defined by Fayol, Urwick, and others have been accepted as the principal functions of managers. Managing means accomplishing the goals of the group through effective and efficient use of resources. The *manager* creates and maintains an internal environment in an enterprise in which individuals work together as a group. *Managing* is the art of doing, while *management* is the body of organized knowledge underlying the art. In modern management, staffing is frequently separated from the planning function, directing has been labeled "leading" or "supervising," and "controlling" is used interchangeably with "evaluating."

Theories, Concepts, and Principles

The knowledge base of management science includes theories, which in turn include concepts, methods, and principles. The principles are related and can be observed and verified to some degree when they are translated into the art or practice of management. *Concepts* are thoughts, ideas, and general notions about a class of objects that form a basis for action or discussion. *Principles* are fundamental truths, laws, or doctrine on which other notions are based. Principles provide guidance to concepts and to thought or action in a situation.[7] In nursing management, research—Urwick's "investigation of facts"—becomes part of the theory of the field.

If nursing is going to base its theories on laws, nurses will need to validate principles through research. This is a difficult task, as theorists in the social sciences have discovered. It is difficult to reduce human behavior to laws. Nurses deal with human behavior in all roles, but particularly so in nursing management.

White explores a viewpoint on nursing theories in which she addresses "prescriptive theories." She notes that their use as practical guidelines "must be broad enough to encompass a wide range of practice situations but not so broad as to be meaningless." A theory of decision making might be more beneficial than a theory of nursing in the practice arena. Nurses believe that for nursing to be a real profession, it should have a scientific and theoretical base. Nursing is thus a practice profession based on the physical and social sciences.[8]

Nurse managers learn to merge the disciplines of human relations, labor relations, personnel management, and industrial engineering into a unifying force for effective management. Many nurse managers would add the theory of nursing to this list. A successful synthesis of these disciplines would promote employee commitment, increased productivity, good labor relations, and competitiveness in health care. If these goals are not achieved, the work force is poorly managed.

There are contradictions in management theory because of a lack of agreement about sets of ideas and concepts among and within disciplines.[9] Two common approaches are described in the following sections.

Critical Theory

Steffy and Grimes note that a strict natural science approach to the social sciences is naive because subjective or qualitative analysis is important to quantitative research. This holds true for management and, consequently, for nursing management. Health care organizational models are not objective and value-free. The authors suggest a critical approach to organizational science rather than a phenomenological or hermeneutic approach.

A phenomenological approach uses second-order constructs or "interpretations of interpretations." It requires researchers to become participants in the organization and to suspend all judgments and preconceived ideas of possible meanings. The nurse manager would interpret the meaning of nursing management experiences or observations and arrive at a nursing management theory from the aggregate of meanings.

Hermeneutics is the art of textual interpretation. The nurse manager as researcher would view herself or himself as an historically produced entity and would recognize personal biases when doing research. She or he would consider the specific context and historic dimensions of data collected and would reflect on the relationship between theory and history.[10]

Critical theory is an empirical philosophy of social institutions. Theories are translated into practice by decision makers, in this case nurse managers. "Theories in use" are behavioral technologies that include Organizational Development (OD), Management by Objectives (MBO), performance appraisal, and other practice-oriented activities performed by managers. Critical theory aims to (1) critique the ideology of scientism, "the institutionalized form of reasoning which accepts the idea that the meaning of knowledge is defined by what the sciences do and thus can be adequately explicated through analysis of scientific procedures"; and (2) "to develop an organizational science capable of changing organizational processes." These aims are compatible with a theory of nursing management. Nurses are using science to legitimize the practice of clinical nursing and nursing management.[11]

More descriptive research studies are needed in nursing management. This will require more nurse managers be trained in nursing research and suggests that the members of the nursing community ought to unify to implement a critical theory of nursing management. Nursing administration researchers could validate organizational knowledge against objectively verifiable criteria of "purposive-rational" action or through consensus of "communicative" action. Nurses construct and possess a language of nursing (shared symbols). Critical theory will include the cognitive intent, or aim of research, and the values and beliefs of the researcher. Nurse managers employing a critical theory approach would determine how their subordinates interpret organizational phenomena. They would discuss possible falsities of interpretations with them, bringing out illusions and delusions.[12]

General Systems Theory

General systems theory is an organismic approach to the study of the general relationships of the empirical universe of an organization and human thought. It grew out of biology as an analogy between an organism and a social organization. Boulding describes nine levels of a general systems theory.[13] They are given here with nursing management applications.

1. *A static structure or level of frameworks.* Nursing is a discipline with an aggregate population of registered nurses (educated at several levels, including those with hospital diplomas and associate through doctoral degrees), licensed practical nurses, and nonlicensed persons (for example, aides, orderlies, attendants, nursing assistants, and clerks). They function within an organizational structure of superior-subordinate relationships with a top administrator, middle managers, and practitioners. Usually these persons function in an environment where the focus of attention is the client. One approach to a framework in nursing is that nurses apply the nursing process in giving care to patients. There are many similarities between nursing process and nursing management. See Figure 1–1.

2. *A moving level of predetermined necessary motions or clockworks.* Nurse managers process the knowledge and skills of nursing management—nursing planning, organizing, leading, and evaluating—to produce nursing care through nursing management. The function of nursing management is the use of personnel, supplies, equipment, and clinical knowledge and skills to give nursing care to clients within varying environments. One of these environments is the hospital physical plant. Nursing planning (NP) plus nursing organizing (NO) plus nursing leading (NL) plus nursing evaluating (NE) equals nursing management (NM):

$$NP + NO + NL + NE = NM$$

To this we may add that nursing management (NM) plus nursing practice (NP) equals nursing care of clients (NCC). The move is toward equilibrium.

FIGURE 1–1. An Open System

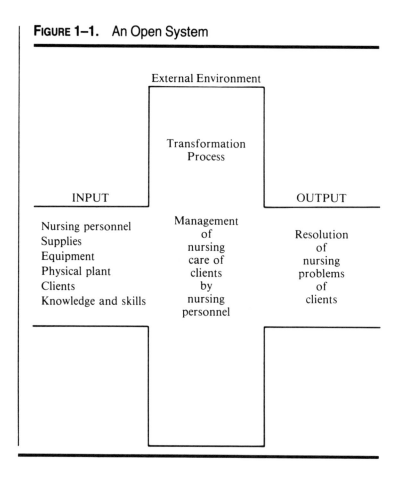

External Environment

Transformation Process

INPUT

Nursing personnel
Supplies
Equipment
Physical plant
Clients
Knowledge and skills

Management
of
nursing
care of
clients
by
nursing
personnel

OUTPUT

Resolution
of
nursing
problems
of
clients

3. *A control mechanism level—the thermostat.* In nursing administration this thermostat could be the top administrator or any subordinate manager. This person maintains a management information system that transmits and interprets information and communication to and from employees. Production of nursing care of satisfactory quality and quantity depends upon the manager maintaining an environment satisfactory to employees.

4. *The level of the open-system or self-maintaining structure—the cell.* Nursing management will survive and maintain the nursing organization by being open to new ideas, new techniques of management, and the input of human and material resources to produce the nursing care needed by clients. It will reproduce itself by keeping up to date and by developing replacements.

5. *The genetic-societal level.* There is a division of labor even within nursing management, but especially among nursing personnel who produce the nursing care of patients. The raw materials—human and material resources—are *input.* They are processed as *throughput* by a group of nursing personnel with varying knowledge and skills. The *output* is the nursing care of clients produced.

6. *The "animal" level.* This level has increased mobility, teleological (designing or purposeful) behavior, and self-awareness. Some evidence is emerging that nursing management is reaching this level. As nurse managers learn the knowledge and skills of the business and industrial world, they are adapting them to the management of nursing services. This puts nursing management and nursing practice on a much more scientific basis, the end result of which may be that nurses will be able to demonstrate how what they do affects the clients' outcomes: from empiricism to theory.

7. *The "human" level.* The nurse manager develops a self-consciousness and knows that he or she can

process the knowledge and skills of management to produce specific results.

8. *The level of social organization.* Nurse managers at this level distinguish themselves from other groups of managers. Nurse managers operate within complex roles; their functions are made effective by communication.

9. *Transcendental systems.* At this level nurse managers ask questions for which there are as yet no answers. Theoretical models of nursing management extend to level 4, the level of application of most other models. Empirical knowledge is deficient at nearly all levels. Descriptive models are needed to catalogue events in nursing. The movement toward decentralization and participatory management is still a very simple system. General systems theory is the skeleton of a science.

Disciplines and sciences have bodies of theory (or knowledge) that grow with meaningful information. The empirical universe provides general phenomena relevant to many different disciplines including nursing. These phenomena can be built into theoretical models, including one for nursing management. Nursing as a discipline has varied populations (phenomena) that have dynamic interactions among themselves. These include professional nurses, technical nurses, practical nurses, and nonlicensed nursing personnel, as well as professional nursing teachers, researchers, and managers. Individuals within the discipline interact with the environment (another phenomenon). Through knowledge and experience they grow, growth being a universally significant phenomenon. The media for growth are information and communication, other phenomena.[14]

Another version of the key concepts of general systems theory is summarized in Figure 1–2.

NURSING MANAGEMENT

In nursing, management relates to performing the functions of planning, organizing, staffing, leading (directing) and controlling (evaluating) the activities of a nursing enterprise or division of nursing departments and departmental subunits. A nurse manager performs these management functions to deliver health care to patients. Nurse managers or administrators work at all levels to put into practice the concepts, principles, and theories of nursing management. They manage the organizational environment to provide a climate optimal to provision of nursing care by the clinical nurses.

Management knowledge is universal; so is nursing management knowledge. It uses a systematic body of knowledge that includes concepts, principles, and theories applicable to all nursing management situations. A nurse manager who has applied this knowledge successfully in one situation can be expected to do so in new situations. Nursing management occurs at the head nurse, supervisor, and director or executive levels. At the director or executive level, it is frequently termed "administration." The theories, principles, and concepts remain the same. They can all be classified under the major functions of nursing management or nursing administration.

Nursing administration is the application of the art and science of management to the discipline of nursing. Nursing management is also the group of nurse managers who manage the nursing organization or enterprise. Finally, nursing management is the process by which nurse managers practice their profession. Although many nursing management jobs do not require special certification, such certification is available. The American Nurses' Association awards two levels of management certification: Certified Nurse Administrator and Certified Nurse Administrator, Advanced. The American Organization of Nurse Executives has in the past certified nurse managers at the nominee, candidate, and fellow levels. Both programs require education, experience, and examinations.

Who Needs Nursing Management?

All types of health-care organizations, including nursing homes, hospitals, home health-care agencies, ambulatory care centers, student infirmaries, and many others, need nursing management. Even the nurse working with one client and family needs management knowledge and skills to help people work together to accomplish a common goal. A primary nurse working with several clients prioritizes their care to assist them to improved health or, sometimes, peaceful death.[15]

FIGURE 1–2. Key Concepts of General Systems Theory

Subsystems or Components. A system by definition is composed of interrelated parts or elements. This is true for all systems—mechanical, biological, and social. Every system has at least two elements, and these elements are interconnected.

Holism, Synergism, Organicism, and Gestalt. The whole is not just the sum of the parts; the system itself can be explained only as a totality. Holism is the opposite of elementarism, which views the total as the sum of its individual parts.

Open-Systems View. Systems can function in one of two ways: (1) closed or (2) open. Open systems exchange information, energy, or material with their environments. Biological and social systems are inherently open systems; mechanical systems may be open or closed. The concepts of open and closed systems are difficult to defend in the absolute. We prefer to think of open–closed as a continuum; that is, systems are relatively open or relatively closed.

Input-Transformation-Output Model. The open system can be viewed as a transformation model. In a dynamic relationship with its environment, it receives various inputs, transforms these inputs in some way, and exports outputs.

System Boundaries. It follows that systems have boundaries that separate them from their environments. The concept of boundaries helps us understand the distinction between open and closed systems. The relatively closed system has rigid, impenetrable boundaries, whereas the open system has permeable boundaries between itself and a broader suprasystem. Boundaries are relatively easily defined in physical and biological systems but are harder to delineate in social systems such as organizations.

Negative Entropy. Closed physical systems are subject to the force of entropy, which increases until eventually the entire system fails. The tendency toward maximum entropy is a movement to disorder, complete lack of resource transformation, and death. In a closed system, the change in entropy must always be positive; however, in open biological or social systems, entropy can be arrested and may even be transformed into negative entropy—a process of more complete organization and ability to transform resources—because the system imports resources from its environment.

Steady State, Dynamic Equilibrium, and Homeostasis. The concept of a steady state is closely related to that of negative entropy. A closed system eventually must attain an equilibrium state with maximum entropy—death or disorganization. However, an open system may attain a state in which the system remains in dynamic equilibrium through the continuous inflow of materials, energy, and information.

Feedback. The concept of feedback is important for understanding how a system maintains a steady state. Information concerning the outputs or the process of the system is fed back as an input into the system, perhaps leading to changes in the transformation process or in future outputs. Feedback can be positive or negative, although the field of cybernetics is based on negative feedback. Negative feedback is informational input that indicates that the system is deviating from a prescribed course and should readjust to a new steady state.

Hierarchy. A basic concept in systems thinking is that of hierarchical relationships among systems. A system is composed of subsystems of a lower order and is also part of a suprasystem. Thus, there is a hierarchy of the components of the system.

Internal Elaboration. Closed systems move toward entropy and disorganization. In contrast, open systems appear to move in the direction of greater differentiation, elaboration, and a higher level of organization.

Multiple Goal–Seeking. Biological and social systems appear to have multiple goals or purposes. Social organizations seek multiple goals, if for no other reason than that they are composed of subunits and individuals with different values and objectives.

Equifinality of Open Systems. In mechanistic systems there is a direct cause-and-effect relationship between the initial condition and the final state. Biological and social systems operate differently. Equifinality suggests that certain results may be achieved with different initial conditions and in different ways. This view suggests that social organizations can accomplish their objectives with diverse inputs and with varying internal activities (conversion processes).

SOURCE: F. E. Kast and J. E. Rosenzweig, "General Systems Theory: Applications for Organization and Management," *Academy of Management Journal*, December 1972, 447–464. Reprinted with permission.

General Principles of Nursing Management

Nursing Management Is Planning. Planning is primary to all other activities or functions of management. Planning is a thinking or conceptual act that is frequently committed to writing. Although many people in nursing make plans informally, the commitment of plans to paper is essential to their accomplishment. If plans are not written down, they probably will not be implemented.

Planning is the forecasting of events—the building of an operational plan. Planning is also a management function of every nursing leader—from professional clinical nurse to head nurses, supervisors, directors, and administrators.

Planning is an important management function that helps reduce the risks of decision making, problem solving, and effecting planned change. The nursing manager who learns to plan will aim for maximum utilization of all resources—money, supplies, equipment, and, of course, personnel.

Planning will help workers achieve job satisfaction. All people plan their activities to some extent. Individual plans may include a weekly schedule of personal events, a sequential list of daily activities, or an appointment calendar. A predetermined fire evacuation route is a special kind of plan—a disaster plan.

Planning requires a knowledge of the characteristics of the planning processes and the relationships within a system; planning elements; planning standards; knowledge of and skill in, implementing the planning process, including applying standards to the work situation; and acquisition of the skills necessary to bring the planning process up to the set standards. Planning makes the utilization of time effective. During the planning function, nurse managers analyze and assess the system, set organizational and personal long-range (strategic) and short-range (tactical or operational) objectives, assess present organizational resources and capabilities, and specify and prioritize activities, including alternatives.

Management plans are business plans. They specify goals, strategies, responsibilities, policies, and budgets. They use directions, progress, adjustments, and measurement. Management planning forces nurse managers to analyze unit activities and structure. It is a process of human action and interaction, the work environment being a microcosm of society.

Health-care organizations are social entities in which cooperation and competition conflict. They have life and character as well as patterns of behavior that become entrenched. Personal success is tied to organizational success in the form of paychecks, promotions, careers, and job security. Peer pressure among nurses may create conflict with the goals of the organization.

Ratcliffe and Logsdon specify six stages in the planning process:

1. Design stage
2. Delegation stage
3. Education stage
4. Development stage
5. Implementation stage
6. Follow-up stage (performance evaluation and feedback)

Personnel are involved in goal setting, performance evaluation, and feedback on a continual basis. Business planning takes into account the behavioral process.[16]

Nursing Management Is the Effective Utilization of Time. Because management is the effective utilization of time, successful nurse managers plan in order to use their time effectively. In nursing, management is affected by the abilities and limitations of the nurse manager, who has a theory or systematic set of management principles and methods that relate to the larger institution and the nursing organization within it. Such a theory will include knowledge of the mission or purpose of the institution but may require development or revision of the mission or purpose of the nursing division. From a clearly defined mission statement, the nurse manager develops clear and realistic objectives for nursing services. This theory will also provide the foundation on which the nurse manager makes operational or management plans, sets priorities, formulates strategies, and assigns work. Managerial jobs and structures are designed from this theory. Decisions of top managers—at least those of the chair of the nursing division—will be affected by input from lower levels of highly knowledgeable and skilled personnel. It is good management practice to seek this input rather than block or discount it, because it is often a source of imaginative proposals that can be incorporated into improvements in personnel management and, ultimately, nursing practices and patient care services. Application of knowledge of a theory or systematic set of principles and methods of nursing management is necessary for the effective utilization of time. See Figure 1–3.

Nurse managers' decisions will be influenced by time elements, as all management decisions are so influenced. Management decisions take into account the future, particularly with regard to human resources. Nursing management performs in the present while planning for future performance, growth, and change.

All resources are finite, including nursing personnel and the supplies and equipment used. Resources are managed for efficiency and effectiveness to achieve productivity—output of a given amount during a specified time that generates enough income to exceed expenses and realize a profit. Effective utilization of time requires the implementation of plans by an organization directed toward productivity.

Nursing Management Is Decision Making.   Nursing management requires decisions to be made by nurse managers at every level, from division to depart-ment to ward or unit. This is especially true where a service is provided 24 hours a day. The process of decision making will vary depending on whether traditional patterns of communication are followed or decision making is decentralized to the level of its implementation; see Figure 1–4.

Meeting Patients' Nursing Care Needs Is the Business of the Nurse Manager.   The patient is the starting point at which the business of nursing is defined, and it is the patient who is to be satisfied. Nursing management performs the activities needed to determine what patients see, think, believe, and want. Part of the performance is to be sure patients are asked, because they buy their care and therefore buy satisfaction of wants. Anticipatory management means building into objectives a determination of what the business of nursing is, will be, and should be, discarding the obsolete through systematic abandonment.

To achieve these objectives nurse managers perform three major tasks in which they manage human and material resources. These are:

1. Perform to achieve a specific purpose or mission for the division, department, and ward or unit.
2. Make work productive.
3. Manage social impacts and social responsibilities.

Management and practice are involved in all three tasks of nurse managers. The end product,

FIGURE 1–3.   Examples of Effective Utilization of Time

1. The chief nurse executive keeps an appointment schedule that relates to management plans. This schedule is followed for all activities—organizational meetings, divisional meetings, professional meetings, travel, rounds, individual appointments, and so on.

2. The head nurse of a home health-care agency has planned staff meetings at the beginning and end of each week. Schedules of individual nurses are reviewed at each meeting and are compared with productivity goals that balance the budget.

3. A home health-care nurse reviews the schedule each day. It must be tightened so that five more patient visits can be added during the 40-hour workweek. Otherwise, a merit pay increase will not materialize.

FIGURE 1–4.   Examples of Managerial Decision Making

1. A staff nurse decides whether to apply for a clinical promotion. If the application is accepted, a performance results contract will require additional productivity, including continuing education and increased participation on committees and in special nursing activities such as discharge planning and quality assurance studies. It will also result in higher pay.

2. The chief nurse executive makes a decision as to whether to increase the number of clinical nurse III positions in the budget or allocate more funds to head nurse development. Both are needed and the pros and cons of splitting limited resources have to be weighed.

the work of the personnel other than managers, is the practice of nursing. The social impact and social responsibilities of nursing have been highly visible when nurses have gone on strike or serious shortages of nurses have occurred.

Professional nurses are primarily knowledge workers, applying their knowledge to the gathering of data, the making of nursing diagnoses and nursing prescriptions, the supervision of the implementation of the nursing care plan by skilled workers, and the evaluation and adjustment of the plan. They are clinical decision makers. Their work involves skills and the training of skilled workers; however, nurse managers recognize that the primary functions of professional nurses are based on expert, in-depth knowledge. Nurses earn their livelihood and probably gain their greatest job satisfaction with knowledge gained in an educational institution and put to work in a service institution. That same knowledge is used to build the society within which those institutions exist and to achieve institutional goals. According to Drucker, "to make our institutions perform responsibly, autonomously, and on a high level of achievement is thus the only safeguard of freedom and dignity in the pluralistic society of institutions."[17]

Nursing as an institution does not make decisions; nurse managers do. Management is essential to the institution of nursing. It is independent of ownership, rank, or power, being an objective function that ought to be grounded in responsibility for performance. Nurse managers are the professionals who practice the discipline of nursing management, carry out its functions, and discharge its tasks.

Nursing performance results in care that will meet patients' needs, the care being a product potentially desired by all people at a cost they can afford. Care given is the end product of management of a division of nursing. Nurse managers design a model organization that will provide this product. Nursing workers see themselves as resources who have the opportunity of producing nursing care services. Nurse managers will build and manage new nursing organizations and at the same time manage the old or existing ones.

People are the true resource of the division of nursing, and people are made productive by effective nursing management. Through the nursing function they earn their livelihood and find access to their needs for social status, community and individual achievement, and satisfaction. Nurse managers make the work environment suitable for practicing nurses to meet needs related to their personalities, to controls over quantity and quality of work, and to citizenship. The satisfaction of these needs requires opportunity for the individual to assume responsibility, to be an active participant in planning work, to gain satisfaction, to receive incentives and awards, to give leadership to others, to achieve status, to be motivated, and to fulfill a function. See Figure 1–5.

Nursing Management Is the Formulation and Achievement of Social Goals. Social innovation is essential in dealing with the health needs of poor people, people who live in large cities, and people confronted by environmental pollution. The goal of

---

FIGURE 1–5. Examples of Nursing Personnel, Nursing Functions, and Nurse Managers

1. Nursing personnel—Human resources with expert knowledge and skills, they practice nursing to produce patient care.

2. Nursing functions—Ms. Williams practices clinical nursing to earn a living. Other functions of nursing are management, teaching, and research.

Ms. Allen proudly tells people that she works as a registered nurse at the general hospital. Through her work she is satisfying social needs, community needs, and personal needs.

3. Nurse managers—Ms. George tries to place personnel where they desire to work. This is a function of management, and Ms. George is working to satisfy needs related to employee personalities and controls over quantity and quality of work.

Mr. St. Clair makes full use of the recognition program. He sees all performance appraisals and has supervisors make recommendations for recognition of all personnel who are outstanding or who perform unique humanitarian acts. Through his leadership workers will receive incentives and awards, achieve status, and be motivated to provide health care to patients.

meeting such needs is also partly dependent on the nurse manager. The nurse manager manages the institution's social impacts and discharges its social responsibilities relative to nursing. Formulating these goals and supporting clinical nurses in achieving them are managerial tasks; see Figure 1–6.

Professional nurses being knowledge workers, the goal of nurse managers is to make their knowledge productive. To do so requires drastic changes in job structure, careers, and organizations. Knowledge workers learn to plan so that they can be productive. To find out who they are, the kind of work for which they are fitted, and how they work best, clinical nurses are assisted, guided, counseled, and assigned by nurse managers. Nurse managers hold themselves accountable for the quality of work life. Individuals who are fulfilled are able to achieve peak production. Nursing organizations adapt to the needs, aspirations, and potentials of individual members. Development results from human energies as well as from economic wealth.

The nurse manager is often an entrepreneur who recognizes that low-productivity activities are in need of change. One creates new activities to produce new, improved, or better services. The question one might ask is, "Is this activity producing the desired results in terms of patient and personnel satisfactions?" The public wants total health care services at a cost individuals can afford. Managers seek to deliver these services.

Innovation provides better and more economical services. They are marketed so that the patient will be ready to receive them. In the area of staff development the goal of the nurse manager is to make investments in knowledge productive.

Nursing Management Is Organizing.   Organizing is identifying the organizational needs from mission statements and objectives and from observations of work performed, and adapting the organizational design and structure to meet these needs. Like planning, organizing primarily involves thinking.

There are four building blocks for organizational structures:

1. Unit
2. Department
3. The top; the division or executive level of organizational management
4. The operational level, including all phases of work within the organizational structure

During the organizing process, activities are grouped, responsibility and authority are determined, and working relationships are established to enable both the organization and the employees to realize their mutual objectives. The organizational structure relates to the effectiveness of communication. Organizing is a continual process that may take from 1 week to 5 or 10 years. Organizing for decentralization and the participatory management process could fall in the strategic planning category of 3 to 10 years.

Nursing Management Is One Primary Function of the Division of Nursing.   In addition to the main function of nursing management, another main function is the practice of nursing. Both functions have goals of modification or improvement of patient

---

FIGURE 1–6.   Examples of Areas of Goals of Nurse Managers

1. *Health needs of poor people.* A director of nursing in a rural area has sponsored a meeting with other nurse managers from institutions in the area. Their agenda will include discussion of "people who have no health insurance and cannot afford it: identification of their health needs and of ways to meet them." Invited guests include the State Medicaid director and other public health officials.

2. *Health needs of people in large cities.* A nurse manager of an institution in a large city has asked the local nurses' association to assist with a project to identify elderly people with fixed incomes who are in need of health care. Their goal will be to find ways of providing needed health care that is affordable through negotiating with HMOs, PPOs, physicians, hospitals, and other agencies.

3. *Health needs of people confronted with environmental pollution.* After much publicity about lead poisoning of children from local industrial pollutants, the chair of the division of nursing consults with the hospital administrator on determining the health-care needs of children involved. As a consequence nurses are being educated to assist with providing this needed health service to these children.

status. Nursing management must be effective if a health-care organization and the organization of nursing are to function efficiently and effectively.

Nursing Management Denotes a Social Position or Rank, a Discipline, and a Field of Study. A division of nursing has a management function, a management task, and management work. These activities are performed by nurse managers with titles denoting increasing responsibilities using nursing management theory. As in leadership, a title does not make a nurse a manager. A title indicates the position is one of management; see Figure 1–7.

As a discipline, management is a branch of knowledge or learning. The discipline of nursing management draws from the generic discipline of management. Through adoption and application of the methods of the discipline of management, nurse

FIGURE 1–7. Examples of Nursing Management as Function, Social Position or Rank, Discipline, Field of Study, Task, and Work

1. *Nursing management function.* Several of the positions within the organization do not fulfill the purpose for which they exist. The nurse administrator will review the organization and functions of the entire division.

2. *A social position or rank.* Ms. Joliet is assistant chair of a division of nursing.

3. *A discipline.* Ms. Fisk has learned management theory and has been trained to be proficient in all the management skills that make her a strong charge nurse. She is strong in the discipline of nursing management.

4. *A field of study.* Mr. Wilbur is majoring in the management of nursing services in his university program.

5. *Nursing management task.* One of the pieces of work to be done by the charge nurse was to plan a holiday schedule based on the expected workload.

6. *Nursing management work.* Ms. Zeller's primary nursing team gives good nursing care to their patients. They produce under Ms. Zeller's management.

managers are able to extend their knowledge or learning in the discipline of nursing management. Thus they develop a field of study.

Nursing Management Is the Active Organ of the Division of Nursing, the Organization, and the Society in Which It Functions. Every health-care institution is an organ of society and exists for society. The division of nursing exists for the good of people—clients or patients. The organization, through the division head, has power and authority over its employees. It has an effect on the community as a source of services, jobs, and waste products and pollutants. It has a concern for the quality of life and may be seen by consumers as ethically above that of economic institutions of the business world. It must have the support of society, which needs its services.

In business and industry it takes a profitable organization to make a social contribution, as a bankrupt one can neither employ personnel nor provide services to patients. Patients or consumers keep the health-care institution and the division of nursing in existence and people employed. Their use of nursing services makes the institution a success and keeps it operational. Nurse managers work to have the organization through its personnel produce what these patients need and want. Nursing management functions to manage the nursing business or industry and make nursing profitable in fulfilling its social contribution.

The chair of the division of nursing manages the total nursing operation, and each nurse manager manages the nursing activities of a department or unit. Although it is often carried on the overhead rather than the profit side of the ledger, the division of nursing performs for society and as a business. Nursing care provides for some of human beings' needs and wants. Nursing management recognizes that nursing as an institution exists for its contribution and performance rather than for the convenience of employees. To accomplish this nurse managers show a contribution by nursing personnel, who they manage for performance.

Nurse managers satisfy clients, physicians, nurses, technicians, clients' families, employers, labor unions, and numerous professional entities.

Nurse managers look to managers in business and industry as exemplars who have built sound institutions. Following their example means learning to provide needed primary nursing care services to clients on an economically feasible basis.

Nursing practice is the means by which nurses use their knowledge to practice their skills and use supplies, equipment, and other resources effectively to give satisfactory health care to people. As an organ of the nursing organization, nursing management acts to accomplish the nursing work and ultimately clients' health goals.

Organizational Cultures Reflect Values and Beliefs. The institutional culture within which nursing management is performed is built up over a number of years in all organizations. Managers in nursing have a common purpose of making productive the values, aspirations, and traditions of employees who are individuals as well as members of communities and of society. Social and economic development of nursing will thus take place, resulting in satisfactory services to clients; see Figure 1–8.

Responses to change reflect the values inherent in an organization's culture and the behavior of its members. Nurse managers are assessed against values and responses to change. Values include autonomy for nursing's practitioners, prestige, and a regard for advanced preparation.[18]

Shared values create bonds among nurse managers and nurse workers. Nurse managers articulate moral values and beliefs, basic attitudes and loyalties, concepts, and policies as shared entities, value

being placed on both process and results. Maidique indicates that strategy and strategic planning are overintellectualized, indicating they are overvalued. Workers who attend to product, customer, and marketplace produce better results than does a grand strategy. To achieve success one coordinates and integrates workers and specialized talents.[19]

Maidique questions the value of a Master of Business Administration (MBA) degree and its content, noting that persons with MBAs have not managed U.S. industries to ascendancy. Management education is followed with performance in which basic values are laid down by a strong leader over 10 to 20 years. It takes a long time and a strong leader to make an organization great.[20]

Nursing Management Is Directing or Leading. Directing is an action element of nursing management—the interpersonal process by which nursing personnel accomplish the objectives of nursing. It is the process of applying the management plans to accomplish the objectives of nursing.

Directing is often called the leading function of nursing management. It includes the processes of delegating, supervising, coordinating, and controlling the implementation of the organized plan. The nurse administrator's philosophy will determine whether directing is authoritarian or democratic.

A Well-Managed Division of Nursing Motivates Employees to Give Satisfactory Performance. Nurse employees provide health-care services for an institution within an institutionalized society dependent on its members' performances. Health-care institutions are among the most complex social institutions. Their members or employees will give satisfactory performances in return for their livelihood, opportunities for advancement, opportunities for status within society, self-esteem, and self-actualization. Satisfactory performance results from job satisfaction, a condition requiring that nurse managers stimulate motivation of nurse employees; see Figure 1–9.

Nursing Management Is Effective Communication. Effective communication assures that all levels of personnel know the mission or purpose, the philosophy or beliefs, and the specific objectives of the institution and the division of nursing. Effective communication will result in fewer misunderstand-

FIGURE 1–8. Examples of Nursing Management as a Culture and a System of Values and Beliefs

1. Clients place high value on nursing care they recognize as good.
2. Nursing management is well developed in an organization where professional nurses have equal status with physicians, dentists, pharmacists, and members of other disciplines.
3. All nursing workers have values and beliefs, which an effective nurse manager will learn to use.
4. It is important for a charge nurse to know and support the needs of all nursing workers, including their desire to have time to participate as citizens, how they see their jobs, and what they hope to become.

FIGURE 1–9. Examples of Directing or Leading

1. Employees are rewarded for satisfactory performance by a system of merit pay increases and chances for promotion.
2. Personnel policies provide for time off with pay for continuing education related to the job.
3. Salary compensation provides for annual or biannual longevity pay increases, during an entire span of employment.
4. A public relations program provides for publicity that tells the story of nursing and of contributions made by people in different nursing jobs.
5. The chief nurse executive hires a consultant to assist nurses interested in writing for publication.

FIGURE 1–10. Examples of Nursing Management as Effective Communication

1. As an exercise, the charge nurse had clinical nurse staff read the written statements of mission and specific objectives for their units and for the division and departments of nursing. They then discussed how their work related to each objective at each level. They wrote a summary of their discussion, including some recommended revisions of the specific unit objectives for the charge nurse to implement and to forward to senior nursing management as applicable. People working here achieved a common vision, a common understanding, and unity of direction and effort as a result of the exercise.

2. The nursing practice committee prepared an article to tell why the division of nursing existed, what its personnel believed in, and what their goals were. They took it to the local paper, where it was printed in the Sunday edition.

3. All new employees joining the division of nursing receive orientation that teaches them the mission, the philosophy, and the objectives of the division of nursing and of the department or unit to which they are assigned. When they transfer to another department or unit, they are taught its mission, philosophy, and objectives.

ings and will give employees a common vision, common understanding, and unity of direction and effort. Compatible decisions can then be made. Poor communication results in failures and frustrations due to lack of clear purpose, philosophy, and objectives; see Figure 1–10.

Nursing Management Is Staff Development. Staff development is important to nurse managers from two perspectives: staff development for employees and staff development that prepares clinical nurses for management positions. Clinical nurses may become angry if they are placed in management positions without preparation or consultation. At first they may feel exultation and anticipation for being promoted and for moving up the career ladder. Once confronted with all of the intricacies of interpersonal relationships and management of resources, they begin to feel angry at not being prepared.[21]

A few hospitals use assessment center techniques. These include a thorough job analysis and a series of activities, including weighted interviews designed to evaluate the qualifications of the candidate for the particular job. Once the candidates are selected they are trained for the job using simulation techniques, including simulations of job performance. In-house managers are educated to teach in the program. Pretests and post-tests, in-basket exercises, role playing, leaderless group discussion, and outside exercises related to the particular nurse manager role are all used in the training program. Most materials require content validity. The candidates are usually evaluated using a Likert scale.[22]

Management development is big business: 500,000 managers take management education programs at least once every year; 7,800 minicourses for executives are conducted at the University of Pennsylvania Wharton School in one year; and 14,000 managers are enrolled in management seminars at AT&T annually. In the new health-care environment, home health-care agencies, ambulatory care centers, and similar health-care agencies are increasing. They are no less complex than hospitals and need cost controls and increased productivity to thrive. Unless nurses are educated to manage them they will either lose out to other professions or will manage them poorly and be unhappy and unsuccessful.[23]

Nurses require preparation for their management jobs, including synthesis of nursing and management knowledge. The nurse manager is prepared to manage other nurses who will provide the clinical care. Education of nurse managers will provide human resource management skills, including preceptor and mentor assignments. A model of progression from nursing expertise to management expertise is illustrated in Figure 1–11.[24]

To prepare clinical nurses for beginning management roles, the Mount Sinai Medical Center of Greater Miami designed a voluntary 2-day "Taking Charge" course. Goals included greater competence, confidence, and continuity; preparation for problem solving; job satisfaction; and a positive leadership experience. A guidebook was prepared for use during the learning experience and for reference. Topics covered included communication, leadership styles, time management, managing stress, staffing, assignments, rounds, reports, ordering supplies, unit operations, position description, policies, patient care assessment, quality assurance, conflict management, and counseling. A posttest and 3-month follow-up indicated the course to be successful. The clinical nurses were more effective, showing improved self-concept, self-esteem, and assertiveness. The morale and climate both improved.[25]

At Mount Sinai, management development of nurses is taken seriously. Recognizing that nurse managers have onstage and backstage roles to perform, one management program focused on communication skills. These skills are required for onstage management in which different "hats" are put on for each role: negotiator, counselor, director, delegator, collaborator, or controller. The nurse manager is a "hands-on-the-organization" person.

The communication course is one 2-hour session each week for 10 weeks. It covers such topics as communication style, nonverbal communication, listening, conflict management, verbal messages, rumors, committees, team-building, and communication climate. It helps prepare the nurse manager to respond to multiple issues from multiple sources. Backstage, it provides the nurse manager with the ability to communicate in the business world with other executives. These nurse managers must also be well-versed in management theories, with a knowledge of economics, finance, and accounting. They must be assertive, proactive, and collegial.[26]

A system for developing nurse administrators has been published by Fralic and O'Connor. They make frequent reference to the work of Katz and of Charns and Schaefer. Katz classifies management skills into three categories:

1. Conceptual skills that are an innate ability, or thinking skills.
2. Technical skills that include methods, processes, procedures, or techniques.
3. Human skills that relate to leadership ability and intergroup relations.

In nursing, technical skills are divided into nursing management technology and nursing practice technology. Fralic and O'Connor relate the conceptual, human, and technical skills to three management levels with the chief nurse executive needing the highest level of conceptual competence and the head nurse needing the highest level of nursing practice technology. The needed staff development is evident in the role requirements.[27]

Spicer indicates that scientific management knowledge is the base of the nurse manager's role, including knowledge of a model role and the ability to conceptualize it. Preparation for management and support during the transition are needed for the change from clinical nurse to nurse manager. This role model would demonstrate the relationships between politics and strategy, between power and influence.[28]

Preparation of nurse managers includes knowledge of legal labor practices and institutional policy in managing employees. It includes preparation for in-service training, including principles of adult education, performing a needs survey, and preparing, presenting, and evaluating programs. Money matters concern all levels of nurse managers and include budgeting, managing cost and revenue centers, and productivity. Nurse managers use performance appraisal as a continuum directed toward results. Preparation of nurse managers assists them in becoming self-directed.[29]

Nursing Management Is Controlling or Evaluating. Controlling is an action element of nursing management. It includes the processes of evaluating the carrying out of the adopted plan, the given orders, and the established principles through establishing standards, comparing performance with standards,

FIGURE 1–11.   Management Progression for Nursing

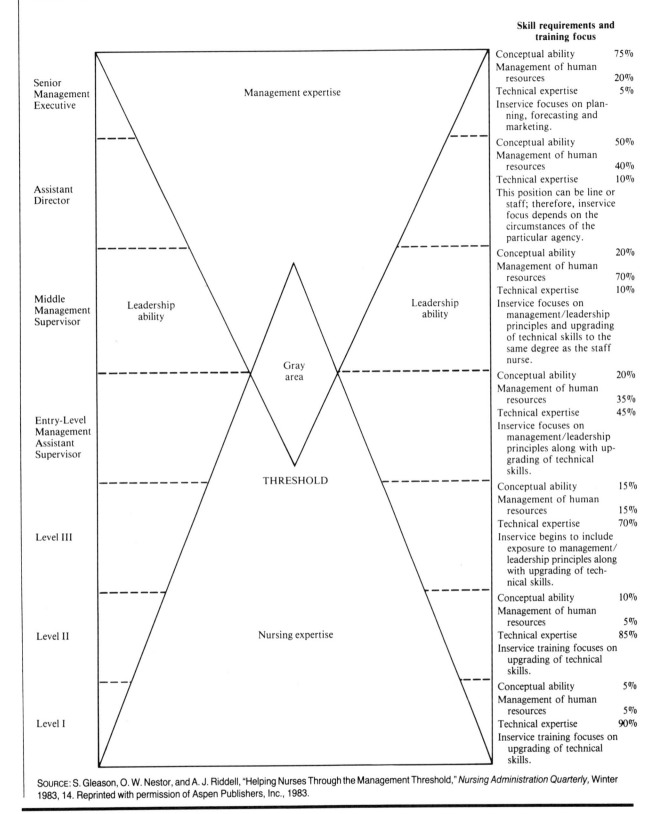

Skill requirements and training focus

Senior Management Executive — Management expertise		
Conceptual ability		75%
Management of human resources		20%
Technical expertise		5%

Inservice focuses on planning, forecasting and marketing.

Assistant Director

Conceptual ability		50%
Management of human resources		40%
Technical expertise		10%

This position can be line or staff; therefore, inservice focus depends on the circumstances of the particular agency.

Middle Management Supervisor — Leadership ability — Gray area

Conceptual ability		20%
Management of human resources		70%
Technical expertise		10%

Inservice focuses on management/leadership principles and upgrading of technical skills to the same degree as the staff nurse.

Entry-Level Management Assistant Supervisor

Conceptual ability		20%
Management of human resources		35%
Technical expertise		45%

Inservice focuses on management/leadership principles along with upgrading of technical skills.

THRESHOLD

Level III

Conceptual ability		15%
Management of human resources		15%
Technical expertise		70%

Inservice begins to include exposure to management/leadership principles along with upgrading of technical skills.

Level II — Nursing expertise

Conceptual ability		10%
Management of human resources		5%
Technical expertise		85%

Inservice training focuses on upgrading of technical skills.

Level I

Conceptual ability		5%
Management of human resources		5%
Technical expertise		90%

Inservice training focuses on upgrading of technical skills.

SOURCE: S. Gleason, O. W. Nestor, and A. J. Riddell, "Helping Nurses Through the Management Threshold," *Nursing Administration Quarterly,* Winter 1983, 14. Reprinted with permission of Aspen Publishers, Inc., 1983.

and correcting deficiencies. The controlling function of nursing management is frequently called evaluating.

A theory of nursing management evolves from the theory of nursing and the nursing process. Just as data are collected and analyzed by the clinical nurse to make the nursing care plan, so does the nurse manager collect and analyze data to do planning. The clinical nurse organizes the care of individual patients as well as the care of a group of patients (a total practice). Likewise, the nurse manager organizes work at division, department, or unit level. While the clinical nurse performs the directing or leading function with other nursing personnel, patients, and families (applies nursing orders), the nurse manager performs the directing or leading function of larger groups of personnel and the use of more material resources. Controlling or evaluating is performed by the clinical nurse in assessing the results of nursing advice in terms of patients' outcomes. The clinical nurse also evaluates those personnel who assist or work for him or her. Nurse managers perform the controlling or evaluating function at division, department, and unit levels. They evaluate programs, personnel performance, and outcome (qualitatively and quantitatively). Development of nursing management theory will transform theory of nursing and theory of management. Research in nursing management will validate the theory of nursing management.

All of these major functions of nursing management operate independently and interdependently. They will be examined in detail in succeeding chapters.

NURSING MANAGEMENT AND ROLES

Role Development

The nurse manager draws from the best and most applicable theories of management to create an individual management style and performance. This requires knowledge and the skill to use it. The nurse manager continues to acquire management knowledge and to use it to solve managerial problems. This requires a contingency approach, as no single approach works for all situations. The nurse manager acts with the assumption that clinical nurses and other personnel want to be competent and that with managerial support they will be motivated to achieve competence. With achievement of each competence goal, a higher one is set. Clinical nurses will seek out the organization that fits their needs.[30]

McClure vividly points out that nurse managers are managing a clinical discipline performed by professional nurses. Nurses are predominantly female, with conflicts between being nurses and being homemakers. The nurse manager devises strategies to deal with these conflicts. There are blue-collar nurses who lack knowledge of nursing research and do not read to keep up to date. They want the nurse managers to do everything, while white-collar nurses want to be treated differently. White-collar nurses want job enrichment with primary nursing and professional autonomy. They want to be organized like the medical staff with staff appointments and peer review. The nurse manager manages these two groups differently.[31]

Freund surveyed chief executive officers (CEOs) and directors of nursing (DONs) of 250 university-affiliated hospitals. The sample based DON effectiveness on:

1. General management/health/nursing knowledge, including finance, accounting, computer literacy, nursing, health-care field, and productivity.
2. Human management skills, including communication, interaction with people, sensitivity, and humor.
3. Total organization view (theory and behavior) with nursing as part of management team and nursing's interests blended with the entire organization's interests.
4. Support by CEOs. DONs did not think CEOs viewed this as important.
5. Medical staff relations. Smooth and peaceful nursing–medical staff relationships were more important to CEOs, while DONs desired a collegial relationship.
6. Flexibility/negotiation/compromise. CEOs cited flexibility for DON effectiveness while negotiation and compromise were cited by DONs.
7. Political savvy. DONs indicated the political nature of their jobs required political savvy, while CEOs did not view this as crucial to DONs.
8. Knowledge of advanced clinical practice.

Figure 1–12. Characteristics of the Rational and Intuitive Modes of Thought

Aspect	Rational Mode	Intuitive Mode
Ordering of the mode	Linearity, sequence Discrete steps	Iteration, cycles Simultaneity, interaction, association
Elements and their relationships	Discrete entities Logically interrelated categories	Gestalts, integrated wholes Many experience forms (difficult to categorize) Integration through meaning and significance
Reliance on context	Little reliance on context Assumption of boundaries Explicitness	Strong reliance on context Unbounded or difficult to bound Large amount of implicitness
Movement and control of the process	Finalization of one step before passing to another Relative inflexibility Great control over process	Emergence and evolution of gestalts Relative flexibility Little control over the process

Source: P. S. Nugent, "Management and Modes of Thought," *The Journal of Nursing Administration,* February 1982, 19–25. Reprinted with permission of Lippincott/Harper & Row, © February 1982.

Of the DONs, 73.1 percent had graduate degrees, with 60.2 percent being MSNs, 8.2 percent MBA/MHA, and 4.7 percent Ph.D./DNS. Ninety-two percent of the CEOs had graduate degrees, with 81.6 percent being masters degrees and 10.4 percent doctorates. Management experience averaged 19 years for CEOs and 13 years for DONs. DONs began in clinical practice.[32]

Cognitive Styles: Intuitive Thinking versus Rational Thinking

Nugent states that management science is based on the assumption that reason or rational thinking is the only form of thought. Rational modes of thought are based on a cognitive style of learning, deciding, and solving problems that is systematic, analytic, reflective, and field-independent.

There is also an intuitive mode of thought. Intuitive modes of thought are based on a different cognitive style of learning, deciding, and problem solving that is intuitive, global-relational, active and field-dependent.[33]

Differences between rational and intuitive modes of thought are summarized in Figure 1–12.[34]

Rational and intuitive modes alternate in real life. Intuitive thinkers are frequently blocked when confronted by rational thinkers. They have to think in causal terms rather than in terms of meaning and significance and this stifles and frustrates them, making them inarticulate. Rational thinkers, in turn, can become frustrated and uncomfortable when confronted with intuitive thinkers. Many people do not know that these different cognitive domains exist.[35]

How can knowledge of cognitive styles work for nurse managers? They should acknowledge that both rational and intuitive thinkers are needed in nursing. Both are needed to solve problems and make decisions by generating and structuring ideas. The intuitively thinking nurse generates ideas and the rational nurse orders and analyzes them. They complement each other.

Nurse managers and clinical nurses can benefit from having both intuitive and rational thinkers who set and evaluate goals. One type will formulate goals that are flexible, generating ideas and images of hopes, desires, and expectations. They will describe the future. The resulting gestalt can then be translated by the other type into structure with specificity of goals, objectives, means, and actions. The processes can alternate, with new ideas and goals emerging. Knowledge of intuitive and rational thinking should be applied to the job of managing nurses.[36]

Because the role of the nurse manager at evolving levels is complex, knowledge of cognitive styles can be important to selection of a balanced-ability management team, featuring both intuitive and rational cognitive skills. The ability to select and use such a team involves sound education that can be translated into skills. Didactic learning is combined with experiential learning. As the nurse manager progresses in the role, she or he learns to go to the source of new knowledge and to synthesize it with the old, eventually applying it to new situations. This evolution occurs as nurse managers progress through management levels.

Management Levels[37]

Nurse managers perform at several levels in the health-care organization. These include first line patient care management at the head nurse level, middle management at the department level, and top management at the division and executive levels. In some organizations decentralization places the head nurse at middle management level and redistributes department level functions to staff functions under a matrix or other organizational structure. The roles of middle managers and executive managers are developmental, building upon knowledge and skills as the scope of the nurse manager's role increases in breadth and depth.

Middle Nurse Managers.   The following are some of the knowledge and skills needed by nurses in middle management roles:

1. Financial management—knowledge and skills to prepare and defend a budget for expenses of unit personnel, supplies, capital equipment, and revenues to meet expenses. Ability to manage scarce and expensive resources for performance.

2. Ability to consider moral choices related to human needs, moral principles for behavior, and individual feelings in making decisions.

3. Recognition of and advocacy for patients' rights.

4. Active and assertive effort to share power within the organization, including shared power for nursing practitioners. This includes nursing autonomy, which is threatened by authoritarian management. In turn, practicing nurses are involved in solving managerial problems.

5. Ability to communicate and to promote effective communication among nursing staff and others.

6. Knowledge of internal factors related to purpose, tasks, people, technology, and structure.

7. Knowledge of external factors related to economy, political pressures, legal aspects, sociocultural characteristics, and technology.

8. Ability to study situations and use knowledge of management concepts and techniques, analyze them, make correct diagnoses of problems, and tie the process together as decisions.

9. Ability to provide for staff development.

10. Ability to provide climate in which nurses clearly perceive that they are pursuing meaningful and worthwhile goals through their individual efforts.

11. Ability to effect change through an orderly process.

12. Knowledge of how to empower clinical nurses through committee assignments, quality circles, primary nursing, and even titles. At Mount Sinai Medical Center of Greater Miami, head nurses are department heads who write goals and objectives, prepare and manage the unit budget, and prepare plans. They are encouraged to be organized and unified, to network, and to be community leaders in the health-care field, including working with legislators.[38]

13. Commitment to maintain self-development through reading and attending workshops and other educational programs.

While this list is in no way complete, it is a beginning and will be built upon in succeeding chapters. A list of management competencies identified as being needed by head nurses in Alabama acute care hospitals is given as Appendix 1–1.

Executive Nurse Managers. Executive nurse managers increase their knowledge and skills, building on what they learned as middle managers. Nurse managers at this level should be able to:

1. Understand financial management as it applies to costing and pricing nursing care. They must be able to convey this knowledge to the nurses providing care.
2. Empower middle nurse managers.
3. Undertake corporate self-analysis of what nursing can do (skills, capabilities, weaknesses), assumptions about itself, its environment, and its beliefs.
4. Specify, weigh, interrelate, and accomplish multiple goals simultaneously.
5. Abandon obsolete principles of standardization, centralization, specialization, and concentration.
6. Share authority and power through decentralization with participatory management, employee involvement, and quality-of-worklife programs.
7. Establish and use a matrix organization with task forces and project teams with project leaders.
8. Set the stage for clinical nursing practice. This does not necessarily require that the nurse executive be clinically competent.
9. Advise nursing educators on content of nurse administration programs.
10. Set depth and breadth of nursing research programs.
11. Anticipate future of health care and of nursing.
12. Manage strategic planning.
13. Serve as mentors, role models, and preceptors to lower-level managers, graduate students, and others.
14. Recognize and use authority and power potential.
15. Coordinate the division budget.

SUMMARY

A theory of nursing management evolves from a generic theory of management governing effective use of human and material resources. Four major elements of management are planning, organizing, directing or leading, and controlling or evaluating. All management activities, cognitive, affective and psychomotor, fall within one or more of these major functions that are operational simultaneously.

A main thrust of nursing management is that the focus is on human behavior. Nurse managers educated in the knowledge and skills of human behavior manage professional nurses, as well as nonprofessional nursing workers, to achieve the highest level of productivity in patient care services. To do this they acquire the management competencies of leadership to stimulate motivation through communication with the workforce.

General principles of nursing management include the following:

1. Nursing management is planning.
2. Nursing management is the effective utilization of time.
3. Nursing management is decision making.
4. Meeting patients' nursing care needs is the business of the nurse manager.
5. Nursing management is the formulation and achievement of social goals.
6. Nursing management is organizing.
7. Nursing management is one primary function of the division of nursing.
8. Nursing management denotes a social position or rank, a discipline, and a field of study.
9. Nursing management is the active organ of the division of nursing, the organization, and the society in which it functions.
10. Organizational cultures reflect values and beliefs.
11. Nursing management is directing or leading.
12. A well-managed department of nursing motivates employees to give satisfactory performance.
13. Nursing management is effective communication.
14. Nursing management is staff development.
15. Nursing management is controlling or evaluating.

The primary role of the nurse manager is to manage a clinical practice discipline. To accomplish this requires numerous competencies that are supported by a theory of nursing management.

NOTES

1. H. Fayol, trans., *General and Industrial Management*, by C. Storrs (London: Pitman & Sons, 1949), 3.
2. Ibid., 5–6.
3. R. M. Hodgetts, *Management: Theory, Process, and Practice* (Orlando, FL: Academic Press, 1986), 40.
4. Fayol, op. cit., 8–9.
5. Ibid., 19–20.
6. L. Urwick, *The Elements of Administration* (New York: Harper & Row, 1944), 14–15.
7. L. C. Megginson, D. C. Mosley, and P. H. Pietri, Jr., *Management, Concepts and Applications*, 2d ed. (New York: Harper & Row, 1986), 15. They define theories as part of knowledge and as statements of cause-effect relationships involved in a set of phenomena. They include principles, rules, methods, and procedures that form the knowledge base of science. According to them a principle is a general belief or proposition sufficiently applicable to a situation to provide a guide to thought or action in that situation. A concept is "an abstract or generic idea generalized from particular instances that serves as the basis for an action or discussion. . . . a law is a statement of an order or relation of phenomena, that, so far as is known, is invariably true under the given conditions."
8. V. White, "Nursing Theory: A Viewpoint," *The Journal of Nursing Administration*, July-August 1984, 6, 15.
9. W. Skinner, "Big Hat, No Cattle: Managing Human Resources, Part I," *The Journal of Nursing Administration*, July-August 1982, 27–29.
10. B. D. Steffy and A. J. Grimes, "A Critical Theory of Organizational Science," *Academy of Management Review*, April 1986, 322–336.
11. Ibid.
12. Ibid.
13. K. E. Boulding, "General Systems Theory: The Skeleton of Science," *Management Science*, April 1956, 197–208.
14. Ibid.
15. V. Henderson, *The Nature of Nursing* (New York: MacMillan, 1966), 15.
16. T. A. Ratcliffe and D. J. Logsdon, "The Business Planning Process—A Behavioral Perspective," *Managerial Planning*, March-April 1980, 32–38.
17. P. F. Drucker, *Management: Tasks, Responsibilities, Practices* (New York: Harper & Row, 1973, 1974), x.
18. M. A. Poulin, "Future Directions for Nursing Administration," *The Journal of Nursing Administration*, March 1984, 37–41.
19. M. A. Maidique, "Point of View: The New Management Thinkers," *California Management Review*, Fall 1983, 151–160.
20. Ibid.
21. B. A. Taylor and A. deSimone, "Taking the First Steps to Become a Nurse Manager," *Nursing Administration Quarterly*, Winter 1983, 17–22.
22. S. DeWeese and D. Satecki, "Combining Management Education with an Assessment Center," *Nursing Management*, August 1986, 80–81.
23. S. Gleeson, D. W. Nestor, and A. J. Riddell, "Helping Nurses Through the Management Threshold," *Nursing Administration Quarterly*, Winter 1983, 11–16.
24. Ibid.
25. B. A. Taylor and A. DeSimone, op. cit.
26. D. M. Reeves and N. Underly, "Nurse Managers and Mickey Mouse Marketing," *Nursing Administration Quarterly*, Winter 1983, 22–27.
27. M. F. Fralic and A. O'Connor, "A Management System for Nurse Administrators, Part 1," *The Journal of Nursing Administration*, April 1983, 9–13; ibid., "A Management Progression System for Nurse Administrators, Part 2," *The Journal of Nursing Administration*, May 1983, 32–33; ibid., "A Management Progression System for Nurse Administrators, Part 3," *The Journal of Nursing Administration*, June 1983, 7–12.
28. J. G. Spicer, "Dispelling Illusions with Management Development," *Nursing Administration Quarterly*, Winter 1983, 46–49.
29. Ibid.
30. M. L. McClure, "Managing the Professional Nurse: Part I, The Organizational Theories," *The Journal of Nursing Administration*, February 1984, 15–21; ibid., "Managing the Professional Nurse: Part II, Applying Management Theory to the Challenges," *The Journal of Nursing Administration*, March 1984, 11–17.
31. Ibid.
32. C. M. Freund, "Director of Nursing Effectiveness: DON and CEO Perspectives and Implications for Education," *The Journal of Nursing Administration*, June 1985, 25–30.
33. P. S. Nugent, "Management and Modes of Thought," *The Journal of Nursing Administration*, February 1982, 19–25.
34. Ibid.
35. Ibid.
36. Ibid.
37. J. O'Leary, "Do Nurse Administrators' Values Conflict with the Economic Trend?" *Nursing Administration Quarterly*, Summer 1984, 1–9; M. L. McClure, "Managing the Professional Nurse: Part I. The Organizational Theories," op. cit.; M. A. Maidique, op. cit.; M. A. Poulin, op. cit.; M. A. Fralic and A. O'Connor, "A Management Progression System for Nurse Administrators, Part I," op. cit.; G. Gentleman, "Power at the Unit Level," *Nursing Administration Quarterly*, Winter 1983, 27–31; M. A. Poulin, "The Nurse Executive Role: A Structural and Functional Analysis," *The Journal of Nursing Administration*, February 1984, 9–14.
38. C. Gentleman, "Power at the Unit Level."

REFERENCES

Arndt, C. and Huckabay, L. M. D., *Nursing Administration: Theory for Practice with a Systems Approach*, 2d ed. (St. Louis: Mosby, 1980).

Clark, M. D., "Loss and Grief Behavior: Application to Nursing Managerial Practice," *Nursing Administration Quarterly*, Spring 1984, 53–60.

Drucker, P. F., *The Frontiers of Management* (New York: Truman Talley Books, 1986).

Hillestad, E. A., "Is It Lonely at the Top?" *Nursing Administration Quarterly*, Spring 1984, 1–13.

Koontz, H. and Weihrich, H., *Management*, 9th ed. (New York: McGraw-Hill, 1988).

Kroner, K., "If You're Moving Into Management . . ." *Nursing 80,* November 1980, 105–114.

Marriner, A., "Development of Management Thought," *The Journal of Nursing Administration,* September 1979, 21–31.

Swansburg, R. C., *Management of Patient Care Services* (Saint Louis: Mosby, 1976).

Ibid., *Nurses and Patients: An Introduction to Nursing Management* (Hattiesburg, MS: Impact III, 1978).

Wagner, L., Henry, B., Giovinco, G., and Blanks, C., "Suggestions for Graduate Education in Nursing Administration," *Journal of Nursing Education,* May 1988, 210–218.

APPENDIX 1–1. Abstract: Management Competencies Desired of Head Nurses

---

SWANSBURG, RUSSELL CHESTER. B.S.N., Western Reserve University, 1952. M.A., Teachers College Columbia University, 1961. Ph.D., University of Mississippi, 1984. Dissertation directed by Professor Robert B. Ellis.

Head nurses of wards or units are one of the largest components of management in the health care system in the United States. They manage immense resources of personnel, supplies, and equipment at a time when the health care industry accounts for more than 10 percent of the gross national product and the price tag is rising. The objective of this study was to identify a list of management competencies which will define the role of the head nurse.

To accomplish the purpose of this study the sample was confined to Type 1A hospitals that were members of the Alabama Hospital Association. From the literature and job descriptions a questionnaire was developed that contained 205 management competencies under the headings of the four major functions of management: planning, organizing, directing, and controlling or evaluating. This questionnaire was submitted to a panel of authorities including two hospital administrators, two nurse supervisors, and two head nurses. They rated each competency and the top eighty, twenty for each major management function, were selected for the final questionnaire.

A total of 272 questionnaires was mailed and 203 were returned for a rate of 74.6 percent. The data were coded and statistically manipulated to obtain arithmetic means, analyses of variance, and results from the Scheffé post-hoc comparison test.

While the findings indicated that there were significant differences on eighteen of the eighty head nurse management competencies when analysis of variance was used, the Scheffé post-hoc comparison test and the arithmetic mean indicated that the hypothesis could be accepted for all eighty competencies. There are no significant differences in the ratings of competencies needed by head nurses among hospital administrators, nurse supervisors, and head nurses in fourteen Alabama hospitals.

It was concluded that management competencies of head nurses can be identified and codified under the primary management functions of planning, organizing, directing, and controlling (evaluating). They can be used for educational preparation, recruitment, selection, placement, and development of professional nurses for head nurse positions.

Findings

Analysis of variance revealed no significant differences between the highest and lowest mean ratings on sixty-two management competencies. A list of these competencies follows:

Management Competencies Indentified as Expected of Head Nurses in Alabama Hospitals by a Majority of Hospital Administrators, Nurse Supervisors and Head Nurses from the Sample

Planning Competencies

1.1 Develops and keeps up-to-date written statements of objectives, both short-range and long-range, for the ward or unit.

1.2 Develops management plans that operationalize each objective of the ward or unit, and that specify activities or actions, persons responsible for accomplishing them, target dates or time frames, and provide for evaluation of progress.

1.3 Develops a staffing plan that is based on timing nursing activities, acuity rating of patients, and patient census.

1.4 Plans for nurses to practice a modality of nursing (functional, team, primary, modular, or joint practice).

(continued)

APPENDIX 1-1.   Abstract: Management Competencies Desired of Head Nurses (*continued*)

1.5 Plans to use the nursing process to gather data, assess, diagnose, set goals, prescribe, intervene and apply nursing care, evaluate, provide feedback, make changes and be accountable to the consumer.

1.6 Participates on organizational and department committees.

1.7 Assists staff development department in planning educational activities, including orientation.

1.8 Plans for education of students in the health-care field through collaboration between faculty of the educational institutions and unit personnel.

1.9 Develops management plans to handle unit emergencies.

1.10 Uses job descriptions for each employee that are performance based and that state results to be achieved.

1.11 Uses time effectively setting priorities for workloads.

1.12 Plans for effective directing and coordinating activities that will make personnel productive.

1.13 Makes evaluation plans for evaluating personnel performances, management activities, and quality assurance of patient care.

1.14 Develops and interprets policies, rules, regulations, methods and procedures specific to the ward or unit and that support those of the department or organization, soliciting input from personnel.

Organizing Competencies

2.1 Groups or organizes activities to attain goals and sustain the enterprise.

2.2 Groups activities to effect intradepartmental and interdepartmental coordination.

2.3 Designs roles of individual personnel to fit capabilities and motivation of persons available.

2.4 Designs roles of individual personnel to help employees contribute to objectives.

2.5 Groups activities for full use of resources, people, material, and to fulfill time demands of shifts.

2.6 Groups activities to facilitate nursing services that will promote health of individuals and groups.

2.7 Groups activities to achieve priorities, allow for change, and for flexibility in achievement of objectives.

2.8 Groups activities to facilitate training of employees.

2.9 Groups activities to facilitate communication.

2.10 Develops and maintains a unit or ward organizational chart that depicts line and staff authority relationships within the ward or unit, within the department, and between units; it serves as a reference for delegation of authority, for depicting responsibility and accountability, for supervision, and for channels of communication.

2.11 Updates organizational plan to fit changes in plans, goals and objectives.

2.12 Maintains the principle of unity of command.

2.13 Organizes to recruit, train, and retain personnel.

2.14 Maintains the principle of span of control.

2.15 Coordinates all activities of the unit.

2.16 Organizes to use a modality of nursing care: functional, modular, team, primary, or joint practice.

Directing Competencies

3.1 Provides clearly stated, current, written directions in the form of policies, procedures, standards of care, job descriptions, and rules.

3.2 Works with personnel to achieve unit or ward objectives and their personal objectives.

3.3 Applies human relations knowledge and skills of leadership, group dynamics, labor relations, motivation, and change theory.

3.4 Demonstrates knowledge of personnel and a belief and trust in their productive abilities.

3.5 Works to create harmony of all activities to facilitate achieving the objectives, building staff morale (esprit de corps).

3.6 Encourages self-direction and self-discipline of employees, working all shifts periodically to supervise and evaluate personnel.

3.7 Makes self available to staff members for assistance, teaching, counsel and evaluation.

3.8 Works to identify and direct activities to meet the needs of nursing personnel and satisfaction of patients.

3.9 Serves as a model of professional nursing behavior for nursing staff.

3.10 Coordinates activities of all groups providing patient services.

3.11 Provides for safety of employees and patients.

3.12 Interprets procedures to be followed in emergency situations.

APPENDIX 1–1. Abstract: Management Competencies Desired of Head Nurses (*continued*)

3.13 Uses effective and satisfactory staffing patterns and schedules.

3.14 Maintains discipline.

3.15 Maintains expert and up-to-date knowledge of nursing and hospital policies.

3.16 Reports to nursing supervisor on ongoing basis.

Controlling (Evaluating) Competencies

4.1 Uses professional and accreditation standards (such as ANA and JCAH) in developing all phases of a control or evaluation plan.

4.2 Evaluates the performance of nursing personnel using a process and standards that define expected results, and that are measurable.

4.3 Makes an evaluation plan for each employee and discusses it with him/her. This includes agreement about satisfactory versus unsatisfactory performance.

4.4 Puts the evaluation plan into effect, making and recording observations and meeting and discussing results that provide immediate feedback to nursing personnel.

4.5 Evaluates nursing care plans.

4.6 Evaluates emergency routines, such as cardio-pulmonary resuscitation, and disaster plans.

4.7 Evaluates forms on which nurses record nursing data.

4.8 Uses a comprehensive and effective quality assurance program as part of the evaluation plan.

4.9 Keeps the evaluation process continuous for all areas of control.

4.10 Uses nursing rounds as part of the control or evaluation plan.

4.11 Plans and develops a high degree of mutual trust and support with employees.

4.12 Establishes a cycle of continuing the evaluation process.

4.13 Provides for summaries that identify exceptions to the standards.

4.14 Uses facts and direct contact to settle issues that arise from controlling.

4.15 Controls the budget for personnel, supplies, minor and capital equipment.

4.16 Evaluates absenteeism and turnover for the purpose of reducing them.

Data on the remaining eighteen management competencies were subjected to the Scheffé test to determine whether significant differences existed *other than* between the highest and lowest means. A list of these competencies follows.

Management Competencies on Which Hospital Administrators, Nurse Supervisors, and Head Nurses Were Not in Agreement

1. Develops and keeps up-to-date a mission or purpose statement that tells the reason for existence of the ward or unit, and that supports those of the department and organization.

2. Develops and keeps up-to-date a philosophy statement that supports those of the department and organization.

3. Assists in recruiting, selecting, assigning, retaining, and promoting competent nursing personnel based on individual qualifications and capabilities without regard to race, national origin, creed, color, sex, or age.

4. Prepares budget for personnel, supplies, equipment, and revenues of the ward or unit.

5. Has thorough knowledge and skills in the planning process and uses them to assess planning needs of the ward or unit.

6. Maintains up-to-date knowledge and skills of the planning functions of nursing management.

7. Groups activities for optimal correlation for decision-making and problem solving.

8. Groups activities to achieve a level of management that delegates responsibility and authority to the lowest competent operational level.

9. Maintains a written management or operational plan that defines functions and relationships of personnel or positions depicted on the organizational chart.

10. Keeps all employees informed of the organizational structure and functions.

11. Communicates effectively giving clear concise directions.

12. Applies management plans to effect the mission, philosophy, and objectives statements.

13. Does hiring interviews.

14. Directs personnel in carrying out assignments involving registered nurses in directing activities.

(continued)

APPENDIX 1-1. Abstract: Management Competencies Desired of Head Nurses (*continued*)

15. Uses evaluation standards that are accurate, suitable, objective, flexible, economical, and mirror the organizational pattern of the ward or unit.
16. Evaluates staff development activities.
17. Keeps up-to-date in knowledge and skills of all phases of evaluation, including helping others improve.
18. Uses the results of a patient acuity rating system to control or evaluate staffing.

Application of the ANOVA and the Scheffé test indicated a significant difference in the grand mean between head nurses and nurse supervisors on management competency number 16. There were significant differences between hospital administrators and nurse supervisors on numbers 1, 2, 5, 6, 7, 8, 9, 10, 11, 12, 14, 15, 17, and 18. Significant differences were indicated between hospital administrators and head nurses on numbers 1, 2, 3, 4, 5, 12, 13, 15, and 17. All eighteen of these management competencies were accepted using arithmetic means on a point scale of 0 to 4 points. They all fell in a range above 2.5 points and were selected by the sample of respondents at the *usually expected* or *always expected* levels.

Conclusions

Completion of the study resulted in the following conclusions:

1. Management competencies of head nurses can be identified and codified. They can be codified under the primary management functions of planning, organizing, directing, and controlling (evaluating).

2. There is significant agreement on these management competencies among three groups of Alabama hospital personnel, administrators (chief executive officers), nurse supervisors, and head nurses.

3. A composite job description of these management competencies can be developed for head nurses working in Alabama hospitals. While it is not inclusive, the entire eighty head nurse management competencies validated in this study can be used. They can be used for educational preparation, recruitment, selection, placement, and development of professional nurses for head nurse positions.

4. The list of head nurse competencies could be expanded and tested using others listed on the original questionnaire submitted to the panel of six experts. Also, the validated list could be tested on a random sample of hospitals in other states to validate management competencies desired of head nurses on a national level.

Recommendations

Based upon the findings of the study, the following recommendations are submitted:

1. Administrators and faculties of nursing education programs at the bachelor's and master's degree levels should compare the competencies developed from this study with those established as goals or objectives for their students with the purpose of making programs more relevant.

2. Hospital and nursing service administrators should examine job descriptions of their head nurses and revise them to reflect those management competencies identified in the study which they consider relevant for their organizations.

3. Hospital and nursing service administrators should evaluate the in-house management development programs in light of the head nurse management competencies identified in this study. They should develop programs that incorporate those competencies they consider relevant for their organizations.

4. Organizations such as the Alabama Hospital Association, the Alabama Society for Nursing Service Administrators, and the Alabama State Nurses' Association should examine their objectives and programs in the area of nursing management. They should modify them based on the results of this study and the needs of their organizations.

5. Officials responsible for accreditation and certification of nursing management functions should examine their standards and procedures in these areas and modify them according to their goals.

The Planning Process

2

INTRODUCTION

Definition

Planning, a basic function of management, is a principal duty of all managers within the division of nursing. It is a systematic process and requires knowledgeable activity based on sound managerial theory. The first element of management defined by Fayol was planning. He defined it as making a plan of action to provide for the foreseeable future. This plan of action must have unity, continuity, flexibility, and precision. Fayol outlined the contents of a plan of action for his business, a large mining and metallurgical firm. This plan included annual and 10-year forecasts. Forecasting takes advantage of input from others. It improves with yearly experience, gives sequence in activity, and protects a business against undesirable changes. Fayol's concept was that planning facilitates wise use of resources and selection of the best approaches to achieving objectives. Planning facilitates the art of handling people; it requires moral courage, since it can fail. Effective planning requires continuity of tenure. Good planning is a sign of competence.[1]

Urwick wrote that research in administration provides needed information for forecasting. According to Urwick, investigations should be carried out and their results expressed in terms of the concrete. Planning should be based on objectives, which should be framed in terms of making a product or providing a service that the community needs. Simplification and standardization are basic to sound planning procedures. The product or service should be of the right pattern. Planning provides information to coordinate work effectively and accurately. A good plan should be based on an objective, be simple, have standards, be flexible, be balanced, and use available resources first.[2]

Douglass stated that "planning is having a specific aim or purpose and mapping out a program or method beforehand for accomplishment of the

25

goal."[3] She further defined planning as being "a continuous process of assessing, establishing goals and objectives, and implementing and evaluating or controlling them, which is subject to change as new facts are known."[4]

Alexander stated that planning "is deciding in advance what to do, how to do it, when to do it, and who to do it."[5] She dealt with long- and short-term planning, decision making, strategies, policies, programs, rules, and procedures as elements of planning.[6]

Steiner defined planning as a process beginning with objectives; defining strategies, policies, and detailed plans to achieve them; achieving an organization to implement decisions; and including a review of performance and feedback to introduce a new planning cycle.[7]

Planning is an administrative function that takes some of the risk out of decision making and problem solving. It ensures that the probable outcome will be a desirable one that will be effective in terms of use of human and material resources and production of the product or service. In nursing, planning helps to ensure that clients or patients will receive the nursing services they want and need and that these services are delivered by satisfied nursing workers.[8]

Ackoff describes four orientations to planning: reactivism, inactivism, preactivism, and interactivism.

Reactivism. Looks to the past and considers technology an enemy. It supports the old organizational forms of an authoritarian paternalistic hierarchy. Control operates from the top, with plans submitted from the bottom. Problems are addressed separately, with immediate supervisors adjusting, editing, and adding to plans as they proceed through the hierarchy to the top. Reactive planning is ritualistic; in such systems planning is considered a prerogative of management. Experience is considered the best teacher and age gives knowledge, understanding, and wisdom. Products and services of organizations oriented to reactive planning are replaced by the technological advances of other organizations. Reactive organizations support the arts and humanities, people and values, a sense of history, feelings of continuity, and preservation of traditions. Reactivists do tactical (short-range or operational) planning.

The present health care environment does not always support reactive planning by nurse managers. It is too technical, both for patients and for scarce professional nurses. Also, the latter resist authoritarianism and paternalism, as they want to participate.

Inactivism. Inactivism as a planning orientation prevents change. It operates by crisis management, where the goal is to control discomfort without addressing its cause. Managers are kept busy with red tape and bureaucracy. The effective instrument is the committee, which operates to keep people busy until the work is outdated or success is thwarted by insufficient resources. Knowledge of current events plus connections are more important than competence. Manners are valued. This orientation is prevalent among subsidized government agencies, service departments in corporations, or universities. Nurse managers will participate in such planning in these institutions. Inactivists do tactical or operational planning.

Preactivism. Dominant in U.S. organizations, preactivistic managers accelerate change to exploit the future. They believe that technology causes change and is therefore a panacea. Values associated with preactivism include management by objectives (MBO), inventiveness, growth, permissiveness, decentralization, and informality. Planning is done from the top down, with objectives. The appeal of preactivism is that planning is associated with science and technology, the future. Because it is based mainly on long-term forecasting it is often full of errors.

Nurse managers fall into the technological traps of preactivism. Plans are frequently made, but many are never made operational. Preactivists concentrate on strategic (long-range) planning.

Interactivism. Interactivists believe the future can be created, so they design a desirable future and invent ways of achieving it. In this view, technology is valued depending on how it is used; and experience reveals problems and experiments lead to their solutions. The focus is on development, learning, and adaptation. Interactivistic planners may establish a planning period for achieving goals, objectives, and ideals. Goals are considered ends to be attained within the planning period. Objectives are ends hoped for eventually, but progress is expected within the planning period. Ideals are ends that are not entirely attainable, but progress is expected within and after the planning period. Interactivists emphasize normative planning.[9]

Which type of planning is best for a nursing organization? Many nurse managers would opt for interactivism, as it is proactive. Some of the characteristics of reactivism, inactivism, and preactivism are also useful to present-day nurse managers. One could assess the working environment, decide which orientation to planning is most productive, and attempt to move in that direction. A nurse manager could select a style of planning that blends reactivism, inactivism, preactivism, and interactivism.

Purposes of Planning

Douglass listed the following as reasons for planning:

1. It leads to success in achieving goals and objectives.
2. It gives meaning to work.
3. It provides for effective utilization of available personnel and facilities.
4. It helps in coping with crisis situations.
5. It is cost-effective.
6. It is based on past and future, thus helping reduce the element of change.
7. It can be used to discover the need for change.
8. It is needed for effective control.[10]

Among the activities of planning that Douglass addresses are assessment by collection, classification, analysis, interpretation, and translation of data; strategic planning; development of standards; identification of needs and priority setting; management by objectives; and formulation of policies, rules, regulations, methods, and procedures.[11]

Donovan wrote that planning has several benefits, among which are satisfactory outcomes of decisions; improved functions in emergencies; assurance of economy of time, space, and materials; and the highest use of personnel. She included decision making, philosophies, and objectives as key elements in planning.[12]

Several factors relative to successful planning should be known and put into action by successful managers. These are:

1. A knowledge of the characteristics of planning.
2. A knowledge of the elements of the planning process.
3. A knowledge of the strategic or long-range planning process.
4. A knowledge of the tactical or short-range planning process—functional versus operational.
5. A knowledge of planning standards.
6. A knowledge of and skill in applying the planning processes, including standards, to the work situation.
7. Skill in bringing the planning process up to the standard set, when there are deficiencies.[13]

Characteristics of Planning

What is the nature of planning? What is so distinctive about it that requires a nurse administrator to have the knowledge and skills requisite to engage in planning? In an environment of changing technology, mounting costs, and multiple activities, there is a need for the chief nurse administrator and subordinate managers to plan. The forecasting of events and the laying out of a system of activities or actions for accomplishing the work of nursing and of the organization are prerequisites to success. Koontz and Weihrich defined planning as "selecting missions and objectives and the actions to achieve them; it requires decision making, that is, choosing future courses of action from among alternatives."[14] They view planning as an elementary function of management. In planning, the nurse administrator would avoid leaving events to chance; she would apply an intellectual process to consciously determining the course of action to take in accomplishing the work of the total nursing organization. Donovan stated that the planning process must be deliberate and analytic to produce carefully detailed programs of action that will achieve objectives.[15]

The nurse manager plans effectively to create environments in which nursing personnel will provide the nursing care desired and needed by clients. In this environment clinical nurses will make decisions about the form or modality of practice and nurse managers will work with nursing personnel to establish and meet their personal objectives while meeting the objectives of the organization. According to Hodgetts, planning establishes a path to where managers and subordinates want to go.[16] It should be comprehensive, with nurse managers carefully determining objectives and making detailed plans to accomplish them. It has generally been implied that top administrators in nursing focus on long-range or strategic planning, while operational nurse managers focus on short-range or tactical planning. This process is outmoded. All managers and representative clinical nurses should have input into strategic planning.

Rowland and Rowland state that planning begins with a philosophy about nursing. They list the phases of planning as being determining objectives, collecting data, developing a plan of action, setting goals, and evaluating.[17]

Planning involves the collection, analysis, and organization of many kinds of data (the *how*) that will be used to determine both the nursing care needs of patients and the management plans that will provide the resources and processes to meet those needs. Accepting the fact that nursing is a clinical practice discipline providing a human service, nurse managers plan in order to nurture the practitioners who provide the service.

Some of the kinds of data that will need to be collected and analyzed for planning purposes include:

1. Daily average patient census.
2. Bed capacity and percent of occupancy.
3. Average length of stay.
4. Number of births.
5. Number of operations.
6. Trends in patient populations.
   a. Diagnoses.
   b. Age groups.
   c. Acuity of illness.
   d. Physical dependency.
7. Trends in technology.
   a. Diagnostic procedures.
   b. Therapeutic procedures.
8. Environmental analysis.
   a. Forces impacting upon nursing from within: availability of nurses, turnover, other departments.
   b. Forces impacting upon nursing from outside: government, education, accreditation bodies, and others.

c. Trends in health care and in nursing, including changes in characteristics.
d. Threats to the nursing profession.
e. Opportunities for the nursing profession.

Figure 2–1 demonstrates examples of data that would be collected and analyzed for planning purposes by nursing managers.

Data on diagnostic and therapeutic procedures will be used to plan for new procedures, to revise old procedures, and to make new procedures known to nursing personnel. This is certainly not an exhaustive list of sources of data that will be used for planning purposes. Other sources will be listed in this chapter.

Planning has the characteristics of an open system, being a dynamic organizational process. It leads to success rather than failure. It prevents crisis and panic that are costly, unrealistic, chaotic, distorting of achievement, and dominated by a single person. Planning thus improves nursing division performance. Planning identifies future opportunities and expectations based on conditions, through forecasting techniques that range from simple to

FIGURE 2–1. Planning Data for Nurse Managers

- Live births have decreased 30 percent in the 3 years since the institution of a family planning program.
- Sixty-three percent of live births are discharged within a 24-hour period.
- The number of deliveries with complications has increased from 210 to 257 in one year.
- A new cardiac catheterization laboratory has been completed.
- The hospital planning board has decided to coordinate with other hospitals in the area to consolidate specialty services for newborn care, cardiovascular surgery, and neuroscience services.
- Enrollment of students for clinical nursing affiliation has decreased from 450 to 392 in one year.
- Enrollment of students in the nursing cooperative education program has decreased from 102 to 87 students.
- Medicare reimbursement pays $____ per patient for days of home care.

complex. Simple forecasting techniques follow the process of gathering data and analyzing them to determine alternative decisions and what effects each will produce. Strengths, weaknesses, opportunities, and threats are part of this analysis, which leads to decision, choice, and implementation. In complex forecasting, computer-based mathematical models are available. They are high in cost, require a lot of time and specialized skills, and extend from 3 to 15 years.

Planning is viewed as resting on logical, reflective thinking that is neither cast in concrete nor all encompassing. If needed, leadership or top management will effect change to do effective planning. They will obtain input from all levels to ensure success through format, procedures, time frames, maintenance, and input review.

Planning is the key element of nursing that gives it direction, cohesion, and thrust. It causes all nursing personnel to focus on goals and objectives and stimulates their motivation. Through the planning process nurse managers select and retain the elements of past and present plans that work. They focus on the future and they implement. Thus they successfully manage nursing personnel and material resources to achieve the objectives of the nursing enterprise.

Elements of Planning

While planning is characterized as being a conceptual or thinking process, it produces specific elements or constituent parts that are readily identifiable. These include written statements of mission or purpose, philosophy, objectives, and detailed management or operational plans—the blueprints by which the purpose, philosophy, and objectives are put into measurable actions. Management or operational plans include decision-making and problem-solving processes. They include strategies, policies, and procedures.

The nursing division's strategic and operational plans are road maps that describe the business by name and location. Nurse managers will make them informative by including a description that is a summary of the work of the division.

The summary describing the nursing division will include enough information to give outsiders a bird's-eye view of its totality. This will include the nursing products and services provided by quantity, which can be admissions, discharges, patient days, number of patients by acuity categories, research projects, education programs, students, outpatient visits, and other products and services. The description will summarize marketing activities of the nursing division, including total revenues and expenses. It will describe the managerial style of the division and its impact on employees. This will be related to the organizational plan of the division of nursing.

Planning is the assessment of the nursing division's strengths and weaknesses, covering factors that affect performance and facilitate or inhibit the achievement of objectives. This assessment process will have objectives of its own, both long-range and short-range. As an example, if the clinical promotion ladder is a strength in nurse retention but is weakly applied by selective nurse managers, the problem will be addressed by written objectives.

Planning entails formulation of planning premises by extrapolating assumptions from the information analyzed.[18] If data indicate nurses will be in shorter supply because of decreased enrollments in schools of nursing and increased opportunities for women to enter other fields, this finding should be translated into a premise. Other premises evolve related to increased salaries and fringe benefits and improved conditions of work. These will lead to further premises for marketing a career in nursing to high school students.

Planning implies writing specific, useful, realistic objectives (the *why*) that will reflect both strategic and operational goals for the division of nursing and its personnel. Objectives become the reasons for an operational nursing management plan (the *what*) that will detail activities to be performed, the target dates or time frames for their accomplishment (the *when*), the persons responsible for accomplishing them (the *who*), and strategies for dealing with technical, economic, social, and political aspects. These operational plans will have control systems for monitoring performance and providing feedback. Objectives and operational plans are discussed in detail in chapter 3.

Good management, according to Meier,

starts with a coordinated purposeful organization of people who collectively on a functional responsibility basis are responsible for:
1. Setting objectives
2. Planning strategy

3. Setting goals—short term objectives
4. Developing company philosophy
5. Setting policies—the plan
6. Planning the organization
7. Providing personnel
8. Establishing procedures
9. Providing facilities
10. Providing capital
11. Setting performance standards
12. Initiating management programs.
13. Developing of management information systems
14. Activating people.[19]

Good management keeps the nursing division successful, ensuring its growth, success, and direction and a return on investment in the future.

STRATEGIC PLANNING

Nursing administrators can increase effectiveness through strategic planning, which can promote professional nursing practice and the long-range goals of the organization and the division of nursing. Strategic planning is defined as "a continuous, systematic process of making risk-taking decisions today with the greatest possible knowledge of their effects on the future; organizing efforts necessary to carry out these decisions and evaluating results of these decisions against expected outcome through reliable feedback mechanisms."[20]

Strategic planning in nursing is concerned with what the division of nursing should be doing. Its purpose is to improve allocation of scarce resources, including time and money, and to manage the division of nursing for performance. Strategic planning provides strategic forecasting from 3 years up to more than 20 years. It should involve top nurse managers and can effectively involve representatives of all levels of nursing management and practice. It will include analysis of projected technological advances, the internal and external environments, the nursing and health care market and industry, the economics of nursing and health care, availability of human and material resources, judgments of top management, and other factors.[21]

In today's world the strategic planning process is used to acquire and develop new health care services and product lines. These include new nursing services and products. Strategic planning is also used to divest outdated services and products. Both

activities present moral and ethical dilemmas for the managers and practitioners of nursing. Strategic planning can foster better goals, better corporate values, and better communication about corporate direction. It can lead to changes in operating management and organization. Strategic planning can produce better management strategy and analysis and can forecast and mute external threats.

Figure 2–2 lists ways in which strategic planning can be used to improve management.

Strategic or long-range planning came into vogue after World War II and is prevalent in business and industry. It is becoming prevalent in the health care world because of technological progress, modernization of the industry, increased government roles, and increased complexity of nursing management. It requires nurse managers to manage in the future tense by defining the future of

---

FIGURE 2–2. How Strategic Planning Can Be Used to Improve Nursing Management

To provide accountability and monitoring of performance, tie merit to performance.

To set up more formal planning programs and require divisional and unit planning.

To integrate strategic plans with operational and financial plans.

To think more and concentrate on strategic issues.

To improve knowledge of and training in strategic planning.

To increase top management involvement and commitment.

To improve focus on competition, market segments, and external factors.

To improve communication from top administration and nursing management.

To allow better execution of plans.

To use more realism and less rationalizing and vacillating.

To improve the development of nursing management strategies.

To improve the development and communication of nursing management goals.

To put less emphasis on raw numbers.

nursing in many areas. These areas include the setting of objectives, the study of forces affecting objectives, the development of an organization to achieve the objectives, the allocation of resources, the implementation of objectives through specific policies and plans, the evaluation and provision of feedback related to accomplishing these objectives, and finally the development of a new strategic plan with new objectives.[22]

A strategic plan is coldly objective in evaluating what nursing business is and will be. It does not leave success to chance and prevents the status quo from paralyzing nursing progress. Strategic planning leads to strategic management becoming an integral part of thinking in all management operations, including budgeting, information, compensation, and organization.[23]

Critical thinking about the past, present, and future state of affairs helps in developing, implementing, and evaluating a well-formulated strategic plan. During this process sensitivity to the needs of the institution, its personnel, and its clientele is required. The plan will be flexible and adaptable to environmental changes. Quantifiable outcomes increase the accuracy of a strategic plan. Each day the nurse manager makes sound decisions that can be positively related to advanced planning and can range from the simple to the complex.

Participants in the strategic planning process will range from top nursing management to a cross-section of all levels of management. Including input from clinical nursing personnel promotes professional satisfaction throughout the nursing division.

Among the benefits of strategic planning is the giving of a sense of direction to all managers and practitioners of nursing within the organization. The strategic plan becomes a flexible control mechanism that can be modified to deal with variables, conservation of resources, and professional satisfaction. The strategic plan deals concretely with complex projects or programs in multistage time sequences.[24]

Human Resources Planning

Human resource strategic planning is undertaken as part of the strategic planning process. This is essential to retention of outstanding professional talent. It is not enough to address only the business activities of nursing such as management processes and functions, budgets, objectives, staffing, and the like. The goals of the division are accomplished through its people. Nurse managers serve in dual roles, as managers of human resources and managers of nursing operations. Nurse managers need to enlist the good offices of the human resource department and use it. They also need to develop an understanding between other operational departments and nursing.[25]

Strategic human resources planning decides how the full spectrum of human resources will affect the strategic and operational plans. If the human resources do not fit the strategic plan, the nurse manager decides what action to take. This can include locating new people with special skills or upgrading the skills of senior personnel. There will be a statement of objectives for the human resource program in the strategic plan. It can be developed with input from clinical nurses.[26]

Other elements of strategic human resource planning will include:

1. Projection for future growth, changes in the employment market, external demographics, balancing human resources against finances, and other limitations.
2. Development of a strategic human resource planning approach that describes actions, roles, authorities, and responsibilities of the human resource department, line management, and individual employees.
3. Inventory of human resource planning skills that include future issues, a system for translating strategic business plans into human resource requirements and programs, career development, two-way communication, attitude surveys, employee sensings, group feedback sessions, and exit interviews.
4. Analysis of current and future macro issues of major world influences that will affect the strategic business plan (SBP) and the human resources plan (HRP). These will include the age of the population, productivity in U.S. industry, inflation, politics, unions, technology, expectations of nurses, and other factors.
5. Analysis of current and future micro issues of major organizational influences. These include geographic location, availability of skills, potential in-house promotions, living costs, and unions.
6. Development of programs to support the SBP and the HRP.

7. Provision for periodic and timely audits.
8. Support and commitment of all management levels.[27]

As part of strategic planning nurse managers will develop goals and objectives that:

1. Address increased automation of nursing information systems.
2. Project changes that will occur in nursing products and services.
3. Project the organization and types of employees that will be needed for changed products and services.
4. Trace trends in the corporate culture: values, cultural rituals, social processes, learning patterns of clients and employees.
5. Address retraining of employees with outmoded jobs.
6. Explore future leads through content analysis, extrapolation of trends simulation forecasting, modeling, scenario projection, and trend impact analysis. These are complex techniques that can improve forecasting.
7. Assess new management techniques that include open work systems, quality of work life programs, quality circles, and participatory management techniques.
8. Promote job security and career development, including management of nurses who are "fast burners," the top 5 to 10 percent of the nurse force.
9. Lower barriers to women, minorities, older workers, new workers, immigrants.
10. Keep employees updated in knowledge and skills and provide more resources to learning and development.
11. Develop policies for dual careers of employees, changing careers and life values, changes in the work ethic related to personal and leisure activities, downgrading and demoting employees.[28]

Conclusions about the Strategic Planning Process

Strategic planning is considered to be a goal-setting process that is largely carried out by top management. There are many instances of long-range plans being made, with fewer instances of their having been put to use. In truth, many operating nurse managers have need to be trained in the strategic planning process. This training would include techniques to involve operational managers and thereby commit them to decisions. Development of global goals and strategies broaden the identification and solution of problems, thereby reducing threats to and unveiling opportunities for the organization.

The demonstrated usefulness of scientific planning will influence the behavior of operating managers. Rewards, in the form of both pay and praise, will motivate these operating managers.

There are phases and stages in the process of strategic planning, as summarized in Figure 2–3.

FUNCTIONAL AND OPERATIONAL PLANNING

Some nursing planning is performed at a service or departmental level and is referred to as "functional planning." It generally relates to a specialty service within a nursing division. For example, the staff development director would be included in development of the strategic plan, but would develop operational plans for staff development as a whole and for specific services or units. Likewise, the director of surgical nursing would assist in developing the strategic plan but would develop departmental goals, objectives, and operational plans related to the surgical nursing units.

Operational plans are everyday working management plans. They are plans developed from both long-range objectives and the strategic planning process and short-range or tactical plans. In development of operational objectives, new strategic objectives can emerge or old ones can be modified. Strategic and tactical plans are made into operational plans and carried out at all levels of nursing management, not just at the patient-care level.

Operational managers develop goals, objectives, strategies, and targets to set the strategic plan in motion. They match each unit goal or objective to a strategic goal or objective. Their objectives can be much more detailed and specific than the strategic objectives. There can be numerous operational objectives that support one strategic objective.

All aspects of an operational plan are based on goals and on achieving them. The individual leadership style determines whether goal setting will be of the top-down or bottom-up variety. Bottom-up

FIGURE 2–3. Summary of Phases of Strategic Planning Process

Phase 1
The Mission and the Creed
Develop statements that define the work, the aims, and the character of the division of nursing. These include idea statements of values and beliefs. They are called mission (or purpose) and creed (or philosophy).

Phase 2
Data Collection and Analysis
Collect and analyze data about the health-care industry and nursing. Such data should include internal forces that define the work and affect employees, clients, stockholders, creditors; technological advances; threats; opportunities to improve growth and productivity; external forces such as competition, communities, government and political issues, and legal requirements; marketing and public relations or image; trends in the physical and social work environments; and communication. Use simple and complex forecasting techniques, including trend lines, group consensus, nominal group process, and a qualitative decision matrix that uses probabilities based on conditions of certainty, risk, and uncertainty. Refer to Appendix 18-1 for definitions.

Phase 3
Assess Strengths and Weaknesses
Define those factors from the data analysis that influence the management of the division of nursing. List them as strengths that will facilitate effectiveness and achievement of goals and objectives or as weaknesses that will impede achieving goals and objectives.

Phase 4
Goals and Objectives
Write realistic and general statements of goals. Break the goals down into concrete written statements of objectives the division of nursing intends to accomplish in the next 3 to 5 years.

Phase 5
Strategies
Identify untoward conditions that could develop in achieving each objective. Note administrative actions to avoid or manage them. Use this information to modify goals and objectives, making contingency plans for alternative actions.

Phase 6
Timetable
Develop a timetable for accomplishing each objective. Identify by geographic units as well.

Phase 7
Operational and Functional Plans
Provide guidelines or general instructions that lead the functional and operational nurse managers to develop action plans to implement the goals and objectives. These will include detailed actions, policies, practices, communication and feedback, controlling and evaluation plans, timetables and persons to be held accountable.

Phase 8
Evaluation
Provide for formative evaluation reports before, during, and after the operational plan is implemented. Provide for summary evaluation that is quantified. Report actual versus expected results.

goal setting is participatory, using guidelines from the operational manager.[29] Participatory goal setting is believed to increase commitment and achievement. Increased participation leads to greater group cohesiveness, which in turn fosters increased morale, increased motivation, and increased achievement and productivity. Individuals, including nurse managers, can ensure greater success in achievement of their goals by building in some slack in terms of projected resources and time.

Nurse managers who reject goals of participating staff should explain reasons for rejection. Participation in goal setting does not alone ensure success. Figure 2–4 illustrates the concepts of strategic and operational planning. Like the plan itself, such planning should be flexible.

The concept that goals are global in nature while objectives are more detailed is confusing to some participants in the planning process. This has been particularly true in nursing, where written

FIGURE 2–4. Timetable for Strategic and Operational Planning

1. Organization
   Mondays 7–9 A.M. Conference room. Breakfast.
   Attendees: chief executive officer (CEO), assistants (including for division of nursing), and understudies.
   Agenda: CEO, with input from all others, relates each item to strategic plan. CEO updates and develops written operational plans at meeting or immediately following, then reviews them for next agenda for progress and for strategic plan development.
   Minutes: Prepared and distributed to attendees.

2. Division of Nursing
   Monday 3–4 P.M. Nursing Conference Room.
   Attendees: chief nurse executive (CNE), associates, department heads, chairs of clinical consultants, nursing management, and staff nurse committees.
   Agenda: Chairs, with input from CNE and all others, relate each item to strategic plan of division of nursing. These goals and objectives have already been coordinated with the organizational strategic plan. CNE and others update operational plans of division and departments during meeting or immediately following, then review them for next agenda, for progress, and for nursing strategic plan development.
   Minutes: Prepared and distributed to attendees, to CEO and to selected others.

3. Service and Unit
   Department heads meet with their head nurses at mutually determined times and places. The groups have agendas, keep minutes, update written operational plans, and provide feedback to functional managers and the CNE.

organizational goals have seldom been in evidence. They probably did not exist in many hospitals. There is more activity in this aspect of management today. External influences create a demand for a strategic plan, and more nurse managers have had management education and training.[30]

Some organizations do not develop separate goals and objectives. Instead, they develop objectives and from the objectives develop management plans. In actual practice, organizational objectives are often goals labelled as objectives. As they are developed into operational plans, specific goals and objectives are written for each major activity.

The goal is to plan, to assess progress toward goals and objectives at all levels, and to provide feedback to all levels of management. Efficiency is also a goal; all levels of management should guard against unnecessary time spent in meetings. At the same time organizational changes are occurring, controlling activities are in operation and activities are being evaluated.

PLANNING NEW VENTURES

In an era of competitiveness, each nurse manager can be called upon to develop ideas for new ventures, be they nursing products or services. For example, continuing education courses can be packaged, marketed, and presented within the organization or taken on the road. Hospitals are moving into home health care, durable medical goods, wellness and fitness programs, and many other ventures. The basic rule for undertaking new ventures is to do sound planning.

Any new venture should have a separate marketing plan. The nurse manager will consult with marketing department personnel and develop a marketing operational plan that will:

1. Define problems and opportunities that may confront the new enterprise and product.
2. Define the competitive position of the product and set objectives to meet anticipated problems and opportunities.
3. Detail work steps, schedules, assignment of responsibilities, budgets, and other elements of implementation.
4. Describe the monitoring (control) plan.[31]

The marketing plan should be separate from a primary operational plan. This plan will include gathering and analysis of data related to the product or service as it already exists in the area. If the product is continuing education, who will the customers be? They could be nurse managers, nurse educators, R.N.s, or L.P.N.s. What is the competition in the market area? Is it local or imported from educational institutions and for-profit companies? Who will pay for the course—Employers or individuals?

In addition the operational plan will gather and analyze data that pinpoint possible strengths and weaknesses, problems, and opportunities. It will identify strategies for taking competitive advantages. Each opportunity, problem, strength, and weakness should be addressed by definitive objectives developed into operational plans for advertising, product development, and even personal selling.

Before any new venture is launched, a control plan is developed. This plan will include measures of performance such as numbers or amounts of products or services to be sold within specific time frames. Managers will be assigned responsibility for comparing expected with actual results and for making corrections in all elements of the plan and its implementation. This plan can be achieved with marketing and operational plan checklists.[32] Figure 2–5 illustrates an operational plan for development of an intermediate cardiac rehabilitation program.

Nursing service planning supports the mission and objectives of the institution. For this reason the nurse administrator needs to know the plans and programs of the health facility administrator and of other departments where personnel contribute to the joint effort of providing health care services. The nurse administrator should be a voting member of all important committees of the institution. This will include committees dealing with budgets, planning, credentialing, auditing, utilization, infection control, patient care improvement, library, and all others concerned in any way with nursing service, nursing activities, or nursing personnel.

The nurse administrator who participates in institutional committee work achieves an overall view of hospital problems and activities and is in a position to interpret problems, policies, and plans of the hospital to nursing personnel. He or she can also interpret nursing needs and problems to hospital personnel of other departments. This planning integrates the nursing care program into the total program of the health care institution.

OPERATIONAL HUMAN RESOURCE PLANNING

Planning encompasses the writing of personnel policies that will assist in recruiting and maintaining a qualified staff. Data for development of these policies will need to be collected and analyzed in cooperation with the personnel division and representatives of the nursing staff. It is an ethical responsibility of nursing management to inform nurses about information compiled on them and to ensure that only needed information is retained. This information should be used to develop jobs and to recruit, select, assign, retain, and promote nursing personnel based on individual qualifications and capabilities and without regard to race, national origin, sex, age, creed, or color. The information will be used to develop personnel policies to classify personnel according to competence and to establish salary scales commensurate with qualifications and positions of comparable responsibility within the community and agency. Written copies of personnel policies, job descriptions, and job standards will be made available to all nursing personnel.

PRACTICAL PLANNING ACTIONS

Practical day-to-day planning actions of value to the nurse administrator include the following:

1. At the beginning of each day, make a list of actions to be accomplished for the day. Cross off the actions as they are accomplished or at the end of the day. At the beginning of the next workday, carry over actions not accomplished; either do them first or decide whether they are actions that really need to be done. Do not hold tasks over from one day to the next indefinitely.

2. Plan ahead for meetings. If the meeting is a nursing responsibility, prepare and distribute the agenda in advance. Have a secretary call members for their items to be listed on the agenda. Forward nursing items for the agenda of organizational meetings to the appropriate chair in advance. Prepare for the presentation.

3. Identify developing problems and put them in the appropriate portion of the division's operational or management plans.

4. Review the operational or management plan on a scheduled basis. Do this with key managers so that

FIGURE 2–5.   Division of Nursing—Cardiac Rehabilitation Program

Strategic Objective.   The patient is provided with an effective patient and patient-family teaching program, which will include guidance and assistance in the use of medical center resources and community agencies that can contribute support to the patient's total needs.

Operational Objectives	Actions	Target Dates and Persons Responsible	Accomplishments
Meet with the cardiologist to determine his perception of the program: goals, resources to be used, breadth of services to be provided, etc.	1. Prepare an agenda for meeting with the cardiologist.	Do by July 1, 1989; Swansburg and Perry.	The following agenda was developed: ■ Need for new services. ■ What will it be? ■ What will it cost? ■ What will be charged? ■ Who will pay? ■ Where will it be done? ■ Who will do it? ■ How many patients? ■ What equipment and supplies are needed?
	2. Make appointment with the cardiologist.	May 3, 1989 at 11 A.M. in Dr. C's office; S and P.	May 3, 1989. Had a meeting with Dr. C, the cardiologist. The purpose of this program is to rehabilitate patients following open heart surgery, angioplasty, and post-MI. It is the intermediate phase between acute care and when they enter "bounce back." The following decision evolved from the meeting: 1. We will undertake this program on a limited basis as there is no other such service available. 2. The service will include: physical exercises, monitoring, progress report by patient, counseling as indicated.

FIGURE 2–5. Division of Nursing—Cardiac Rehabilitation Program (*continued*)

Operational Objectives	Actions	Target Dates and Persons Responsible	Accomplishments
			3. Only patients with insurance or with ability to pay will be accepted.
			4. It will be done in P.T. on Mon., Weds., and Fri. from 7 to 9 A.M.
			5. Equipment and supplies will be in-house.
			6. The CV clinical nurse specialist will be the project director.
Meet with the CV clinical nurse specialist and plan the program.	3. Make appointment with nurse D to plan the program.	May 4, 1989 at 8 A.M.; S and P with D.	Plan: 1. D will coordinate with PT director. 2. P will figure cost of program by the hour and set charges with accounting office. 3. D will borrow equipment to run the program until the next capital budget. 4. Accomplish this by May 12, 1989.
Have plan completed by May 31, 1989.	4. Set up a control chart to identify when each phase of project will be completed.	May 12, 1989; P.	May 10, 1989: Done. Posted.
	5. Write policy and procedure for the program. Include admission and discharge procedures and emergency plan.	May 31, 1989; D.	May 29, 1989; Draft presented; minor changes needed. May 31, 1989: Done.
	6. Obtain equipment and supplies.	May 31, 1989; D.	May 17, 1989: Done.
	7. Coordinate with PT director.	May 12, 1989; D.	May 17, 1989: Done.

(continued)

FIGURE 2–5.   Division of Nursing—Cardiac Rehabilitation Program (*continued*)

Operational Objectives	Actions	Target Dates and Persons Responsible	Accomplishments
	8. Meet with cardiologist when all of this is done.	June 1, 1989; P, S, and D.	Met with cardiologist June 2, 1989. Dr. C is happy with plan and will be ready to start on July 1, 1989.
Provide for third-party reimbursement.	9. Discuss with insurance companies.	June 15, 1989; P.	June 15, 1989: Insurance reps will visit the program and make decision. Appointment made.
Develop marketing plan.	10. Prepare a detailed marketing plan.		Marketing plan is already in operation with announcements mailed to all area cardiologists.
Develop an evaluation plan.	11. Prepare evaluation plan.	June 30, 1989; P and D.	D has a good evaluation plan.
	12. Implement the program.	July 1, 1989; D.	July 1, 1989: Had our first patient today. Cardiologist was there as required by insurance companies. All went well.
	13. Evaluate the program weekly until stabilized.	D, beginning July 8, 1989.	

each knows personal responsibilities for accomplishment of activities.

5. Review the appropriate portions of the division operational or management plan with subordinate nurse managers when they are being counseled. Department, unit, or clinic plans will be reviewed at the same time.

6. Plan for discussion of ideas gleaned from professional publications. This can be part of a job standard, with different managers assigned specific topics or journals. This may help to integrate research results into practice.

7. Suggest similar practical planning actions to nursing department heads and other nurse managers.

Planning will also be necessary to provide programs for orientation and continued learning of nursing personnel, so that all will have current knowledge and be current in practice. Improvement of patient care and of other administrative and hospital services necessitates initiation of, utilization of, and participation in studies or research projects in the health care field.

Two additional large and important areas for planning are, first, educational programs that include student educational experience in the division of nursing and, second, evaluation of clinical and administrative practices to determine if the objectives of the division are being achieved.

WHY DIVISIONAL PLANNING?

There are many good reasons for planning, and avoidance of duplicated efforts is one of them. Planning will also improve communication throughout the division and the institution and will reduce fragmentation by helping functional units to head in the same direction. Planning is good management training for all nurse managers, including charge nurses and supervisors. During its initial phases, planning will use an objective analysis of the division to determine its current status. This will include an analysis of mission, strengths and weaknesses, and environment, as well as a survey of how all employees feel about the division. The analysis will also assess the future of the division and the major threats and opportunities it will face during the next year and the next 5 or 10 years. Planning will engineer a design for monitoring and evaluating divisional performance. This design will involve as many people as possible in planning and managing their own areas of responsibility.

Once manager and employee have agreed on objectives, programs and projects, and schedules, employees can control their own jobs and report only when things turn out better or worse than planned.

Planning is such a primary and essential element of management that managers cannot be effective without it.

Problems with Divisional Planning

All planning requires discipline and organization on the part of managers, and managers, being human, usually prefer short-range solutions to problems. They prefer to "shoot from the hip," and some even enjoy management by crisis. Many managers are threatened by the change produced by planning; they resist it even to the point of sabotage.

Planning must be approached logically and calmly. Planning will threaten the insecure and may even threaten the nurse administrator who must provide total support in terms of giving or obtaining the resources to accomplish divisional planning. Strategies must be developed to address these problems and to ensure that representative nurse managers participate on all planning teams.

Provision of nursing care to patients is the purpose of a division of nursing. The standards of the Joint Commission on Accreditation of Healthcare Organizations for nursing services state that there will be an organized nursing department or service; that this organization must meet nursing care needs of patients according to established standards of nursing practice; and that "individualized, goal-directed nursing care is provided to patients through use of the nursing process."[33]

To Make Planning Successful

Rather than creating a separate planning staff of nurses, it is better to keep the responsibility for planning a line management function. The people who make plans effective and productive, the people who use them, are the ones who should write them. Nurse managers should be sure plans are based on data from all sections and not biased by a few. Some people see planning as a management style; it is a tool as well. Plan for what the health care of the future will be: with inflation and recession, the impact of the local economy on health care needs will become greater than it already is. Economics is forcing us to teach people to do more for themselves and their families. Nurse managers will certainly have to plan for changes in value systems.

Make decisions about the kind of planning to be undertaken. Which management level should perform specific aspects of planning? Involve personnel in planning activities they are going to carry out. Teach personnel the elements of planning and mesh it with other management functions. Ensure that all managers are involved. Accept outcomes different from those originally planned, since activities may quickly become outdated and require modified plans.

UNIT PLANNING

Planning must extend to the operational units. The processes involved are the same. It is here that the work for which the division of nursing exists takes place. Planning must be done on a daily, weekly, and long-range basis. Daily planning is related to patient care and includes history taking, assessment, and nursing diagnosis and prescription. It involves matching people to jobs, developing policies and procedures specific to the types of clients cared for, identifying training needs, preparing and conducting training programs, coordinating all patient care activities, supervising personnel, and evaluating.

Unit objectives must be clearly defined, and a sound management or operational plan must be made to achieve them. An operating instruction from one division of nursing states, "The division of nursing has a stated philosophy and objectives. Personnel of each unit within the division will have their own philosophy and will set up their own objectives. The objectives will be continuously evaluated, and a written statement as to progress will be sent to the chairman's office each August and February."

Figure 2–6 is a plan for accomplishing objectives related to management improvement and resource management for an intensive care unit.

RELATIONSHIPS TO ORGANIZATION

Planning within the division of nursing is intended to assist in fulfilling the mission of the health care facility. It supports the organization's objectives and meshes with the plans of all other departments contributing to provision of total health care needs, whether direct or indirect (such as planning for the environment). Planning includes delineation of the responsibilities of nurse managers in relation to activities in other departments in which nursing participates. The organizational chart will show the relationship of the division of nursing to the board of control, the administrator, and other departments.

FIGURE 2–6. Ward Operational Plan—Intensive Care Unit

1. Management Improvement: Unit Objectives   February 1, 1989
   1.1 Precipitate imaginative thinking to improve existing procedures, capitalize on time expenditure, and introduce modern concepts and materials that directly enhance unit accomplishment.
   1.2 Promote creativity in improving the existing patient environment.
   1.3 Provide more modern concepts of total patient care by constant review and revision of unit administrative/managerial policies.

Plans for Achievement of Objectives	Actions	Target Dates	Accomplishments
1.1–1.2 Plan and implement a continuing unit improvement program.	1. Conduct a continuous review and analysis of unit improvement efforts through:	February	Reviewed and found current for following reasons: Turnover in personnel is fast. All objectives were not adequately met; We need to establish a better way of accomplishing them.
	1.1 Monthly unit conferences to review and update philosophy and objectives. Strive to accomplish more in each objective area.	February–July	

FIGURE 2–6. Ward Operational Plan—Intensive Care Unit (*continued*)

Plans for Achievement of Objectives	Actions	Target Dates	Accomplishments
	1.2 Patient suggestions.	Review each month.	
	1.3 Suggestions of superiors.	Daily	
	1.4 Revise unit procedures.	April	Done
	1.5 Brief all personnel. Discuss philosophy, objectives, job descriptions, performance standards, hospital and nursing service policies and procedures, and unit procedures.	February	Done. In addition all nurses were counseled by the charge nurse. Nursing technicians are presently receiving counseling and all is being documented. Counseling had not been documented in 6 years except for remarks such as, "Things went well and we did our job, so no counseling was needed."
	2. Review equipment and supplies for improvement by addition or deletion.		
	2.1 Submit work order to alter a locker as a drying cabinet for respirator parts, since moisture provides a growth medium for *Pseudomonas* bacteria.		Disapproved. Disposable tubing was approved, ordered, and in use by June.
	2.2 Check on status of new floor, piped-in compressed air system, and cardiac monitors.	February–April	New floor to be done by Aug. 1. Compressed air started by March 15. Cardiac monitors arrived April 3. Patient units 1, 3, and 4 were equipped. Unit 4 was designated the maximum monitoring site and is to be used to monitor patients with Swan-Ganz arterial lines and questionable cardiac conditions.

(continued)

FIGURE 2–6.　Ward Operational Plan—Intensive Care Unit (*continued*)

Plans for Achievement of Objectives	Actions	Target Dates	Accomplishments
1.3 Review standardized policies and procedures for implementation of more current concepts of improved care accomplishments	3. Evaluate all areas of management for current standardized efficiency.		
	3.1 Check all areas of infection sources.		
	3.1.1 Culture floors and equipment to check cleaning procedures.	February	This was done, and cleaning procedures were looked at and improved when they appeared poor. Adhesive
	3.1.2 Clean air conditioning filters.	February	floor mats were placed at entrance and exit areas in an effort to control
	3.1.3 Check wall suction, since filters do not appear to be doing the job.	February	dust carried in by personnel and visitors. Air conditioning filters were replaced in February. Wall suction valves were
	3.1.4 Eliminate messy bedside stands.	February	replaced. Pipelines were found to be clogged with secretions and system had
	3.2 Improve safety.		to be purged. Shelves were mounted on wall by four
	3.2.1 Secure equipment.	April	units to replace bedside stands. Respirators,
	3.2.2 Isolate oxygen nebulization units from suction.	April	nebulizers, and blenders were mounted on wall above each patient unit.
	3.2.3 Send all equipment to central supply for processing.	April	Suction bottles were relocated and outlets changed in an effort to isolate them from the
	3.2.4 Improve efficiency of Ambu resuscitators.	April	oxygen nebulization units. Swan-Ganz catheters were standardized and requisitioning was transferred from the unit to central supply. Ambu bags were equipped with corrugated tubing to serve as an oxygen reservoir and deliver a maximum concentration of 99% to 100%. The disposable Aqua-pack nebulizer was deleted, resulting in a $40-per-case saving.

FIGURE 2–6. Ward Operational Plan—Intensive Care Unit (*continued*)

Plans for Achievement of Objectives	Actions	Target Dates	Accomplishments
	Projected: an anesthesiologist will be assigned to the intensive care unit. All bronchoscopies will be done here. Open heart surgery is still an open and current topic.		

Myra C. Breck, R.N.
Charge Nurse, ICU

2. Resources management
   2.1. Provide, secure, and maintain the appropriate and economical use of supplies and equipment that will permit unit personnel to devote maximum time and care to patient activities.
   2.2. Provide the unit with adequate tools for safe and effective patient care.
   2.3. Provide the unit with conservative utilization and centralization of unit supplies and equipment, thus promoting peak efficiency in meeting patients' needs.

Plans for Achievement of Objectives	Actions	Target Dates	Accomplishments
2.1 Plan, evaluate, and project needed supplies and equipment that will enhance effective and safe nursing care.	Identify projected needs with unit manager through review of: 1. Unit inventories of equipment and budgetary estimate. 2. Standards for supplies. 3. Availability of supplies and equipment. 4. Economical use of supplies and equipment.	February	Items ordered (projected replacements for 1988–1989): 1 Thermometer—electronic, $300. 1 IV pump, $700. 5 transducers, $385. 1 respirator, $2750. 1 sphygmomanometer, $655. 1 Wright respirometer, $275. 4 metal storage cabinets
2.2–2.3 Plan and execute appropriate utilization of materials	1. Economical use of expendable supplies and adequate safeguards to prevent misuse and loss. 2. Knowledge of principles of operation of appropriate mechanical equipment and procedures for effecting prompt servicing and repairs.		4 Ambu bags Vertical venetian blinds 1 blood gas analyzer, $7455. New cubicle curtains Items replaced: ECG and defibrillator, portable ECG machine, MA1 filters, spirometers, suction regulators. Items deleted: 1 electronic thermometer, 1 internal/external defibrillator (to dog lab), 2 compressor units.

(continued)

FIGURE 2–6.   Ward Operational Plan—Intensive Care Unit (*continued*)

Plans for Achievement of Objectives	Actions	Target Dates	Accomplishments
			Miscellaneous: file card supply system revamped, shelving obtained for lower doors. Personnel turnover—projected losses: Ms. Speich, R.N., June; Ms. Ullman, R.N., Aug.; Ms. Urbom, R.N., May; Ms. Malloy, R.N., June; Mr. Falco, ward clerk, April. Projected gains: Ms. Tishoff, R.N., May; Mr. Robertshaw, R.N., May; Mr. Angelus, R.N., April; Mrs. Figuera, unit secretary, April.

Myra C. Breck, R.N.
Charge Nurse, ICU

SOURCE: R. C. Swansburg, *Management of Patient Care Services* (Saint Louis: Mosby, 1978), 49–53.

Plans will provide for optimum support of the nursing division by other departments providing services, supplies, and equipment used by the nursing service. There will be plans for regular meetings with the hospital administrator for participation on all hospital committees concerned with general administrative policies and activities and the total program of the organization. There will also be plans for periodic reports to the board of control, through administrators, concerning the programs, major plans, and problems of the division of nursing.

SUMMARY

Planning is a mental process by which nurse managers use valid and reliable data to develop objectives and determine the resources needed and a blue-print for their use in achieving the objectives. The major purpose of planning is to make the best possible use of personnel, supplies, and equipment.

Strategic planning sets objectives for long-range nursing activities of 3 to 5 years. While traditionally done by top managers, it is an important skill for all nurse managers to develop. It ensures survival. Human resource planning will ensure effective use of a scarce commodity, the professional nurse. Strategic planning has a mission; collects and analyzes data; assesses strengths and weaknesses; sets goals and objectives; uses strategies; operates on a timetable; gives operational and functional guidance to nurse managers; and includes evaluation.

Tactical planning is short range planning. Operational planning puts strategic and "tactical planning" in operation. It includes goals, objectives, strategies, actions, a timetable, identification of responsible persons, and note of accomplishments. Operational planning is daily, weekly, and monthly planning and can provide data for further strategic and tactical planning.

NOTES

1. H. Fayol, trans. by C. Storrs, *General and Industrial Management* (London: Isaac Pitman & Sons, 1949), 43–50.
2. L. Urwick, *The Elements of Administration* (New York: Harper & Row, 1944), 26–34.
3. L. M. Douglass, *The Effective Nurse: Leader and Manager* (3d. ed., Saint Louis: C. V. Mosby, 1988), 92–93.
4. Ibid., 94.
5. E. L. Alexander, *Nursing Administration in the Hospital Health Care System*, 2d ed. (Saint Louis: C. V. Mosby, 1978), 132.
6. Ibid., 134–150.
7. G. A. Steiner, *Top Management Planning* (New York: Macmillan, 1969), 1.
8. M. Beyers and C. Phillips, *Nursing Management for Patient Care*, 2d. ed. (Boston: Little, Brown, 1979), 41–48.
9. R. L. Ackoff, "Our Changing Concept of Planning," *The Journal of Nursing Administration*, Oct. 1986, 35–40.
10. Douglass, op. cit., 95–96.
11. Ibid., 96–106.
12. H. M. Donovan, *Nursing Service Administration: Managing the Enterprise* (Saint Louis: C. V. Mosby, 1975), 50–64.
13. P.F. Drucker, *Management: Tasks, Responsibilities, Practices* (New York: Harper & Row, 1973), 121–129.
14. H. Koontz and H. Weihrich, *Management* (New York: McGraw-Hill, 1988), 16.
15. Donovan, op. cit., 63–64.
16. R. M. Hodgetts, *Management: Theory, Process, and Practice*, 4th ed. (Orlando, FL: Academic Press, 1986), 97.
17. H. S. Rowland and B. L. Rowland, *Nursing Administration Handbook*, 2d ed. (Rockville, MD.: Aspen, 1985), 24–27.
18. W. E. Reif and J. L. Webster, "The Strategic Planning Process," *Arizona Business*, Apr. 1976, 14–20.
19. A. P. Meier, "The Planning Process," *Managerial Planning*, July/Aug. 1974, 1–5, 9.
20. P. F. Drucker, op. cit., 125.
21. D. H. Fox and R. T. Fox, "Strategic Planning for Nursing," *The Journal of Nursing Administration*, May 1983, 11–16; R. N. Paul and J. W. Taylor, "The State of Strategic Planning," *Business*, Jan.-Mar. 1986, 37–43.
22. Z. C. Mercer, "Personal Planning: An Overlooked Application of the Corporate Planning Process," *Managerial Planning*, Jan./Feb. 1980, 32–35.
23. Ibid.
24. D. H. Fox and R. T. Fox, op. cit.
25. E. J. Metz, "The Missing 'H' in Strategic Planning," *Managerial Planning*, May/June 1984, 19–23, 29.
26. E. C. Smith, "How to Tie Human Resource Planning to Strategic Business Planning," *Managerial Planning*, Sept./Oct. 1983, 29–34.
27. Ibid.
28. E. J. Metz, op. cit.
29. R. Cushman, "Norton's Top-Down, Bottom-Up Planning Process," *Planning Review*, Nov. 1979, 3–8, 48.
30. When the terms "goals" and "objectives" are used, their meaning should be defined. Some references cite goals as being strategic and objectives as being tactical or operational; others use the opposite definitions.
31. D. W. Nylen, "Making Your Business Plan an Action Plan," *Business*, Oct.-Dec. 1985, 12–16.
32. E. K. Singleton and F. C. Nail, "Guidelines for Establishing a New Service," *Journal of Nursing Administration*, Oct. 1985, 22–26.
33. Joint Commission on Accreditation of Healthcare Organizations, *Accreditation Manual for Hospitals* (Chicago, IL.: American Hospital Association, 1989), 133–139.

REFERENCES

Bryan, E. L. and R. E. Welton, "Let Your Business Plan be a Road Map to Credit," *Business*, July-Sept. 1986, 44–47.

Forman, L., "Which Comes First, the Planning Process or the Planning Model?," *Business Economics*, Sept. 1979, 42–47.

Gray, D. H., "Uses and Misuses of Strategic Planning," *Harvard Business Review*, Jan.-Feb. 1986, 89–97.

Palesy, S. R., "Motivating Line Management Using the Planning Process," *Planning Review*, Mar. 1980, 3–8, 44–48.

Paul, R. N., and J. W. Taylor, "The State of Strategic Planning," *Business*, Jan.-Mar. 1986, 37–43.

Pearce, W. H., "I Thought I Knew What Good Management Was," *Harvard Business Review*, Mar.-Apr. 1986, 59–65.

Redman, L. N., "The Planning Process," *Managerial Planning*, May/June 1983, 24–30, 40.

Mission, Philosophy, Objectives, and Management Plans

3

INTRODUCTION

Statements of mission or purpose, of philosophy or beliefs, of objectives, and of an operational or management plan have already been referred to; in this chapter, these basic tools of management are discussed in greater detail. Knowledge of their use is part of the theory of nursing management. They are part of the planning function of nursing management and skill in using them successfully is part of the strategy of nursing management planning.

Written statements of purpose, philosophy, and objectives and written operational plans are the blueprints for effective management of any enterprise, including a health-care institution. They are a component of planning at each management level. Statements at the corporate level serve the top managers of the organization. Those at the division level serve the managers of major divisions such as nursing, operations, or finance. These statements evolve from and support those of the institution. Services, departments, and units each have written statements of purpose, philosophy, and objectives and written operational plans that are developed from and support the documents at the division and corporate levels;[1] see Figure 3–1.

MISSION OR PURPOSE

Each organization exists for specific purposes or missions and to fulfill specific social functions. For health-care organizations this means providing health-care services to maintain health, cure illness, and allay pain and suffering. Business enterprises and government provide most of the economic resources to pay for these services. Although nursing has not been considered a profit-making enterprise, this condition is changing as third-party payers require better cost-accounting procedures.

Defining a mission or purpose allows nursing to be managed for performance. It describes what it

FIGURE 3–1. Evolution of Mission, Philosophy, and Objectives Statements and Operational Plans

Operational plans
Mission (purpose) statements
Philosophy (beliefs) statements   Corporate →
Objectives statements   Division →
Operational (management)   Department →
  plans   Unit.

will be and what it should be. It describes the constituencies to be satisfied. It is the professional nurse manager's commitment to a specific definition of purpose or mission.

One purpose of a nursing entity is to provide nursing care to clients. This can include promotion of self-care concepts. Thus the statement should include definitions of nursing and self-care as defined by professional nurses.

Virginia Henderson has defined nursing as follows:

The unique function of the nurse is to assist the individual, sick or well, in the performance of those activities contributing to health or its recovery (or to peaceful death) that he would perform unaided if he had the necessary strength, will or knowledge. And to do this in such a way as to help him gain independence as rapidly as possible.[2]

Yura and Walsh describe the nursing process as

an orderly, systematic manner of determining the client's health status, specifying problems defined as alterations in human need fulfillment, making plans to solve them, initiating and implementing the plan, and evaluating the extent to which the plan was effective in promoting the optimum wellness and resolving the problems identified.[3]

King defined nursing as

a process of action, reaction, interaction, and transaction whereby nurses assist individuals of any age group to meet their basic human needs in coping with their health status at some particular point in their life cycle. Nurses perform their functions within social institutions and they interact with individuals and groups. Therefore, three distinct levels of operation exist: (1) the individual; (2) the group; and (3) society.[4]

Orem defined nursing as follows:

Nursing is an art through which the nurse, the practitioner of nursing, gives specialized assitance to persons with disabilities of such a character that more than ordinary assistance is necessary to meet daily needs for self-care and to intelligently participate in the medical care they are receiving from the physician. The art of nursing is practiced by 'doing for' the patient with the disability, by 'helping him to do for himself,' and/or by 'helping him learn how to do for himself'. Nursing is also practiced by helping a capable person from the patient's family or a friend of the patient learn how 'to do for' the patient. Nursing is thus a practical and didactic art.[5]

Kinlein suggested that "nursing is assisting the person in his self-care practices in regard to his state of health."[6] Emerging from these and other theories of nursing is a commonality of terms central to the definition of nursing: nurse, patient or client, individual, group, society, nursing process, self-care, and health.

A further mission of nursing is to provide a public good and this should be indicated in the statement of mission or purpose. The statement of mission or purpose tells why the nursing entity exists. It is written so that it can be known by all people working within the organizational entity, since it states the reason for their employment. An ultimate strategy is to have nursing personnel participate in developing mission statements and in keeping them updated, so that they will know, understand and support them.

The mission should be known and understood by other health care practitioners, by clients and their families, and by the community. A statement of purpose must be dynamic, giving action and strength to evolving statements of philosophy, objectives, and management plans. Statements of purpose can be made dynamic by indicating the relationship between the nursing unit and patients, personnel, community, health, illness, and self-care. Figures 3–2, 3–3, and 3–4 represent examples of mission statements from three different levels: the organization, the division, and the unit, respectively.

Use Figure 3–5 to develop or evaluate the mission statements of your employer or organization.

Mission statements are used in successful business and industrial organizations to provide a clearly defined reason for being. They are simple statements to move the organization forward and are formulated for performance, products, and services. They contain statements of ethics, principles, and standards that are understood by workers. Workers who clearly perceive that they are pursuing meaningful and worthwhile goals through their individual efforts are more committed and dedicated than those who do not.[7]

FIGURE 3–2.   Mission and Purpose of the University of South Alabama Medical Center

1. It is the mission of the University of South Alabama Medical Center to provide the best possible health care services and resources for the people of the community and the state and to provide a high-quality setting conducive to the medical education and research activities of the College of Medicine.
2. To provide good quality and cost-effective acute care services to patients to get them discharged to self-care as safely and quickly as possible.
3. To provide a dynamic innovative setting for clinical experiences for postgraduate education, medical students, nursing students and allied health students.
4. To provide a setting for the conduct of funded medical, nursing, and allied health research.
5. To establish and maintain sound financial practices and procedures, recognizing the patient care and education missions will only be achieved through the protection and growth of hospital assets.
6. To provide a safe and comfortable environment that is conducive to learning and which provides an environment that allows the patient and family to feel their emotional and medical needs are being satisfied.

SOURCE: Courtesy of the University of South Alabama Medical Center, Mobile, Alabama.

FIGURE 3–3.   Purposes—Division of Nursing

The purposes of this organization shall be:

1. To assess, plan, implement, and evaluate nursing care in keeping with the standards for professional nursing practice, as defined by professional nurses of the staff and the ANA Standards of Nursing Practice. Believing that health is not merely the absence of disease or infirmity but a state of optimum physical, mental, and social well-being, nursing care promotes self-care concepts and enables clients to meet their basic human needs in coping with their health status throughout their life cycles.

2. To develop and continuously evaluate systems and methods of nursing management with open channels of communication between all levels of practitioners and other disciplines. This system holds final authority and accountability for the quality of nursing care delivered by each professional practitioner at every level.

3. To strive to constantly improve the quality of nursing care delivered by providing and promoting staff development programs, ongoing nursing research programs, and formal mechanisms for evaluating the level of care provided, including quality assurance, patient classification systems, and a quality monitoring system. In addition, to develop and implement formal client education programs fostering self-care abilities.

4. To be accountable for providing quality nursing care at the lowest cost to our clients utilizing the nursing process to set attainable self-care goals for them.

5. To evaluate, make changes and additions as needed.

SOURCE: Courtesy of the University of South Alabama Medical Center, Mobile, Alabama.

Proprietary changes have brought change and competition to the hospital industry. They have also brought business techniques, moving the hospital industry from being facilities-dominated to being market-driven. The corporate structures of for-profit hospitals consider product line and function. They focus on mission. This focus has been adopted by not-for-profit hospitals that now look at mission

FIGURE 3–4. Purpose—Sixth Floor

The purpose of the sixth floor is consistent with the purpose of the Division of Nursing.

1. To assess the physical, emotional, and spiritual needs of patients, their families, and/or significant others so as to provide optimal care.

2. To provide each patient with an individualized plan of care, in regard to their needs, in a cost-effective manner to the patient and the hospital.

3. To serve as the patient's, family's, and/or significant other's advocate to assure complete care with regard to the patient's, family's, and/or significant other's needs.

4. To provide and promote continuing education through in-services, research projects, and patient care conferences to improve the quality of our health care.

5. To incorporate all disciplines related to patient's care, in evaluating the needs of the patient, family, and/or significant others.

6. To assess and evaluate our quality of nursing care on an ongoing basis through quality assurance and monthly audits.

SOURCE: Courtesy of the University of South Alabama Medical Center, Mobile, Alabama.

statements relative to new markets, market share, and diversification. These new not-for-profit corporate structures are organized like chains and look at regionalization and integration as linkages. Their leadership is dynamic and future-oriented rather than being focused on maintenance.[8]

PHILOSOPHY

A written statement of philosophy sets out values and beliefs that pertain to nursing administration and nursing practice within the institution or organization. It verbalizes the nurse manager and nurse practitioners' visions of what they believe nursing management and practice are. It states their beliefs as to how the mission or purpose will be achieved, giving direction toward this end. Statements of philosophy are abstract and contain value statements about human beings as clients or patients and as workers, about work that will be performed by nursing workers for clients or patients, about self-care, about nursing as a profession, about education as it obtains to competence of nursing workers, and about the setting or community in which nursing services are provided. The character and tone of service are set by planning that evolves purpose and philosophy statements, one from the other, for the organization, division, department or service, and ward or unit.

Hodgetts indicates that all managers in any organization have a set of values, each generation being different from the preceding one.[9] Predictions of future values for the 1990s will reflect the future values of society. Nurse managers will be involved and will reflect the values of the times in their statements of philosophy. The philosophy of an organization is very often implicit and is not written down.

As with mission statements, philosophy statements evolve from higher levels of management and practice. Figures 3–6, 3–7, and 3–8 are exam-

FIGURE 3–5. Standards for the Evaluation of Mission Statements of the Nursing Division and Its Departments, Services, and Units

1. The mission statement tells the reason for the existence of the nursing division, department, service, or unit in relation to the practice of nursing and of self-care as defined by the nursing staff and in relation to the service being provided to the community of clients. Once definitions of nursing and self-care have been developed by the nursing staff and ratified by the nursing administration, they may be quoted in the mission statement.

2. The mission statement supports the mission of the organization, within the nursing division.

3. It indicates that the nursing organization exists to provide a public good.

4. You may add to these standards.

FIGURE 3–6.   Philosophy of the University of South Alabama Medical Center

---

Policy   We believe that:

- The University of South Alabama Medical Center is dedicated to excellence in the fields of patient care, teaching, and research.
- We are dedicated to providing the most effective and efficient patient care.
- We are committed to provide services for patients requiring highly specialized and unique medical treatment.
- We are committed to providing a safe environment for patients, staff, and guests. We assure the rights of patients to confidentiality, full disclosure of risks involved in care, and involvement in decision making.
- Continuing education is essential to competence of staff. Professional growth and development is both a personal and organizational responsibility.
- Research should be fostered to the extent possible and should follow acceptable guidelines for protection of human subjects.
- We have an obligation to monitor all activities through quality assurance and to initiate corrective measures when indicated.
- Everyone should be treated with dignity.
- There are fiscal limits to what we can do, therefore every employee must market the hospital to obtain revenues to maintain financial stability.
- Health care for the medically indigent is the responsibility of society and the community from which they come. Our capacity and obligation for providing indigent care is limited to what the community supports.
- We have an obligation to use our finances and limited resources responsibly and maintain and improve the fiscal integrity of our institution.
- Health care should focus on wellness as well as illness. We promote and plan for patients to care for themselves from time of admission.
- We are the leaders in health care in this community. We believe in supporting laws and regulations and in working to make changes that benefit our mission.
- Our staff are our best asset and they will be treated with respect.
- Our staff have a responsibility to provide learning experiences for all students in the health care field, including providing appropriate clinical settings and role models.

SOURCE: Courtesy of the University of South Alabama Medical Center, Mobile, Alabama.

FIGURE 3–7.   Philosophy of the Division of Nursing

We believe that:

- The philosophy of the Division of Nursing is consistent with the philosophy of the University of South Alabama Medical Center.
- We are dedicated to excellence in patient care, teaching, and research and to providing the most effective and efficient care.
- Everyone should be treated with dignity.
- Health is not merely the absence of disease or infirmity but a state of optimum physical, mental, and social well-being.
- Nursing care promotes self-care concepts, enabling patients to meet their basic human needs in coping with their health status throughout their life cycles. Nursing involves a broad approach of health care aimed at a healthy society through education of the public.
- Professional nursing care at University of South Alabama Medical Center is provided equally to all patients accepted for treatment.
- Patients and their families have a right to be kept informed about all aspects of their health status and to participate in decisions affecting their care to the fullest extent possible.
- The physical, mental, spiritual, and social needs of our patients can be achieved by striving to maintain goal-directed multidisciplinary plans of care.
- The highly specialized care offered at the Medical Center requires qualified staff for all positions. The most important assets of the institution are the staff and they will be treated with respect.
- We have an obligation to manage personnel and finances to achieve maximum productivity.
- Improvement of the quality of nursing is assured by the continuous evaluation of nursing care and positive modifications to nursing techniques and activities.
- Continuing education is essential to the delivery of quality professional nursing and is both a personal and organizational responsibility.
- We have a responsibility to provide appropriate learning experiences and role models for all students in the health care field.
- We accept the responsibility of being involved in nursing research.

SOURCE: Courtesy of the University of South Alabama Medical Center, Mobile, Alabama.

Figure 3–8. Philosophy of Sixth Floor

- We believe that all patients should be given equal, individualized care by all nursing staff incorporating physical, emotional, and spiritual needs.
- We believe the goal of health care should be assisting the patient to progress toward a level of optimal health.
- We believe that the patient should be encouraged by all nursing staff to progress toward self-care and independence.
- We believe that it is the responsibility of all nursing staff to act as a patient advocate to provide quality care according to the wishes of the patient, family, and/or significant others.
- We believe that continuing education is a necessary component of continuing improvement in health care.
- We believe that nursing is an integral part of health care and the nurse is an important member of the health care team.
- We believe that patients, their families, and/or significant others have the right to be well informed about the patient's state of health, prognosis, and care.

Source: Courtesy of the University of South Alabama Medical Center, Mobile, Alabama.

ples of philosophy statements for the organizational, divisional, and unit levels, respectively.

Use Figure 3–9 to develop or evaluate philosophy statements of your employer or organization.

OBJECTIVES

Objectives are concrete and specific statements of the goals that nurse managers seek to accomplish. They are action commitments through which the mission will be achieved and the philosophy or beliefs sustained. They are used to establish priorities. They are stated in terms of results to be achieved and focus on the provision of health care services to clients. Like the statements of mission and philosophy, they must be functional and useful. They must be alive. Moore has stated, "If objectives are presented in terms of what can be observed, they can serve as useful tools for evaluation of nursing care and personnel performance, and as a basis for planning educational programs, staffing, requisi-

tion of supplies and equipment, and other functions associated with the nursing department."[10]

According to Moore, there should be objectives for evaluation of patient care, evaluation of personnel performance, planning educational programs, staffing, and requisition of supplies and equipment.

Drucker indicates that mission and purpose, as well as the basic definition of a business, have to be translated into objectives if they are to become more than insight, good intentions, and brilliant epigrams never to be achieved. Objectives are concrete statements that become the standards against which performance can be measured. Objectives are the basic tactics of any business, including the business of nursing management. Objectives must be selective rather than global and they must be multiple rather than single, so as to balance a wide range of

Figure 3–9. Standards for Evaluation of Philosophy Statement of the Nursing Division, Department, Service, or Unit

1. A written statement of philosophy should exist for the nursing division or department or service or unit.
2. A written statement of philosophy should be developed in collaboration with nursing employees, the consumers, and other health-care workers.
3. Nursing personnel should share in an annual (or more frequent) review and revision of the written statement of philosophy.
4. The written statement of philosophy should reflect these beliefs or values:
   4.1 The meaning of the clinical practice of nursing.
   4.2 Recognition of rights of individuals and of the responsibility of nursing personnel to serve as advocates for those rights.
   4.3 Selective other statements about humanity, society, health, nursing, nursing process, and self-care relevant to external forces (community, laws, etc.) and internal forces (personnel, clients, material resources, etc.), research, education, and family as are deemed appropriate to accomplishing the mission of the division, department, service, or unit.
5. The nursing philosophy should support the philosophy of the organization as expressed at all levels above the nursing division.
6. The statement of philosophy should give direction to the achievement of the mission.
7. You may add to these standards.

needs and goals related to nursing services to clients or patients; productive use of people, money, and material resources; updating through innovation; and the discharge of a social responsibility to the community. Objectives must be used, and one way to use them is to develop them into specific management and operational plans.[11]

The nursing staff—specifically, the nurse manager—must decide where efforts will be concentrated to achieve results. Some areas of concentration have already been mentioned. Others may be similar to those related to business and industry. They include marketing and the development of health care services in areas of need. As an example, there has recently been increased activity in the area of physical and mental wellness or fitness. There is potential for much more in the area of prevention of disease and injury.

Another area for objectives is innovation. This would include the introduction of new methods and particularly the application of new knowledge.

Organization and use of all resources—human, financial, and physical—are areas for objectives. They address the need to develop managers, the needs of major groups within the division including nonmanagerial workers, labor relations, the development of positive employee attitudes, and maintenance and upgrading of employee skills. Objectives provide for attractive job and career opportunities. They provide activities to control worker assignment and productivity. Objectives are the means by which productivity in nursing is measured.

Objectives are also needed in the area of social responsibility. Society must believe that nursing is useful and productive and that it does a desired job; see Figure 3–10.

Management balances objectives. Some will be short-range, with their accomplishment in easy view or reach. Others will be long-range, and some may even be in the "hope to accomplish" category. The budget is the mechanical expression of setting and balancing objectives. The nurse manager plans two budgets, one for operations and one for future capital expenditures. Some priorities will be set with the budget, as illustrated in Figure 3–11.

Objectives are the fundamental strategy of nursing, since they specify the end product of all nursing activities. They must be capable of being converted into specific targets and specific assignments so that nurses will know what they have to do

FIGURE 3–10.   Examples of Categorical Areas for Writing Objectives

- *Evaluation of patient care.* To develop methods of measuring the quality of patient care.
- *Evaluation of personnel performance.* The patient benefits from close nursing supervision of all nonprofessional personnel who give patient care and from continuous appraisal of the nursing care given and the performance of all nursing personnel based on professional standards.
- *Planning educational programs.* The patient benefits from a continuous, flexible program of in-service education for all division of nursing personnel, adapted to orientation, skill training, continuous education, and leadership development.
- *Staffing.* To establish a systematic staffing pattern for patient care so that all members of each department can function in accordance with their skill levels for the maintenance of continuity of nursing care and management of nursing service.
- *Requisition of supplies and equipment.* To supply nursing personnel with adequate resources to facilitate patient care; to anticipate future nursing needs and plan for the acquisition of needed resources.
- *Marketing.* To collaborate and consult with intradepartmental health team members for maximal effectiveness in promoting health care and disease prevention. New programs will be developed to meet identified needs.
- *Innovation.* To influence progressive nursing practices and research training programs in supporting changing trends that improve the quality of patient care.
- *Organization and use of all resources (human, financial, and physical).* To apply standards for decentralization of decision making and increase efficiency and effectiveness of staffing and budgeting.
- *Social responsibility.* To support, publicize, and sustain service to the community in health endeavors.

Some of these objectives are not as clearly stated as they could be; however, each was fully developed in the operational plan for its accomplishment.

to accomplish them. Objectives become the basis and motivation for the nursing work necessary to accomplish them and for measuring nursing achievement. They make possible the concentration of human and material resources and of human

FIGURE 3–11. Examples of Balanced Objectives

- *Long-range objective.* Write a plan to develop patient teaching guides for all areas.
- *Short-range objective.* Establish procedures for safe nursing care by having fire department personnel hold classes on fire evacuation procedures for all nursing personnel on all three shifts.
- *Future budget.* Plan with the budget director to have funds allocated to repaint patients' rooms and replace worn and torn furniture.
- *Current budget.* Implement the classes for expectant parents for which funds have been allocated.

efforts. Objectives are needed in all areas on which the survival of nursing and health care services depend. In nursing all objectives should be performance objectives that provide for existing nursing services for existing patient groups. They provide for abandonment of unneeded and outmoded nursing services and health care products. They provide for new nursing services and health care products for existing patients. They provide for new groups of patients, for the distributive organization, and for standards of nursing service and performance.

Objectives are the basis for work and assignments. They determine the organizational structure, the key activities, and the allocation of people to tasks. Objectives make the work of nursing clear and unambiguous, with measurable results, deadlines, and specific assignments of accountability. They give direction and make commitments that mobilize the resources and energies of nursing for the making of the future. Objectives are needed for the organization, division, and all wards or units. They should be changed as necessary, particularly when there is a change of mission or when current objectives are no longer functional.[12] Refer to Figure 3–12 for a breakdown of the elements of objectives.

Figures 3–13, 3–14, and 3–15 are examples of objectives for an organization, a nursing division, and a nursing unit, respectively. Use Figure 3–16 to develop or evaluate the objectives of your own organization.

THE OPERATIONAL PLAN

Objectives must be converted into actions: activities, assignments, and deadlines, all with clear accountability. The action level is where nurse managers eliminate the old and plan for the new. It is where time dimensions are put into perspective and new and different methods can be tried. It is where nurse managers answer these questions over and over again: What is it? What will it be? What should it be?

An operational plan is the written blueprint for achieving objectives. It specifies the activities and procedures that will be used to achieve them and sets timetables for their achievement. It tells who the responsible persons are for each and every activity and procedure. It describes ways of preparing people for jobs and procedures for evaluating

FIGURE 3–12. The Elements of Objectives

- *A performance objective.* The patient receives individualized care in a safe environment to meet the total therapeutic nursing needs—physical, emotional, spiritual, environmental, social, economic, and rehabilitative (also illustrates next provision).
- *Existing nursing services for existing patients.* Nurse consultants have been made available from medical nursing, surgical nursing, mental health nursing, and maternal and child health nursing. Their services can be requested by any professional nurse or physician.
- *Abandonment of outmoded nursing services and products.* New isolation procedures have been implemented and the old handwashing basins have been discarded.
- *New nursing services for new groups of patients.* Plans are being made to offer consultative nursing services from the general hospital to nursing homes in the area. In the future this will be extended to retirement homes. Both actions are the result of market surveys.
- *Distributive organization for new nursing services.* The nurse manager has evaluated the necessity of restructuring the organization of the division of nursing to provide new nursing services.
- *Standards of nursing service and performance.* The nurse manager has decided to use the Standards of Nursing Practice developed by the ANA Congress for Nursing Practice for all nurses within the division.

FIGURE 3–13.　Goals of the University of South Alabama Medical Center

Global Goals

Increase paying patients.

Increase awareness of resources among public.

Short-term plan of what we sell.

Long-term plan of what we sell.

Increase in services.

Educate the staff to sell the hospital formal plan to build hospital on campus.

Research provision of differently priced services.

Market hospital to university employees.

Improve access to hospital.

Improve intelligence.

Residents to use Medical Center for private practice.

Improve managing of patients for maximum reimbursement.

Create new markets.

Improve efficiency.

Recognize hospital as a business.

Reconcile difference in goals between Foundation and hospital.

Definitive Goals

1. Increase paying patients.
   1.1 Plan for incentive for M.D.'s (Steve).
   1.2 Who are private M.D.'s using hospital? (Pat).
   1.3 Survey private M.D.'s in town (John).
   1.4 Market HMO (internal) (Susie and John).
   1.5 Input from department heads (Brookley meeting).
   1.6 Create new markets and identify opportunities through money arrangements.
      1.6.1 Where are they? (Dept. Heads).
      1.6.2 Maintain ROA.
      1.6.3 Maintain Keesler arrangement.
      1.6.4 Surrounding counties.
      1.6.5 HHC.
      1.6.6 Public service (plan for industry—Pat)
      1.6.7 Organizations and involvement (clinic and campus).
      1.6.8 Student organizations on campus.
   1.7 Market hospital to university employees.
2. Increase awareness of resources among public.
   2.1 P.R. plan.
   2.2 Short-term marketing plan of what we sell (identifying what we are selling now).
3. Long-term marketing plan of what we sell.
   3.1 What new products can we sell (or divert)?
   3.2 Formal plan to build hospital on campus.
4. Educate the staff to sell the hospital.
   4.1 Just for the pride of it.
   4.2 Management people in civic organizations.
   4.3 Reference 1.4.
   4.4 Employees identify with P.R. and marketing people.
   4.5 Recognize hospital as a business.
5. Research provision of differently priced services.
   5.1 Innovative ways to bill for services.
6. Improve access to hospital.
   6.1 Parking.
   6.2 Waiting areas.
   6.3 Emergency Department.
7. Improve intelligence (above board).
   7.1 Professional groups.
   7.2 Reference 4.2.
   7.3 Internal network.
8. Residents to use Medical Center for private practice.
9. Improve efficiency.
   9.1 Improve managing of patients for maximum reimbursement.
      9.1.1 Audit bills with charts.
10. Improve cooperative relationship between Foundation (C of M) and Medical Center.

SOURCE: Courtesy of the University of South Alabama Medical Center, Mobile, Alabama.

FIGURE 3–14. Objectives of the Division of Nursing

The objectives of this Division of Nursing shall be to provide the patient:

1. Individualized care in a safe environment to meet the patient's total needs as assessed by the professional nurse, utilizing the nursing process. This care covers physical, emotional, spiritual, environmental, social, economic, and rehabilitational needs involved in planning total patient care.

2. An effective teaching program which will include guidance and assistance in the use of medical resources and community agencies.

3. Benefits of effective communication, cooperation, and coordination with all professional and administrative services involved in the planning of total patient care.

4. Benefits of a continuous, flexible program of in-service education for all departments of nursing personnel adapted to orientation, in-service, continuing education and leadership development.

5. Benefits from nursing services' participation in education of students.

6. With cost-effective care by the timely procurement, effective utilization, and proper handling of equipment and supplies.

7. Benefits through a positive work atmosphere in which nurses' job satisfaction is attained.

8. Benefits from a close association between division of nursing personnel and community nursing organizations and groups to keep abreast of current trends and advancements in nursing.

9. Maximum nursing care hours, by relieving nursing personnel of non-nursing duties.

10. Benefits from the development of a cost-effective balanced budget for the division of nursing.

11. Benefits from close supervision by an R.N. of all personnel who give patient care and from continuous evaluation of the care given.

12. Benefits from implementation of the results of nursing research.

SOURCE: Courtesy of the University of South Alabama Medical Center, Mobile, Alabama.

care of patients. It specifies the records that will be kept and the policies needed. It gives individual managers freedom to accomplish their own objectives as well as those of the institution, division, department, ward, or unit. The operational plan is sometimes called a management plan; refer to Figures 3–17 and 3–18.

STRATEGY

Planning is the strategy of an organization. It is essential to any and all businesses including those providng health care.

Top management has to answer planning questions like these:

1. Where do we go and what do we want to become? Such questions seek to define the organization's mission and objectives.
2. What and where are we now? The purpose here is to examine and define the organization's philosophy and objectives.
3. How can we best get there? The answer to this question will take the form of ongoing plans that include organizing, directing, and controlling concepts.

Such activities constitute the strategy of top management. They are developed into the strategy of the nursing division's top management and subsequently into the strategy of nursing and other business units of the organization. Planning is nei-

FIGURE 3–15.   Objectives of Sixth Floor

The objectives of the Sixth Floor shall be to provide the patient, family, and/or significant others:

1. Individualized total patient care based on an assessment by an R.N., considering all needs, physical, emotional, and spiritual, of the patient, family, and/or significant others.

2. The nursing process will be the basis of all care given by the professional nurse.

3. To provide quality care in a cost-effective manner to patient and hospital.

4. To coordinate information from all disciplines, to plan for optimum care while hospitalized and after discharge.

5. To involve the patient's family and/or significant others in caring for the patient to meet their needs.

6. To identify problem areas in nursing care through monthly audits to ensure the quality of our nursing care.

7. To provide a variety of in-service [training] from all departments involved in the care of the patient to increase knowledge and improve nursing care.

SOURCE: Courtesy of the University of South Alabama Medical Center, Mobile, Alabama.

ther a top-down nor a bottom-up proposition. Each level must harmonize their strategies with those below and above.[13]

Focusing on development and use of planning strategies is a key element that gives direction, cohesion, and thrust to the nursing division. Nurse employees involved in achieving objectives and goals are motivated. They should be clearly defined and focus on the future without losing sight of the present. Successful implementation of management plans to achieve mission objectives and goals while sustaining philosophy results in productivity, profitability, and achievement. This process is managing and it is performed by managers.[14]

Cavanaugh relates strategy to power, indicating that organizational power gives nurse administrators the power to do their jobs better. Her suggestions for nurse managers to strategize are summarized as follows:

1. Use the political system to turn personal power into organizational power.
2. Recognize the self-interests of others in the organization and use them in a win-win manner.

FIGURE 3–16.   Standards for Evaluation of Statements of Objectives for a Nursing Division, Department, Service, or Unit

1. The objectives for the nursing division, or department, or service, or unit should be in written form.
2. The objectives should be developed in collaboration with the nursing personnel who will assist in achieving them.
3. Nursing personnel should share in an annual (or more frequent) review and revision of the written statements of objectives.
4. The written statements of objectives should meet these qualitiative and quantitative criteria:
   4.1 They operationalize the statements of mission and philosophy; they can be translated into actions.
   4.2 They can be measured or verified.
   4.3 They exist in a hierarchy or sequence that is by priority.
   4.4 They are clearly stated.
   4.5 They are realistic in terms of human and physical resources and capabilities.
   4.6 They direct the use of resources.
   4.7 They are achievable (practical).
   4.8 They are specific.
   4.9 They indicate results expected from nursing efforts and activities; the ends of management programs.
   4.10 They show a network of desired events and results.
   4.11 They are flexible and allow for adjustment.
   4.12 They are known to the nursing personnel who will use them.
   4.13 They are quantified wherever possible.
   4.14 They exist for all positions.
5. You may add to these standards.

FIGURE 3–17.   Management Plan

Objective.   The client receives skilled nursing services to meet his total individual needs as diagnosed by professional nurses. This process is systematic, beginning with the gathering of base data and it is planned, implemented, evaluated, and revised on a continual basis. It covers physical, emotional, spiritual, environmental, social, economical, and rehabilitational needs and includes health teaching involved in the planning of total client care. Its ultimate goal is to assist clients to, or return them to, optimal health status and independence as quickly as possible.

Actions	Target Dates	Accomplishments
1. Institute primary care nursing.	January 1–June 30	Assigned to Ms. Scott. Decision made to attempt to use self-care concepts of Orem: (1) definition, and
1.1 Assign problem of overall development of a plan.	January 31	(2) nursing systems.
1.2 Assign development of a self-care concept for application using Orem and Kinlein as references.	February 15	Assigned to Ms. Longez January 19. In discussion with Ms. Scott and Ms. Longez a decision was made to investigate application of self-care using the nursing process as described by Kinlein. The nursing staff were particularly interested in the nursing history process described by Kinlein. Ms. Longez has added this dimension to her assignment. She has requested Mr. Jarmann be assigned to assist her and he has agreed.
1.3 Organize resources.	February 28	February 5; Ms. Scott has just updated me on the project. A good portion of her plan has been developed. They are now doing a staffing plan including job descriptions and job standards. February 27; The plan is completed and has been discussed with me. A few minor adjustments are being made.
1.4 Coordinate plan.	March 31	
1.4.1 Nursing personnel.		Done. All want to participate.
1.4.2 Administrator.		Done.
1.4.3 Public relations.		Announcements made to community through news media.
1.4.4 Physicians.		Done and well received.
1.4.5 Other as needed.		Presented to board per request of administrator. They want progress reports.
1.5 Select and train staff.	April 30	Assigned to Ms. Finch for training. Will be assisted by Ms. Scott and Ms. Longez. I will select staff with their recommendation.
1.6 Implement.	June 30	Ms. Scott wants to direct implementation and I have concurred.

FIGURE 3–18. Standards for Evaluation of Management Plan of Nursing Division, Department, Service, or Unit

1. The written management plan should operationalize the objectives of the nursing division, department, service, or unit. It should specify activities or actions, persons responsible for accomplishing them, and target dates or time frames, as well as providing for evaluation of progress. Each activity or action should be listed in problem-solving or decision-making format, as appropriate.

2. The management plan is personal to the incumbent, who should select the standards for developing, maintaining, and evaluating it. The nurse manager should solicit desired input from appropriate nursing persons and others.

3. The actions listed should reflect planning for:

   3.1 Nursing care programs to ensure safe and competent nursing services to clients.

       3.1.1 The nursing process, including data gathering, assessment, diagnosis, goal setting and prescription, intervention and application, evaluation, feedback, change, and accountability to the consumer.

       3.1.2 A process and outcome audit.

       3.1.3 Promotion of self-care practices.

   3.2 Establishment of policies and procedures for employing competent nursing personnel: recruitment, selection, assignment, retention, and promotion based on individual qualifications and capabilities without regard to race, national origin, creed, color, sex, or age.

   3.3 Integration of nursing-care programs into the total program of the health-care organization and community through committee participation in professional and service activities, and credentialing of individuals in organizations, including nursing organizations.

   3.4 A budget that is evaluated and revised as necessary.

   3.5 Job descriptions that include standards stated as objectives, outcomes, or results and that are known to the incumbents.

   3.6 Specific utilization of personnel. This part of the plan should:

       3.6.1 Conform to a staffing plan that is based on timing nursing activities and rating of patients.

       3.6.2 Match competencies of people to total job requirements.

       3.6.3 Place prepared people in practice.

       3.6.4 Place prepared people in administration.

       3.6.5 Place prepared people in education.

       3.6.6 Place prepared people in research.

       3.6.7 Foster identification of non-nursing tasks and their assignment to appropriate other departments or non-nursing personnel.

       3.6.8 Recognize excellence in all fields: administration, education, research, and practice.

   3.7 Provision of needed supplies and equipment for nursing activities.

   3.8 Provision of input into remodeling and establishing required physical facilities.

   3.9 Orientation and continuing education of all nursing personnel.

   3.10 Education of students in the health-care field according to a written agreement and collaborative implementation between faculty of the educational institutions and personnel of the service organization.

   3.11 Development of nursing research staff, research activities, and application of the research findings of others.

   3.12 Evaluation of all objectives—organizational, divisional, departmental, and at the service and unit level, as well as those stated in the individual's job description and standards.

4. The management plans should have mileposts that are reasonable and attainable, with deadlines included.

5. Management plans should be based on complete information.

6. You may add to these standards.

3. Diagnose, plan, and execute an effective political campaign to achieve a well-thought-out, purposeful goal.
4. Define ways to achieve objectives while helping others. Know people and their goals.
5. Disengage from losing issues and from issues in which you have to defend yourself on someone else's turf. A technique for doing this is placing it at the end of an agenda or leaving it out of minutes.
6. Defend your territory.
7. Plan and carry out an offense on issues of your own choosing and commitment.
8. Build coalitions.
9. Exploit opportunities using situations to advantage. Go after winning issues.
10. Set situations to benefit persons who can benefit you, then deliver the goods at a cost-effective price.[15]

A political climate exists in any organization and its democratic nature requires compromise, trade-offs, favors, and negotiation. Nurse managers must be political to gain their goals and objectives in this climate. Ehrat identifies four considerations of political strategy:

1. Structural considerations. The first major political concept is to learn the history of the organization, including its past struggles and their outcomes. Budgets reflect one of these political outcomes. What is valued by the organization? The successful nurse manager identifies this valued data and operates within its constraints and boundaries.
2. Economic considerations. What are the costs versus the benefits? Give something in return for gaining something better. All departments expect to gain a fair share of an increased budget. To ensure that nursing has equity, nurse managers develop clientele, confidence, a meaningful network, administrative support, and effective platform skills, and they exploit their opportunities. In gaining and sustaining this influence they do not go beyond tolerated limits.
3. Process considerations. Timing is important and is learned from managerial experience and maturation. Resolution is needed to prepare for and carry out negotiation and compromise. Impact must be considered from the viewpoint of oppo-

sition, support, risks, price, and trade-offs. All require strategies.
4. Outcome considerations. The outcome must meet minimum standards of satisfaction and avoid trouble. It must meet some needs of everyone. Consensus means 70 to 80 percent approval, agreement, and support.

Resources in the health care field are scarce, causing political conflicts and power struggles. Nurse managers must learn the strategy associated with political knowledge and skills.[16]

The nurse manager moving into a new nursing management position plans strategies for success. From day one, this person arrives early, listens, is polite, and does not criticize the predecessor. This nurse manager makes friends with the boss, assumes authority, eliminates nonessentials, trains subordinates, and delegates decision making to them. She or he establishes a psychological distance; avoids gripers and treats all employees as adults; maintains an open mind; and follows good communication skills by keeping people informed and accepting input.

When conflicts occur the nurse manager does not take sides. This individual attends to actions that produce quick results, affect the organization, are favorable to employees, and require a small investment. Vision is provided by giving a sense of nursing's mission, its importance, its relevance, and the meaningfulness of nursing work. This is done by listening, sharing, developing mutual ideas, and enlisting support of informal leaders.

Clear, complete plans are developed in seven key results areas of management:

1. Client satisfaction.
2. Productivity.
3. Innovation.
4. Staff development.
5. Budget goals.
6. Quality.
7. Organizational climate.

These will include standards of performance that challenge and inspire. The nurse manager follows the rules. Rewards are given, including praise to relieve anxiety and for accomplishments and the best pay possible. Back talk, disobedience, insubordination, and malcontents are not tolerable.

They are won over or neutralized. Decisions are made on test data and judgment.[17]

SUMMARY

The basic tools of management planning are statements of mission or purpose, philosophy or beliefs, and objectives and an active operational or management plan. All managers use such documents to accomplish the work of nursing.

The statement of mission or purpose tells the reason an entity exists, be it the organization, division, department, or unit. The nursing mission statement pertains to the clinical practice of nursing supported by research, education, and management.

The statement of philosophy reflects the values and beliefs of the organizational entity. It is translated into action by nursing personnel.

Objectives are concrete statements describing the major accomplishments nurses desire to achieve. Major categorical areas for objectives include:

1. Organization and use of all resources, human, financial and physical.
2. Social responsibility.
3. Staffing.
4. Requisition of supplies and equipment.
5. Planning educational programs.
6. Innovation.
7. Marketing.
8. Evaluation of patient care.
9. Evaluation of personnel performance.

Operational or management plans convert objectives into action and include activities, assignments, deadlines, and provision for accountability. A major strategy of an organization is the planning process and the formulation and use of statements of mission, philosophy, and objectives and organizational plans developed with the broadest possible input.

Statements of mission, philosophy and objectives support each other at different management levels, from the unit up to the service or department, then to the division, and finally to the organization.

NOTES

1. For a classic article on purpose, philosophy, and objectives, refer to M. A. Moore, "Philosophy, Purpose, and Objectives: Why Do We Have Them?," *Journal of Nursing Administration*, May-June 1971, 9–14.
2. V. Henderson, *The Nature of Nursing* (New York: Macmillan, 1966), 15.
3. H. Yura and M. B. Walsh, *The Nursing Process*, 5th ed. (New York: Appleton-Century-Crofts, 1988), 1.
4. I. M. King, "A Conceptual Frame of Reference in Nursing," *Nursing Research*, Jan.-Feb. 1968, 27–31.
5. D. E. Orem, *Nursing: Concepts of Practice* (3d. ed., New York: McGraw-Hill, 1985), 18.
6. M. L. Kinlein, *Independent Nursing Practice with Clients* (Philadelphia: J. B. Lippincott, 1977), 23.
7. S. D. Truskie, "The Driving Force of Successful Organizations," *Business Horizons*, May-June 1984, 43–48.
8. G. E. Sussman, "CEO Perspectives on Mission, Healthcare Systems, and the Environment," *Hospital and Health Services Administration*, Mar./Apr. 1985, 21–34.
9. R. M. Hodgetts, *Management: Theory, Process, and Practice*, 4th ed. (Orlando, FL.: Academic Press, 1986), 277–280.
10. Moore, op. cit., 13.
11. P. F. Drucker, *Management: Tasks, Responsibilities, Practice* (New York: Harper and Row, 1978), 99–102.
12. *Report on the Project for the Evaluation of the Quality of Nursing Service* (Ottawa, Ontario: Canadian Nurses Association, 1966), 47–48.
13. R. Cushman, "Norton's Top-Down, Bottom-Up Planning Process," *Planning Review*, Nov. 1979, 3–8, 48.
14. A. P. Meier, "The Planning Process," *Managerial Planning*, July/Aug. 1974, 1–5, 9.
15. D. E. Cavanaugh, "Gamesmanship: The Art of Strategizing," *The Journal of Nursing Administration*, Apr. 1985, 38–41.
16. K. S. Ehrat, "A Model for Politically Astute Planning and Decision Making," *The Journal of Nursing Administration*, Sept. 1983, 29–35.
17. V. C. Sherman, "Taking Over: Notes to the New Executive," *The Journal of Nursing Administration*, May 1982, 21–23.

Staffing and Scheduling

4

STAFFING PHILOSOPHY

Staffing is certainly one of the major problems of any nursing organization, whether it be a hospital, nursing home, home health care agency, ambulatory care agency, or another type of facility. Aydelotte has stated, "Nurse staffing methodology should be an orderly, systematic process, based upon sound rationale, applied to determine the number and kind of nursing personnel required to provide nursing care of a predetermined standard to a group of patients in a particular setting. The end result is prediction of the kind and number of staff required to give care to patients."[1]

The staffing process is complex. Components of the staffing process as a control system include a staffing study, a master staffing plan, a scheduling plan, and a nursing management information system (NMIS). The NMIS includes these five elements:

1. Quality of patient care to be delivered and its measurement.
2. Characteristics of the patients and their care requirements.
3. Prediction of the supply of nurse power required for items 1 and 2.
4. Logistics of the staffing program pattern and its control.
5. Evaluation of the quality of care desired, thereby measuring the success of the staffing itself.[2]

West adds a position control plan and a budgeting plan; see Figure 4–1.[3]

Nurse staffing must meet certain regulatory requirements. Among these are legal requirements of Medicare. The Medicare Survey report is excerpted in Figure 4–2.

This legal standard is further supported by other standards such as Nursing Services (NR) Standard NR4 of the *Accreditation Manual for Hospitals, 1989,* given in Figure 4–3.

FIGURE 4–1. Components of the Staffing Process

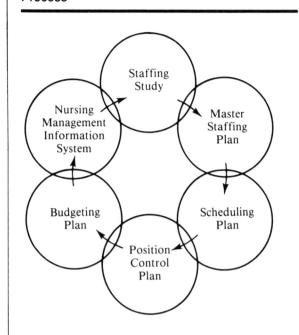

SOURCE: Reprinted from *Topics in Health Care Financing*, Vol. 6, No. 4, p. 15 with permission of Aspen Publishers, Inc. © Summer 1980.

Other standards include the ANA *Standards for Organized Nursing Services and Responsibilities of Nurse Administrators Across All Settings,* ANA *Standards of Nursing Practice,* and state licensing requirements. From all of these and from the expectations of the community, of nurses, and of physicians, the nurse administrator will develop a staffing philosophy as a basis for a staffing methodology. Community expectations will be related to economic status, to local value and belief systems, and to local standards of culture. Nurses' expectations will be related to the same community standards and in addition to their perceptions of the practice of nursing and its components, to the results desired, and to the workload tolerated. See Appendix 4.1, "Staffing—Assignment Principles for Nursing Personnel."

Nurse managers can discern from the nursing division's existing statements of purpose, philosophy, and objectives various values related to staffing. A staffing philosophy may encompass beliefs about using a patient dependency system or patient classification system for identifying patient care needs. It may cover beliefs about use of skilled personnel as a core staff with a float pool for supplemental staffing. It may also specify who will be responsible for hiring.[4]

Objectives of nurse staffing are excellent care and high productivity. Professional nurses can develop a statement of purpose that is comprehensive in stating the quality and quantity of performance it is intended to motivate. Purpose statements should be quantified.[5] Examine those in Chapter 3.

STAFFING STUDY

A staffing study should gather data about environmental factors within and outside the organization that affect staffing requirements.

Aydelotte listed four techniques drawn from engineering to measure the work of nurses. All involved the concept of time required for performance.[6] These techniques are:

1. Time study and task frequency.
   1.1 Tasks and task elements (procedures).
   1.2 Point and time started.
   1.3 Point and time ended.
   1.4 Sample size.
   1.5 Average time.
   1.6 Allowance for fatigue, personal variation, and unavoidable standby.
   1.7 Standard time = steps 1.5 + 1.6.
   1.8 Frequency of task × standard time = the measurement of nursing activity.
   1.9 Total of all tasks × standard time = volume of nursing work.
2. Work sampling (variation of task frequency and time). Procedure is as follows:
   2.1 Identify major and minor categories of nursing activities.
   2.2 Determine number of observations to be made.
   2.3 Observe random sample of nursing personnel performing activities.
   2.4 *Analyze observations.* Frequency occurring in a specific category = percent of total time spent in that activity. Most work sampling studies sample direct care and indirect care to determine ratio.
3. Continuous sampling (variation of task frequency and time). Technique is the same as for work sampling except that:

FIGURE 4–2.   Medicare and Medicaid Regulations

482.23 *Condition of participation: Nursing services.*

The hospital must have an organized nursing service that provides 24-hour nursing services. The nursing services must be furnished or supervised by a registered nurse.

(a) *Standard: Organization.* The hospital must have a well-organized service with a plan of administrative authority and delineation of responsibilities for patient care. The director of nursing service must be a licensed registered nurse. He or she is responsible for the operation of the service, including determining the types and numbers of nursing personnel and staff necessary to provide nursing care for all areas of the hospital.

(b) *Standard: Staffing and delivery of care.* The nursing service must have adequate numbers of licensed registered nurses, licensed practical nurses (vocational), and other personnel to provide nursing care to all patients as needed. There must be supervisory and staff personnel for each department or nursing unit to ensure, when needed, the immediate availability of a registered nurse for bedside care of any patient.

(1) The hospital must provide 24-hour nursing service furnished or supervised by a registered nurse and have a licensed practical nurse or registered nurse on duty at all times, except for rural hospitals that have in effect 24-hour nursing waiver granted under §405.1910(c) of this chapter.

(2) The nursing service must have a procedure to ensure that hospital nursing personnel for whom licensure is required have valid and current licensure.

(3) A registered nurse must supervise and evaluate the nursing care for each patient.

(4) The hospital must ensure that the nursing staff develops, and keeps current, a nursing care plan for each patient.

(5) A registered nurse must assign the nursing care of each patient to other nursing personnel in accordance with the patient's needs and the specialized qualifications and competence of the nursing staff available.

(6) Non-employee licensed nurses who are working in the hospital must adhere to the policies and procedures of the hospital. The director of nursing service must provide for adequate supervision and evaluation of the clinical activities of non-employee nursing personnel which occur within the responsibility of the nursing service.

(c) *Standard: Preparation and administration of drugs.* Drugs and biologicals must be prepared and administered in accordance with Federal and State laws, the orders of the practitioner or practitioners responsible for the patient's care as specified under §482.12(c), and accepted standards of practice.

(1) All drugs and biologicals must be administered by, or under supervision of, nursing or other personnel in accordance with Federal and State laws and regulations including applicable licensing requirements and in accordance with the approved medical staff policies and procedures.

(2) All orders and biologicals must be in writing and signed by the practitioner or practitioners responsible for the care of the patient as specified under §482.12(c). When telephone or oral orders must be used, they must be—

  (i) Accepted only by personnel that are authorized to do so by the medical staff policies and procedures, consistent with Federal and State law;

  (ii) Signed and initialed by the prescribing practitioner as soon as possible; and

  (iii) Used infrequently.

(3) Blood transfusions and intravenous medications must be administered in accordance with State law and approved medical staff policies and procedures. If blood transfusions and intravenous medications are administered by personnel other than doctors of medicine or osteopathy, the personnel must have special training for this duty.

(4) There must be a hospital procedure for reporting transfusion reactions, adverse drug reactions, and errors in administration of drugs.

SOURCE: Commerce Clearing House, Inc., Medicare and Medicaid Regulations. As adopted, 51 F.R. 22010 (June 17, 1986, effective September 15, 1986), 8551-4 to 8551-5.

FIGURE 4–3.   Nursing Services (NR) Standards NR4 JCAHO

NR4 Nursing department/service assignments in the provision of nursing care are commensurate with the qualifications of nursing personnel and are designed to meet the nursing care needs of patients.*

Required Characteristics

NR.4.1 A sufficient number of qualified registered nurses are on duty at all times to give patients the nursing care that requires the judgment and specialized skills of a registered nurse.*

NR.4.2 Nursing personnel staffing also is sufficient to assure prompt recognition of any untoward change in a patient's condition and to facilitate appropriate intervention by the nursing, medical, or hospital staffs.*

NR.4.3 In striving to assure quality nursing care and a safe patient environment, nursing personnel staffing and assignment are based on at least the following:*

NR.4.3.1 A registered nurse plans, supervises, and evaluates the nursing care of each patient;

NR.4.3.2 To the extent possible, a registered nurse makes a patient assessment before delegating appropriate aspects of nursing care to other nursing personnel;

NR.4.3.3 The patient care assignment minimizes the risk of the transfer of infection and accidental contamination;

NR.4.3.4 The patient care assignment is commensurate with the qualifications of each nursing staff member, the identified nursing needs of the patient, and the prescribed medical regimen; and

NR.4.3.5 Responsibility for nursing care and related duties is retained by the hospital nursing department/service when nursing students and nursing personnel from outside sources are providing care within a patient care unit.

NR.4.4 The nursing department/service defines, implements, and maintains a system for determining patient requirements for nursing care on the basis of demonstrated patient needs, appropriate nursing intervention, and priority for care.*

NR.4.4.1 Specific nursing personnel staffing for each nursing care unit, including, as appropriate, the surgical suite, obstetrical suite, ambulatory care department/service, and emergency department/service, are commensurate with the patient care requirements, staff expertise, unit geography, availability of support services, and method of patient care delivery.*

NR.4.4.2 The hospital admissions system allows for participation from the nursing department/service in coordinating patient requirements for nursing care with available nursing resources.

NR.4.5 Only qualified registered nurses are assigned to head nurse/supervisor positions in the surgical and obstetrical suites.*

The asterisked items are key factors in the accreditation decision process. For an explanation of the use of the key factors, see "Using the Manual," page ix.

SOURCE: JCAHO, "Nursing services (NR)," *Accreditation Manual for Hospitals, 1989* (Chicago, 1989), 137–138. Copyright 1988 by the Joint Commission on Accreditation of Healthcare Organizations, Chicago. Reprinted with permission.

3.1 Observer follows one individual in the performance of a task.

3.2 Observer may observe work performed for one or more patients if they can be observed concurrently.

4. Self-reporting (variation of task frequency and time). Procedure is as follows:

4.1 The individual records the work sampling or continuous sampling on himself or herself.

4.2 Tasks are logged using time intervals or time tasks start and end.

4.3 Logs are analyzed.

Many work sampling studies focus on procedures, ignore standards, and are lacking in objectivity, reliability, and accuracy. The techniques themselves are sound; see Figure 4–4.

According to West, "There are three cardinal rules for forecasting staffing requirements."[7] The first is to base staffing projections upon past staffing history; Figure 4–5 is designed as a data sheet for this purpose. The data can be collected from the patient classification system reports and census reports. Such data are readily available in most hospitals; some NMISs, such as Medicus, provide numbers of personnel required, including the mix of R.N.s, L.P.N.s, and N.A.s. Other data needed are sick time, overtime, holidays, and vacation time. The attrition rate is also important and will be discussed elsewhere. In some patient classification systems these are built into the staffing formula. For example, at the University of South Alabama Medical Center, the Medicus system provides the following formula for staffing:[8]

$$\frac{\text{Average Census} \times \text{Nursing Hours} \times 1.4 \times 1.14}{7.5}$$

The second cardinal rule for staffing is to review current staffing levels. Review of future plans for the institution is the third cardinal rule.[9] When clinical nurses are involved in staffing plans they will have confidence in them. These staffing studies can be made with electronic spreadsheets.

Staffing requires much planning on the part of the nurse administrator. Data must be collected and analyzed. These data include facts about the product—patient care. They include diagnostic and therapeutic procedures performed by both physicians and nurses. They include the knowledge elements of professional nursing translated into professional nursing skills of history taking and assessment, nursing diagnosis and prescription, application of care, evaluation, record keeping, and all other actions related to the primary health care of patients.

Basic to planning for staffing of a division of nursing is the fact that qualified nursing personnel must be provided in sufficient numbers to ensure adequate, safe nursing care for all patients 24 hours a day, 7 days a week, 52 weeks a year. Each staffing plan must be tailored to the needs of the hospital and cannot be arrived at by a simple worker/patient ratio or formula.

Planning for staffing requires judgment, experience, and thorough knowledge of the require-

ments of the organization in which the individual nurse administrator is employed. It requires support of hospital administration, physicians in charge of clinical services, and the nursing staff.

The basic requirement is unchanging, regardless of the type or size of the institution: plan for the kinds and numbers of nursing personnel that will give safe, adequate care to all patients and will ensure the work of nursing is productive and satisfying.

Changing, expanding knowledge and technology in the physical and social sciences, in the medical field, and in economics influence planning for staffing. Health care institutions are treating more clients on an outpatient basis. New drugs, improved diagnostic and therapeutic procedures, and reimbursement charges have decreased the lengths of hospitalization. Standards of the Joint Commission on Accreditation of Healthcare Organizations, the American Nurses Association, and other professional and governmental organizations have required upgrading of health care.

Planning for staffing is influenced by changing concepts of nursing roles for clinical nursing practitioners and specialists. Decision making is being delegated to the lowest practical level. Ward clerks and unit managers have assumed duties formerly done by nursing personnel.

Patient populations are changing as birth rates decline and longevity increases. Staffing plans are influenced by institutional missions and objectives related to research, training, and many specialties. They are influenced by personnel policies and practices related to vacations, time off, overtime, holidays, and other factors. They are influenced by policies and practices related to admission and discharge times of patients, assignment of patients to wards, and intensive and progressive care practices.

The amount and kind of nursing staff required will be influenced by the degree to which other departments carry out their supporting services. This is particularly true during weekends, evenings, nights, and holidays. Plans must be made to furnish staffing requirements for nursing personnel to perform non-nursing duties such as dietary functions, clerical work, messenger and escort activities, and housekeeping. Whether these services should or should not be carried out by nursing personnel is not the point here; the point is that the degree to which the situation exists must be considered in any plan. Nurse managers must avoid assuming respon-

FIGURE 4–4. Work Sampling Study

RN, LPN, NA (*circle one*)

Task or Procedure	Time Started	Time Ended	Minutes
1.			
2.			
3.			
4.			
5.			
6.			
7.			
8.			
9.			
10.			

(A) Total number of tasks and procedures = _____
(B) Total minutes = _____

Average Time

(B) Total minutes	÷	(A) Total number of tasks and procedures	=	(C) Average time per procedure or task
(B) _____	÷	(A) _____	=	(C) _____

Standard Time

Average time	+	Time allowed for fatigue, personal variation, and unavoidable standby	=	Standard time in minutes
(C) _____	+	(D) _____	=	(E) _____

Measurement of Nursing Activity

Standard time	×	Frequency of an individual task or procedure	=	Measurement of nursing activity
(E) _____	×	(F) _____	=	(G) _____

Volume of Nursing Work

Standard time	×	Total number of tasks and procedures	=	Volume of nursing work
(E) _____	×	(A) _____	=	(H) _____

SOURCE: Adapted from: M. K. Aydelotte, *Nurse Staffing Methodology: A Review and Critique of Selected Literature.* (Washington, D.C.: U.S. Government Printing Office, January, 1973).

FIGURE 4–5. Staffing History Data Sheet

Year _____ Month _____ Cost Center _____

Day	ADC	Patient Acuity	Personnel				
			Sick Hours	Overtime Hours	Holiday Hours	Vacation Hours	Other
1							
2							
31							
Average							

SOURCE: Constructed from: M. E. West, "Implementing Effective Nurse Staffing Systems in the Managed Hospitals," *Topics in Health Care Financing,* with permission of Aspen Publishers, Inc. © Summer, 1980, 16.

sibility for non-nursing services and encourage the appropriate departments to perform such services. When they do not, nurse managers should have a system of charging the provided services to the appropriate other cost center. They will then become revenue to the nursing cost center.

Staffing plans will be influenced by the number and composition of the medical staff and the medical services offered. Nursing requirements will be affected by characteristics of patient populations determined by the size and capability of the medical staff. Special requirements of individual physicians, time and length of their rounds; time, complexity, and number of tests; medications and treatments; and kind and amount of surgery will all affect the quality and quantity of nursing personnel required and influence their placement.

Arrangement of the physical plant has a large impact on staffing requirements. Fewer personnel are needed for a modern, compact facility equipped with labor-saving devices and efficient working arrangements than for one that is spread out and has few or no labor-saving devices. Different staffing is required for a facility that is arranged functionally than for one that is not. If, for example, the operating suite is not next to the labor and delivery rooms, recovery room, and intensive care units, more staff will be needed to meet acceptable standards of quality and safety. Many other architectural features must be considered, such as location of patient rooms in relation to the nursing stations; the location of specialized units, work rooms, and storage space; and the time required to transport patients to other sections of the hospital for diagnostic or therapeutic services such as radiography and nuclear medicine.

Staffing is further affected by the organization of the division of nursing. Plans must be reviewed and revised to organize the department to operate efficiently and economically, with written statements of mission, philosophy, and objectives; sound organizational structure; clearly defined functions and responsibilities; written policies and procedures; effective staff development programs; and planned periodic evaluation. Staffing plans for such a department will be different from those for one that is loosely organized with overlapping functions and responsibilities, vague or conflicting policies, and poorly defined standards of nursing practice.

STAFFING ACTIVITIES

Price identified seventeen different staffing activities and suggested that the nurse administrator identify by names the persons responsible for each of the seventeen activities. She further suggested:

1. The one person ultimately responsible for each activity should be identified.
2. The category and position of the person who *should* be responsible for each activity should be identified.

3. The activity should be specified as requiring nursing or non-nursing personnel.
4. This review be performed for the day shift, evening shift, night shift, and weekend and holiday shifts.

A modified Price format for gathering data and analyzing responsibility for staffing activities is depicted in Figure 4–6.[10]

Orientation Plan

A main purpose of orientation is to help the nursing worker adjust to a new work situation. This should be a planned program that includes orientation—whether through a "buddy" system, a special orientation unit, or other method. Those nursing tasks and skills required of each nursing worker who is not proficient in them should be the focus of this program. Productivity is increased, since fewer personnel are needed when they are fully oriented to the work situation.

Staffing Policies

Written staffing policies should be readily available in at least the following areas:

1. Vacations.
2. Holidays.
3. Sick leave.
4. Weekends off.
5. Consecutive days off.
6. Rotation to different shifts.
7. Overtime.
8. Part-time personnel.
9. Use of "float" personnel.
10. Exchangeability of staff.
11. Use of special abilities of individual staff members.
12. Exchanging hours.
13. Requests of personnel.
14. Requests of management.
15. The work week.

Work Contracts

There should be a work contract between each employee and the institution. The contract should state the date employment is to commence, the job classification, the hours of work, the rate of pay, whether the job is full time or part time, and any

FIGURE 4–6. Responsibility for Staffing Activities

Staffing Activity	Person Responsible Day Shift	Person Responsible Evening Shift	Person Responsible Night Shift	Person Responsible Weekend Shift	Person Responsible Holiday Shift
Recruitment					
Interviewing and screening					
Hiring: Registered nurses					
Licensed practical nurses					
Nurse aides					
Orderlies					
Assignment to clinical units					
Assignment to shifts					
Preparing work schedule in advance					
Maintaining daily schedule					
Adjusting: Staff absence, patient needs					
Calculating turnover					
Calculating hours of care					
Checking time cards, payroll					
Policy development					
Telephone communication					
Contract compliance					

SOURCE: Adapted from: E. M. Price, Staffing for Patient Care (New York: Springer, 1970), 12. Used with permission.

other specific points agreed upon between employee and institutional representative. Both should sign it. See Figure 4–7.

Staffing Function

The staffing function should probably be centralized, as this removes a clerical burden from first-line nurse managers and provides more time for their attention to direct patient care and nursing practice activities. All of the activities related to staffing should be developed into policies and procedures that reflect the thinking of nursing administration and can be performed by non-nurse employees. Obviously, nurse managers will remain involved in hiring, firing, and promotions, in consultation with

FIGURE 4–7.   El Camino Hospital Nursing Service Work Agreement

I accept employment at El Camino Hospital with the following understanding. That I:

1. Must have Health Service clearance prior to hire.

2. Am being hired to work as a Staff Nurse _____ Step _____ at _____ (salary) starting _____ (orientation date). My employee time category will be _____ .

3. Am being assigned to _____ (unit) on _____ (shift) and committ myself to work on this unit and shift for a minimum of _____ months before requesting a transfer or status change.

4. Will float from my assigned area as required.

5. Am being employed on a trial basis for ninety days and that during this period a preceptor will be designated to oversee my orientation and will discuss my progress with me.

6. Will abide by the Job Description for my position, the rules of conduct as stated in the Employees Handbook and the Nursing Department dress code.

7. Understand that because of fluctuating patient census, the hospital cannot guarantee that I will work the full number of hours assigned in my category and that there may be times when it will be necessary for me to reschedule holidays or vacations or take time off without pay.

8. Can obtain information regarding retirement and employee benefits from the Personnel Department.

9. (Optional) We mutually agree to the following: _____

_____

_____

_____

_____

_____

Signature of applicant _____

Date _____

Original to Personnel
Copy to Employee
PA/hds   10/77

Signature of Head Nurse _____

Date _____

SOURCE: Reprinted from *Nursing Decentralization: The El Camino Experience* by J. N. Althaus et al., p. 50, with permission of Aspen Publishers, Inc., © 1982.

top nurse managers and human resource specialists.

A sign of maladministration in nursing is too many levels of supervision. There is often a professional nurse employed at the department or division level to perform the function of scheduling. Scheduling is time consuming and can be done by non-nursing personnel. Price recommends that a non-nurse perform the staffing function, advised by professional nurses as needed. The staffing employee should be a very competent person: "a good business person, mature, effective in interpersonal relations, objective in dealing with personnel, fair and firm; one who can communicate effectively orally, by phone, and in writing; and finally, one who has above average mathematical ability."[11]

STAFFING THE UNITS

Each patient care unit should have a master staffing plan. This should include the basic staff needed to

FIGURE 4–8. Formula for Estimating a Core Staff per Shift

The average daily census for a 25-bed medical-surgical unit over a 6-month period is 19 patients. The basic average daily hours of care to be provided are 5 hours per patient per 24 hours. How many total hours of care will be needed on the average day to meet these standards? 19 × 5 = 95 hours. If the work day is 8 hours, this means 95 ÷ 8 = 11.9 or 12 full-time-equivalents (FTE) staff are needed to staff the unit for 24 hours. An FTE is one person working full time (40 hours a week) or several persons who together work a total of 40 hours a week. A total of 12 FTE × 7 days per week = 84 shifts per week, if the staffing is to be the same each day. If each employee works 5 8-hour shifts per week, 84 ÷ 5 = 16.8, the number of FTEs needed as basic staff for this unit.

The number of nursing personnel to cover sick leave, vacations, and holidays or other absences can also be determined and added to the basic staff. This information is determined from a study of personnel policies and use. It is frequently included in patient classification system formulas. Such additional staff may be provided from a float pool.

The next determination to be made is the ratio of R.N.'s to other nursing personnel. If the ratio is determined as 1:1,

how many of the basic staff of 16.8 should be R.N.s? One half of the total, which would be 8.4 R.N.s and 8.4 others (L.P.N.s, nurse's aides, orderlies, or nursing assistants). A study of staffing patterns in 80 med/surg, pediatrics, and post-partum units in twelve Salt Lake City Community hospitals recommends a mix of 58% RNs, 26% LPNs and 16% aides.[12]

The final determination is how many personnel are needed for each shift. Warstler recommends proportions of day—47%, evening—35%, and night—17%.[13] This means that for a total staff of 16.8 personnel, 8 would be assigned to days, 6 to evenings, and 2.8 to nights. This is obviously approximate; other patterns could also be chosen by the nurse administrator.

The number of complementary nursing personnel would be added to this basic staff. They could be a group of one R.N., one L.P.N., and one other and assigned accordingly. They are entered into the following table as numbers in parenthesis added to the figure for basic staff.

In today's reimbursement environment complementary personnel may be budgeted as a pool. They may even exist only as a portion of basic personnel assigned to a pool.

Basic Staffing Plan for 25-Bed Medical-Surgical Unit

Category	Day	Evening	Night	Totals
R.N.s	4 + (1)	3	1.4	8.4 + (1)
L.P.N.s	2	2 + (1)	1.4	5.4 + (1)
Others	2	1	0 + (1)	3 + (1)
Totals	8 + (1)	6 + (1)	2.8 + (1)	16.8 + (3)

staff the unit each shift. Basic staff is the minimum or lowest number of personnel needed to staff a unit. It includes fully oriented, full- and part-time employees. The number may be based on examination of previous staff records and the expert opinion of nurse managers. It includes all categories: registered nurses, licensed practical nurses, and nursing technicians or assistants for each shift. See Figure 4–8 for a formula for determining a core staff per shift.

Next the number of *complementary* personnel are determined. The are scheduled as an addition to the basic group, but the total number in both groups

will be controlled by financial resources and the availability of personnel. They provide the flexibility needed to meet short-range and unexpected changes. Complementary personnel are not ensured a permanent pattern and are usually scheduled for 4-week periods.

Float personnel are employees who are not permanently assigned to a station. They provide flexibility to meet increased patient loads as well as unexpected personnel absences. The number and kinds of float personnel can be accurately determined from general monthly records that show absence rates, personnel turnover, and fluctuations in patient care workloads. Float personnel may be assigned to a pool.

Some nurse administrators do not hire part-time nursing personnel. They may be an economic or cost-control factor in staffing since they usually do not receive the same benefits as full-time personnel. Part-time personnel will be better motivated if they receive some benefits, such as a number of holidays and vacation days proportionate to days worked and pay increases when they complete the aggregate days worked by full-time personnel. Their total hours worked can be controlled to fill actual shortfalls.

Whatever the staffing policy, it should be arrived at through consultation with clinical nurses. The nursing department personnel budget is also a master staffing plan. The process for developing a master staffing plan is depicted in Figure 4–9.

STAFFING MODULES

Cyclic Scheduling

Cyclic scheduling is one of the best ways of staffing to meet the requirements of equitable distribution of hours of work and time off. A basic time pattern for a certain number of weeks is established and then repeated in cycles.

Advantages of cyclic scheduling include the following:

1. Once developed, it is a relatively permanent schedule, requiring only temporary adjustments.
2. Nurses no longer have to live in anticipation of their time off-duty, as it may be scheduled for as long as six months in advance.
3. Personal plans may be made in advance with a reasonable degree of reliability.
4. Requests for special time off are kept to a minimum.
5. It can be used with rotating, permanent, or mixed shifts and can be modified to allow fixed days off and uneven work periods, based on personnel needs and work period preferences.
6. It can be modified to fit known or anticipated periods of heavy workload and can be temporarily adjusted to meet emergencies or unexpected shortages of personnel.

Since it is relatively inflexible, cyclic scheduling only works with a staff that rotates by policy and personal choice.

An infinite number of basic cyclic patterns can be developed, tailored to suit the needs of each unit. Samples are shown in Figure 4–9. Patterns should reflect policy, workload factors, and staff preferences. Nursing personnel may use a staffing board (Figure 4–10) to develop a pattern and cycle satisfactory to them.

Patterns should be reviewed periodically to see that they meet the purpose, philosophy, and objectives of the organization and the division of nursing, that they are practical with regard to the numbers and qualifications of personnel, that they are satisfactory to nursing personnel, that they are meeting patient needs, and that they are using people effectively.

Scheduling records should be retained for a specific time, probably one year. They provide valuable statistical information for planning staffing as well as historical information for questions related to personnel on duty when specific events occurred.

It has been stated previously that staffing policies should be established in specific areas. Policies that may be considered are:

1. Personnel are scheduled to work their preferred shift as much as possible.
2. Personnel choices are balanced to meet the needs of the unit and of other employees.
3. An employee is allowed to make her/his own arrangements for special time off or exchange within specific personnel policies.
4. Policies have been established for making schedule changes.
5. Each employee has a copy of his or her work schedule.
6. Consideration has been given to staffing during hours of clinical experience for students.
7. There is a weekend and holiday schedule policy; it is a common practice in many organizations throughout the United States to plan alternate weekends off for nursing personnel. Weekend coverage can be by "weekends only" employees; staffing levels needed can be influenced by hospital policies on admissions and discharges and weekend staffing policy.

FIGURE 4–9. Cyclic Schedules

week	1							2							3							4						
	S	M	T	W	T	F	S	S	M	T	W	T	F	S	S	M	T	W	T	F	S	S	M	T	W	T	F	S
1	N	N	N	N	N	–	–	–	–	E	E	E	E	E	E	–	–	D	D	D	D	D	D	–	–	N	N
2	D	D	D	–	–	N	N	N	N	N	N	N	–	–	–	–	E	E	E	E	E	E	E	–	–	D	D	D
3	E	E	–	–	D	D	D	D	D	D	D	–	–	N	N	N	N	N	N	–	–	–	–	E	E	E	E	E
4	–	–	E	E	E	E	E	E	E	–	–	D	D	D	D	D	D	–	–	N	N	N	N	N	N	N	–	–
charge	–	D	D	D	D	D	–	–	D	D	D	D	D	–	–	D	D	D	D	D	–	–	D	D	D	D	D	–
N	1	1	1	1	1	1	1	1	1	1	1	1	1	1	1	1	1	1	1	1	1	1	1	1	1	1	1	1
D	1	2	2	1	2	2	1	1	2	2	1	2	2	1	1	2	2	1	2	2	1	1	2	2	1	2	2	1
E	1	1	1	1	1	1	1	1	1	1	1	1	1	1	1	1	1	1	1	1	1	1	1	1	1	1	1	1

Minimum Basic Schedule

week		1							2							3							4						
		S	M	T	W	T	F	S	S	M	T	W	T	F	S	S	M	T	W	T	F	S	S	M	T	W	T	F	S
Permanent shifts	1	N	N	N	–	–	N	N	N	N	N	–	–	N	N	N	N	N	–	–	N	N	N	N	N	–	–	N	N
	2	N	N	N	N	N	–	–	–	–	N	N	N	N	N	N	N	N	N	N	–	–	–	–	N	N	N	N	N
	3	E	E	E	E	E	–	–	E	E	E	E	E	–	–	E	E	E	E	E	–	–	E	E	E	E	E	–	–
	4	–	–	E	E	E	E	E	–	–	E	E	E	E	E	–	–	E	E	E	E	E	–	–	E	E	E	E	E
	5	E	E	–	–	D	E	E	E	E	–	–	D	E	E	E	E	–	–	D	E	E	E	E	–	–	D	E	E
Rotate	6	D	–	–	N	N	N	N	N	N	N	N	–	–	D	D	D	D	D	D	–	–	–	D	D	D	D	D	–
	7	–	D	D	D	D	D	–	–	D	D	D	–	D	D	D	–	–	N	N	N	N	N	N	N	–	–	–	D
	8	–	D	D	D	–	D	D	D	D	D	D	D	–	–	–	D	D	D	D	D	–	–	D	D	D	–	D	D
	9	D	D	D	D	D	–	–	–	D	D	D	D	D	–	–	D	D	D	–	D	D	D	D	D	D	D	–	–
Leave relief	10	–	–	D	D	D	D	D	D	D	D	–	D	D	D	–	–	–	D	D	D	D	D	D	–	–	D	D	D	–
assistant	11																												
charge	12																												

week		5							6							7							8						
		S	M	T	W	T	F	S	S	M	T	W	T	F	S	S	M	T	W	T	F	S	S	M	T	W	T	F	S
	1	N	N	N	–	–	N	N	N	N	N	–	–	N	N	N	N	N	–	–	N	N	N	N	N	–	–	N	N
	2	N	N	N	N	N	–	–	–	–	N	N	N	N	N	N	N	N	N	N	–	–	–	–	N	N	N	N	N
	3	E	E	E	E	E	–	–	E	E	E	E	E	–	–	E	E	E	E	E	–	–	E	E	E	E	E	–	–
	4	–	–	E	E	E	E	E	–	–	E	E	E	E	E	–	–	E	E	E	E	E	–	–	E	E	E	E	E
	5	E	E	–	–	D	E	E	E	E	–	–	D	E	E	E	E	–	–	D	E	E	E	E	–	–	D	E	E
	6	–	D	D	D	–	D	D	D	D	D	D	D	–	–	–	D	D	D	D	D	–	–	D	D	D	–	D	D
	7	D	D	D	D	D	–	–	–	D	D	D	D	D	–	–	D	D	D	–	D	D	D	D	D	D	D	–	–
	8	D	–	–	N	N	N	N	N	N	N	N	–	–	D	D	D	D	D	D	–	–	–	D	D	D	D	D	–
	9	–	D	D	D	D	D	–	–	D	D	D	–	D	D	D	–	–	N	N	N	N	N	N	N	–	–	–	D
	10	–	–	D	D	D	D	D	D	D	D	–	D	D	D	–	–	–	D	D	D	D	D	D	–	–	D	D	D	–
	11																												
	12																												

Eight-Week Cycle—Mixed Shifts

SOURCE: Department of the Air Force, *USAF Hospital Nursing Service Manual* (Washington, D.C.: U.S. Government Printing Office, 1971), 4-4 to 4-14.

(continued)

FIGURE 4–9.   Cyclic Schedules (*continued*)

Weeks 1–5

week	1 (S M T W T F S)	2 (S M T W T F S)	3 (S M T W T F S)	4 (S M T W T F S)	5 (S M T W T F S)
1	N N N N N – –	E E E E E – –		– N N N N N – –	– E E E
2	– N N N N N – –	– E E E E E –			– N N N N N
3	N N N N N – –	– N N N N N – –	– E E E E E –		
4	E E –		– N N N N N – –	– E E E E E –	
5	– – E E E E E –			– N N N N N – –	– E E E E E –

Weeks 6–10

week	6	7	8	9	10
1	E E – –		– N N N N N – –	– E E E E E –	
2	– – E E E E E –		– N N N N N – –	– E E E E E –	
3	N N N N N – –	E E E E E –		– N N N N N – –	– E E E
4	– N N N N N – –	– E E E E E –			– N N N N
5	– N N N N N – –	– E E E E E – –			

Weeks 11–15

week	11	12	13	14	15
1	– N N N N N – –	E E E E E – –			– N N N N N
2	– N N N N N – –	– E E E E E – –			
3	E E –	– N N N N N – –	– E E E E E –		
4	– – E E E E E – –	– N N N N N – –	– E E E E E –		
5	N N N N N – –	E E E E E – –	– N N N N N – –	– E E E	

Weeks 16–20

week	16	17	18	19	20
1	– – E E E E E –		– N N N N N – –	– E E E E E – –	
2	N N N N N – –	E E E E E – –	– N N N N N – –	– E E E	
3	– N N N N N – –	– E E E E E – –		– N N N N N	
4	– N N N N N – –	– E E E E E –			
5	E E –		– N N N N N – –	– E E E E E –	

Weeks 21–25

week	21	22	23	24	25
1		– N N N N N – –	E E E E E –		
2	E E –	– N N N N N –	– E E E E E –		
3	– – E E E E E – –		– N N N N N – –	– E E E E E – –	
4	N N N N N – –	E E E E E –		– N N N N N – –	– E E E
5	– N N N N N – –	– E E E E E – –			– N N N N

Twenty-Five-Week Cycle

FIGURE 4–9. Cyclic Schedules (*continued*)

week	1							2						
	S	M	T	W	T	F	S	S	M	T	W	T	F	S
1	N	N	N	N	N	–	–	–	–	N	N	N	N	N
2	D	D	D	–	–	N	N	N	N	D	D	D	–	–
3	E	E	–	–	D	D	D	D	D	D	D	–	–	D
4	–	–	E	E	E	E	E	E	E	–	–	D	D	D
5	D	D	D	D	D	–	–	–	–	E	E	E	E	E
charge	–	–	D	D	D	D	D	D	D	–	D	D	D	–
N	1	1	1	1	1	1	1	1	1	1	1	1	1	1
D	2	2	3	2	3	2	2	2	2	2	3	3	2	2
E	1	1	1	1	1	1	1	1	1	1	1	1	1	1

week	3							4						
	S	M	T	W	T	F	S	S	M	T	W	T	F	S
1	N	N	–	–	N	N	N	N	N	N	–	–	N	N
2	–	–	E	E	E	E	E	E	E	–	–	D	D	D
3	D	D	D	D	D	–	–	–	–	E	E	E	E	E
4	D	–	N	N	–	D	D	D	D	D	D	D	–	–
5	E	E	–	–	D	D	D	D	D	–	N	N	–	D
charge	–	D	D	D	D	D	–	–	D	D	D	D	D	–
N	1	1	1	1	1	1	1	1	1	1	1	1	1	1
D	2	2	2	2	3	3	2	2	3	2	2	3	2	2
E	1	1	1	1	1	1	1	1	1	1	1	1	1	1

Cyclic Schedule—Permanent Nights

week	1							2						
	S	M	T	W	T	F	S	S	M	T	W	T	F	S
1	–	–	E	E	E	E	E	E	E	–	–	E	E	E
2	N	N	N	N	N	–	–	–	–	E	E	E	E	E
3	D	D	D	–	–	N	N	N	N	N	N	N	–	–
4	–	–	D	D	D	D	D	D	D	D	–	–	N	N
5	D	D	–	D	D	D	–	–	–	D	D	D	D	D
6	E	E	E	E	–	–	D	D	D	–	D	D	D	–
7	E	E	–	–	E	E	E	E	E	E	E	–	–	D
charge	–	D	D	D	D	D	–	–	D	D	D	D	D	–
N	1	1	1	1	1	1	1	1	1	1	1	1	1	1
D	2	3	3	3	3	3	2	2	3	3	3	3	3	2
E	2	2	2	2	2	2	2	2	2	2	2	2	2	2

week	3							4						
	S	M	T	W	T	F	S	S	M	T	W	T	F	S
1	E	E	E	E	–	–	D	D	D	–	D	D	D	–
2	E	E	–	–	E	E	E	E	E	E	E	–	–	D
3	–	–	E	E	E	E	E	E	E	–	–	E	E	E
4	N	N	N	N	N	–	–	–	–	E	E	E	E	E
5	D	D	D	–	–	N	N	N	N	N	N	N	–	–
6	–	–	D	D	D	D	D	D	D	D	–	–	N	N
7	D	D	–	D	D	D	–	–	–	D	D	D	D	D
charge	–	D	D	D	D	D	–	–	D	D	D	D	D	–
N	1	1	1	1	1	1	1	1	1	1	1	1	1	1
D	2	3	3	3	3	3	2	2	3	3	3	3	3	2
E	2	2	2	2	2	2	2	2	2	2	2	2	2	2

week	5							6							7						
	S	M	T	W	T	F	S	S	M	T	W	T	F	S	S	M	T	W	T	F	S
1	–	–	D	D	D	D	D	D	D	D	–	–	N	N	N	N	N	N	N	–	–
2	D	D	–	D	D	D	–	–	–	D	D	D	D	D	D	D	D	–	–	N	N
3	E	E	E	E	–	–	D	D	D	–	D	D	D	–	–	–	D	D	D	D	D
4	E	E	–	–	E	E	E	E	E	E	E	–	–	D	D	D	–	D	D	D	–
5	–	–	E	E	E	E	E	E	E	–	–	E	E	E	E	E	E	E	–	–	D
6	N	N	N	N	N	–	–	–	–	E	E	E	E	E	E	E	–	–	E	E	E
7	D	D	D	–	–	N	N	N	N	N	N	N	–	–	–	–	E	E	E	E	E
charge	–	D	D	D	D	D	–	–	D	D	D	D	D	–	–	D	D	D	D	D	–
N	1	1	1	1	1	1	1	1	1	1	1	1	1	1	1	1	1	1	1	1	1
D	2	3	3	3	3	3	2	2	3	3	3	3	3	2	2	3	3	3	3	3	2
E	2	2	2	2	2	2	2	2	2	2	2	2	2	2	2	2	2	2	2	2	2

Seven-Week Rotating Cycle

FIGURE 4–10. Staffing Board

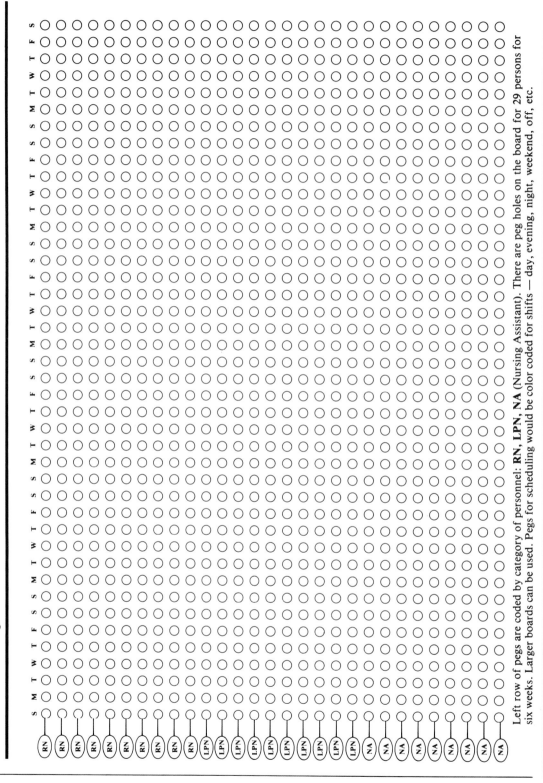

Left row of pegs are coded by category of personnel: **RN, LPN, NA** (Nursing Assistant). There are peg holes on the board for 29 persons for six weeks. Larger boards can be used. Pegs for scheduling would be color coded for shifts — day, evening, night, weekend, off, etc.

Nursing Decentralization of El Camino Hospital

In the El Camino Experience in nursing decentralization, head nurses rotated to an advisory position named "complex captain." Their staffing function included:

1. Gathering and using data for determining staffing numbers from patient-census figures; average length of stay; discharges and admissions by days of week, months of year, and season; emergency room cases; seasonal fluctuations; and the influence of such factors as physician vacations, medical conventions, business layoffs, school vacations, and the demographics of the community.

2. Forecasting admissions, surgeries, vacations, conventions for 2 to 3 weeks in advance.

3. Performing utilization reviews of staffing to assist with forecasting and planning.

4. Forecasting core staffing for 2-week periods. Core staff reflects the number of staff needed to care for the number of patients forecasted for a given unit.

5. Matching patient-dependency system with staffing. Reports are sent to nursing staffing office 3 times a day; information is sent to admitting offices for use in placing patients.

6. Maintaining central staffing board.

7. Maintaining float pool with cross-trained personnel.

8. Reviewing float position with budget and staffing coordinators.

9. Hiring and signing work agreements with new personnel.[14] See Figure 4–7 on p. 70.

Staffing secretaries can type the schedule, assign floats, call additional staff, and supply the head nurse with data for scheduling paid time off or excused absences. Secretaries will use the nursing management information system for this if one exists.

PATIENT CLASSIFICATION SYSTEMS

A patient classification system (PCS) is essential to staffing nursing units of hospitals. It quantifies the quality of nursing care. In selecting or implementing PCS a representative committee of nurse managers and clinical nurses should be used. The committee can include a representative of hospital administration. Inclusion of the latter will decrease skepticism about the PCS.

Purposes

The committee will identify the purposes of the PCS to be purchased or developed. Among these purposes are:

1. Staffing. The system will establish a unit of measure for nursing: *time*. This unit of measure will be used to determine both numbers and kinds of staff needed. Perceived patient needs can be matched with available nursing resources.

2. Budgeting. The predescribed unit of time will be used to determine the actual cost of nursing service. Profits and losses of nursing can then be determined.

3. Tracking changes in patient care needs. A PCS gives nurse managers the ability to moderate and control delivery of care services, adjusting intensity and cost.

4. Determining values for the productivity equation, which is output divided by input. Reducing input costs reduces costs of each output (time unit). In the prospective payment system (PPS), this output measure has been the discharged patient. Outputs become the criteria for measuring nursing productivity, regardless of quality. PCSs provide workload indexes as productivity measures.

5. Determining quality. Once a standard time element is established, staffing is adjusted to meet the aggregate times. A nurse manager can elect to staff below the standard time to reduce costs. Thus the nurse manager makes a decision to reduce quality by reducing times and cost. It is best to do this in

collaboration with clinical nurses. They are the personnel who are continually present and can assist with developing and applying more efficient procedures and protocols. This can involve rearrangement of the physical setting and the assembling of equipment and supplies. Their involvement will increase their trust and respect, improve their attendance and work habits, improve work force stability, and reduce errors. Their input into decision making can be through product evaluation and selection, identification of non-nursing tasks to be performed by lower-priced workers, increased mechanization, and job evaluation.[15]

Nursing Management Information Systems for PCSs

Nursing Management Information Systems (NMISs) are described in more detail in chapter 18. A good one is basic to a sound PCS. It will provide shift reports of personnel needed and assigned, by type. It will provide staffing and productivity data by unit and area. It will provide average data on the intensity of care needed by class of patient. It will provide the cost per time unit of patient care by class of patient.[16]

Characteristics Desired of PCSs

The following characteristics are desirable for PCSs. Such systems should:

1. Differentiate intensity of care among definitive classes.
2. Measure and quantify care to develop a management engineering standard.
3. Match nursing resources to patient care requirements.
4. Relate to time and effort spent on the associated activity.
5. Be economical and convenient to report and use.
6. Be mutually exclusive, counting no item under more than one work unit.
7. Be open to audit.
8. Be understood by those who plan, schedule, and control the work.
9. Be individually standardized as to the procedures needed for accomplishment.
10. Separate requirements for registered nurses and other staff.[17]

Components of PCSs

The first component of a PCS is a method for grouping patients or the classification categories. Johnson indicates two methods of categorizing patients. Using "factor evaluation," each patient is rated on independent elements of care; each element is scored (weighted); scores are summarized and the patient placed in a category based on the total numerical value obtained. Using "prototype evaluation," each patient is categorized to a broad description of care requirements.[18]

Johnson describes a prototype evaluation with four basic categories and one category for a typical patient requiring 1:1 care. Each category addresses activities of daily living, general health, teaching, emotional support, treatments, and medications. Data are collected on average time spent on direct and indirect care; see Figure 4–11.

A second component of a PCS is a set of guidelines describing the way in which patients will be classified, the frequency of classification, and the method of reporting the data; see Figure 4–12. The third component of a PCS is the average amount of time required for care of a patient in each category; see Figure 4–13.

A method for calculating required staffing and required nursing care hours is the fourth and final component of a PCS.

The formula is "the sum of the standard times for each category multiplied by the number of patients in that category plus the indirect care time equals required hours of patient care. Dividing this value by 7.0 (number of hours staff actually work each shift) results in the number of staff required to work early shift."[19]

The Commission for Administration Services in Hospitals (CASH) system of patient classification appears to be of the "prototype evaluation" type. CASH is a patient classification design that rates patients by intensity of care and establishes a category relating to nursing hours required based on patients' ability to feed and bathe themselves with supervision, mobility status, special procedures and treatments, and observational, institutional, and emotional needs. This design is quantified by determining the nursing care time associated with the critical indicators. The GRASP® system of patient classification uses a workload measurement design to evaluate the categories of tasks that nurses perform in providing patient care and identifies how

FIGURE 4–11. Classification Categories— Medical Surgical Units

Category I—Self Care

1. Activities of daily living.
   a. Eating—feeds self or needs little assistance.
   b. Grooming—almost entirely self-sufficient.
   c. Excretion—goes to bathroom alone or almost alone. Not incontinent.
   d. Comfort—Self-sufficient.
2. General health—good—admitted for a diagnostic procedure, simple procedure, or surgery that is simple or minor.
3. Teaching and emotional support—routine teaching for simple procedures, follow-up teaching or discharge teaching. No unusual or adverse emotional reactions. Patient may require orientation to time, place, and person once a shift.
4. Treatments and medications—none or simple medications or treatment.

Category II—Minimal Care

1. Activities of daily living.
   a. Eating—needs help in preparing food, positioning, or encouragement to eat. Can feed self.
   b. Grooming—can do majority of care unassisted or with minimal assistance.
   c. Excretion—needs help getting to bathroom or using urinal. Not incontinent or experiences occasional stress incontinence or dribbling.
   d. Grooming—can do majority of care unassisted or with minimal assistance.
2. General health—mild symptoms including more than one mild illness. Requires monitoring of vital signs, diabetic urines, uncomplicated drainage, or infusion.
3. Teaching and emotional support—needs 5–10 minutes a shift for teaching or emotional support. Patient may be mildly confused, belligerent, or agitated but is well controlled by medications, frequent orientation, or restraints.
4. Treatments and medications—Requires 20–30 minutes a shift. Needs evaluation of effectiveness of medication or treatment frequently. May require observation q2h for mental status.

Category III—Moderate Care

1. Activities of daily living.
   a. Eating—needs to be fed but can chew and swallow.
   b. Grooming—unable to do much for self.
   c. Excretion—needs bedpan or urinal placed or removed. Can only partially turn or lift self. Incontinent two times each shift.
   d. Comfort—completely dependent and needs turning but can be turned by one person.
2. General health—acute symptoms may be impending or subsiding. Requires monitoring and evaluation of physiological or emotional state q2–4h. Has continuous drainage or infusion which requires monitoring q1h.
3. Teaching and emotional support—requires 10–30 minutes a shift. Very apprehensive or mildly resistive to teaching. Patient may be confused, agitated, or belligerent but is fairly well controlled by medications, frequent orientation, or restraints.
4. Treatments and medications—requires 30–60 minutes a shift. Requires frequent observation for side effects or allergic reaction. May require observation q1h for mental status.

Category IV—Extensive Care

1. Activities of daily living.
   a. Eating—cannot feed self. Difficulty chewing and swallowing. May require tube feeding.
   b. Grooming—complete bath, hair care, oral care. Patient cannot assist at all.
   c. Excretion—incontinent more than two times a shift.
   d. Comfort—cannot turn self or assist with turning. May require two people to turn.
2. General health—seriously ill. Exhibits acute symptoms such as bleeding and/or fluid loss, acute respiratory episodes, or other episodes requiring frequent monitoring and evaluation.
3. Teaching and emotional support—requires more than 30 minutes a shift. Teaching of very resistive patients or care and support of patients with severe emotional reactions. Patient may be confused, belligerent, or agitated and is not controlled by medications, frequent orientation, or restraints.
4. Treatment and medication—requires more than 60 minutes a shift. Elaborate treatments done more than one time in a shift or requiring two persons. May require observation more frequently than q1h for mental status.

Category V—Intensive Care Requires one-to-one observation or continuous monitoring each shift.

SOURCE: K. Johnson, "A Practical Approach to Patient Classification," *Nursing Management,* June 1984, 40. Reproduced by permission.

FIGURE 4–12. Directions for Classifying Patients

1. Patient classification will be reviewed one time each shift by the charge nurse or her designee on the 7–3 and 3–11 shifts.
2. Classification is made by comparing the individual patient with each of the categories. If a charge nurse is unsure as to what category a patient belongs she should refer to the ADL indicator only and classify by those guidelines.
3. The cue sheet is only a guideline. It is not expected that every patient will be classified in the same category by disease entity alone.
4. After the category is selected, the charge nurse will place a number on the Kardex to denote that patient's classification

    Self Care   — I   Extensive Care — IV
    Minimal Care   — II   Intensive Care — V
    Moderate Care — III

5. The charge nurse (or designee, i.e., secretary) will tally the number of patients in each category. The nursing office will call for the tallies at approximately 1 p.m.–9 p.m.
6. Patients who have private duty nurses and sitters are classified according to the level of care the staff on the unit must provide to the patients.

SOURCE: K. Johnson, "A Practical Approach to Patient Classification," *Nursing Management,* June 1984, with permission.

much nursing time is required for each task. The time is then totalled.[20] GRASP® is a "factor evaluation" design, as is Medicus.

There is only general agreement that three to five categories of patient acuity are sufficient for a PCS. Alward argues that four categories are best to reduce variance and statistical probability of error. She also states that the factor evaluation instrument is better than the prototype system as it prevents ambiguity or overlap among the categories.[21]

Examples

Nursing Model. PCSs based on a model of nursing are rare. Auger and Dee[22] describe one based on the Johnson Behavior System Model. It is based on

eight behavioral subsystems: ingestive, eliminative, sexual, dependency, affiliative, achievement, aggressive-protective, and restorative; see Figure 4–14.

Patent behaviors and nursing interventions were rank-ordered for four categories of patient acuteness; see Figure 4–15.

Patient behaviors and nursing intervention categorization criteria for eliminative and affiliative subsystems are given in Figure 4–16.

Fourteen pairs of observers were used to rate each subsystem of behavior for all patients present on the unit during the shift. Observers agreed on independent ratings of patient behavior for the eight subsystems. Employees were trained to do patient ratings. New employees rate patients differently, indicating a need to develop a common frame of reference for all observer-raters. This system

FIGURE 4–13. Data Collection—Standard Care Hours per Patient Category

DIRECTIONS: Consider a patient for whom you have cared for today in each of the following categories. Indicate, to the best of your ability, the amount of time that is required to care for the patient. If you did not care for a patient in one of the categories this shift, please leave that category blank. Your cooperation in completing these forms is appreciated.

Category I   — Self Care   _____ Minutes
Category II   — Minimal Care   _____ Minutes
Category III — Moderate Care _____ Minutes
Category IV   — Extensive Care _____ Minutes

CHECK ONE: FILL IN BLANK:

RN   _____   _____ Shift
LPN   _____   _____ Unit
Aide/Attendant _____   _____ Date

Please leave this form in the area designated for that purpose on the nursing unit.

SOURCE: K. Johnson, "A Practical Approach to Patient Classification," *Nursing Management,* June 1984, with permission.

FIGURE 4–14. Definitions and Behavioral Characteristics of Behavioral Subsystems

Subsystem	Definition	Critical Behavioral Characteristics
Ingestive	Behaviors associated with the intake of needed resources from the external environment, including food, information, and objects, for the purpose of establishing an effective relationship with the environment	Food/fluid intake: sensory perception: mental status
Eliminative	Behaviors associated with the release of physical waste products	Bowel/bladder patterns; hygiene
Affiliative	Behaviors associated with the development and maintenance of interpersonal relationships with parents, peers, authority figures; establishes a sense of relatedness and belonging with others	Attachment behaviors; interpersonal relationships; communication skills
Dependency	Behaviors associated with obtaining assistance from others in the environment for completing tasks and/or emotional support; includes seeking of attention, approval, recognition	Basic self-care skills; emotional security
Sexual	Behaviors associated with a specific gender identity for the purpose of pleasure and procreation	Knowledge and behavior congruent with biological sex
Aggressive-Protective	Behaviors associated with real or potential threat in the environment for the purpose of ensuring survival	Protection of self through direct or indirect acts; identification of potential danger
Achievement	Behaviors associated with mastery of one-self and one's environment for the purpose of producing a desired effect	Problem-solving activities; knowledge of personal strengths and weaknesses
Restorative	Behaviors associated with maintaining or restoring energy equilibrium; relief from fatigue, recovery from illness, and so on.	Sleep behavior; leisure/recreational activities; sick role behavior

Source: J. A. Auger and V. Dee, "A Patient Classification System Based on the Behavioral System Model of Nursing: Part 1," April, 1983, 40. Reprinted with permission.

applies to psychiatric patients but indicates the necessity for rating psychosocial factors on all patients.[22]

Auger and Dee list four advantages to relating nursing models to PCSs:

1. Providing a frame of reference for the systematic assessment of patient behaviors and the development of nursing intervention.

2. Providing a frame of reference for all practitioners in the clinical setting.

FIGURE 4–15.   General Framework for Categorization of Nursing
Care Requirements

Patient Behaviors		Nursing Interventions
Behaviors that are a) Healthy; b) Appropriate to developmental stage; c) Adaptive to environment. Behavioral subsystems that are currently inactive. Physical health status: normal	I	Maintain and support healthy, developmentally appropriate behaviors. Reinforce independent behaviors in adaptive areas. Provide general supervision.
Behaviors that are a) Inconsistent; b) In process of being learned; c) May or may not be appropriate to developmental stage; d) Maladaptive to the environment. Physical health status: chronic or acute health problem of minor significance, such as cold.	II	Provide moderate/periodic supervision. Maintain behavioral programs designed to modify maladaptive behaviors and maintain new adaptive behaviors. Structure environment as needed to provide limits on behaviors. Provide care in the context of group setting. Provide nursing care appropriate to illness and handicaps. Implement medical regime.
Behaviors that are a) Severely maladaptive to the environment; b) Not appropriate to developmental stage. Physical health status: chronic or acute health problem of major significance, such as seizures.	III	Provide direct supervision. Implement behavioral programs designed to modify maladaptive behaviors. Initiate teaching of new behaviors. Reinforce healthy adaptive behaviors. Structure environment to provide limits on behaviors. Provide intensive nursing care appropriate to illness and handicaps. Critical activities: new admissions, seclusion and restraint, Electroconvulsive Therapy.
Category III and IV behavior in one or more subsystems of acute intensity and/or frequency: includes self destructive acts and aggression toward others	IV	Care provided on a one-to-one basis for eight (8) hours per shift, that is, suicide observation.

Source: J. A. Auger and V. Dee, "A Patient Classification System Based on the Behavioral System Model of Nursing: Part I," *The Journal of Nursing Administration*, April, 1983, 41. Reprinted with permission.

3. Providing a theoretical framework of knowledge and behavior.
4. Providing for consistency and continuity of care.
   Auger and Dee emphasize orientation and teaching of all new personnel so the system will be used effectively. This is true of all PCSs, including their use to make decisions about admissions.[23]

In-House versus Purchased PCSs.   Purchased PCSs are very expensive and must be modified for spe-

FIGURE 4–16. Samples of Level III Categorization Criteria for Two Behavioral Subsystems

Eliminative Subsystem	
Patient Behaviors	Nursing Interventions
1. Absence of bowel control.	1. Implement behavioral program for toilet training, bedwetting, and encopresis.
2. Absence of bladder control.	2. Total care of eliminative needs: diapers, colostomy care, drains, and so on.
3. Absence of established pattern of elimination or disruption of established pattern resulting in dehydration.	3. Teach self-care, independent skills related to hygiene/eliminative tasks.
4. Failure to dispose of body wastes in sanitary manner: for example, fecal smearing.	4. Direct supervision of hygiene care.
5. Excessive diaphoresis.	5. Attend closely to changes in elimination pattern for signs and symptoms of physical problems.
	6. Provide medications, as ordered by physician.

Affiliative Subsystem	
Patient Behaviors	Nursing Interventions
1. Absence of emotional attachment to others or excessive intense attachments.	1. Provide regular, intensive one-to-one interactions to establish relationship.
2. Failure to establish or maintain relationships on an individual basis.	2. Implement behavioral program to increase frequency of interactions with staff/family/peers.
3. Failure to establish or maintain relationships in group interactions.	3. Implement behavioral program to increase participation in group activities.
4. Failure to initiate/maintain effective communication: verbal, nonverbal, and written.	4. Promote adaptation to change by planning and limiting number of changes.
5. Indiscriminate attachment to others.	5. Limit contact with family when indicated; provide information regarding denial of rights.
6. Resistant to change in milieu or daily routine.	6. Implement behavioral program to develop basic communication skills and role model interactional techniques.
7. Lack of awareness of personal space.	7. Assist in identification and expression of positive/negative feelings.
8. Unable to express positive/negative feelings in direct way; denial of feelings.	

SOURCE: J. A. Auger and V. Dee, "A Patient Classification System Based on the Behavioral System Model of Nursing: Part I," *The Journal of Nursing Administration,* April, 1983, 41. Reprinted with permission.

cific hospitals. In-house PCSs can be developed by using work analysis techniques. Methods for developing such systems are described in several references. Most use observation or self-recovering of activities in which personnel are trained to list activities they perform at timed intervals. Observation on a continuous or internal basis can be costly in time and money. Self-reporting is cheaper but employees must be trained.[24]

Alward states that it is more realistic to use the budget to determine staffing. She suggests selecting a prototype or factor evaluation classification instrument and revising it to conform with the division's nursing practice.[25]

Nybert and Wolff describe a PCS that calculates the total time, direct and indirect, needed to care for each patient by unit, shift, and job classification. The required time is compared with actual and budgeted nursing time per patient. This system has been used for over 5 years and has been found to identify patient care trends, improve efficiency of staffing, and justify budgeting changes. It is used for utilization review: using access to admitting and working diagnosis, surgical procedures, physican consultants, patient classification category, and a listing of all the daily nursing care activities. If hospitalization is not justified, a chart review is done. This computerized system determines nursing costs per patient by unit, Medicare patients and non-Medicare patients by diagnosis, and average and total costs of Medicare and non-Medicare patients. In one 2-week period, Medicare patients required 10 percent more nursing resources per day and 40 percent more nursing time for their entire hospitalization. If this finding holds true in other hospitals, nurse managers can use the data to petition for increased Medicare reimbursement.[26]

Microcomputer Models. Microcomputer models of PCSs exist. One of these described by Gragmen has modules for planning nursing care and dealing with the budget. This system projects the number of hours of care for each of four patient levels that will meet budgetary and program delivery constraints of the staffing parameters. It is a staffing system that addresses the "demand" function based upon planning and the "management" function based upon a blending of planning and actual situations. Thus the input variables can be changed and the budget renegotiated. This model plans nursing time and resource allocation daily, based upon patient case

mix and census. It gives the head nurse control over resource use.[27]

Adams and Duchene describe a PCS that includes nursing diagnosis with related etiology, nursing care goals, and potential patient outcomes. It is an in-house system, the advantages of which include:

1. Knowledge of the data tool.
2. Capability for altering the system to accommodate changes in procedural time standards.
3. Ability to make changes in staffing levels of care.
4. Ability to make percentage alterations of time given to indirect activities.

It produces a plan of care with acuity as a by-product for determining nurse staffing needs.[28]

Problems with PCSs

One of the major problems of PCSs is to maintain reliability and validity. This can be done through continuing education and quality assurance (QA) checks. A calendar can be established to have external personnel from staff development or another nursing department or unit develop a classification following that done by unit personnel (interacter reliability). This can be done monthly or more often, depending upon the results. Patients can be monitored on different days and different shifts, with a stratified random sample of about 15 or 20 percent of the patient census. Simple percentage agreement of 90 percent or higher indicates satisfactory reliability. If agreement is below 80 percent, the system should be reviewed and adjusted.

A calendar can also be established to take a unit rotation work sample to determine whether procedures or tasks change with time and technology. This can be an annual spot check. Validation of PCSs varies. A questionnaire can be used to evaluate nursing staff's satisfaction with hours of care. Validity can also be tested by using an expert panel of nurses. Patient category descriptions or critical indicators of nursing intervention and patient requirement lists should be reviewed annually by using standards. The PCSs must be altered if results of QA checks or work samples so indicate.

Orientation and continuing education are the best methods of assuring reliability and validity. The nursing staff must find the PCS credible. If they believe that the classifications are accurate and useful they will try to rate patients accurately. They need periodic classes to update them and keep them well informed. Managers must support the use of a valid and reliable PCS since it indicates the institution's commitment to quality patient care.

Nursing should orient other department heads and physicians to the use of PCSs. Admissions and placements of patients are related to PCS outcomes.[29]

Practicing nurses want the PCS to provide more staff. Managing nurses want to use it to validate staffing and scheduling and permit variable staffing. These objectives must be kept in harmony.

MODIFIED APPROACHES TO NURSE STAFFING AND SCHEDULING

Many different approaches to nurse staffing and scheduling are being tried in an effort to satisfy the needs of employees and meet workload demands for patient care. These include game theory, modified work weeks (10- or 12-hour shifts), team rotation, "premium day" weekend nurse staffing, and "premium vacation" night staffing. Such approaches should support the underlying purpose, mission, philosophy, and objectives of the organization and the division of nursing and should be well defined in a staffing philosophy and policies. Nurses are like other workers in one respect: they would like to live as normal a home life as possible. Shifts have to be staffed and patient care needs met. The successful nurse executive will try to accommodate both by using the best administrative staffing methodology available. It must be considered from the economic or cost/benefit viewpoint.

Staffing and scheduling are reasons for turnover and retention. Understaffing has a negative effect on staff morale, delivery of quality care, and the nursing practice modality. It can close beds. It causes absenteeism from staff fatigue, burnout, and professional dissatisfaction. On the other hand, nurse managers want to receive value for their money. There are economic constraints that are further stretched by the costs of recruiting, hiring, and orienting new nurses and for overtime and temporary hires when the environment creates turnovers and absenteeism. Overstaffing is expensive and has a negative effect on staff morale and productivity. Staffing and scheduling must balance the personal needs of nurses with the economic and productivity needs of organizations.[30]

Modified Work Weeks

Modified work-week schedules using 10- and 12-hour shifts and other methods are commonplace. A nurse administrator should be sure they are fulfilling the staffing philosophy and policies, particularly with regard to efficiency. Also, they should not be imposed upon the nursing staff, but should show a mutual benefit to employer, employee, and ultimately the clients served.

The 10-Hour Day. One modification of the work week is four 10-hour shifts per week in organized time increments. A problem of this model is time overlaps of 6 hours per 24-hour day. The overlaps can be used for patient-centered conferences, nursing care assessment and planning, and staff development. Also the overlap can be scheduled to cover peak workload hours. Peak workload demands can be identified by observation, consensus, or self-recording by professional nurses. It can be done by hour or by a block of 3 to 4 hours. The staffing board in Figure 4–10 can be used to solve these problems.

Longer work days can decrease overtime because of overlapping shifts. Absenteeism and turnover are decreased because nurses have more days off. All of these factors decrease costs. Such a system can increase staffing needs if mechanisms are not used to maintain productivity. Some organizations use a 7-days-on, 7-days-off schedule but only pay for 70 hours in two weeks.[31]

The 4-day, 10-hour work schedule for night nurses was studied in a hospital that had difficulty recruiting qualified nurses to the night shift. It had been perceived that 10-hour shifts had stabilized staffing in intensive care with increased productivity and decreased turnover.

Turnover on the night shift had been 70 percent for an 8-month period. Positions stayed vacant longer than for other shifts and sick time was higher. This increased recruitment and orientation time. Nurses were involved in planning the 4-day, 10-hour night shift schedule. Night nurses agreed to use overlap hours to assist with day shift care. The day shift agreed to reduce staff by one FTE. Plans were discussed with and accepted by the union. Assignment of personnel and meeting schedules

FIGURE 4–17.   A Comparative Graph of Casual Absenteeism on One Unit with Different Schedules

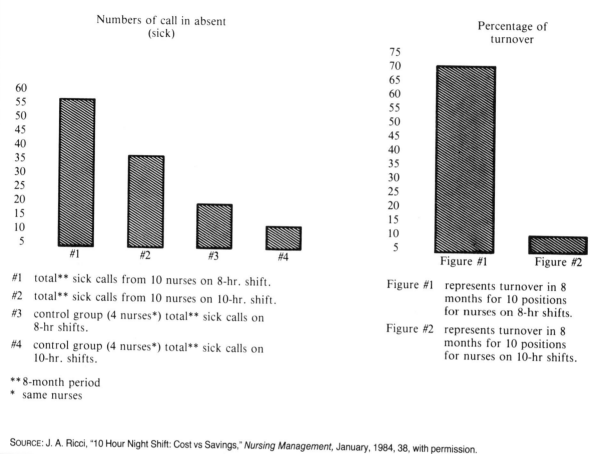

#1   total** sick calls from 10 nurses on 8-hr. shift.

#2   total** sick calls from 10 nurses on 10-hr. shift.

#3   control group (4 nurses*) total** sick calls on 8-hr shifts.

#4   control group (4 nurses*) total** sick calls on 10-hr. shifts.

** 8-month period
* same nurses

Figure #1   represents turnover in 8 months for 10 positions for nurses on 8-hr shifts.

Figure #2   represents turnover in 8 months for 10 positions for nurses on 10-hr. shifts.

SOURCE: J. A. Ricci, "10 Hour Night Shift: Cost vs Savings," *Nursing Management*, January, 1984, 38, with permission.

were addressed and resolved through participatory management.

The results included reduced sick time on the 10-hour shift, reduced turnover, increased incentive, increased requests for night shift, and decreased labor hours;[32] see Figure 4–17.

The 12-Hour Shift.   A second scheduling modification is the 12-hour shift in which nurses work seven shifts in 2 weeks: three on, four off; then four on, three off. They work a total of 84 hours and are paid 4 hours overtime. Twelve-hour shifts and flexible staffing have been reported to have improved care and saved money because nurses can manage their home and personal lives better.[33]

Vik and MacKay report a study of the quality of care by nurses who worked 12-hour versus 8-hour shifts. It was a matched study of three units each. The Quality Patient Care Scale was used as the measuring instrument. The "quality of care received by patients on the 8-hour shift units was significantly higher than that received by patients on the 12-hour shift units."[34] Shift patterns worked by nurses do affect the care received by patients. However, recruitment and retention of nurses can balance out reduced quality of care when vacancies are high. This was a limited study needing replication.

There is a break-even point for costs. It is the point at which recruiting, absenteeism, retention, and overtime cost savings equal the shift losses from 12-hour scheduling.[35]

The Weekend Alternative.   Another variation of flexible scheduling is the weekend alternative. Nurses work two 12-hour shifts and are paid for 40 hours plus benefits. They can use the weekdays to go to school or for other personal needs. There are several variations of the weekend schedule. Monday-through-Friday nurses have all weekends off.

Metcalf reports a test of the 12-hour weekend plan of two shifts on Saturday and Sunday, 7:00 A.M. to 7:00 P.M. and 7:00 P.M. to 7:00 A.M. The day shift were paid at rate of 36 hours of pay for 24 hours worked. The night shift were paid at the rate of 40 hours of pay for 24 hours worked.

The sample included R.N.s, L.P.N.s, and nurses' aides. Employed staff could volunteer for the shift and new staff were required to work it, as this was not a "weekends only" schedule. Full-time staff participating in it had two weekends out of three off. Results showed that only 3 percent of the total sample wanted the schedule discontinued, while 75 percent perceived weekend staffing as better.

While illnesses and other absences increased by 19 percent, this negative finding was outweighed by positive ones. Recruiting improved, with vacancy rates dropping from 13 to 7 percent of budgeted positions. Use of agency personnel was cut in half and salary costs did not increase. Staffing and morale both improved. Problems were addressed to improve the plan.[36]

Other Modified Approaches

Team rotation is a method of cyclic staffing in which a nursing team is scheduled as a unit. It would be used if the team nursing modality were being practiced by a team.[37]

"Premium day" weekend nurse staffing is a scheduling pattern that gives a nurse an extra day off-duty, called a "premium day," if he or she volunteers to work one additional weekend within a four-week scheduling block. This staffing technique could be modified to give the nurse a "premium day" off for every additional weekend worked beyond those required by nurse staffing policy. This technique does not add directly to hospital costs.[38]

"Premium vacation" night staffing follows the same principle as "premium day" weekend staffing. An example would be the policy of giving an extra five working days of vacation to every nurse who works a permanent night shift for a specific period of time—3 months, 4 months, or 6 months. This would be in addition to regular vacation time.

A study by Imig, Powell, and Thorman indicated that while flexible staffing filled vacant positions, it did not increase payroll costs, hours per patient day, or overtime, and decreased absenteeism by 60 percent. The hospital in this study returned to 8-hour shifts because primary nursing was threatened. In this particular study there was *no change* in medication errors, patient and staff injuries, quality of care plans, complaints, recruitment, and staff attitudes from before to 6 months after flexible staffing. Also, use of agency nurses was not reduced.[39]

Positive Aspects

Nurses of the 1980s want flexible scheduling to better accommodate their personal lives. Flexible time (frequently called "flextime") schedules have become an increasingly important aspect of employment practices generally, with 11.9 percent of all nonfarm wage and salary workers on such schedules in 1980. They have improved attitudes and increased productivity as employees have gained more control over their work environment. There have been adjustments to their own "bioclock" by employees. Transportation has become more efficient and flexible. Employees have better control of work activities.[40]

A study was done by the New York state government to control weaknesses of previous studies. Staggered work hours were compared to fixed work hours. The study showed that:

1. The greatest level of satisfaction and the least dissatisfaction with the workday was expressed by employees in the agency with the greatest flexibility in scheduling.
2. Those in the agency with fixed schedules expressed the strongest dissatisfaction and lowest level of satisfaction.
3. Statistically, there were no significant differences in job satisfaction among these groups.
4. Decreased commuting time may improve satisfaction with flextime.[41]

Flexible scheduling improves recruiting, absenteeism, and retention. There are many flexible scheduling variations available. Before using them, nurse managers should establish philosophy and set objectives.

Negative Aspects

Among the disadvantages of 10- and 12-hour days are:

1. Minimum weekend staffing (or excess staff on weekends).
2. Unsafe travel times.
3. Shift overlaps that decrease total number of personnel on duty.
4. Costs for overtime.
5. Fatigue.
6. Strain on family life.
7. If the schedule is not carefully planned, the loss of shifts can require increased staffing.
8. State law may require overtime pay for hours worked in excess of 8 in a day and 40 in a week.
9. Less continuity of care.
10. Less communication among staff.
11. Developing, maintaining, and explaining the master schedule.
12. Modification of primary assessing.[42]

Cross-Training

Cross-training of nursing personnel can improve flexible scheduling. Nurses need to be prepared to function effectively in more than one area of expertise. They can be kept in similar clinical specialties or families of clinical specialties. They require complete orientation and ongoing staff development to prevent errors and increase job satisfaction. This can be done for both unit-assigned nurses and pool nurses. There should be policies, job descriptions, and performance evaluations. Pools can be in-house supplemental staffing agencies that use full-time and part-time nurses. Benefits can be prorated or employees can have choice of increased pay instead of benefits.

Scheduling with NMIS

Planning the duty schedule does not always match personnel with preferences. This is one major dissatisfaction among clinical nurses. Their satisfaction can be improved by posting the number of nurses needed by time slots and allowing them to put colored pins in slots to select their own times. The staffing board can be used; refer to Figure 4–10.

Staffing is a major reason for having an NMIS. A microcomputer can be used to show via menus and printouts: nurses required by time slots, restrictions, off-duty policy, days-off paired, and cyclical schedule as well as single rotation.[43]

Hanson defines a management information system (MIS) as "an array of components designed to transform a collective set of data into knowledge that is directly useful and applicable in the process of directing and controlling resources and their application to the achievement of specific objectives."[44]

Information stimulates action through management decision making. Data do not; they must be processed to be useful. Information must be timely to be useful. The process for establishing any MIS is:

1. State the management objective clearly.
2. Identify the actions required to meet the objective.
3. Identify the responsible position in the organization.
4. Identify the information required to meet the objective.
5. Determine the data required to produce the needed information.
6. Determine the system's requirement for processing the data.
7. Develop a flow chart.[45]

Refer to Chapter 18, Nursing Management Information Systems, for a more detailed discussion.

Productivity

Definition

Productivity is commonly defined as

$$\frac{Outputs}{Inputs}$$

Hanson translates this definition into:

$$\frac{Required\ staff\ hours}{Provided\ staff\ hours} \times 100 = Productivity$$

To illustrate,

$$\frac{380.50\ required\ staff\ hours}{402.00\ provided\ staff\ hours} \times 100 = 94.7\ percent\ productivity$$

Productivity can be increased by decreasing the provided staff hours while holding the required staff hours constant or increasing them. This data becomes information when related to an objective that indicates variances.[46] Since resources for health care are limited, the nurse manager is faced with the task of motivating clinical nurses to increase productivity.

Productivity in nursing is related to both efficiency of use of clinical nursing in delivering nursing care to avoid waste and the effectiveness of that care relative to its quality and appropriateness. Brown indicates that productivity in the United States has declined. He cites as evidence of this claim increased labor costs without corresponding increases in performance. This is due to such factors as inexperienced workers, technological slowdown due to outdated equipment and lessened research and development, government regulations, a diminished work ethic, increased size and bureaucracy in business and industry, and erosion of the managerial ethic.[47]

Measuring Productivity

In developing a model for an MIS, Hanson indicates several formulas for translating data into information. In addition to the productivity formula, he indicates that hours per patient day (HPPD) is another data element that can provide meaningful information when provided for an extended period of time. HPPD is determined by the formula

$$\frac{\text{Staff hours}}{\text{Patient days}} = \text{HPPD}$$

For example,

$$\frac{52,000 \text{ staff hours}}{2883.5 \text{ patient days}} = 18.03 \text{ HPPD}$$

$$52,000 \text{ staff hours} = 25 \text{ FTEs} \times 2080 \text{ work hours per year;}$$

$$2883.5 \text{ patient days} = 7.9 \text{ average daily census (ADC)} \times 365 \text{ days per year.}$$

No allowance is made for personal time such as coffee breaks, meals, vacations, holidays, sick time, or decreased census time. The figure of 18.03 HPPD may be a high provision of HPPD even for intensive care.

Another useful formula is

$$\frac{\text{Provided HPPD}}{\text{Budgeted HPPD}} \times 100 = \text{Budget utilization}$$

$$\frac{18.03 \text{ provided HPPD}}{16.0 \text{ budgeted HPPD}} \times 100 = \begin{array}{l} 112.7 \text{ percent} \\ \text{budget} \\ \text{utilization} \end{array}$$

This would be over budget if the provided hours had been net of personal time. Since they were not, the HPPD provided may be highly productive. The adequacy of the budget is determined as:

$$\frac{\text{Budgeted HPPD}}{\text{Required HPPD}} \times 100 = \text{Budget adequacy}$$

$$\frac{16.0 \text{ budgeted HPPD}}{18.03 \text{ required HPPD}} \times 100 = \begin{array}{l} 88.74 \text{ percent} \\ \text{budget} \\ \text{adequacy} \end{array}$$

Obviously, if the required HPPD is equal to the provided HPPD and exceeds the budgeted HPPD, productivity is high because of the budget inadequacy. According to Hanson, all data become information when related to the objective.[48] Staffing should be defined in terms of the goal of HPPD to be provided. This will relate to productivity, budget utilization, and budget adequacy. Whether it will be effective or not depends upon measurement of quality of outcomes.

Artinian, O'Connor, and Brock measured nursing productivity by using the number of physicians' orders written during a specific period as an estimate of nursing services provided for a particular patient. They counted the number of patient contacts generated by each physician order and separated them for licensed and unlicensed nursing personnel. Nurses summarized and enumerated changes in nursing care during the preceding five years. These changes were examined and those related to physicians' orders were selected. They did not measure independent nursing function or indirect care, assuming the latter to be similar to direct care. A pilot study to show whether the sickest patients generated the most nursing contacts indicated these results:

1. Three *not* acutely ill patients had 59.5 licensed nurse contacts and 47.5 nonlicensed nurse contacts in 5 days.

2. Three acutely ill patients had 302.7 licensed nurse contacts and 58.3 nonlicensed nurse contacts in 5 days.

3. There was a 103 percent increase in licensed nurse–patient contact from 1975–76 to 1981–82. This was statistically significant. It converted to a 27 percent increase in the nursing productivity index.[49]

One would conclude that the more acutely ill patients are, the more licensed nurse contacts they require.

Davis indicates that productivity in nursing is the volume and quality of products divided by the cost of producing and delivering them. It is directly related to what nurses do and how they do it. Systems have been developed to determine nursing cost per patient per shift. For example, at University Hospitals of Cleveland, the following formula is used: nurse competence rank × hourly salary rate × required nursing hours × care acuity = the nursing cost per patient. For example,

$$\text{Clinician III} \times \$12.50 \times 3 \text{ hours} \times 5 = \$562.50 \text{ per shift.}[50]$$

Smith, Mackey, and Markham developed a Productivity Monitoring System for the recovery room. The performance ratio was the required FTEs divided by worked FTEs. The data were used to decide whether to fill vacant positions and to develop a budget.[51]

Mailhot reported an analysis of problems in an operating room: poor physical environment, inadequate financial support, poor systems, and low morale. The department was overstaffed by ten FTEs. Task forces were formed that used brainstorming and open forums to solve the problems. They used Lewin's Force Field analysis, putting complex decision alternatives through an outcome matrix, developing needed evaluation tools, and using pilot projects to test all changes. They made eighty-seven changes in one year; see Figure 4–18.

In addition they marketed services to patients and surgeons, provided management training for operating room managers, analyzed operating room procedures, and held an open day between director and staff once every 6 weeks in which each person saw the director. They reduced the staffing by 38 FTE positions and the budget by $1.5 million

in three years. Job satisfaction surveys indicated improvement.[52]

Differences among Productivity Models

Producers of services do not fit the same productivity models as do producers of material goods. There is marked discretion in determining both expected and actual role performances of nurses who do not produce physical outputs. This is a reason why such nursing prescriptions as "emotional support" are difficult to measure. Patient outputs or outcomes can be measured by client satisfaction as well as by client condition upon discharge. There has been greater emphasis upon nursing process than upon nursing outcome. Haas defines efficiency as the relationship of personnel assigned and time spent to materials expended, as well as capital and management employed, for the greatest economy in use. The productive nurses must balance their personal energies and their institution's resources with their effectiveness.[53]

Curtin indicates that productivity in nursing is related to the application of knowledge. Professional productivity must be measured by means of efficacy, effectiveness, and efficiency in applying knowledge. She indicates that these processes can be objectively measured by using:

1. Objective measures of efficacy: years of formal education, levels of academic achievement, evidence of continuing education and skill development, and years of experience.
2. Objective measures of effectiveness: demonstrated ability to execute job-related procedures, correctly prioritized activities, performance according to professional and legal standards, appropriate information clearly and concisely recorded, and cooperative working with others.
3. Objective measures of efficiency: promptness, attendance, reliability, precision, adaptability, and economical disposition of resources.[54]

Curtin and Zurlage acknowledge that human services such as nursing are difficult to test, return, or exchange if unsatisfactory. They propose a system for measuring nursing productivity that includes a nursing productivity equation, an equation relating nursing productivity to hospital revenue, and a Nursing Productivity Index.[55]

FIGURE 4–18. Examples of Major Operating Room Department Changes

Renovation	Restructuring of Department	Communication	Systems	Strategic Plan
Instrument room	Reorganized management team	Nurse-physician committee	Materials management (established 5-7 day inventory)	Attained voting privileges on OR medical committee
Lounge locker room	Implemented RN specialization	OR delay reporting form	Equipment preventative maintenance program	Reallocated block time
Office space	Developed clinical ladder for RNs	House-wide staff exchange program	Established consignment program	Developed satellite ORs for same-day surgery
Fail-Safe electrical project	Reclassified eight positions	Provide internal external consultation	Held vendor faires	Developed five-year goals
Storage area	Revised job descriptions for all staff	Publish in OR and general nursing journals	Resolved phantom scheduling	Developed P.E.R.T. chart for 1½ year master plan
Hospital modernization plan	Redesigned staff nurse orientation	Staff Development programs	OR computer scheduling	Marketed new procedures/ equipment
	Developed and implemented management education series	Sought and attained medical director	Computerized utilization statistic program	Attained treatment room
	Assessed and modified all policies and procedures	Brought perfusionists under OR management	Computerized room delay program	Established health faires
	Hired staff specialists	Developed patient teaching tools	Restructured pricing	Initiated annual department/ get-together
	Evaluated and purchased new scrubs	Developed staff teaching tools	Modified billing process	
	Initiated "open door" policy	Developed audio-visual modules for basic programs	Color-coded scrub clothes	
	Implemented director's "open days" with staff every six weeks	Initiated monthly meetings with staff and assistant head nurses	Established cost containment committee	
	Supported 11 managers in their return-to-school		Established quality assurance committee	
	Initiated written commendations		Developed FTE control mechanism	
			Restructured for DRGs	
			Developed equipment education plan	
			Began instrument repair/replacement program	
			Initiated environment rounds	

SOURCE: C. B. Mailhot, "Setting OR's Course Toward Greater Productivity," *Nursing Management*, October 1985, with permission.

A Nursing Intensity Index has been developed and tested in all departments at Johns Hopkins Hospital. A pilot study was done in which records of eight major services were examined. These records were scored by three raters each for average agreement which varied from 82 to 95 percent. Modifications were made in the index as a result of the pilot study. A full study was then done using 784 records, each scored by two nurses. The results:

1. Nursing intensity levels varied widely within every clinical department and nursing unit.
2. The full study sample included 239 diagnostic-related groups (DRGs). Of these, 64 percent consist of only one level of nursing intensity, 31 percent contain two levels of nursing intensity, 4 percent contain three levels of nursing intensity, and 1 percent contain four levels of nursing intensity.
3. A weighted average coefficient of variation for total charges across all clinical departments was computed.
4. Average interraters' agreement across all clinical departments was 84 percent.
5. The Nursing Intensity Index is both a valid and reliable instrument for patient classification.
6. The Nursing Intensity Index correlates strongly (.61) with the Severity of Illness Index.
7. It can be used to systematize cost allocation for nursing and do variable billing, establish sound nurse staffing systems, monitor quality of patient care delivery, trace patient population trends, and do case mix analysis.[56]

Improving Nursing Productivity

Nursing productivity is being improved and the reported knowledge and skills are adding to the theory of nursing management. Rabin indicates that professionals can impose productivity values upon themselves. Managers should develop managerial goals and values. They need a standard of performance for themselves. Professionals can commit themselves to fostering innovative attitudes and technologies, stimulating performance by commitment to constructive action and follow-ups, living up to standards of practice, keeping up to date, and being receptive to public review. Almost any profession can develop measurable standards of performance and productivity.[57]

Employers should measure nursing output objectively and pay for it accordingly in salary, benefits, and promotions. There has been some progress in nursing in the form of standards of practice, clinical ladders, and models of peer review, among others. These need to be supported in the workplace, along with respect for the individual dignity of nurses, support for their personal commitment to professional goals, and support for the integrity of their professional judgments.[58]

Productivity can be managed and improved through:

1. Planning that increases the variations between inputs and outputs by:
   1.1 Outputs increasing, inputs decreasing.
   1.2 Outputs increasing, inputs remaining constant.
   1.3 Outputs increasing faster than inputs.
   1.4 Outputs remaining constant, inputs decreasing.
   1.5 Outputs decreasing more slowly than inputs.
2. Soliciting staff's ideas and recommendations.
3. Creating challenges.
4. Managers showing interest in staff's achievement and concerns.
5. Praising and rewarding good performances.
6. Involving staff.
7. Having a meaningful set or family of outcome measures for which data are available or easy to gather and over which workers have some control. Such measures should be easily understood.
8. Selecting measures compatible with white-collar functions and corporate measures.
9. Monitoring workload changes in staffing requirements with established standards.
10. Combining support with employees' understanding, motivation, and recognition.
11. Increasing ratio of professional to nonprofessional staff.
12. Placing admitted patients based on resource availability.
13. Improving skill, energy, and motivation through staff development, books, tuition reimbursement, paid meals, yoga lessons, bonuses and vacation days, and other incentives.
14. Work simplification, work flow analysis, and other approaches.

15. Making an organizational diagnosis of problems, resources, and realities.
16. Setting the climate for productivity by asking nurses what makes them productive and then doing it. Measure before and after.
17. Decreasing waiting and stand-by time, coffee klatches, social breaks, meal times.
18. Stimulating nurse managers and clinical nurses to want to achieve excellence.
19. Setting targets for increasing output on an annual basis without additional capital or employees.
20. Having personnel keep and analyze time diaries to determine personal improvement actions.
21. Setting personal objectives and measuring performance against them.
22. Making a commitment to improved productivity, effectiveness (doing the right things), and efficiency (doing things right).
23. Seeking new products and services and new methods and ways of producing them.
24. Seeking new and useful approaches to old problems.
25. Improving quality of nursing products, emphasizing such ideas as consistency, longevity, riskiness, perfectibility, and value.
26. Maintaining concern with the process and method of producing nursing care.
27. Improving use of time.
28. Reducing the cost of what nurses do by returning unused budgeted funds.
29. Improving esthetics: the quality of work life and the pleasantness and beauty of the environment.
30. Applying the ethical policy statements of professional nursing organizations.
31. Gaining the confidence of peers.
32. Recognizing the need to do better.[59]

SUMMARY

Staffing and scheduling are major components of nursing management. Traditional patterns have been slavishly adhered to until recent years. A nursing division needs a practical and written philosophy that guides all staffing and scheduling activities and that is acceptable to the staff.

Staffing studies can be used to determine staffing needs related to personnel skills, numbers of personnel, and time/workload requirements. Staffing can be planned by using computer models that calculate workload requirements from patient classification data or patient classification systems (PCSs). There are many modified approaches to nurse staffing and scheduling, including modified work weeks, team rotation, permanent shifts, and permanent weekends. While some consultants advise against mixing modified work weeks, they are in practice frequently mixed.

Productivity, the unit of output of nursing, is of increasing interest to nurse managers. It must include quality care indicators that can be observed and measured. Productivity is commonly defined as the outputs of production, divided by the inputs of production. Research needs to be undertaken to determine the key to increased productivity by professional nurses. Is it money or some other aspect of job satisfaction? One theory is that a combination of work, environment, and rewards will maintain or increase productivity.

NOTES

1. M. K. Aydelotte, *Nurse Staffing Methodology: A Review and Critique of Selected Literature* (Washington, DC: U.S. Government Printing Office, Jan. 1973), 3.
2. Ibid, p. 26.
3. M. E. West, "Implementing Effective Nurse Staffing Systems in the Managed Hospital," *Topics in Health Care Financing*, Summer 1980, 11–25.
4. J. N. Althaus, N. M. Hardyck, P. B. Pierce, and M. S. Rodgers, "Nurse Staffing in a Decentralized Organization: Part I," *The Journal of Nursing Administration*, March 1982, 34–39.
5. R. C. Minetti, "Computerized Nurse Staffing," *Hospitals*, July 16, 1983, 90, 92; P. P. Shaheen, "Staffing and Scheduling: Reconcile Practical Means with the Real Goal," *Nursing Management*, Oct. 1985, 64–69.
6. Aydelotte, op. cit., 26–31.
7. West, op. cit., 16.
8. The figure of 1.4 represents 1.4 workweeks of 5 days to cover a 7-day week; 1.14 represents the built-in holidays, sick leave, annual leave; 7.5 represents 7.5 productive hours on an 8-hour shift.
9. West, op. cit., 17.
10. E. M. Price, *Staffing for Patient Care* (New York: Springer, 1970), 12.
11. Ibid, 21–22.
12. "Study Questions All-RN Staffing," *RN* November, 1983, 15–16.
13. M. E. Warstler, "Some Management Techniques for Nursing Service Administrators," *Journal of Nursing Administration*, Nov.-Dec. 1972, 25–34.

14. J. N. Althaus, N. M. Hardyck, P. B. Pierce, and M. S. Rodgers, op. cit.; Ibid., "Nurse Staffing in a Decentralized Organization: Part II," *The Journal of Nursing Administration*, April 1982, 18–22.

15. T. P. Herzog, "Productivity: Fighting the Battle of the Budget," *Nursing Management*, Jan. 1985, 30–34; T. Porter-O'Grady, "Strategic Planning: Nursing Practice in the PPS," *Nursing Management*, Oct. 1985, 53–56; K. Johnson, "A Practical Approach to Patient Classification," *Nursing Management*, June 1984, 39–41, 44, 46; R. E. Schroeder, A. M. Rhodes, and R. E. Shields, "Nurse Acuity Systems: CASH Versus GRASP," *Nursing Forum*, Feb. 1984, 72–77; R. R. Alward, "Patient Classification Systems: The Ideal Versus Reality," *The Journal of Nursing Administration*, Feb. 1983, 14–18; J. Nyberg and N. Wolff, "DRG Panic," *The Journal of Nursing Administration*, April 1984, 17–21.

16. E. J. Halloran and M. Kiley, "Case Mix Management," *Nursing Management*, Feb. 1984, 39–41, 44–45.

17. R. E. Schroeder, A. M. Rhodes, and R. E. Shields, op. cit.

18. K. Johnson, op. cit.

19. Ibid., 41.

20. R. E. Schroeder, A. M. Rhodes, and R. E. Shields, op. cit.

21. R. R. Alward, op. cit.

22. J. A. Auger and V. Dee, "A Patient Classification System Based on the Behavioral System Model of Nursing: Part I," *The Journal of Nursing Administration*, Apr. 1983, 38–43.

23. V. Dee and J. A. Auger, "A Patient Classification System Based on the Behavioral System Model of Nursing: Part II," *The Journal of Nursing Administration*, May 1983, 18–23.

24. R. R. Alward, op. cit.

25. Ibid.

26. J. Nyberg and N. Wolff, op. cit.

27. T. E. Grazman, "Managing Unit Human Resources: A Microcomputer Model," *Nursing Management*, July 1983, 18–22.

28. R. Adams and P. Duchene, "Computerization of Patient Acuity and Nursing Care Planning," *The Journal of Nursing Administration*, April 1985, 11–17.

29. P. Giovannetti and G. G. Mayer, "Building Confidence in Patient Classification Systems," *Nursing Management*, Aug. 1984, 31–34; R. R. Alward, op. cit.

30. American Hospital Association, "Strategies: Flexible Scheduling," 1985, 12 pp.

31. Ibid.

32. J. A. Ricci, "10-Hour Night Shift: Cost Versus Savings," *Nursing Management*, Jan. 1984, 34–35, 38–42.

33. C. M. Fagin, "The Economic Value of Nursing Research," *American Journal of Nursing*, Dec. 1982, 1844–1849.

34. A. G. Vic and R. C. Mckay, "How Does the 12-Hour Shift Affect Patient Care?," *The Journal of Nursing Administration*, Jan. 1982, 12.

35. T. W. Lant and D. Gregory, "The Impact of 12-Hour Shift: An Analysis," *Nursing Management*, Oct. 1984, 38A, B, D–F, H.

36. M. L. Metcalf, "The 12-Hour Weekend Plan—Does the Nursing Staff Really Like It?," *The Journal of Nursing Administration*, Oct. 1982, 16–19.

37. D. Froebe, "Scheduling: By Team or Individually," *Staffing: A Journal of Nursing Administration Reader* (Wakefield, MA.: Contemporary Publishing, 1975).

38. D. W. Fisher and E. Thomas, "A 'Premium Day' Approach to Weekend Nurse Staffing," *Staffing: A Journal of Nursing Administration Reader* (Wakefield, MA.: Contemporary Publishing, 1975).

39. S. I. Imig, J. A. Powell, and K. Thorman, "Primary Nursing and Flexi-Staffing: Do They Mix?," *Nursing Management*, Aug. 1984, 39–42.

40. J. B. McGuire and J. R. Liro, "Flexible Work Schedules, Work Attitudes, and Perceptions of Productivity," *Public Personnel Management*, Spring 1986, 65–73.

41. Ibid.

42. American Hospital Association, op. cit.; B. Arnold and E. Mills, "Care-12: Implementation of Flexible Scheduling," *The Journal of Nursing Administration*, July-Aug. 1983, 9–14; A. Mech, M. E. Mills, and B. Arnold, "Wage and Hour Laws: Their Impact on 12-hour Scheduling," *The Journal of Nursing Administration*, March 1984, 24–25; M. L. Metcalf, op. cit.

43. B. Moores and A. Murphy, "Planning the Duty Rota; One, Computerized Duty Rotas," *Nursing Times*, July 4, 1984, 47–48; D. Canter, "Planning the Duty Rota; Two, Back to Basics," *Nursing Times*, July 4, 1984, 49–50.

44. R. L. Hanson, "Applying Management Information Systems to Staffing," *The Journal of Nursing Administration*, Oct. 1982, 5–9.

45. Ibid.

46. R. L. Hanson, "Staffing Statistics: Their Use and Usefulness," *The Journal of Nursing Administration*, November, 1982, 29–35.

47. D. S. Brown, "The Managerial Ethic and Productivity Improvement," *Public Productivity Review*, Sept. 1983, 223–250.

48. R. L. Hanson, "Staffing Statistics: Their Use and Usefulness," op. cit. The formulas are Hanson's; applications are the author's.

49. B. M. Artinian, F. D. O'Connor, and R. Brock, "Comparing Past and Present Nursing Productivity," *Nursing Management*, Oct. 1984, 50–53.

50. D. L. Davis, "Assessing and Improving Productivity in the Operating Room," *AORN Journal*, Oct. 1984, 630, 632, 634.

51. J. L. Smith, M. K. V. Mackey, and J. Markham, "Productivity Monitoring: A Recovery Room System for Economizing Operations," *Nursing Management*, May 1985, 34A–D, K–M.

52. C. B. Mailhot, "Setting OR's Course Toward Greater Productivity," *Nursing Management*, Oct. 1985, 42I, J, L, M, P.

53. S. A. W. Haas, "Sorting Out Nursing Productivity," *Nursing Management*, Apr. 1984, 37–40.

54. L. Curtin, "Reconciling Pay with Productivity," *Nursing Management*, Feb. 1984, 7–8.

55. L. L. Curtin and C. L. Zurlage, "Nursing Productivity: From Data to Definition," *Nursing Management*, June 1986, 32–34, 38–41.

56. J. A. Reitz, "Toward a Comprehensive Nursing Intensity Index: Part I, Development," *Nursing Management*, Aug. 1985, 21–24, 26, 28–30; Ibid., "Part II, Testing," *Nursing Management*, Sept. 1985, 31–32, 34, 36–40, 42.

57. J. Rabin, "Professionalism and Productivity," *Public Productivity Review*, Sept. 1983, 217–222.

58. L. Curtin, op. cit.

59. M. F. Fralic, "The Modern Professional and Productivity," Annual Meeting of the Alabama Society for Nursing Service Administrators, Huntsville, AL, 1982; R. L. Hanson, "Man-

aging Human Resources," *The Journal of Nursing Administration*, Dec. 1982, 17–23; G. H. Kaye and J. Utenner, "Productivity: Managing for the Long Term," *Nursing Management*, Sept. 1985, 12–13, 15; S. A. W. Haas, op. cit.; D. L. Davis, op. cit.; D. S. Brown, op. cit.

References

Bermas, N. F. and A. Van Slyck, "Patient Classification Systems and the Nursing Department," *Hospitals,* Nov. 16, 1984, 99–100.

Evans, C. L. S., "A Practical Staffing Calculator," *Nursing Management,* Apr. 1984, 68–69.

Gebhardt, A. N., "Computers and Staff Allocation Made Easy," *Nursing Times*, Sept. 1, 1982, 1471–1473.

Henney, C. R. and R. N. Bosworth, "A Computer-Based System for the Automatic Production of Nursing Workload Data," *Nursing Times,* July 10, 1980, 1212–1217.

Jecmen, C. and N. M. Stuerke, "Computerization Helps Solve Staff Scheduling Problems," *Nursing Economics,* Nov.–Dec. 1983, 209–211.

Jelinek, R. C., T. K. Zinn, and J. R. Brya, "Tell the Computer How Sick the Patients Are and It Will Tell How Many Nurses They Need," *Modern Hospital,* Dec. 1973, 81–85.

Price, E., *Simplified Staffing: The Price Plan for Effective Scheduling,* Hospital Workshops, 30951 Cole Grade Road, Valley Center, CA 92082.

Stuerke, N., "Computers *Can* Advance Nursing Practice." *Nursing Management,* July 1984, 27–28.

Appendix 4–1. University of South Alabama Medical Center Hospital Staffing-Assignment Principles for Nursing Personnel

Staffing standards and patterns are used to ensure optimum care for the patients over a 24-hour period. Each patient care unit has a position Kardex listing their approved budget positions. Vacancies are filled according to this list.

Staffing will be done to support the mission, philosophy and objectives of the USA Medical Center and the Department of Nursing.

Nursing Service personnel will be employed and assigned according to experience, education, demonstrated performance and choice.

Charge Nurses of shifts will be designated by the head nurse of the unit on a daily basis when there is no permanent charge nurse.

Nursing personnel may at any time request reassignment by communication with their head nurse. Their requests will be referred to the Director of Nursing and to the Assistant Administrator for Nursing as appropriate. They will be expected to give reasons and their requests will be honored on the basis of staffing needs and vacancies. Their names will be maintained on a waiting list on a priority preference basis. Transfers may be negotiated between departments. A transferring employee is expected to work out a 2-week transfer notice in assigned unit.

Avoid personnel doubling back on duty with only an 8-hour break. When possible avoid more than two (2) different shifts in a week's period, except in emergencies. The fewer the shift changes the better. Personnel should be consulted before scheduling of doubling back, i.e. 3–11 –

7–3. After schedule has been posted no change should be made without consulting employee and agreement by both parties.

Variable staffing patterns may be used, such as 4-10 hour days or combinations that adapt to the workload, wage and hour laws and staff satisfaction.

Personnel who are planning extensive dental work or elective surgery must coordinate with their supervisor.

Vacations may be taken any time during the year. Request should be submitted for approval to Head Nurse/Supervisor with consideration for patients' needs being met. Each unit will maintain a vacation request procedure. Vacation requests will be honored in the order in which they have been submitted. A master vacation plan should be made for each calendar year. The Head Nurse is responsible for planning vacation coverage. Vacations may be scheduled over holidays, however, no employee will be scheduled for vacation during more than one of the three holidays, Thanksgiving, Christmas and New Years.

Nursing personnel will not be penalized for taking earned vacation, with prior approval. Normal scheduled weekends off are not altered when vacation is scheduled. With 5–10 days vacation a person is entitled to one extra weekend off.

Staffing Policy

1. Personnel may elect to work a permanent evening shift, a permanent night shift or rotating shifts.

(continued)

APPENDIX 4–1.   University of South Alabama Medical Center Hospital Staffing-Assignment Principles for Nursing Personnel (*continued*)

2. Personnel should be scheduled to have at least every third weekend off. Weekends for 11–7 personnel will be scheduled for Friday and Saturday if desired.
3. Part-time personnel will work according to the needs of the unit.
4. Head Nurses/Supervisors will work weekends according to unit and department needs. Head Nurses/Supervisors are expected to adjust their schedules to meet the needs of the patients and staff on a 24-hour basis.

Scheduling

Personnel time schedules are to be made out for each unit for a six week period.

The time will be finalized and posted two (2) weeks prior to expiration of current time schedule and a copy forwarded to Nursing Service Administration.

Weekly staffing sheets are to be turned in each Friday for the following week. (Week Monday through Sunday).

Changes in Schedules

Any change in time requested after posting must be coordinated with Head Nurse and the corrections made in the office of the Assistant Administrator for Nursing. Changes may be made by telephone. Schedule changes will be negotiated between Head Nurse/Supervisor and Employee.

Special Requests

Special requests for time will be submitted to the Head Nurse/Supervisor at least two (2) weeks in advance of posting time schedules. These requests will be honored as long as patient care needs can be met.

Supervisors will make every effort to arrange duty schedules so personnel who desire to do so, may attend off-duty classes. However, overtime cannot be incurred when scheduling for non-mandatory classes.

Working Overtime

All scheduled "overtime work" will be approved by the Head Nurse, Supervisor or Director in advance. Directors, Supervisors and Head Nurses are ultimately responsible to monitor overtime records, indicate area worked and cost center to which overtime is to be charged. RN's cannot leave the unit without adequate RN relief for the on-coming shift.

Calling in Absent

"Calling in" close to one's scheduled "work shift" for unexpected crisis, illness, may happen on occasion; however, adequate coverage of patient care needs is a serious obligation and personnel are expected to meet it.

All call-in's for absences or for lateness must be called directly to the Director of Staffing or page the Directors on weekends, 3–11 or 11–7 through the operator. Nursing Service secretary will notify the Head Nurse or Director. "Call-in's" must be received by Nursing Service at least two (2) hours before the scheduled shift. Employees not adhering to the two hour rule will be considered absent and will not receive sick pay for that day. Exceptions to this rule will be made for emergencies as determined by the department director. The reasons for absence should be indicated. Personnel are expected to estimate the length of time of the anticipated absence, and/or the expected return to work date, at the time of the initial call. If this is not possible, it is expected that the individual will call Nursing Service daily until a return to work date is known. For abuse of call-ins, see absenteeism and tardiness policy.

No Shows

"No shows" i.e., not showing up for a scheduled work day are not acceptable at any time. An attempt will be made by the Head Nurse or Supervi-

APPENDIX 4–1. University of South Alabama Medical Center Hospital Staffing-Assignment Principles for Nursing Personnel (*continued*)

sor or Director to contact the scheduled employee at the time of the "no show", in order to clarify the reasons, etc. Not "showing up" for work is subject to disciplinary action. Three (3) incidents and/or shifts of "no shows" will result in immediate dismissal.

Late to Work

All individuals are expected to be "on duty" and "ready" for report at the beginning of a shift, i.e. 7:00 A.M., 3:00 P.M. and 11:00 P.M. Employees who abuse tardiness should be referred to the absenteeism and tardiness policy. Difficulty in getting to work on time should be discussed with the Head Nurse or Supervisor.

"Reports" will begin on time and all scheduled personnel are expected to be present to listen to report and clarify assignments.

Mandatory Meetings

Mandatory meetings of nursing personnel are an extreme inconvenience to off-duty personnel. Personnel will be paid for hours worked. However, off-duty personnel will only be *mandated* to return for a meeting when patient care is threatened. They will be approved by the Assistant Administrator prior to *announcement*.

Reassignments

The staffing is adjusted to meet the patient's needs as effectively as possible. At times it is necessary to reassign nursing personnel on a daily basis or temporary basis to meet these needs. Whenever possible nursing personnel will be reassigned to a unit within their nursing department, or to a like unit.

Nursing personnel will be floated based on their qualifications. Refusal to be reassigned will result in disciplinary action. Negotiations between personnel is encouraged.

Personnel scheduled for overtime have the option of going home rather than being reassigned.

SOURCE: Courtesy of the University of South Alabama Medical Center, Mobile, Alabama.

Personnel Management

5

INTRODUCTION

While professional nurses' dissatisfactions with work have been widely studied, the long-term solutions have been largely ignored. The theory of nursing management includes knowledge of personnel management related to recruiting, selecting, credentialing, assigning, retaining, promoting, and terminating personnel. Recruiting has two facets, recruiting students into generic programs and recruiting RNs into service institutions and agencies. Credentialing includes licensing.

RECRUITING

Recruiting Students into Nursing

In 1980 the American Hospital Association published a package of materials entitled *Hospital Nurse Recruitment and Retention: A Source Book for Executive Management.* It indicated there was a national shortage of 100,000 hospital nurses.[1] A flood of publicity on this shortage led to the formation of a National Commission on Nursing. This commission listed "eight top themes in descending order of importance" that it considered important in reducing the shortage:

1. Nursing leadership should be an integral part of senior management.
2. Nursing should be more involved in all levels of hospital decision making.
3. Nurses' management skills should be developed and nurses should be provided more opportunities for leadership positions.
4. The organizational structure should be decentralized to facilitate communication and decision making.
5. Collaborative or joint practice programs between nurses and physicians should be established.

6. The nursing educational system needs to be rationalized in terms of entry-level requirements and clinical practice preparation.
7. Career development programs for clinical practice and administrative positions should continue to be developed and implemented.
8. Nursing leaders should be appointed to key committees to foster and strengthen nurses' interaction with medical staff and the board.[2]

By 1983 the entire situation had changed, with every major nursing journal focusing on a glut of nurses in many (but not all) areas. The reasons were many, varied, and speculative. All related to economics. People were out of work so they did not have health insurance because of its cost and could not be hospitalized short of an emergency. Hospitals were downsizing as occupancy decreased due to DRGs. A few hospitals reported layoffs of nurses. Nursing publications attempted to analyze the job market and supply the information to nurses.[3]

The 1990s are projected to produce acute shortages of nurses. Enrollments in schools of nursing are declining and the decline is expected to continue. Enrollment in professional (R.N.) nursing programs dropped 13 percent, falling from a high of 251,000 in 1983 to 218,000 in 1985.[4] The 1987 enrollment was 193,712.[5] Only the part-time R.N. to B.S. student nursing education programs expanded enrollments.[6]

A decline in the number of high school graduates is projected through the mid-1990s. There will be a concurrent increasing growth in persons over 65 years of age, the prime consumers of nursing services.[7] Thus the pool from which nursing students are recruited is diminishing at a time when the need is increasing.

There will be other significant changes evinced by the 3.6 million 4-year-olds of 1986, who will be college age in the year 2000. According to Hodgkinson:

1. Twenty-four percent of them live below the poverty line. In 1984 there were 3,330,000 poor people over 65—but 11,455,000 poor children under 15.
2. Far fewer of these 4-year-olds are white, suburban, and middle class than was the case in 1970. (The group with the most rapid decline in birthrate is the group that normally makes up most of the college freshman class.)
3. One third of these 4-year-olds are nonwhite, though minority can no longer be considered synonymous with poor. (Blacks, Hispanics, and Asians have large and growing middle classes and span almost as broad a socioeconomic range as whites. Colleges have yet to realize that they can recruit Blacks from a ghetto, or they can go to Shaker Heights for top-notch minority students. Indeed, today many inner-city high schools are turning out excellent students.)
4. Eighteen percent of today's 4-year-olds were born out of wedlock.
5. More than 45 percent of them will be raised by a single parent before they reach 18 years of age.
6. A higher percentage of 4-year-olds today than in the past do not speak English. Instead they speak a dazzling array of languages, from Urdu to Mandarin. Spanish is only one of these many languages.
7. An increasing number of today's 4-year-olds have physical and emotional handicaps.
8. Fifty-four percent of them have mothers who work outside the home and the children receive some form of day care. By the time they reach school age, two thirds of their mothers will be working, most of them full-time.
9. Twenty percent of the girls among today's 4-year-olds will become pregnant during their teen years.[8]

From the forgoing the implications for nursing can be forecast as:

1. Schools of nursing should now begin to profile their students. Who are they? Where do they come from? What is the level of their achievement in high school?

2. More adults should be recruited into nursing. These include both men and women seeking second careers and women entering a career field after their children have entered school.

3. Collaboration with the public schools should be proactive. Nursing educators, managers, researchers, and clinical practitioners should all be part of the recruitment effort. They can advise school counselors on program requirements and support the schools to meet those requirements. Such mea-

sures might include financial assistance to keep students in school through graduation and to enable them to enter nursing programs after graduation.

4. Support should be given to potential dropouts in the Black, Hispanic, and Asian middle classes to maintain them in high school through graduation and into college. They will require assistance with language, culture, and finances. Schools of nursing will need to make accommodations to the language and customs of these persons. They are the workers who will be paying Social Security for future retirees.

5. Nurses should give proactive support to public education at all levels. The future of nursing and of our society depends upon it, since public school students are potential future nurses and productive workers of all occupations.

6. With over 14 million immigrants to socialize into U.S. culture, nurses should become a part of the process. Again, they must be proactive in encouraging nursing students to take elective courses in liberal arts that reflect the cultures of these people.

7. Higher education needs to be adapted to assimilate minorities. This is a challenge to nursing educators. They will have to begin the process at the high-school level, by helping to initiate programs of study that prepare minorities to enter nursing programs, including supplemental and remedial programs. Such efforts will need to be continued throughout the nursing education program.

8. Support for high-school graduates of lower ability is essential.

9. Attention to retention of college and university students can be of value to schools of nursing. A plan should be made to recruit the 50 percent of 4-year degree candidates who do not graduate. These include students in twenty-four major academic fields of study, with 1300 different academic majors in undergraduate education.

10. Employers will need to prepare minorities, including nurses, for promotion, thus giving them visibility to potential nursing students. The military services have been doing a better job of this than have civilian institutions. One has only to look at the hierarchy of educational institutions, health-care institutions, and business and industrial institutions to discern this.

11. While community colleges handle most students who are considered outside the mainstream because of their ethnicity, age, and cultural background, this can be changed. Baccalaureate faculty can initiate the changes. Otherwise the number of nursing graduates with associate degrees will increase while baccalaureate nursing graduates will continue to decrease. Both need to be maintained at levels to meet market demand.

12. Emphasis on research and publication should not diminish. However, faculty should be promoted and tenured based on teaching excellence as well.

13. Teaching methodology should focus upon wide use of teaching strategies and less on lectures that keep students passive.[9]

Of late, women have been entering other career fields such as medicine, law, business administration, dentistry, and so forth. These have traditionally been predominantly male fields with higher pay and better working conditions than nursing. Although there are numerous studies of dissatisfaction among nurses, there appears to be only sporadic progress in improving pay and working conditions.

Nurse managers are the people who can change the work environment. They are not the only ones, however. An all-R.N. staff may not be financially possible. The professional nurse practitioner is highly qualified in terms of knowledge and skills and the decision maker in the nursing process. She or he can direct the work of others without continual direct involvement in such procedures as bathing, making beds, feeding patients, and other procedures. The professional nurse should do the history, make the nursing diagnosis, direct the application of nursing care, evaluate the results, and make changes as needed. The debate on entry into practice needs to be redesigned and realigned to focus upon the professional nurse as the clinical decision maker.

Every major agency or institution employing nurses should have a committee that focuses on the recruitment of students into nursing education pro-

FIGURE 5–1. Strategies to Recruit Students into Nursing Education Programs

1. Form committee to make plan.
   1.1 Include clinical nurses.
   1.2 Set goals.
   1.3 Make management plan for each goal.
2. Obtain recruitment materials from organizations.
   2.1 National League for Nursing (NLN).
   2.2 American Nurses' Association (ANA).
   2.3 American Organization of Nurse Executives (AONE)/American Hospital Association (AHA).
   2.4 National Student Nurses' Association (NSNA).
   2.5 American Association of Colleges of Nursing (AACN).
   2.6 State.
   2.7 Local.
3. Prepare additional recruitment materials.
   3.1 News stories for newspapers, TV, and radio.
   3.2 Posters for schools.
   3.3 Speakers bureau.
   3.4 Model speeches.
   3.5 Tours.
4. Coordinate with other nurse education programs and prospective employers of nurses.
   4.1 Associate degree programs.
   4.2 Diploma programs.
   4.3 BSN programs.
   4.4 Hospitals.
   4.5 Public health.
   4.6 Staffing agencies.
   4.7 Ambulatory care facilities.
   4.8 Nursing homes.
   4.9 LPN programs.
   4.10 Other.
5. Prepare and offer consultation programs for junior and senior high schools.
   5.1 Administrators.
   5.2 Teachers.
   5.3 Guidance counselors.
   5.4 Students.
6. Coordinate activities of recruiters in schools of nursing.
   6.1 Sources of information by telephone and mail.
7. Involve community agencies in recruitment efforts.
   7.1 Professional organizations.
   7.2 Social organizations.
   7.3 Service organizations.
   7.4 Others.
8. Evaluation of results accomplished.
   8.1 Number and locations of programs presented.
   8.2 Number of students counselled.
   8.3 Number of follow-ups.
   8.4 Number of applicants to local or other programs.
   8.5 Home rooms visited.
   8.6 Career days held by high schools.
   8.7 Career days held by schools of nursing.
   8.8 Career days held by employers.
   8.9 Inquiries to source persons by telephone or letter.
9. Work/study programs.
   9.1 High school with employer.
   9.2 High schools with schools of nursing.
   9.3 Schools of nursing with employers.
   9.4 Cooperative education.

grams. Small organizations can form recruitment consortiums. Clinical nurses should be well represented. They will provide ideas that will give an authentic and positive image of professional nursing practice. The focus should be realistic but positive for men and women, for minorities, and for a cross-section of high school students.

A survey of nearly 1,000 hospitals was done by the American Organization of Nurse Executives and the American Hospital Association in December 1986. Participation in high school and college career days was found to be a major recruitment strategy. Most activities were aimed at recruiting student nurses into jobs. A few efforts were directed to junior high school or high school students or guidance personnel.[10]

Figure 5–1 lists activities to pursue in recruiting students into nursing education programs.

The business of recruiting students into nursing will require long-term strategies for all educators and providers. Recruitment will be more effective if the consumers are activated. The profession tends to lose sight of this source of support. Professional nurses can work through community organizations to involve the community in changing the image of nursing and in the recruitment effort.

State nurses' associations are gearing up to address the nursing shortage. Their efforts should lead to results rather than pronouncements such as resolutions passed at conventions or meetings catalogued in publications.

Efforts should be made to provide education at times convenient to students, most of whom have to work. Little has been done to provide evening and weekend courses for basic or generic students. This could be a major area of breakthrough in recruitment, particularly for older adults. There are no reasons for the lack of evening and weekend courses, including Sundays, except the will and efforts of faculty and clinical facility personnel.

Nurses can do more to obtain financing for student education. Many service organizations would provide scholarships if asked. Minority students should be targeted and marketed, then supported once they are recruited.

Recruiting Nurses into Employment

Employers of registered nurses are competing for available personnel. How do they capture their attention? The channels include newspaper ads, journal ads, professional placement agencies, placement bureaus at universities, and special publications. Professional nurses seeking jobs have personal contacts and obtain information at job fairs, career days, professional meetings, and conventions. The business of recruiting clinical nurses into jobs should be managed with planning, organization, direction, and a method of evaluating its effectiveness.

Clinical nurses, the foundation of nursing care of patients, are the sector of nurses in shortest supply. There are few vacancies for top nurse executives. First line and middle managers are frequently promoted from within—many without management preparation, although this is changing with increased emphasis on the development of graduate programs in nursing management. Colleges and universities with baccalaureate programs are fast upgrading their faculty, requiring doctorates rather than master's degrees. Jobs are developing for nursing researchers.

Jobs for nursing managers, educators, and researchers have specific requirements for specialization, education, and experience. Many are filled through search committee procedures that attempt to fit the applicant to the organization. In times of critical shortages, clinical nurses are frequently hired without attempts to achieve such a fit.

The Recruiter.   Many large organizations employ a nursing recruiter. This can be a professional nurse or a personnel recruitment specialist. Both should work from a management plan that includes input from clinical nurses working within the organization.

The objective of the recruiter is to induce qualified professional nurses to apply for jobs. First, information about the organization's job openings must be made known to the target population. This is done through advertisements in Sunday newspapers and in issues of nursing journals. The ads should be broad enough to give potential applicants knowledge of particular positions, salaries and fringe benefits, and the organizational climate. Results of studies of factors that attract nurses can be used as a basis for developing job advertisements.

In 1983 an American Academy of Nursing study depicted both nurse administrators and staff nurses as agreeing on what factors attracted nurses to come to hospitals and stay there. Among those factors are "adequate and competent colleagues, flexibility in scheduling, educational programs that allow for professional growth, and recognition as individuals."[11]

During 1985–86 Kramer and Schmalenberg resurveyed 16 of these magnet hospitals, comparing them with the best-run corporate communities as described by Peters and Waterman in their book *In Search of Excellence.* Many similarities were found. Magnet hospitals "are infused with values of quality care, nurse autonomy, informal, nonrigid verbal communication, innovation, bringing out the best in each individual, value of education, respect and caring for the individual, and striving for excellence."[12]

A well-thought-out ad can be a successful method of recruiting nurses. It is better to spend money to develop an effective advertisement than to save money on an ineffective one. A successful ad will win attention when it focuses upon its subject: the professional nurse. It will obtain results when it piques the interest of the professional nurse in seeking more information. Figure 5–2 lists criteria for developing an effective newspaper or nursing journal advertisement.

Professional nurses should be recruited just like other professionals. If clinical nursing is important, clinical nurses will be recruited, as are nursing managers, educators, and researchers.

In recruiting nurses from outside the commu-

FIGURE 5–2. Criteria for Developing an Effective Nurse Recruitment Advertisement

1. Target the population.
2. Catch the reader's attention.
3. Consider a picture that depicts a professional nurse in action, the kind of action nurses say they want.
4. List several factors that attract nurses.[13] These may include:
    4.1 Opportunity for self-fulfillment.
    4.2 Knowledge of helping others.
    4.3 Intellectual stimulation.
    4.4 Educational opportunity.
    4.5 Fellowship with colleagues.
    4.6 Adequate income.
    4.7 Opportunity for innovation.
    4.8 Opportunity to choose hours.
    4.9 Opportunity for advancement.
    4.10 Chance to be a leader.
    4.11 Adequate support systems.
    4.12 Child-care facilities.
    4.13 Good fringe benefits.
5. Involve clinical nurses in developing the advertisement.
6. Test the advertisement on the clinical nurse staff.
7. Run the ad in the Sunday newspapers. Select those that are read by the target population.
8. Run the ad in nursing journals read by the target population.
9. Provide for telephone and mail replies from applicants.
    9.1 Free telephone numbers.
    9.2 Specific address.
10. Provide for effective telephone and mail replies to be returned from organization.
    10.1 The phone should be answered with positive responses that elicit interviews. It can be effective if clinical nurses make immediate follow-up calls to prospective applicants.
    10.2 Effective packages of recruitment materials mailed to prospective applicants. (Depict and detail factors listed under number 4.)
11. Arrange for interview, including a visit to the organization.
    11.1 Contact person and sponsor.
    11.2 Travel reimbursement.
    11.3 Paid room and meals.
    11.4 Interviews with person doing hiring, personnel specialists including recruiter, and clinical nurses.
12. Follow-up offer in writing.

nity area, efforts should be directed toward those factors that would attract professional nurses to move. These might include geographic attractions: winter sports such as skiing or sunshine and beaches. They also might include cultural attractions such as museums, symphony orchestras, and operas, or educational opportunities.

Recruitment Tips. There are a number of important tips for recruiting clinical nurses.[14]

Tip 1. Keep potential applicants and employees from making mistakes when using private employment agencies.

1. Make sure they understand everything they sign and that they agree only to terms they want, including jobs.
2. Be sure they know the employer is paying the finder's fee.

Tip 2. When possible, prospective employees should talk with nurses who are already employed and are involved in the recruitment process. Questions that might come up include:

1. How does management differentiate among associate degree, diploma, and B.S.N. graduates?
2. Can a good salary be negotiated?
3. Are opportunities provided for continuing education, advancement, increased responsibility, and input into the work environment?
4. Is there dissatisfaction among nursing staff?
5. Is the management/administrative staff competent/capable? What are its qualities/abilities?
6. Will nurses be required to rotate shifts or work overtime?
7. Is there a rapid turnover rate in nursing personnel?

Tip 3. Do not use blind ads (those that give a coded box number). They tend to keep applicants from making personal contacts about jobs as names, telephone numbers, and addresses are omitted. Blind ads also slow down the process of making productive contacts.

Tip 4. Use imaginative recruitment procedures. Explore unusual ways of making contacts, for example through the employed nursing staff, service organizations, community organizations, and professional organizations.

It is important to take every opportunity to catch potential applicants' attention. Form a speakers bureau so nurses can give recruitment presentations before special groups: during meetings of service and professional organizations, on talk shows, at community activities such as Friends of the Art Museum or Friends of the Opera, to political action committees, or even at the local political party organization. Brainstorming can generate a list of imaginative procedures for recruiting nurses. It may even be feasible to form a new organization of Friends of Professional Nurses and involving them with the problem of recruiting students into nursing and nurses into the organization.[14]

Marketing.   Connelly and Strauser recommend a marketing approach to recruitment of nurses. Such an approach would focus upon the nurse as the consumer of employment. They advocate a marketing audit of the nursing environment. Figure 5–3 presents a scheme for a marketing survey for recruiting and retaining nurses that includes some of Connelly and Strauser's ideas. The marketing plan would be a management plan that would determine what needs to be done to sell employment to prospective professional nurses. Data would be analyzed, objectives set, a plan made and promoted, and the objectives evaluated.[15]

Management plans for the long range can include increasing the productivity of local schools. For example, if there is a local associate degree program, can they increase production? What support do they need? Will other organizations cooperate to provide that support—including financial support for a marketing survey, recruitment program, and financial assistance for students?

SELECTING, CREDENTIALING, AND ASSIGNING

Selecting, credentialing, and assigning are all part of the hiring process. While assigning has sometimes been done after the professional nurse was hired, it is unsatisfactory to applicants. They want to know where they will work before reporting for duty and orientation. They do not want surprises and will begin work dissatisfied if they occur.

Selecting

Selecting includes interviewing, the employer's offer, acceptance by the applicant, and signing of a contract or written offer. While the chief nurse executive may interview and hire prospective applicants in small organizations, it is best for the nurse manager who will directly supervise the employee to do the hiring. This person may elect to elicit the input of clinical nurses with whom the prospective employee will be working.

The Interview

The nurse recruiter or a personnel specialist will have completed a personnel folder containing a completed application form, a résumé or curriculum vitae, references, and any documents required by policy or law such as a current valid license to practice nursing, transcripts, and loyalty oaths.

The interviewer should be prepared for the interview by reading the information in the applicant's folder. Figure 5–4 is a check list to use in reviewing this folder.

Notes should be made of questions to be asked about the information contained in the folder.

Adequate time should be set aside for the interview; it should take place in a private office where there will be no interruptions. An interview guide will be helpful in conducting an interview satisfactory to both nurse manager and the applicant; see Figure 5–5.

Thompson defines an interview as "an equal-level, face-to-face discussion between a job seeker and a person with full authority to fill the position under discussion."[16] Nurses are the job seekers and want a face-to-face discussion with the person with hiring authority. They may be looking at several jobs, having narrowed the field down to those that specifically fit their career goals. They know how to make contacts and now want interviews to create opportunities to sell themselves.

The Introduction.   The interviewer should prepare for the interview beforehand. The interviewer should seat the candidate for comfort so that she or he will not be blinded by sunlight and will be facing the interviewer. The interviewer should come out from behind the desk, shake hands with the candidate, call the candidate by name, and introduce

FIGURE 5–3. Marketing Survey for Recruiting and Retaining Nurses

1. Number of vacant positions.
   1.1 Current.
   1.2 Previous month.
   1.3 Percent increase (or decrease).
2. Turnover rate by month and unit.
3. Exit interview results.
   3.1 Number of interviews performed.
   3.2 Number of negative comments (list separately).
       (See Appendix 5–1)
4. New hire demographics.
   4.1 Diploma graduates.
   4.2 A.D. graduates.
   4.3 B.S.N. graduates.
   4.4 Average years of experience.
   4.5 Males.
   4.6 Females.
   4.7 Average age.
   4.8 Percent married.
   4.9 Percent with children of preschool age.
   4.10 Percent with children in school.
   4.11 Percent minorities (nonwhites).
   4.12 Other.
5. Demographics of employed nurses. Profile the "stayers" and target similar recruits.
   5.1 Diploma graduates.
   5.2 A.D. graduates.
   5.3 B.S.N. graduates.
   5.4 Average years of experience.
   5.5 Males.
   5.6 Females.
   5.7 Average age.
   5.8 Percent married.
   5.9 Percent with children of preschool age.
   5.10 Percent with children in school.
   5.11 Percent minorities (nonwhites).
   5.12 Other.
6. Attitude survey (list results separately).
7. Audit of meeting minutes.
   7.1 Staff nurses.
   7.2 Others (list results separately).
8. Audit of performance evaluations (list results separately).
9. Salary levels (list by clinical level and by longevity).
10. Overtime.
    10.1 Hours by month and unit.
    10.2 Costs.
11. Absenteeism data.
    11.1 Daily average.
    11.2 Cause.
    11.3 Monthly total.
12. Agency nurse use.
    12.1 Hours by month and unit.
    12.2 Costs.
13. Monthly budget variances by unit.
14. Utilization of productivity reports (refer to chapter 4).
15. Acuity data by category and unit.
16. Average daily census by day of week and by month (report trends).
17. Recruiting expenses.
18. Major competitors for prospective hires.
19. Analysis of professional literature on recruitment and availability.
20. Analysis of patient relations reports.
21. Reputation and visibility of the organization and division.
    21.1 Community.
    21.2 Employees.
22. Factors causing nurses to avoid organization.
23. Factors that would attract nurses to organization.
24. Sources for recruiting nurses.

himself or herself. This is done to set the candidate at ease.

Questions. Questions should be prepared beforehand. These may include those listed in Figure 5–5. Those specifically desired by the interviewer should be added. The answers should not be written down, as this is distracting and time-consuming. Written notes should be made immediately following the interview.

All candidates for nurse jobs should be treated as professionals. They should not be asked illegal questions, such as those listed in Figure 5–6.

Since information about age and date of birth may be necessary for insurance or other fringe benefits, it can be obtained after the candidate is hired.

FIGURE 5–4. Check List for Reviewing Job Applicant's Folder

1. The application form.
   1.1 Is completed as directed.
   1.2 Written statements are positive.
   1.3 Contains no blanks.
   1.4 Contains no gaps in employment data.
2. References.
   2.1 Are listed.
   2.2 Have been checked.
   2.3 Are satisfactory.
   2.4 Need further checking.
3. R.N. licensure.
   3.1 Has been verified.
   3.2 Is current and valid.
4. Transcripts.
   4.1 Have been verified.
   4.2 Are available.
5. Forms signed.
6. Curriculum vitae or résumé.
   6.1 Is up to date.
   6.2 Lists career goals.
7. Job description provided including blank performance contract.
   7.1 Clinical level established as _____.
   7.2 Years of longevity established as _____.
8. Salary information available.
   8.1 Base salary $_____.
   8.2 Clinical level pay $_____.
   8.3 Longevity pay $_____.
   8.4 Differential $_____.
   8.5 Total pay $_____.
   8.6 Pay days made known.

The candidate will also have questions they want answered. If complete information cannot be given, notes should be made and the information communicated to the candidate as quickly as possible. Figure 5–7 contains possible questions that candidates may ask, which the interviewer should be prepared to answer.

While it is best not to speculate on the course of a job interview, it is possible to prepare for it in such a way that success will be most likely. An interview is simply a conversation between a potential employer and a candidate. There may be a need to modify the interview if the employer wants to hire the nurse to meet the organization's needs, while the candidate seeks to achieve personal goals.

The objective of both interviewer and candidate at the outset of an interview is to create a positive, amicable relationship to the end that a job offer emerges. The interview is the most important factor in gaining this end, as it allows expression of per-

FIGURE 5–5. Interview Guide

Candidate:
Date and time of interview:

1. Arrange seating.
2. Make introductions and establish rapport.
3. Ask prepared questions.
   3.1 Tell me about yourself.
   3.2 What is your present job?
   3.3 What are your three most outstanding accomplishments?
   3.4 What is the extent of your formal education?
   3.5 What three things are most important to you in your job?
   3.6 What is your strongest qualification for this job?
   3.7 What other jobs have you held in this or a similar field?
   3.8 What were your responsibilities?
   3.9 Do you mind irregular working hours? Explain.
   3.10 Would you be willing to relocate? To travel?
   3.11 What minimum salary are you willing to accept?
   3.12 Are you more comfortable working alone or with other people?
4. Answer candidate's questions.
5. Note the following: candidate was—
   5.1 On time.
   5.2 Well dressed.
   5.3 Well mannered.
   5.4 Positive about self.
6. Maintain eye contact.
7. Note candidate's personal values.
8. Close the interview
   8.1 Make an offer.
   8.2 Obtain acceptance.
   8.3 Set timetable for making offer or receiving response to offer.

SOURCE: Adapted with permission from R. C. Swansburg and P. W. Swansburg, *Strategic Career Planning and Development for Nurses* (Rockville, MD: Aspen, 1984), 194.

sonal ideas, abilities, and accomplishments. It adds individual personality to the résumé and completed application forms. To prepare for a job interview, nurse managers should:

1. Decide beforehand that they want the interview to end in a job offer.

2. Know the specific qualifications needed by the organization. Relating them to the candidate will help to identify a fit between candidate and job.

FIGURE 5–6. Questions That Are Illegal

Employment interviewers are forbidden by law to ask the following questions:

1. Your age.
2. Your date of birth.
3. The length of time you have resided at your present address.
4. Your previous address.
5. Your religion; the church you attend; your spiritual advisor.
6. Your father's surname.
7. Your maiden name (of women).
8. Your marital status.
9. Your residence mates.
10. The number and ages of your children; who will care for them while you work.
11. How you will get to work, unless a car is a job requirement.
12. Residence of spouse or parent.
13. Whether you own or rent your residence.
15. The name of your bank; information on outstanding loans.
16. Whether wages were ever garnished.
17. Whether you ever declared bankruptcy.
18. Whether you were ever arrested.
19. Whether you were convicted, unless this is a job-related necessity (for example, in jobs requiring a security clearance.)
20. Hobbies, off-duty interests, clubs.
21. Foreign languages you can read, write, or speak, unless this is a job requirement.

SOURCE: Adapted from conference with Paula Andrews, personnel director, University of South Alabama Medical Center, Mobile, Alabama, 1983. Used with permission.

FIGURE 5–7. Possible Questions from Candidates

1. How much job security does this job have?
2. What previous experience does this type of job require?
3. What is the future of this type of job?
4. What is the growth potential for this particular job?
5. Where will the most significant growth for this type of job in the health care industry occur?
6. What is the starting salary for this job?
7. How do pay raises occur?
8. How does one find out when other job openings occur?
9. What are the fringe benefits of this job?
10. What are the requirements for working shifts and weekends?
11. What are the opportunities for continuing education?
12. What are the opportunities for promotion?
13. What child care facilities are available?
14. What are the staffing and scheduling policies?

SOURCE: Adapted with permission from R. C. Swansburg and P. W. Swansburg, *Strategic Career Planning and Development for Nurses* (Rockville, MD: Aspen, 1984), 196.

3. Decide to win the candidate's liking. The interviewer should come across as someone who respects and values employees. It is important for both interviewer and interviewee to be self-confident and exude the personal chemistry of optimism, good manners, charm, and enthusiasm.

4. Gain a feeling for the values of the candidate. Are they compatible with the organization's mission, philosophy, and objectives?

5. Have expectations about the dress, mannerisms, and other personal characteristics of the candidate. These will be objective. A serious candidate will dress conservatively for the interview. If the applicant is a man, he should be clean-shaven, have his hair neatly cut and styled, be dressed in a business suit and tie, and have appropriate footwear. Beards can be acceptable but should be neatly trimmed. If the applicant is a woman, she should have a neat hairdo, be dressed in a business suit or dress, wear hosiery, and have appropriate jewelry. Makeup should be in good taste and perfume or cologne should be discreet. One's appearance should be

FIGURE 5–8. What Happens During Interviews

The Hiring Executive	The Candidate
1. Gives information about job and institution.	1. Gives information about self.
2. Assesses the competencies the candidate possesses in relation to the job opening.	2. Assesses the opportunity for developing and using competencies on the job.
3. Evaluates the candidate's personal characteristics in relation to the staff members with whom candidate will work (fit to staff).	3. Assesses ability to relate to the employees with whom candidate will work.
4. Assesses candidate's potential to move organization toward its goals.	4. Assesses potential for achieving personal career goals.
5. Assesses candidate's enthusiasm and state of health.	5. Assesses the institution's climate and the morale of the employees.
6. Forms impressions about candidate—behavior, appearance, ability to communicate, confidence, intelligence, personality.	6. Assesses opportunities for promotion and success.
7. Assesses candidate's ability to do the job.	7. Assesses own ability to do the job.
8. Determines facts about candidate.	8. Determines facts about the organization and working conditions.

SOURCE: Adapted with permission from R. C. Swansburg and P. W. Swansburg, *Strategic Career Planning and Development for Nurses* (Rockville, MD: Aspen, 1984), 204.

interpreted as indicating a person of good judgment and impeccable taste. Candidates thus tell the employer they regard the interview as important. The interviewer should dress, act, look, and smell like the right person to be the candidate's manager.

The candidate should come across as a thoroughly pleasant, cooperative, and competent person, one who can deal with the most difficult people problems tactfully, objectively, and successfully. The candidate should be neither blustery and flamboyant nor mouselike and servile. The interviewer should meet the same personal standards. Candidates who disagree with the interviewer's tastes or values should not be rejected unless the disagreement is unacceptable to the good of the organization. They should not be intimidated.

Interviewers should remember that they are human beings responding to human beings during the interviewing process. Both applicant and interviewer are being assessed. The interviewer is deciding from appearance, conversation, and behavior how the nurse will fit the job. The candidate is deciding from similar observation how he or she will like working for the interviewer.[17]

Figure 5–8 summarizes what happens in interviews.

Eye Contact. It is important to maintain good eye contact during an interview. This can be done by following some simple rules. The interviewer should look at the candidate's eyes for about eight seconds, then look away, shifting the body position at the same time. That avoids being thought of as having "shifty" eyes. Also, if eye contact makes one uncomfortable, the focus can be shifted to the bridge of the candidate's nose at a spot between the eyes.

Eye contact tells the candidate the interviewer has trust and credibility.[18]

Establishment of Rapport. At the outset of the interview rapport can be established with the candidate by talking about common friends or interests. This should be kept short, as time is important to both sides.[19]

Closing the Interview. Closing the interview means that the session is at a point where the interviewer is ready to make an offer or has all of the information needed. If ready to make an offer, the interviewer should have all of the information related to salary, fringe benefits, assignment, and scheduling ready for presentation and discussion. If the candidate wants it in writing or wants time to consider the offer, a definite time schedule should be set:

"I want you for this position. I will mail you an offer tomorrow."

"I want you for this position. Please call me and give me your decision between 8 and 10 A.M. Monday."

If the interviewer needs more information, the candidate should be advised of this and told they will be contacted as soon as the information is available. If there are several candidates for a specific job, all will have to be interviewed and a selection made. Candidates should be notified of their rejection. If possible, reasons for rejection should be stated, but in terms that will not destroy candidate's self-esteem or cause legal problems for the employer.

The Assessment Center Process

An assessment center is a method for screening candidates for jobs. It is specific to the job for which candidates are applying. Sullivan, Decker, and Hailstone describe an assessment center for the selection of a head nurse. It has seventeen job dimensions, each being subdivided into abilities that are observed and scored. These job dimensions are:

1. Clinical nursing background.
2. Development of subordinates.
3. Delegation/management control.
4. Planning and organization.
5. Perception/sensitivity.
6. Problem analysis.
7. Problem-solving/decision-making.
8. Risk-taking.
9. Initiation/leadership.
10. Communication skills.
11. Listening skills.
12. Energy level.
13. Stress tolerance.
14. Resilience.
15. Assertiveness.
16. Behavioral flexibility.
17. Accessibility.[20]

Other characteristics of this process include:

1. Exercises are developed to measure dimensions.

2. Assessors are selected and trained to rate the candidates. They are from the supervisor group.

3. The head nurse assessment center (HNAC) is conducted for one day. Each candidate is assessed by at least two persons.

4. Reliability and validity of assessment centers is high. The HNAC has many benefits including selection of competent head nurses, objectivity, broader applicant support, consistency, qualified applicants, head nurse development, and improved management reputation.

5. Among the drawbacks of the HNAC are that it is stressful, time-consuming, and tiring for assessors; it favors outsiders; and it intimidates.

6. The process is job-specific.

7. It is equitable to minorities and women.

8. Supervisors who will work with applicants select them.

9. It has self-development value for participants.

10. It is expensive, stressful, may favor conformity, and may create self-fulfilling prophecies.

11. It diminishes the risk of hiring or promoting inappropriate candidates.

12. It is used in over 2000 companies.[21]

A similar process was described by Battle et al. They developed a master interview tool that categorized content as follows: documented in records, clinical, administration, research, education, and significant factors. Points were assigned according to weight of rating category with various positions. A pool of interview questions was developed to determine the applicant's ability to communicate, organize thoughts, solve problems, and relate to others; to assess the applicant's knowledge, philosophy, experience, and personality traits; and to reveal the applicant's frame of reference, level of expectation, attitudes, feelings, and management style.

Interview panels consist of three members, the chair being appointed by the chief nurse executive. The tool is claimed to have fairly high inter-rater reliability, to decrease interview time, and to assist in selecting the most qualified applicant.[22]

The Search Committee

Almost every job opportunity of any import today will result in the appointment of a search committee. The objective is to obtain input into the hiring process from the people who will be affected by the appointment. Such committees are most widely used in higher education, where faculty members expect (and even demand) to share in the governance of the institution, particularly in the area of hiring.

Composition of Committees. The members of a search committee will come primarily from the specialty area of the position to be filled. In an organization that is filling a key position in obstetrical nursing, for example, the majority of members of the committee will come from the obstetrical nursing staff. This convention, however, is fast disappearing. Since physicians tend not to put nurses on search committees, nurses tend not to put physicians on them. Hospital administrators tend to compromise by including both.

Search committees may include nurses from administration, practice, and the associated school of nursing. Depending upon the nature of the appointment, the committee may also include students, alumni, and persons from related fields or specialties. Some members are appointed by the administration and some by the staff or faculty. The committee will be kept to a manageable size, usually five to ten persons. A chair will be appointed by administration or elected by the search committee and will serve as the liaison between the two.

Responsibilities. A search committee's responsibilities should be clearly laid out by the administration or by the committee itself. Most committees will recruit, screen, interview, and recommend applicants. Final decisions about appointments are generally made by administrators. Members of search committees are committed to their tasks and re-

sponsibilities. They may be committing themselves to five or six months of arduous work.

The search committee usually agrees at the outset to consider all information about applicants as confidential. It will not discuss any individual candidate outside the committee, except in general terms of progress reports to staff or faculty.

Interviewing. Most search committees follow a standard procedure for interviewing. They consider the interview to be a two-way evaluation between them and the interviewee. One or more members are assigned to take each candidate to meals. Introductory questions on unthreatening topics are constructed to set the applicants at ease. Specific questions are predetermined by the committee but are interspersed with spontaneous ones during the interviews. Some committees will supply candidates with their predetermined questions.

If the interview is to be tape-recorded, the applicant's permission will be asked. Once all interviews are completed, the results are tabulated, with each candidate being evaluated separately and then compared with others. Committees do make every attempt at objective comparisons. They weight factors to show differences such as "Candidate 1 has a Ph.D., while Candidate 2 has no doctoral degree but is a tenured professor on a graduate faculty." The candidates then are recommended to the hiring executive on the basis of the three best qualified or a rating system of one to three or more.

Figure 5–9 contains a list of possible search committee interview questions.

Many people wonder what goes on behind the search committee walls. Reres regards the interview as a courtship.[23] Hiller and others describe it as a meeting to determine whether the candidate fits the organization. Information is gained for making decisions and opportunity is provided for candidates to "sell themselves."[24] The atmosphere is expected to be businesslike, not like a social function although the latter are included and are important.

Control is defined as a major factor in the interview process. Candidate nurses will want to have some control of the interview process as will the committee members. Both want it to be positive in achieving its purpose.

Candidates can exert positive control by responding concisely and maintaining a focus on the essential goals of the session. They are communicating well when they give answers in a brief, factual,

FIGURE 5–9. Preparatory Questions for Search Committee

1. What style of management do you follow?
2. What are your personal weaknesses and strengths?
3. What are your perceptions of the role the person in this job will perform?
4. What are your ideas of what the relationships should be between nurses and physicians?
5. What job in nursing would you like most to have?
6. What do you view as the role of nursing in this organization?
7. What do you view as the role of nursing in the community?
8. What do you think of collective bargaining?
9. How would you go about determining that your department operates efficiently and effectively?
10. Why should I (we) hire you?
11. How would you go about meeting the goals of the organization?
12. How would your family adapt to this area?
13. What other jobs are you interviewing for?
14. What are your career goals?

SOURCE: Used with permission from R. C. Swansburg and P. W. Swansburg, *Strategic Career Planning and Development for Nurses* (Rockville, MD: Aspen, 1984), 187.

and friendly manner and their tone of voice is soft and clear, their posture relaxed, and their hands still. They can mainly direct their conversation to one committee member whose background is similar, without excluding any committee members entirely.

Candidates should not bluff answers. They ought to be prepared to ask thoughtful questions at the end of the interview, as this will exert positive control. They can influence the outcome of the interview in part by their appearance, poise, and ability to conduct a fruitful dialogue with search committee members. Candidates have been known to lose through overkill by being too loquacious, bragging too much, being too aggressive, or overestimating their abilities.

Candidates will impress the committee if they have reviewed and can discuss the package of materials sent to them, particularly because questions sometimes will relate to problems in the hiring organization.

Search committees do not interview candidates who are not fully qualified or top contenders. Committees might schedule groups of candidates on the same day. Whether one stands a better chance early or late in the day is anyone's guess. Candidates may face a longer and harder questioning early in the day.

Candidates should be kept from meeting their competitors. Some search committees divide the process so that different candidates are undergoing different interviews or activities simultaneously. Individuals could spend one period with the committee, one period with the faculty, staff, or community groups, and one period touring.

The applicants are meeting people with whom they may work. They are assessing the opportunities and challenges of the job. Nurses are being closely observed for their philosophy and style. They are gathering facts to make the decision as to whether they can work with these people and whether they have the knowledge, skills, and know-how to be productive.

Community representatives on search committees look at abilities related to working with other agencies and local groups, at fiscal management skills, and at reactions to potential conflicts between agencies. Staff members look at clinical and administrative style, decision-making ability, professional goals, and flexibility in working with diverse groups. Top management is interested in fiscal issues, personnel management, and group relationships. These interests help pave the way for nurses to make their decisions about jobs.

Stressful Committee Interviews. Meetings with search committees are potentially stressful. The candidate cannot predict exactly what questions will be asked. Candidates can be stressed by the content of the questions, the manner in which they are asked, or the facial expressions of committee members. Applicants should prepare themselves mentally by taking themselves through the interview in advance. They ought to be confident and not be intimidated.

In addition to the questions cited earlier, they can expect others such as: Do you believe leaders are born or made? Why are you leaving your present job? Why haven't you published? Why haven't you done research? There may be other questions about their professional and personal lives, likes and dislikes about the present job, successes, and so on.

It can be worthwhile to have the committee members do some of the talking by asking them questions related to the topics they introduce in their questions. Nurses should try to discuss their background, accomplishments, and other qualifications during this process.

It is very important to stay away from controversial subjects such as religion, abortion, politics, and confidential matters, although questions about the first two will arise at certain religious institutions as basic doctrinal issues. Candidates are not there to identify problems or offer solutions.

Finally, applicants must be definitive in obtaining a commitment about the job. They should tell the search committee's chair that they need to give adequate notice to a present employer, ask for a definite date for expecting an answer, and be very firm about being interested in the job. A follow-up letter will indicate their seriousness about wanting the position, refreshing the members on the fact that the writer has the competencies to match the job requirements. This should be done while the facts of the interview are current and easily remembered.

Credentialing

Credentialing is the process by which selected professionals are granted privileges to practice within an organization. In health-care organizations this process has been largely confined to physicians. Limited privileges have been granted to psychologists, social workers, and selected categories of nurses such as nurse anesthetists, surgical nurses, and midwives. Generally these categories have been restricted by physican credentialing policies and fall in the category of allied professional staff.

Requirements of the Joint Commission on Accreditation of Healthcare Organizations (JCAHO) require that hospitals investigate, develop recommendations, reach conclusions, and be responsible for their actions in credentialing the medical staff. Licensing and certification provide data to consider in the process.

Components of Credentialing. As with physicians, the components of a credentialing system for nurses would be:

1. Appointment—Evaluation and selection for nursing staff membership.
2. Clinical privileges—Delineation of the specific nursing specialties that may be performed and the types of illness or patients that may be managed within the institution for each member of the nursing staff.
3. Periodic reappraisal—Continuing review and evaluation of each member of the nursing staff to assure that competence is maintained and is consistent with privileges.[25]

Criteria for Appointment. Criteria for appointments would include proof of licensure, education and training, specialty board certification, previous experience, and recommendations. Clinical privileges criteria would include proof of specialty training and of performance of nursing procedures or specialty care during training and previous appointments.

During the credentialing process the committee should look for "red flags" of high mobility, graduation from foreign schools, professional liability suits, and professional disciplinary actions. Each "red flag" is a reason for exercising extra care in reviewing the applicant.

While professional nurses have mostly been hired through personnel offices, nurse managers should give consideration to increasing the professional status of nursing through the credentialing process. See Appendix 5–2.

The American Nurses Association (ANA). A report of the Committee for the Study of Credentialing in Nursing was made in 1979. It included fourteen principles of credentialing related to:

1. Those credentialed.
2. Legitimate interests of involved occupation, institution, and general public.
3. Accountability.
4. A system of checks and balances.
5. Periodic assessments.
6. Objective standards and criteria and persons competent in their use.
7. Representation of the community of interests.
8. Professional identity and responsibility.
9. An effective system of role delineation.
10. An effective system of program identification.
11. Coordination of credentialing mechanisms.
12. Geographic mobility.

13. Definitions and terminology.
14. Communications and understanding.[26]

Credentialing in a hospital relates to appointing health professionals to the staff. Credentialing by professional organizations such as the ANA can be a qualification for such appointments.

Assigning

Assigning professional nurses to jobs is the third part of the hiring process, following selecting and credentialing. During the assignment period the new nurse is oriented to the job description and its use. While assignment to a specific position using the job description may not be possible during the selecting and credentialing processes, candidates should know the possible units to which they may be assigned.

If a candidate wants to work in the operating room, but there are no vacant positions, where can that person be assigned? Offer the candidate a choice of vacant positions. Make a verbal or written contract to transfer the individual to a vacated operating room position when one becomes available. If others are waiting, indicate the order in which they will be assigned to the operating room.

Do not give candidates surprise assignments when they arrive for orientation. Assignment policies should be fair, reasonable, and acceptable to candidates. They will then start work with a positive attitude. A principle to follow is to provide necessary orientation and training to nursing employees to ensure competency, job satisfaction and high productivity in the particular assignments they are accepting.

RETAINING

The retention of competent, professional nurses in jobs is a major problem of the U.S. health-care industry, particularly for hospitals. Most Americans change jobs about fifteen times by age 35, and nurses are no exception. Nurses change and achieve major career goals four or five times in their lifetime, including changing their specialty or the role they plan in the profession.[27] Many do both. Some even retire from two or more systems.

Career Dissatisfaction versus Job Dissatisfaction

There is a difference between career dissatisfaction and job dissatisfaction. A nurse may make a job change because of job dissatisfaction. If dissatisfied with several jobs a professional nurse looks at the work itself, the tasks involved, and the purposes to be served. If they are all distasteful a professional nurse may make a decision to leave the profession.

Turnover

The turnover rate among hospital nurses nationally appears to be between 20 and 70 percent annually. An organization should determine its turnover rate by unit and by organization. It should be done monthly to keep abreast of trends. Leavers should be profiled and defined: average age, marital status, type of program from which graduated, additional education, years of experience, specialty, sex, race, and any other characteristic that will give clues that could decrease turnover and increase retention of competent nurses. Nurse managers should also review the performance of the leavers as well as doing exit interviews.

The crude turnover rate depicts the volume of turnover. It is not a very selective index. An example is given in Figure 5–10. Other data that will give information about turnover and retention are the mean and median service of stayers. These data provide the average tenure of employees. Examples of these data are also illustrated in Figure 5–10, as are mean and median service of leavers, instability rate, wastage rate, and survival of leavers curve.[28]

The sum of the number of months of employment of each nurse as well as other data can be determined by having a good nursing management information system, which will accumulate the data on electronic spreadsheets.

Job Expectations and Satisfactions

The author contends that the high turnover rate in nursing is a result of job dissatisfactions; see Appendix 5–3.

In a survey of nurses' satisfactions and dissatisfactions with their jobs and careers, 6,277 surveys were mailed to nurses in a five-county area around

FIGURE 5–10. Turnover Data

1. Crude turnover rate = $\left[\dfrac{\text{Number (N) of Leavers}}{\left(\dfrac{\text{N at start} + \text{n at end}}{2}\right)}\right] \times 100$

Number (N) of Leavers = number of nurses who left during a year.

N at start = number of nurses employed at beginning of year.

n at end = number of nurses employed at end of year.

Example: (N) = 189
N = 543
n = 529

$\dfrac{189}{\left(\dfrac{543 + 529}{2}\right)} \times 100 = \dfrac{189}{536} \times 100 = 35.26 \text{ percent}$

2. Mean service of stayers = $\dfrac{\text{Sum of the number of months of employment of each nurse}}{\text{Number of nurses employed}}$

Example: $\dfrac{10{,}563 \text{ months}}{529 \text{ nurses}} = 19.97 \text{ months}$

3. Median service of stayers
Rank currently employed nurses by the number of months of employment from the shortest to the longest and choose middle ranking value.

Example:	Months	1–6	7–12	13–18	19–24	25–30	31–36	37–42	43–48	49–54	55–60+
	# of Employees	73	61	55	50	41	39	40	27	39	104
	Total	73	134	189	239	280	319	359	386	425	529

Total nurses (stayers) = 529

$\text{Median} = \dfrac{529}{2} = 265.5$

Median occurs at 25 to 30 months indicating that more than one-half of the nurses have been employed 30 months or less. The median is considered a better measure of central tendency than the mean.

4. Mean service of leavers = $\dfrac{\text{Sum of the number of months of employment of each nurse who left}}{\text{Number of nurses who left}}$

Example: $\dfrac{2417 \text{ months}}{189 \text{ nurses}} = 12.79 \text{ months}$

FIGURE 5–10.   Turnover Data (*continued*)

5. Median service of leavers

Months	1–6	7–12	13–18	19–24	25–30	31–36	37–42	43–48	49–54	55–60	61+
# of Employees	49	35	27	19	14	9	9	10	7	6	4
Total	49	84	111	130	144	153	162	172	179	185	189

Total nurses (leavers) = 189

$$\text{Median} = \frac{189}{2} = 94.5$$

The median occurs at 13 to 18 months. Since the mean and median of leavers are both low, short-term employees are leaving.

6. Instability rate = $\dfrac{\text{Number of leavers who had been employed at beginning of year}}{\text{Number of nurses employed at beginning of year}} \times 100$

Example: $\dfrac{151}{529} \times 100 = 28.54$ percent

Twenty-eight and fifty-four hundredths (28.54) percent of nurses employed at the beginning of the year left during the year.

7. Wastage rate = $\dfrac{\text{Number of newly hired nurses who leave during first year}}{\text{number of nurses newly hired during year}} \times 100$

Example: $\dfrac{40}{113} \times 100 = 35.4$ percent.

Thirty-five and four-tenths (35.4) percent of newly hired nurses, over one-third, leave before the end of one year.

8. Survival of leavers curve

X axis = number of months on job

Y axis = percent of eventual leavers remaining

Period of time = 1 year

Intervals = 6 months

(continued)

FIGURE 5–10.   Turnover Data (*continued*)

Example:

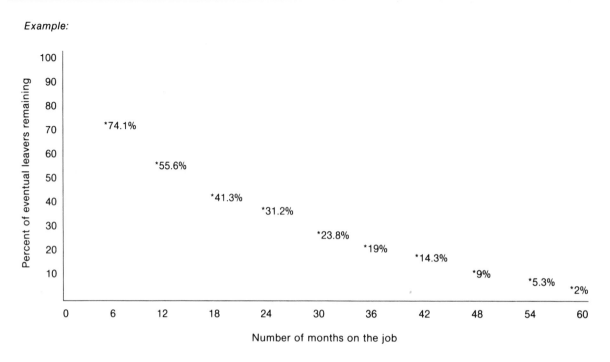

Use data from # 5.

100 percent of 189 leavers were employed at beginning of 12 months period.

$$\frac{189 - 49}{189} = \frac{140}{189} = 74.1 \text{ percent of leavers were employed}$$
6–12 months.

$$\frac{140 - 35}{189} = \frac{105}{189} = 55.6 \text{ percent of leavers were employed}$$
13–18 months.

Since the curve is a sharp drop + a gradual drop, the turnover concentration is among new employees. A straight line would have indicated turnover to be independent of length of service.

SOURCE: Adapted from M. L. Duxbury and G. D. Armstrong, "Calculating Nurse Turnover Indices," *The Journal of Nursing Administration*, March, 1982, 18–24.

Jacksonville, Florida. There were 1,921 responses with the following results:

1. One third of the total reported substantial dissatisfaction with their jobs.

2. One half of the total reported they felt negative about nursing.

3. One half of the total were strongly satisfied with their jobs and careers.

4. *Money was the number one concern and the preferred remedy.*

5. Recognition was the second most serious concern; hours and scheduling were third; too much

responsibility for the money fourth; and stress fifth.

6. The respondents included 337 nurses who were licensed but unemployed in nursing. They planned to return to nursing but considered the hours and pay inadequate.[29]

A study to determine why new graduates select particular settings and why many leave in a short time surveyed 279 nursing seniors in five schools in northern Alabama. The expectations of these new graduates were to:

1. Work full-time.
2. Work days or a desired shift (46 percent of single nurses and 36.5 percent of married nurses would work evenings).
3. Work in a medium-sized to large hospital.
4. Earn a good salary.
5. Have pleasant working conditions.
6. Gain self-fulfillment and a sense of achievement from giving adequate and complete care.
7. Have educational opportunities, intellectual stimulation, and opportunity to develop new skills.
8. Have satisfactory supervision by head nurses.
9. Be recognized and encouraged.
10. Have professional autonomy and power.
11. Work in community that offered higher education opportunities and a good place to raise a family. Factors considered important included good schools, a low crime rate, an economically stable region, a low tax structure, and low cost of living.

In addition, more baccalaureate degree nurses expected to become head nurses, supervisors, and public health nurses than did associate degree nurses. Many would *not* consider working in small hospitals (17.2 percent), Veterans Administration or federally owned hospitals (19.5 percent), investor-owned hospitals (18.8 percent), nursing homes (65.7 percent), doctor's office or clinic (18.6 percent), temporary or private-duty agency (41 percent), or psychiatric or mental health clinic (45.5 percent).[30]

Drucker argues that salaries are not the basic problem with nurse retention and recruitment, a position in opposition to most surveys. He states, "The basic problem is that nurses aren't allowed to do nursing. I've been saying that now for 20 years. The doctors still treat nurses as if they were scullery maids, and that's just not going to work any longer." Drucker believes that hospital administrators must change the attitudes of doctors. Also, focusing nurses' responsibilities on their professional role and increasing their salaries will alleviate the shortage.[31]

Career Planning

Nurse managers will recognize the results of nurse satisfaction surveys. They must now learn to manage professional nurses so they will achieve career and job satisfaction. The first step is to establish a career plan for them within the nursing organization.

To be successful in their careers professional nurses must have a sense of personal fulfillment and job meaningfulness, that they are growing as persons. Nurse managers can create these conditions by determining and correcting the causes of:

- Anxiety and uncertainty.
- Inability to meet personal and organizational goals.
- Lack of clarity about roles played.
- Contradictory demands.
- Dissatisfaction with human relations.
- Rebellion against rules, policies, and regulations.
- The inherent nature of the tasks of the job.
- Competition.
- Being overworked and underutilized.
- Lack of personal and professional growth.
- Dissatisfaction with the quality of associates.

A professional nurse is a reasonable person and reasonable people can accommodate to reality, accept themselves, be interested in others, learn from experience, and be self-actualized.[32]

Nurse managers should restructure nursing services to link assignments and responsibilities to education, experience, and competence. This should be a part of a career program that provides more promotions and pay for clinical nurses, pay for seniority, and increased participation. It should provide for continuing education to upgrade knowledge and skills. It will provide clinical rotation policies that prevent burnout and it should meet professional nurses' scheduling and salary preferences.[33]

When a career structure has been established it will provide for upward mobility for clinical nurses, nurse managers, nursing teachers, and nursing researchers. Professional nurses will decide to take advantage of career advancement opportunities. Jobs for those advancing will be identified and will require advanced knowledge and skills, particularly those related to decision making. Registered nurses who do not want promotion will be rewarded by longevity pay increases and (each year during entire employment) credit for doing their jobs well. Advancing nurses will be rewarded for longevity and for increased responsibility and accountability. Nurses will finally have careers.

The Career Counselor.   A career counselor should be part of the grand strategy for establishing a nursing career program.

Even though an organization might not have a career counselor, every nurse should have one in the person of a superior. This person helps nurses clarify their career goals and make a plan for achieving them. The plan includes work experiences related to off-duty time such as courses, workshops, community service, professional activities, and other activities specifically related to goals. It is a total plan that develops individuals professionally to meet their career aspirations. The career counselor facilitates that program. A supervisor who is not the career counselor can be asked to become one or to provide the opportunity to use someone else.

The counselor should provide nurses with service to advance their careers in nursing, not just within the organization. There should be at least one counselor who can help individuals assess their interests, skills, and values, who can assist with analyzing all of the options open, and who can aid in making the career plans that will lead to achieving career goals.

That individual could be a supervisor, a nurse administrator, a staff development person, or an expert in the chosen field of nursing. In the final analysis, only the individual nurse can develop and direct a career toward achievement of life goals. All others, be they employers, colleagues, peers, counselors, or whoever, can only form a support group.

Staff Development Career Counselor.   One group to contact about career opportunities is the staff development department. There is an awakening notion that staff development can advance the career op-

portunities of professional nurses. Since such counselors traditionally serve in an organizational relationship that provides a staff service to the line of the nursing hierarchy, their role should be identified by the nursing administration. Traditionally, the staff development department fulfills functions of initial orientation and conducts classes in cardiopulmonary resuscitation, intravenous therapy, and the like. On the other hand, some departments are moving toward a career development orientation by involving themselves in such functions as specialty orientation and training and implementing the process of planning, organizing, directing, and evaluating the development of nurses through levels of competency in clinical practice, management, teaching, and research.

Sovie labels the career development functions of the staff development department as professional identification, professional maturation, and professional mastery. These areas can be related to a career ladder program where competencies have been identified for the nurse practicing at several rungs of the ladder. The competencies are stated in the form of job descriptions and increase in complexity. Policies and procedures exist for the process of climbing the ladder. The process is facilitated by a program of staff development for career advancement.

Sovie's model could educate nurses to gain advanced specialized knowledge and skills. This could be achieved through individual plans, with staff development educators acting as counselors and teachers. Nurses could learn to provide the leadership in solving the health-care problems of patients and families. They could develop materials for patient and family education. They could learn to be a primary nurse in practicing the nursing process, not just within the nursing modality. They could learn to engage in professional nursing dialogue with colleagues. Their training could include the competencies of consulting, participation in quality assurance activities, processing and applying reports of research findings, participation in research, and involvement in committee functions. This learning could be part of a personal career plan.[34]

Efforts Outside the Department.   In many organizations these maturation skills are shaped outside the staff development department. Professional nurses who select the management ladder are entered into a continuous program of staff development. As clinical nurses develop the credentials of mastery in a specialty area, they are assigned to that level of practice. All could be encouraged to produce their own staff development functions, including putting on workshops in which they earn a fee. This income could be used to pay for their own continuing education outside their organization. They could provide nurse-to-nurse consultation in their areas of specialization. They could participate on unit, divisional, and organizational committees. Their mastery is rewarded by higher salaries and additional perquisites related to their professional mastery, because they produce more at the same cost.

Nurses in an organization that has a career development program should be moving up the ladder of their choice. The career development program should also provide an opportunity for moving laterally into clinical practice, management, teaching, or research. It should provide job satisfaction and a salary that increases with development and mastery.

If such a career development program does not exist in the organization, nurses can stimulate it. They can first learn about it through research and study, master the knowledge of career development, and then present it to their supervisors and get their support. If attempts to move up fail, nurses may want to move out, but they should not give up easily.[35]

Career Ladders. Clinical nursing offers the most diverse kinds of opportunities. Clinical nursing was largely a nonpromotable area until recent years. There were numerous interesting clinical areas that had been expanded with advanced technology but nurses seldom could be promoted within a clinical area. This is changing fast with the development of clinical career ladders.

A career ladder requires individual effort, assisted by organizational support and reward. It results in career satisfaction to the nurses who participate and in increased productivity for the employer if the program is appropriately conceived and implemented. There must be more results than title changes and increased wages or salaries. The advantages of clinical career ladders are discussed in more detail later.

Among the opportunities are clinical coordinator, clinical specialist, nurse practitioner, primary nurse, patient health educator, and flight nurse.

Advertisements in nursing journals and local newspapers identify these and many more opportunities. Those who want to stay in clinical nursing and advance in terms of all rewards, including money, fringe benefits, professional achievement, and satisfaction, will need to be prepared at the highest level of clinical practice. Clinical nurse specialists are professionals with education and experience at the level of the most complicated patient care problems and needs. Examples are clinical nurse specialists in ostomy care, oncology, or cardiovascular care. They should have the experience and education to perform in a consultative nurse capacity. Most clinical nurse specialists have education beyond the bachelor's level, with either an advanced degree or certificate. They also have had the advanced clinical experience to match the knowledge.

A clinical career ladder is a horizontal development system based on specific criteria used to develop, evaluate, and promote nurses desiring and intending to remain at the bedside. Clinical ladders apply to nurses who want to remain in the clinical setting, whereas career ladders are for those who leave the clinical realm in pursuit of a future in administration, teaching, or research.

A clinical career ladder should:

1. Improve the quality of patient care.
2. Motivate staff in terms of—
   2.1 Job proficiency/expertise (motivate the individual to reach his or her highest level of professional competence).
   2.2 Pursuit of education (an important factor in mobility).
   2.3 Development of career goals.
3. Provide methods of objective and measurable performance evaluation and reward clinical competence for the purpose of advancement.
4. Promote retention within clinical area and reduce turnover rate.

Nurses interested in working under this type of system should understand several points. First, most hospitals have a promotion system of some kind and a few are of the clinical ladder type. Unfortunately, many are based on a seniority system or include seniority as the primary criterion for advancement. Some administrators adopt a form of clinical ladder to help alleviate their recruitment and retention problems. Their ladder may look good on paper but the question is whether it provides the nurses with any significant advantages or is there for administrative advantages. If the system in which a nurse is working promotes to the next higher level according to a time frame without regard for educational status or job performance, then the individual is at a disadvantage. There is no competition or motivation to improve. Everyone will be promoted when they have served their time—both average and above-average nurses.

If the pay differential between levels is not significant, that also will impede motivation. Salary increases should be enough to further motivate the nurses to improve their skills (competence). Responsibility should increase with promotion. If nurses are still performing the same tasks with the same supervision and no additional responsibility after advancement, then they cannot be said to have really advanced professionally.

Performance criteria in any clinical ladder system should be clearly differentiated and specific at each level. The evaluation process must be measurable. Salary differentials must be significant enough to provide motivation. Any system should involve evaluation of educational and leadership criteria as well as skill performance.

Finally, the evaluation of each individual should include input from the direct supervisor and the individuals themselves. A board or panel of three or more nurses may be assembled to review all eligible personnel for promotion. The advantages of such a system are that it increases job satisfaction, improves clinical skills, offers positive motivation for acceptance of continued leadership and educational responsibility, and provides an opportunity for career advancement while remaining in clinical nursing. The disadvantage is that positions may not always be available at higher levels.

Management promotes the system to the end that productivity will be increased. Also, management must assure the maintenance of quality of nursing care.

The following is a basic clinical ladder model that can be added to or fleshed out by management:

A. Clinical/staff nurse I (beginner/novice)
  1. Experience and education
    a. current state licensure with less than one year of experience
  2. Description
    a. needs close supervision.

b. performs basic nursing skills/routine patient care.
    c. begins to develop patient assessment skills/communication skills
B. Clinical/staff nurse II (advanced beginner)
  1. Experience and education
    a. current state licensure with more than one year of experience
    b. B.S.N. with more than six months of experience
    c. M.S.N. without experience
  2. Description
    a. demonstrates adequate/acceptable performance
    b. can differentiate importance of situations and set priorities
    c. requires less supervision
    d. demonstrates interest in continuing education
C. Clinical/staff nurse III (competent)
  1. Experience and education
    a. current licensure with two or more years of experience
    b. B.S.N. with more than one year of experience
    c. M.S.N. with more than six months of experience
  2. Description
    a. demonstrates unsupervised competency using nursing process
    b. is able to plan and organize in terms of short-range and long-range goals
    c. demonstrates direction in actions
    d. accepts leadership responsibility readily
    e. demonstrates well-developed communication skills
    f. shares ideas and knowledge with peers
D. Clinical/staff nurse IV (proficient)
  1. Experience and education
    a. current licensure with three years of clinical experience and pursuit of B.S.N.
    b. B.S.N. with more than two years of experience (preferred)
    c. M.S.N. with more than one year of experience
  2. Description
    a. demonstrates specialized knowledge and skills
    b. continues professional education
    c. assumes leadership/supervisory responsibility

d. recognizes and adjusts to situations that vary from the norm
e. delegates responsibility appropriately; uses wide range of alternatives in solving problems
E. Clinical/staff nurse V (expert)
   1. Experience and education
      a. M.S.N. with more than two years of appropriate clinical experience
      b. B.S.N. required with more than three years of experience; pursuing M.S.N.
   2. Description
      a. demonstrates expertise in clinical practice
      b. assumes/delegates personnel and management responsibility.[36]

Since salary and benefits are the most concrete method of recognizing outstanding performance, valid career ladders should not be undermined with pay practices for certain kinds of nurses, such as those who work in critical care areas. Rewards should be given for levels of responsibility, preparation, experience, and performance. General duty nurses share equal responsibility and greater workload variety than specialty care nurses.

Spitzer and Bolton report the results of a staff survey of 956 career-employed R.N.s. There were 583 respondents who strongly agreed to the following statements on salary and salary equity:

1. When first hired, staff nurses should be paid according to years of experience, acute care experience, and education.
2. Salary adjustments (raises) should be based on clinical performance, additional acquired education, and additional clinical experience (regardless of specialty).[37]

When redesigning a wage and salary structure, nurse managers need to obtain input from the staff. Clinical ladders should be related to productivity. They can be based on a professional practice model and reward competence, knowledge and performance. Essential components are:

1. A number of levels of practice.
2. Differentiation among levels of practice.
3. A job description for performance evaluation.
4. Criteria for placement of new hires.
5. Methods of communication.
6. Identification of development needs of staff.

7. Criteria for measuring effectiveness of ladder relative to quality of care, staff satisfaction/retention, and cost-effectiveness.[38]

Master Plan

A master plan for career development should be developed for the nursing organization and for each unit of the organization. It should include objectives, policies on posting of jobs, development of résumés and curriculum vitae, and strategies for moving up in the organization. It should consider lateral transfers, specialty training and cross-training, and plans for nurses who become physically unable to perform the rigors of acute care nursing.

PROMOTING

Professional nurses have had to turn to management, education, or research for promotion. The development of professional nurse clinical ladders is making some headway, albeit not quickly enough. Many professional nurses want to stay in clinical nursing and will do so if they can be rewarded with promotions that increase their pay and standing within the organization.

One way for nurse managers to assure that all professional nurses have promotion opportunities is to develop a promotion system. The system will indicate all promotion categories within the organization; see Figure 5–11.

Nurse managers should develop specific promotion policies with input from all categories of professional nurses and the human resources department. These policies should include the following:

1. All vacant positions will be posted. This should be true even though change in pay and rank do not occur. Some nurses will want to change units, specialty, shifts, and so on.
2. All interested applicants should file applications for promotion in the human resource department.
3. Human resource department personnel should prepare promotion rosters that rank all candidates by education, experience, performance, and other objective criteria. The best-qualified candidate should be at the top of the list.

FIGURE 5–11. Promotion System

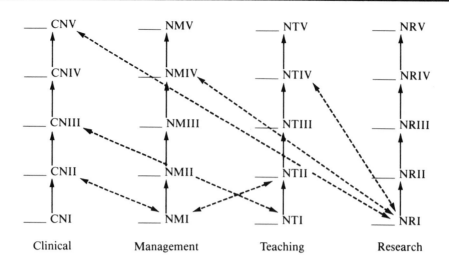

This is a model. Each level would require specific and increasing education, experience and performance accomplishments. The arrows indicate the levels at which nurses from each group could advance laterally. The clinical nurse II (CNII) could advance to nurse manager (NMI) or vice versa. The nurse teacher IV (NTIV) could advance to nurse researcher I (NRI) or vice versa. The blanks in front of each group would have the number of budgeted positions entered. For nurse researchers this could be one position but allow for appointment at, or promotion to higher levels.

4. Applicants should be interviewed and rated by the same set of criteria, a process described previously in this chapter under "Selecting."
5. The best-qualified candidates should be selected for promotion.
6. The results of the promotion process should be announced. Those not selected should be notified and counseled individually rather than learning they were passed over from hearing about or seeing the list of those promoted.
7. The promotion system must be fair and be perceived as fair by professional nurses.

Darling and McGrath write that nurses experience much trauma when moving upward from clinical to managerial nursing. They are unaware of the transition process involved in a promotion, including the fact that their social and professional ties with other clinical nurses are cut. They take on more responsibilities and burdens and soon feel isolated and alone. While they gain visibility and prestige, they get complaints instead of appreciation from their staff.[39]

To prevent promotion trauma, supervisors of promotees can plan a transition program. It will alert them to the changes in their relationships. It will help keep them from blaming their difficulties on personal failings. Such a program will include clear role descriptions and expectations, clear job descriptions, and classes to meet their management knowledge and skills needs. Staff development is as essential for nurses promoted to management as it is for those who stay in the clinical domain. They can know what to expect and how to deal with Darling and McGrath's five stages of promotion: uninformed optimism, informed pessimism, hopeful realism, informed optimism, and rewarding completion. A management development program will keep clinical nurses promoted to management positions from bailing out at the second stage.

TERMINATING

Employees cannot be terminated at will. They are protected by public policy set forth in the National

Labor Relations Act, the Civil Rights Act of 1964, the Discrimination in Employment Act, the Vocational Rehabilitation Act, and the Occupational Safety and Health Act. Also, laws protect "whistle blowers."

Employees should be terminated only after all efforts to retain them have been exhausted. The theory of management includes concepts and principles that, when learned and applied by nurse managers, will assist employees to be competent and productive. Punishment or disciplinary action should be a last resort and should be progressive, moving from a verbal conference, to a recorded conference, to suspension, to discharge. Such action should be covered by written policies and procedures.

Nurse managers including head nurses should have firing authority. They should consult with superior managers and human resource personnel when terminating staff to make sure the action will stand up in court. All policies must be legal and they must be consistently and correctly enforced. Any employee is entitled to a fair hearing and review. The process must allow for appropriate representatives at investigating interviews. When terminated, employees should be paid all benefits they have accrued.[40] Figure 5–12 is a checklist for assessing a legally supportable discharge.

The checklist applies to the discharge of both hourly and salaried employees of union employers. Your answer to any particular question is not necessarily determinative of the legality of the discharge. What is important is that your answers show that you have considered and determined from counsel either that you followed the correct procedure or that it was not applicable in your situation. You should recognize that if you are ignoring the areas covered by this checklist, the discharge may not be supportable in federal or state court, because all of the criteria included are taken from actual cases where an employer's decision was challenged and the court restricted the employer's right to terminate at will.[41]

SUMMARY

A major focus of a theory of nursing management is that personnel should be managed for productivity, for achieving the mission and objectives of the organization. This involves recruiting, selecting, credentialing, and assigning nurses, first into the educational program, then into the division or department of nursing.

Since nursing, a predominantly female occupation, must now compete with all other professions for students, nurse managers should create conditions of work that will be attractive. These include competitive salaries and fringe benefits, flexible schedules, and satisfying conditions of work such as autonomy and recognition.

The population from which all occupations will recruit will change greatly during the next decade. Their demographic makeup will shift, causing recruitment goals to change. Nurse managers should plan student recruitment at early stages of the secondary education process. The poor, minorities, children of single parents, and the physically and emotionally handicapped must be prepared now for careers, including careers in nursing. It is the promise of America.

Each nurse manager should work with other health-care system managers and secondary school teachers and counselors to prepare young men and women for careers in nursing. Once nurses are recruited, selected, credentialed, and assigned, nurse managers should develop strategies to retain them. For high-level positions, search committees are frequently used to recruit. The implication is that professional workers will have input into selecting those with whom they will work and who will give them leadership.

Nurse managers should consider a credentialing process for professional nurses similar to that used for physicians. It is essential that career planning be a major personnel management program within each nursing organization. Employees desire the opportunity to qualify for promotion in clinical, management, education, and research jobs. They are not motivated by dead-end jobs. There should be clear communication of job vacancies and they should be filled by the best-qualified individuals.

Personnel who do not meet acceptable standards of performance should be counseled, warned in writing, and suspended without pay. When all else fails they should be terminated.

NOTES

1. American Hospital Association, "Background on the National Nursing Shortage," *Hospital Nurse Recruitment and*

FIGURE 5–12.   Checklist for Assessing a Legally Supportable Discharge

1. Has the employee been terminated with one of the reasons being—
   a. race
   b. religion
   c. sex
   d. age (over 40)
   e. national origin
   f. children or childbirth
   g. pregnancy
   h. handicap?
2. Did the discharged employee engage in union activity immediately before the discharge or did he/she act in concert (and this is the reason for the discharge) with other employees to—
   a. organize collectively
   b. push for a raise or shorter hours or while protesting ask for changes in other working conditions
   c. support another employee in a protest?
3. Will the discharge violate any type of contract?
   a. Does your employee handbook provide for warnings before an employee may be discharged or that an employee may only be discharged for cause?
   b. Do you have written employee policies that promise "fair treatment"?
   c. Is there a written, signed employment contract?
4. Will the discharge violate any state tort laws?
   a. Have you committed the tort of "outrage"—has the company been abusive in discharging the employee, either through high-handed interrogation methods or through flagrant misrepresentations to the employee as to why he/she is being discharged?
   b. Has the company been negligent in not following its own policies resulting in the employee's discharge?
5. Are you terminating the employee for any of the following?
   a. refusing to do an illegal act
   b. filing a workers' compensation claim
   c. reporting violations of such federal statutes as the Equal Employment Opportunity Act, the Occupational Safety and Health Act, or the Employee Retirement Income Security Act?
   d. whistle blowing over the company's possible violations of state laws, such as anti-trust laws?
6. Is the employee being discharged for refusing to do a job he/she considers unsafe (giving rise to a possible OSHA violation)?
   a. Would doing the job *reasonably* place the employee in imminent danger?
   b. The key to safety cases is: if this job has been performed safely many times in the past, why is it now considered unsafe? Has there been an accident on this job within a short time period giving the employee reason to be concerned for his/her safety?
7. Did you provide a hearing (with company witnesses present) to provide the employee an opportunity to admit or deny the charges?
8. Was the employee given an oral or written warning to correct the conduct?
9. Have you let other employees pass undisciplined for the same conduct you are discharging this employee for?
10. Have you promised the employee, when hiring or subsequently, that the job was there for as long as they wanted? Alternatively, did you promise them an annual contract?
11. Under state and federal laws on disability, is the employee being discharged for a physical condition (e.g., high blood pressure, diabetes, or back conditions)? Have you tried to make reasonable accommodations for that employee to work at another, less strenuous job?
12. Do you have any evidence in writing covering the wrongful conduct (e.g., prior written reprimands) that the employee is being terminated for?
13. Did the employee give up another job or sell his/her home in another city to work for you, and were promises made to secure that employee by having him/her do so?
14. Are you calling the termination one for reduction-in-force (RIF), when in fact the reason you selected this particular employee was for unsatisfactory work performance?
15. If the employee, in the investigatory interview held by the company (if any) to determine the facts, requested a union representative or other employee to represent him/her at the interview, did the company deny the request and proceed with the interview in spite of the request?

SOURCE: Reprinted with permission from *Hospitals,* published by American Hospital Publishing, Inc. Copyright © 1984, Vol. 58, No. 14.

Retention: A Source Book for Executive Management (Chicago: American Hospital Association, Nov. 1980).

2. National Commission on Nursing, *Nursing in Transition: Models for Successful Organizational Change* (Chicago: American Hospital Association, Hospital Research and Educational Trust, and American Hospital Supply Corporation, 1982), 41–2.

3. "Helping Out in Hard Times," *RN* 46, March 1983, 7.

4. N. Miller, *American Organization of Nurse Executives Student Nurse Recruitment Resource Kit* (Chicago: American Hospital Association, 1987), 1.

5. American Nurses Association, "Fact Sheet: Supply and Demand of Registered Nurses," 1988.

6. N. Miller, op. cit.

7. Ibid.

8. H. L. Hodgkinson, "Reform? Higher Education? Don't Be Absurd!" *Phi Delta Kappan*, Dec. 1986, 271–274.

9. Ibid. for the statistics.

10. N. Miller, op. cit.

11. American Academy of Nursing Task Force on Nursing Practice in Hospitals, *Magnet Hospitals: Attraction and Retention of Professional Nurses* (Kansas City, MO: American Nurses Association, 1983), 99.

12. M. Kramer and C. Schmalenberg, "Magnet Hospitals: Part II Institutions of Excellence," *JONA*, February, 1988, 17.

13. These are given different priority by nurses in different surveys. L. Donovan, "What Nurses Want (And What They're Getting)," *RN*, Apr. 1980, 22–30; M. A. Wandelt, P. M. Pierce, and R. M. Widdowson, "Why Nurses Leave Nursing and What Can Be Done About It," *American Journal of Nursing*, Jan. 1981, 72–77.

14. R. C. Swansburg and P. W. Swansburg, *Strategic Career Planning and Development for Nurses* (Rockville, MD: Aspen, 1984), 160–162.

15. J. A. Connelly and K. S. Strauser, "Managing Recruitment and Retention Problems: An Application of the Marketing Process," *The Journal of Nursing Administration*, Oct. 1983, 17–22.

16. M. R. Thompson, *Why Should I Hire You?* (New York: Jove Publications, 1975), 94.

17. R. C. Swansburg and P. W. Swansburg, op. cit., 194–204.

18. Ibid., 205–206.

19. Ibid., 207.

20. E. J. Sullivan, P. J. Decker, and S. Hailstone, "Assessment Center Technology: Selecting Head Nurses," *The Journal of Nursing Administration*, May 1985, 14.

21. Ibid.

22. E. H. Battle, S. Bragg, J. Delaney, S. Gilbert, and D. Roesler, "Developing a Rating Interview Guide," *Journal of Nursing Administration*, 1985, 39–45.

23. M. E. Reres, "Academic Courtship Rites," *Nursing Outlook*, Oct. 1970, 42.

24. B. R. Hiller, R. S. Okolowski, R. M. O'Driscoll, M. Frain, and J. K. Brady, "The Search Interview," *Nursing Outlook*, March 1982, 182–185.

25. H. S. Rowland and B. L. Rowland, *Hospital Legal Forms, Checklists, and Guidelines* (Rockville, MD: Aspen, 1987), 17:1.

26. Committee for the Study of Credentialing in Nursing, "Credentialing in Nursing: A New Approach," *American Journal of Nursing*, Apr. 1979, 674–683.

27. P. E. Norris, *How to Find a Job* (Fairhope, AL: National Job Search Training Laboratories, 1982), 1.

28. M. L. Duxbury and G. D. Armstrong, "Calculating Nurse Turnover Indices," *The Journal of Nursing Administration*, Mar. 1982, 18–24.

29. E. Ginsberg, J. Patray, M. Ostow, and E. A. Brann, "Nurse Discontent: The Search for Realistic Solutions," *The Journal of Nursing Administration*, Nov. 1982, 7–11.

30. C. E. Burton and D. T. Burton, "Job Expectations of Senior Nursing Students," *The Journal of Nursing Administration*, Mar. 1982, 11–17.

31. "Peter F. Drucker and Karl D. Bays Discuss the Toughest Job—Running a Hospital, Part 2," *HMQ*, Summer, 1982, 2–5.

32. A. Levenstein, "Career Dissatisfaction," *Nursing Management*, Nov. 1985, 61–62.

33. E. Ginsberg, J. Patray, M. Ostow, and E. A. Brann, op. cit.

34. M. D. Sovie, "Fostering Professional Nursing Careers in Hospitals: The Role of Staff Development, Part 1," *The Journal of Nursing Administration*, Dec. 1982, 5–10.

35. R. C. Swansburg and P. W. Swansburg, op. cit., 136–138.

36. Ibid., 7–8.

37. R. B. Spitzer and L. B. Bolton, "Attitudes Toward Equitable Pay," *Nursing Management*, June 1984, 32, 36–38.

38. Ibid.

39. L. A. W. Darling and L. G. McGrath, "The Causes and Costs of Promotion Trauma," *The Journal of Nursing Administration*, Apr. 1983, 29–33.

40. B. C. Rutkowski and A. D. Rutkowski, "Employee Discharge: It Depends . . ," *Nursing Management*, Dec. 1984, 39–42.

41. L. L. Curtin, "Pinning the Tail on the NCRB," *Nursing Management*, December, 1984, 7–8.

REFERENCES

Colavecchio, R., "Direct Patient Care: A Viable Career Choice," *The Journal of Nursing Administration*, July-Aug. 1982, 17–22.

"Recruitment and Retention: A Positive Approach," *Nursing Management*, Apr. 1984, 15–17.

APPENDIX 5–1.   University of South Alabama Medical Center Employee Exit Interview

DATE _____

NAME _____ DATE HIRED _____ SHIFT _____

POSITION TITLE _____ DEPARTMENT _____

SUPERVISOR'S NAME _____ DATE SEPARATED _____

CHECK LIST:

_____ ID CARD RETURNED TO PERSONNEL DEPT.
_____ FINAL PAYROLL CHECK FORM COMPLETED
_____ STATE RETIREMENT REFUND FORM COMPLETED
_____ RECEIVED INSURANCE CONVERSION INFORMATION
_____ LOCKER KEYS RETURNED

I. REASON FOR SEPARATION (CHECK APPROPRIATE BOX)

VOLUNTARY RESIGNATION
_____ NEW POSITION
_____ RETIREMENT (VOLUNTARY)
_____ RELOCATION
_____ ILLNESS
_____ PREGNANCY
_____ JOB DISSATISFACTION
_____ RETURN TO SCHOOL
_____ OTHER (SPECIFY)
_____

INVOLUNTARY TERMINATION
_____ RETIREMENT (MANDATORY)
_____ REDUCTION OF STAFF
_____ OTHER (SPECIFY)
_____

II. INTERVIEW

A. SELECTION:

What kind of work have you been doing in our hospital? _____
_____
_____
_____

What kind of work did you do prior to joining our hospital? _____
_____
_____
_____

What type of work do you like best? _____
_____
_____

What type of work do you like least? _____
_____

APPENDIX 5–1. University of South Alabama Medical Center Employee Exit Interview (*continued*)

Why? _____

_____

B. ORIENTATION:

Who explained your job to you? _____

Describe your orientation: _____

_____

_____

Length of time? _____

What did your orientation lack? _____

_____

_____

Were inservice education programs sufficient for your needs? _____

If not, how could programs be improved? _____

_____

C. SUPERVISION:

How do you feel about your Supervisor? _____

_____

_____

_____

Did you take any complaints to your Supervisor? _____ Yes _____ No

If yes, how were they handled? _____

_____

_____

Have you had any problems with your Supervisor? _____ Yes _____ No

If yes, describe: _____

_____

_____

_____

What kind of working relationship did you have with the staff in your department? _____

_____

_____

Was there ample opportunity for communication with co-workers, your Supervisor and Department Head? _____

_____

(continued)

APPENDIX 5–1.   University of South Alabama Medical Center Employee Exit Interview (*continued*)

How could communication be improved? _____

_____

_____

Have you felt administrative support by Hospital Administrators? _____

_____

_____

D. FINANCIAL:

How do you feel about your pay? _____

_____

_____

How do you feel about your progress within this Hospital? _____

_____

_____

E. FOR NURSES:

Was your unit adequately staffed? _____

_____

How do you feel about being pulled to other units? _____

_____

How often were you pulled? _____

_____

F. SUMMARY:

What did you like best about your job? _____

_____

_____

What did you like least about your job? _____

_____

_____

What did you like best about our hospital? _____

_____

_____

What did you like least about our hospital? _____

_____

_____

APPENDIX 5–1. University of South Alabama Medical Center Employee Exit Interview (*continued*)

Why are you really leaving? _____

_____

_____

Would you be willing to stay with our hospital under a more satisfactory arrangement?

_____ Yes _____ No

What changes would be required? _____

Would you return to this hospital if the opportunity existed? _____

_____

G. COMPLETE FOR RESIGNATION:

New Employer: _____ Location: _____

Position: _____ Pay: _____

Hours: _____

III. INTERVIEWER COMMENTS: _____

_____

_____

SOURCE: Courtesy of the University of South Alabama Medical Center, Mobile, Alabama.

APPENDIX 5–2. Procedure for Appointment and Reappointment to the Professional Nursing Staff USAMC

ARTICLE 9

Section 1. Application for Appointment

1.1 All applications for appointment to the professional staff shall be in writing, shall be signed by the applicant, and shall be submitted on a form prescribed by the Executive Nursing Council. The application shall require detailed information concerning the applicant's professional qualifications, shall include the names of at least three like professionals who have had extensive experience in observing and working with the applicant and who can provide adequate references pertaining to the applicant's professional competence and ethical character, and shall include information as to whether the applicant's membership status and/or clinical privileges have ever been revoked, suspended, reduced or not renewed at any other hospital or institution, and as to whether his/her membership in local, state or national nursing societies, or license to practice any profession in any jurisdiction, has ever been suspended or terminated.

1.2 The applicant shall have the burden of producing adequate information for a proper evaluation of his/her competence, character, ethics, and other qualifications, and for resolving any doubts about such qualifications.

1.3 The completed application shall be submitted to the Assistant Administrator who will, after collecting the references and other materials deemed pertinent, transmit the application and all supporting materials to the Credentials Committee for evaluation.

1.4 By applying for appointment to the professional staff, each applicant thereby signifies their willing-

(continued)

APPENDIX 5–2.   Procedure for Appointment and Reappointment to the Professional Nursing Staff USAMC (*continued*)

ness to appear for interviews in regard to the application. Authorization is granted to the hospital for consultation with members of other hospital staffs with which the applicant has been associated and with others who may have information bearing on the applicant's competence, character and ethical qualifications. The applicant releases from any liability all representatives of the hospital and its professional staff for their acts performed in good faith and without malice in connection with evaluating the applicant's credentials. The applicant further releases from any liability all individuals and organizations who provide information to the hospital in good faith and without malice concerning the applicant's competence, ethics, privileges, including otherwise privileged or confidential information.

1.5 The application form shall include a statement that the applicant has received, read and agrees to be bound to the terms and the by-laws of the Division of Nursing at the University of South Alabama Medical Center.

Section 2. Appointment Process

2.1 Within ninety days after receipt of the completed application for membership, the Nursing Credentials Committee shall make a written report of its investigation to the Executive Nursing Council. Prior to making this report the Credentials Committee shall examine the evidence of the character, professional competence, qualifications and ethical standing of the applicant. Every department or section in which the applicant seeks clinical privileges shall provide the Credentials Committee with specific, written recommendations for delineating the applicant's clinical privileges. These recommendations shall be made a part of the report. Together with its report, the Credentials Committee shall transmit to the Executive Nursing Council the completed application and a recommendation that the applicant be either provisionally appointed to the professional staff or rejected.

2.2 At its next regular meeting after receipt of the application and the report and recommendation of the Credentials Committee, the Nursing Executive Council shall determine whether the applicant be provisionally appointed to the professional staff, or be rejected. All recommendations for appointment must specifically recommend the clinical privileges to be granted. These may be qualified by probationary conditions relating to such.

2.3 When the recommendation of the executive committee is favorable to the applicant, the Assistant Administrator shall promptly respond to applicant.

2.4 When the recommendation of the Executive Nursing Council is adverse to the applicant either in respect to appointment or clinical privileges, the Assistant Administrator shall promptly so notify the applicant by certified mail, return receipt requested.

Section 3. Reappointment Process

3.1 At least sixty days prior to the last scheduled meeting of the Credentialling Committee in the calendar year, each individual department or section shall review all pertinent information available on each member scheduled for periodic appraisal and transmit its recommendations in writing to the Executive Nursing Council.

3.2 Reappointment policies must include the periodic appraisal of the professional activities of each member of the professional staff and all other members with clinical privileges in the hospital. Such periodic appraisal should include consideration of physical and mental capabilities. A written record of all matters considered in each member's periodic reappointment appraisal must be made a part of the permanent files of the Division of Nursing at USAMC.

3.3 At least thirty days prior to the last scheduled meeting of the calendar year, the Executive Nursing Council shall make written recommendations to the Assistant Administrator, concerning the reappointment, non-reappointment and/or clinical privileges of each member.

ARTICLE 10: Clinical Privileges

Section 1. Clinical Privileges Restricted

1.1 Every member practicing at this hospital by virtue of professional nursing staff membership or otherwise, shall, in connection with such practice, be entitled to exercise only the granted privileges.

1.2 Privileges granted L.P.N.'s shall be based on their training, experience and demonstrated competence and judgment. The scope and extent of procedures that each LPN may perform shall be specifically delineated and granted in the same manner as all other LPN's within the USAMC. Procedures performed by LPN's shall be under the overall supervision of the Registered Nurse. A

APPENDIX 5–2. Procedure for Appointment and Reappointment to the Professional Nursing Staff USAMC (*continued*)

physician member of the professional staff shall be responsible for the care of any medical problem that may be presented at the time of admission or that may arise during hospitalization.

Section 2. Temporary Privileges

2.1 Upon receipt of an application for professional staff membership from an appropriately licensed practitioner, the Assistant Administrator, upon the basis of information then available and with written concurrence of the chairman of the Executive Nursing Council, shall grant temporary clinical privileges to the applicant.

2.2 Temporary clinical privileges may be granted by the Assistant Administrator for the care of a specific patient to a practitioner who is not an applicant for membership in the same manner and upon the same conditions as set forth in subparagraph (1) of this Section 2, provided that there shall first be obtained such practitioner's signed acknowledgment that she has received and read copies of the professional staff's by-laws, rules and regulations and that she agreed to be bound by the terms thereof in all matters relating to her temporary clinical privileges.

2.3 Specific requirements of supervision and reporting may be imposed by the departmental director concerned on any practitioner granted temporary privileges. Temporary privileges shall be immediately terminated by the Assistant Administrator upon notice of any failure by the practitioner to comply with such special conditions.

2.4 The Assistant Administrator may at any time, upon recommendation of the chairman of either the Executive Nursing Council or the department concerned, terminate a practitioner's temporary privileges. The appropriate departmental chairman or, in his/her absence, the Chairman of the Executive Nursing Council, shall assign a member of the professional staff to assume responsibility for the care of such terminated practitioner's patient(s) until they are discharged from the hospital. The wishes of the patient(s) shall be considered where feasible in selection of such substitute practitioner.

Section 3. Emergency Privileges

3.1 In the case of emergency, any R.N. or L.P.N. member of the professional staff, to the degree permitted by her license and regardless of service or staff or lack of it, shall be permitted and assisted to do everything possible to save the life of a patient, using every facility of the hospital necessary, including the calling for any consultation necessary or desirable. When an emergency situation no longer exists, such R.N. or L.P.N. must request the privileges necessary to continue to treat the patient. In the event such privileges are denied or she does not desire to request privileges, the patient shall be assigned to an appropriate member of the professional staff. For the purpose of this section an "emergency" is defined as a condition in which serious permanent harm would result to a patient or in which the life of a patient is in immediate danger and any delay in administering treatment would add to the danger.

ARTICLE 11: Amendments These By-Laws may be amended by action of the Assistant Administrator upon recommendation of the Executive Nursing Council and Nursing Council, or in keeping with the By-Laws and policies of the University of South Alabama Medical Center.

By: _____
　　　　　　　 Assistant Administrator

Date: _____

Reviewed by: _____

Reviewed by: _____

Approved: _____
　　　　　　　　　 Administrator

Date: _____

Reviewed by: _____

Reviewed by: _____

The author is indebted to Ms. Theo Hawkins, Director of Medical Nursing, the University of South Alabama Medical Center, Mobile, Alabama, for developing this proposal. It was not implemented.

SOURCE: Courtesy of the University of South Alabama Medical Center, Mobile, Alabama.

APPENDIX 5–3.   Response to Identified Factors Causing Job Dissatisfaction

The following are lists of problem factors related to nurses' job dissatisfaction and activities that can be initiated to remedy them. They form the basis for a strategic plan.

1. Problem Factors: Inadequate salaries and fringe benefits

   Remedial Activities:

   a. Establish higher base pay and eliminate gimmicks designed to simply elicit applications and hires.

   b. Establish pay steps based on education, experience, responsibilities (job descriptions), and productivity goals. Use career ladders that include clinical promotions. Include charge nurse responsibility pay.

   c. Extend longevity pay increases to eliminate compaction.

   d. Establish worthwhile pay differentials for shifts, weekends and holidays.

   e. Identify cost of fringe benefits and offer choices: market basket.

   f. Provide child care services.

   g. Provide a strong retirement program.

   h. Include clinical nurses in planning and developing all of these activities including pay policies.

2. Problem Factors: Staffing—philosophy; clerical work; floating; rotating shifts

   Remedial Activities:

   a. Have ad hoc committee of practicing nurses develop a staffing philosophy. Ratify it in nursing administration but explain changes to committee.

   b. Establish float pool with practicing nurse input into policies and procedures.

   c. Allow clinical nurses to make schedules and cover themselves.

   d. Do flexible scheduling.

   e. Expand jobs of clerks and secretaries.

   f. Reassign nonnursing activities to appropriate departments: pharmacy, medical laboratory, dietary, and others.

   g. Do productivity studies and establish a productivity program based on pay per output unit of product.

   h. Support recruitment programs for generic students to enter schools of nursing. Obtain scholarships.

   i. Include clinical nurses in planning and developing all of these activities.

3. Problem Factors: Professionalism—physician-nurse relationships; autonomy; public relations

   Remedial Activities:

   a. Establish multidisciplinary patient care committees.

   b. Put clinical nurses on all hospital committees.

   c. Promote physician-nurse relationships at CEO level.

   d. Promote joint practice with committee of equal numbers of MDs and RNs.

   e. Do an intensive public relations program highlighting nurses. Involve clinical nurses.

   f. Establish primary nursing.

   g. Decentralize decision making.

   h. Establish participatory management.

   i. Implement a nursing theory.

   j. Establish nursing orders.

   k. Establish nursing progress notes or combined physician/nurse progress notes.

   l. Develop a fee-for-service system for supplemental staffing.

   m. Establish a recognition program for excellence in nursing.

   n. Establish a quality assurance program that includes performance evaluation, self, peer and supervisor.

   o. Provide merit awards.

   p. Provide a communication system that informs, that provides avenues for employee expression, and that provides feedback.

   q. Develop market surveys to identify factors that will retain nurses.

   r. Establish employee-management conference committee for resolving grievances.

   s. Establish professional performance committee to discuss professional nursing practice.

   t. Post job openings.

   u. Include clinical nurses in planning and developing all of these activities.

4. Problem Factor: Staff development

   Remedial Activities:

   a. Develop a career development program.

   b. Provide opportunities for continuing education based on employer and employee needs.

   c. Provide orientation and reorientation.

   d. Provide inservice education.

   e. Do communication workshops.

   f. Provide reimbursement for personnel and families.

   g. Provide refresher courses.

   h. Market programs.

   i. Establish preceptorships that reward preceptors.

   j. Do assertiveness training.

   k. Do bicultural training.

   l. Identify incompetent nurses and make them competent or terminate them. Do with peer reviews.

APPENDIX 5–3.   Response to Identified Factors Causing Job Dissatisfaction (*continued*)

m. Work to make continuing education and upward mobility education available.

n. Establish a program for minorities.

o. Do leadership training.

p. Do management development courses.

q. Include clinical nurses in planning and developing all of these activities.

5. Problem Factor: Administration support

Remedial Activities:

a. Teach all staff to follow through on their beliefs and values, going to the top if necessary.

b. Provide system for preventing punitive actions by supervisors.

c. Study nursing productivity system and fix costs of, and revenues from, nursing care.

d. Examine nurse practice act and its rules of implementation. Make written recommendations for change.

e. Have periodic meetings with employees.

f. Provide for interface of nursing education and practice.

g. Recognize the professional nurse as an independent practitioner and a partner to physicians, administrators and other professionals.

h. Improve the safety of patient care.

i. Establish a nurse credentialing system and nursing bylaws.

j. Provide a HIS or NMIS that is dynamic: patient acuity, staff scheduling, order input and results reporting, nursing care plans, and etc.

k. Provide incentive programs including one for unused sick time.

l. Provide fitness programs.

m. Develop nursing managers.

n. Promote unity within nursing.

o. Increase management visibility.

p. Include clinical nurses in planning and developing all of these activities.

Compiled from:

1. Wandelt, Mabel A., et al. Why Nurses Leave Nursing and What Can be Done About It. *American Journal of Nursing,* January, 1981, pp. 72–77.

2. Alabama Hospital Association, *Report from the Task Force to Study Nurse Shortage Situation in State of Alabama,* Prepared, December, 1981.

3. National Commission on Nursing, *Summary of the Public Hearings,* Chicago: American Hospital Association, Hospital Research and Educational Trust, and American Hospital Supply Corporation, 1981, *Nursing in Transition: Models for Successful Organizational Change,* August, 1982.

4. American Academy of Nursing Task Force on Nursing Practice in Hospitals, *Magnet Hospitals: Attraction and Retention of Professional Nurses,* Kansas City: American Nurses' Association, 1983.

5. Alabama Hospital Association, *The Alabama Nurse Study: A Survey of Registered Nurses' Attitudes About Their Profession,* Montgomery, Alabama, 1983.

6. Committee on Nursing and Nursing Education, Institute of Medicine, *"Recommendations: Meeting Current and Future Needs for Nurses,"* Washington, DC.

Principles of Budgeting

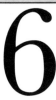

INTRODUCTION

Since the amount and quality of nursing services depend upon budgetary plans, nurse managers must become proficient in related procedures. This proficiency will provide them the resources necessary for safe and effective nursing care. With limited resources and a competitive market, personnel and material resources must be wisely and efficiently used. The enlightened nurse manager knows that the control of a budget determines who controls nursing service. The costs of nursing service have been identified for many years, but the income earned from provision of nursing services has been included with the "bed and board." This practice will cease through the efforts of nurse managers who will not only justify the price put upon this service, but will institute the program and procedures for charging for direct nursing care. To achieve reimbursement for nursing services will mean that government regulations and third-party payer policies will need to be changed to allow for direct payment to nursing providers based upon the amount of care given and the skills of the persons giving it.

Budgeting is an ongoing activity in which revenues and expenses are managed to maintain fiscal responsibility and fiscal health. The nurse manager has responsibility and accountability for managing the nursing budget. The nurse manager makes all of the decisions about adjustment of the nursing budgets to manage programs and costs. These include adding and dropping programs, expanding and contracting programs, and all modifications of revenues and expenses within the nursing unit.

BASIC PLANNING FOR BUDGETING

Planning, discussed in foregoing chapters, yields forecasts for a year and for several years. The budget is an annual plan with an intended outcome that will be effective in terms of the use of human and material resources, of products or services, and of managing the environment to improve productivity. Budgetary planning ensures the best methods are used in achieving financial objectives. It should be based on valid objectives that will produce a product or service that the community needs and will pay for. In nursing, budgetary planning helps ensure that clients or patients will receive the nursing services they want and need from satisfied nursing workers. A good budget should be based on objectives, be simple, have standards, be flexible, be balanced, and use available resources first to avoid increasing cost.

A budget is a best estimate by nurse administrators of nursing revenues and nursing expenses. It should be stated in terms of attainable objectives so as to maintain the motivation of nurse managers at the unit or cost-center level. Nurse managers should be encouraged to have objectives that require considerable management expertise in expending the budget to achieve them. The nursing budget is used for three purposes: (1) to plan the objectives, programs, and activities of nursing service; (2) to motivate nurse managers and nursing workers; and (3) as a standard to evaluate the performance of nurse administrators and managers. Managing the financial end of nursing through an operational budget can obviously create a new dimension for nurse managers. The budget will be a strong support for development and use of written objectives for the nursing division and for each of its units. It will provide strong motivation for effective planning and it will certainly provide standards by which to evaluate the performance of nurse managers. Planning will need to provide for contingencies by indicating what programs or activities can be reduced or eliminated if budget goals are not met.

BUDGETING PROCEDURES

Decentralized budgeting involves the nursing unit managers and their staff in the process. A budgeting model used at El Camino Hospital is depicted in Figure 6–1. Nursing service is labor-intensive, as is reflected in the fact that the first six budget-planning steps pertain to that area:

1. Productivity goal determination: Here the director of nursing services and the head nurse determine the unit's productivity goal for the coming fiscal year.
2. Forecast workload: The number of patient days expected on each nursing unit for the coming fiscal year are forecasted.

FIGURE 6–1.   The Budget Planning Process

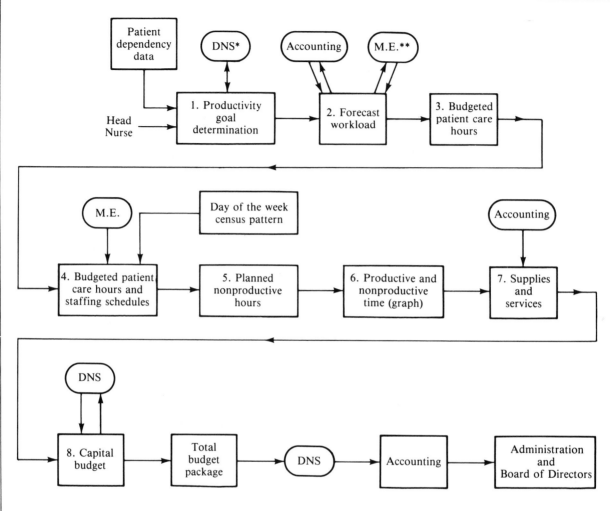

*Director of Nursing Services
**Management Engineer

SOURCE: Reprinted from *Nursing Decentralization: The El Camino Experience* by J. N. Althaus et al., p. 58, with permission of Aspen Publishers, Inc., © 1981.

3. Budgeted patient-care hours: The number of hours expected to be used in patient care for the patient days are forecasted

4. Budgeted patient care-hours and staffing schedules: Here the budgeted patient care hours are reflected in recommended staffing schedules by shift and by day of the week.

5. Planned nonproductive hours: The vacation, holiday, education leave, sick leave, and similar hours are budgeted for the coming year.

6. Productive and nonproductive time: To aid in the planning process, a graph is used to show head and assistant head nurses how the level of forecasted patient days—and therefore the staff-

ing requirements—are expected to move up and down during the year. Productive time is the time spent on the job in patient care, administration of the unit, conferences, educational activities, and orientation.

Only steps seven and eight are concerned with nonlabor expenses:

7. Supplies and services: Here the supplies and purchased services for the year are budgeted.
8. Capital budget: This is where the expected capital investments for the coming year are figured into the budget.

These eight steps result in a total budget package which goes to the nursing administrator for review. Upon preliminary acceptance of this budget, it is sent to the accounting department, where the forecasted patient days are turned into expected revenue. The budgeted productive and nonproductive time is extended into dollars, as are the costs for supplies and services and other operating expenses that will be allocated to a given nursing unit for the coming year. A pro-forma operating statement is then returned to the director of nursing for review with the head nurse. When the director of nursing and the head nurse accept the budget, it is returned to the accounting department and forwarded with the rest of the hospital budgets to administration and the board of directors.[1]

People who pay high prices for health care want accountability of both costs and quality of service. The nursing budget can be a shared responsibility, unit budgeting being prepared with staff involvement at the clinical level. The planning and controlling processes will be ongoing. Through their participation clinical nurses enhance their professional stature. A budget that is prepared and executed as a shared experience becomes an object of ownership to a staff who will put forth effort to work within its framework.

Managing Cost Centers

A cost center is a given area of accountability for both direct and indirect expenditures, for which accountability is assigned. A division of nursing is a cost center, as are each of its units, each clinic, in-service education, surgical suites, and any other section with a nursing mission in which nurses provide services to clients. Each cost center is assigned a code. The American Hospital Association publishes a Uniform Chart of Accounts and Definitions for Hospitals. An organization may use this coding system, which is usually referred to as the patient care system. There have to be workload measurements, sometimes referred to as performance classifications or units of measure. The unit of measure should be identified for each cost center as a specific, quantitative statistic such as inpatient days or relative value units (RVUs). RVUs will define the tangible things done as evidence of production and for measuring quantity, quality, and cost.

Each cost center has a manager called the cost center manager or the responsibility center manager. They are responsible for identifying needs for equipment and programs necessary to maintain progress within the current level of technology at the unit level.

Within a cost center budgeted costs are broken down into subcodes. This promotes better budgetary planning and controlling, as items can be more specifically identified as the budget is being planned. Also, each item purchased can be charged against a specific subcode, with the balance shown for that subcode.

Many hospitals do not credit nursing units as income-producing (revenue) centers; it is time they did so. The same codes will be used for income-producing centers as for cost centers; in fact in some organizations they are known as "activity centers." Nurse managers establish systems for (1) determining that work is being performed by the appropriately skilled person and (2) determining the charges for each hour of care a patient receives. Controlling processes determine that an R.N. is not used continually to perform activities that can be performed by nursing assistants. While minimal downward performance of less skilled activities should be expected as being practical and necessary, upward performance of activities should not be condoned or nursing workers will be performing activities for which they are not educated, skilled, or licensed.

Patient teaching can be charged and paid for by third-party payers when it is planned with initiative. Nordberg and King recognized the need for patient teaching and took action to accomplish third-party payment. They emphasize low-key approaches to financial reimbursement for patient teaching and acknowledge the assistance of their organization's controller. They recommend a thoroughly prepared and documented proposal, covering the program's history, behavioral objectives, operational objectives, chart forms, teaching methods, evaluation tools, follow-up procedures, evidence of cost-effectiveness such as decreased admissions or hospital stays, and teacher qualifications. Such a thorough approach to professional nursing services will often be successful in obtaining third-party payer reimbursement and will help to move these services out of the arena of "room and board" and "staff nursing care service."[2]

Relationship of Budget to Objectives

One of the chief planning activities is to identify the objectives of the nursing division and each of its units. This includes developing each objective into a management plan. One of the first sources of budgetary information is then the nursing objectives. Using these objectives will cause nurse managers to see the benefit of developing pertinent, specific, practical objectives.

Stages of the Budget

For practical purposes there are three stages of development of the nursing budget: (1) the formulation stage, (2) the review and enactment stage, and (3) the execution stage.

Formulation Stage. The formulation stage is usually a set number of months (6 or 7) prior to the beginning of the fiscal year in which the budget will be executed. During this period procedures are used to obtain an estimate of the funds needed, funds available, expenses, and revenue. These procedures and instructions for performing them should be communicated to nursing administrators and unit or cost-center managers by the budget officer.

Financial reports of expenses and revenues will be analyzed by the chief nurse executive, department heads, and cost-center managers.

One of the first steps in writing a budget is gathering data for accurate prediction of expenses (costs) and revenues (incomes). This task can be developed into a system. A primary source of data is objectives for the division of nursing and for each cost center, the objectives of that unit. Programs and activities need to have an estimated cost placed on them. If in-service education personnel want new audiovisual equipment, they should not walk into the nurse administrator's office and expect to have it next week or even next year. It should be planned for six to seven months before the budget for the next fiscal or calendar year will begin and it may be budgeted for any quarter or month within that budgetary year. In surveying the objectives the nurse administrators and managers will evaluate the previous year, review the philosophy, and re-write the objectives for the future.

Other data include programs from other departments that will require use or expansion of nursing resources, expansion of nursing clinics and client-teaching programs, travel costs for attendance at professional and educational meetings, incentive awards, library requirements, clinical and office supplies and equipment, investment equipment and facilities modification on a five-year plan, and contracts for such items as intravenous pumps and oxygen equipment. Data can be obtained from historical financial records of the organization.

Budgeting must be described in terms of programs and activities that are planned to accomplish specified nursing objectives. That is why the writing of objectives is so important and why unit or cost-center budgeting is important. Productivity and accomplishments can be directly related to the unit's programs and activities. This allows financial managers to provide costing or pricing for packages of care. Such a method is referred to as "performance and program budgeting" and causes nurse managers to evaluate deliberately the purposes for which money and resources are being expended. It relates productivity and costs to objectives, making nurse administrators and managers cost-conscious.

Among the cost-center reports that will assist the nurse manager are the following:

Daily staffing reports.

Monthly staffing reports.

Payroll summaries.

Daily lists of financial categories of patients.

Biometric reports of occupancy.

Biometric reports of workload.

Monthly financial summaries of revenues and expenses.

Review and Enactment Stage. Review and enactment are processes of budget development that put all the pieces together for approval of a final budget. Once the cost-center managers present their budgets to the hospital budget council, the chief nurse executive will consolidate the nursing budget. It will then be further consolidated into an organizational budget by the budget officer. Approval will be made by the chief executive officer of the organization and governing board. During this entire process there will be conferences at which budget adjustments are made.

Selling the budget. Nurse managers should be prepared to sell their budgets. These are five steps that help:

1. Be prepared to defend the budget. Every program must be carefully thought through. While each budget committee member will have figures at hand, the nurse administrator and cost-center managers must have a detailed plan for each. This plan will include justification of need, objectives, cost of additional resources (personnel, supplies, equipment, space), and sources of funding.

2. Initiate a marketing strategy. This can include selling programs to budget committee members beforehand. An example would be joint appointments of nursing professors/instructors as nursing staff in a university medical center. The plan should be carefully made, supported by nursing service and nursing college administrators, and sold to the vice-president for academic affairs. Secure the support of interested parties beforehand and decide how to use that support successfully.

3. Anticipate challenges. Who will be against the program? Why will they be against it? Prepare a second defense for each anticipated challenge. When the nursing shortage is less acute, finance personnel are prone to want to cut salaries and fringe benefits. Be prepared to defend call pay, shift differentials, and pay for clinical ladders.

4. Be persuasive without being emotional. If the clinical ladder is under attack, present the differences between the performance requirements for each level and relate them to productivity.

5. Work for win/win situations. Plan fallback positions in the management plan. These could range from optimum to minimally acceptable. Begin with the optimum and if the committee and CEO want cuts, negotiate. They win concessions and the nurse manager wins a program.[3]

Negotiating the budget. Preparation of a sound budget by nurse administrators and cost-center managers will ensure favorable action by the budget committee. The nurse administrator can defend the budget alone or jointly with each cost-center manager. Whichever strategy is used, it should be well planned in advance. When these meetings occur the budget committee will be interested in well-prepared plans. The objective should be clearly stated, the costs should be accurate, and the revenues should be defensible. While some budget requests can be disallowed, there are generally few setbacks when a reasonable and well-prepared budget is ably defended by informed cost-center managers.

Execution Stage. Both the formulation and the review and enactment stages of the budget are planning activities. Execution of the budget involves directing and evaluating activities. The budget is executed by the nurse administrators and managers who planned it. Revisions in execution of the budget may be planned at stated intervals, frequently once or twice during the fiscal year. There will also be procedures for evaluating the budget at cost-center levels. Budgets are prepared for either fiscal years or calendar years, depending upon the policy of the organization.

THE BUDGET CALENDAR

Financial planning is forecasting to ensure resources are allocated to current and projected needs and problems. Resources are the revenues produced to meet expenditures. Budgets are prepared by nurse administrators for policy and management purposes and set out programs of work and finances to pay for them. They include information on objectives of service, function, unit, and client group;

future needs, problems, and trends in demand for services; statistics and unit costs; impact of services and resource allocations; maintenance of existing services; improvement or development of services; and forecasting for a period of several years.

Management should apportion responsibility for budgets among the staff who generate expenditures. Specialties and functions can be compared. Determination of costs is essential to preparing good budgets; nurse managers will be able to determine costs by having knowledge of all direct and indirect costs for a function, unit, or specialty. In general costs and revenues are allocated to cost centers. However, nurse managers should be able to determine costs for individual programs, both those in operation and projected costs for new ones.

All increments in an annual budget should be questioned. These include carry-overs from one budget to the next. There is a common practice of starting with the previous year's expenses without reviewing workload data. When decreases in workload occur the budget should be reduced proportionately.

The entire budgeting process should be translated into a calendar. This can be done by assigning target dates to the steps listed in Figure 6–2.

Cost Accounting

Objectives

Like all other aspects of financial management, cost accounting will be part of the total management plan for all levels of hospital personnel and will be used between hospital and regulator or third-party payer. Nurse managers will develop clear cost-accounting objectives with the hospital administrator and other associate administrators. These will be used in all strategic plans and subsequent operational management plans. They will become an integral part of many management strategies, of communication, of budget negotiations and revisions, of staffing, of cost/price projections, and of cost containment.

Nurse managers will use various objectives pertaining to methodology of cost accounting. They will include methods for measuring the intensity or severity of illness as well as case mix of patients. Nurses have done more in this area than other

FIGURE 6–2.   The Budget Calendar

Formulation Stage

1. Develop objectives and management plans.
2. Gather all financial, historical, and statistical data and distribute to cost-center managers.
3. Analyze data.

Review and Enactment Stage

4. Prepare unit budgets.
5. Present unit budgets for approval.
6. Revise and combine into organizational budget.
7. Present to budget council.
8. Revise and present to governing board.
9. Revise and distribute to cost-center managers.

Execution Stage

10. Direct and evaluate expenses and receipts.
11. Revise budget if indicated.

operational hospital administrators. It is also important to have objectives and methods for measuring performance or outcome against standards. These standards will include short-term expenses related to use of all resources. Information will be relayed to all managers, particularly cost-center managers.

Nurse managers will also have objectives and methods to make maximal use of variable costs, since these fluctuate with volume. They can be controlled more easily through staffing methodologies, inventory control, prices, and practices. All of these objectives for cost accounting need to be coordinated with accounting, data processing, plant management, and other affected departments if they are to be effective in controlling costs. Cost accounting is important to cost management as it describes cost behavior.

Cost Factors

Cost is money expended for all resources used, including personnel, supplies, and equipment. The volume of service provided is the greatest factor affecting costs. Others include length of stay, prices of personnel and material, case mix, efficiencies, and seasonal factors. Although these factors have the greatest influence on cost, still others will have an impact. They include regulation and competition, third-party payers, the age and size of the hospital, services provided, the mission, and physician relationships.

Fixed versus Variable Costs

Fixed costs are not volume-responsive. They remain constant as volume increases or decreases over a given period of time. Among fixed costs are depreciation of equipment and buildings, salaries, fringe benefits, utilities, interest on loans or bonds, and taxes.

Variable costs are volume-responsive and census-controlled. They include such items as meals and linen. Supplies are usually volume-responsive, increasing or decreasing in price with use. If a diagnostic test is used as a unit of activity, it will increase or decrease in cost by volume. For example, if a worker can perform six tests per hour with a given piece of equipment, the cost of the test will increase if fewer than six are done, since the costs of the worker and equipment are fixed. For this reason there should be an established unit for measuring productivity for every cost center. This unit may be numbers of tests, procedures, patients of a specific acuity type, hours or minutes of service, discharges or RVUs. All activities will include fixed and variable costs. Personnel costs and utility costs can be both fixed and variable (mixed), as minimum numbers and amounts are required.

Direct versus Indirect Costs

Direct costs are often considered to be those directly related to patient care. These include the fixed costs of personnel and the variable costs of supplies. Direct costs vary by department; in areas remote from direct patient care these costs would still be considered direct costs of running each department.

Indirect costs include those costs not directly related to patient care, including utilities, administration, and housekeeping. Again they are direct costs within the source department. Some indirect costs are fixed, such as depreciation and administration. Others, such as laundry and accounting, are variable. All indirect costs are allocated or trans-ferred to the using department by a specific methodology.

Every hospital has a method of establishing costs, even if it is the Hospital and Hospital Health Care Complex Cost Report Certification and Settlement Summary, commonly known as the Medicare Cost Report. In a few hospitals the system may be more refined. Nurse administrators must become informed in this activity.

Cost Accounting System

A cost accounting system matches all revenues to costs. This is done by time periods but is not always complete. While monthly reports of revenues and costs are provided to cost-center managers, there are many indirect costs that are only allocated once a year in the Medicare Cost Report. These include the costs of utilities, accounting, administration, data processing, admitting, and other items. Informed and influential nurse managers will use these cost allocations when preparing budgets. They are usually hidden in the operational budget in the form of room costs.

There are two systems of cost accounting, process costing and job order costing. Process costing is a system whereby costs are accumulated and averaged as unit costs within a cost center. They are then added to the product or service. Supply costs are an example that are added as a cost per patient day.

Job order costing accumulates the costs of products or services for an order. Although it is done by averaging, resources are more specifically identified for each product unit or job lot. Better job order costing is done in hospitals now that the diagnostic related group (DRG) system exists. It will become more job- and product-specific as a severity-of-illness index is used and the room rate is unbundled. Costs will then become patient-specific instead of charge-specific. As this occurs, nurse managers will be able to evaluate and compare performance and productivity among cost centers.

Cost assignments to cost centers are made on the basis of direct costing if they are direct costs of patient care. Otherwise they are made by transfer costing from a patient-care support department, or cost allocation if not related to direct patient care or support. Job order sheets are used to account for all services to patients. If direct overhead costs cannot be identified with specific services rendered they are allocated based on some unit of service such as square feet of floor space.

Service Units

Service units are measurable units of productivity or volume that can be used to identify costs. They must be measurable, known to managers, and affected by volume. Productivity is measured by service units produced.

Every cost center should have a measurable service unit. The most common ones are number of visits, treatments, tests or exams, patient days, time in minutes or hours, major or minor operations, team-time concepts, and RVUs. Every cost-center manager should look at the service units being used and determine whether costs are being identified as accurately as possible.

With the increased sophistication of hospital information systems, it is easier for nurse managers to become involved in identifying and costing service units. It can be done by hours of nursing care per category of acuity of illness. To make this an RVU all other direct and indirect costs must be allocated on the basis of hours of nursing care per category of acuity of illness.

Chart of Accounts

A chart of accounts is available from the American Hospital Association. This chart of accounts includes a cost-center number and table for each cost center. It is subdivided into major classifications and subcodes that include salaries and wages, employee benefits, medical and surgical supplies, professional fees, nonmedical and nonsurgical supplies, purchased services, utilities, other direct expenses, depreciation, and rent. These classifications are further divided into subclassifications.

All movement of labor and materials between cost centers must be recorded to be costed to the correct cost center. All fringe benefits must be charged to the appropriate cost center by a system. So must all purchases including those shared. Again, this will be done using allocated shares of service units.

Amortized expenses are deferred but charged to units on a time allocation basis. These include hospital plant and equipment in addition to prepaid items. Usually the prepaid items are charged as service units by the month. Other deferred expenses include unamortized borrowing costs and preopening costs in capital expansion or renovation programs.

Inventory and Cost Transfer

Identifying actual costs of any service unit is improved through an accurate system of inventory control. Based on the number of orders or requisitions, the appropriate proportion of costs can be transferred to the using cost center.

Performance Reporting

Cost-center managers will have performance measured on the basis of those costs under their control. They cannot control building depreciation, the salaries and fringe benefits of administrators and support personnel, or plant and grounds management.

When costs vary, cost-center managers will be able to look at service units and determine the cause. They obviously need a good system of activity reporting to identify and control costs.

Financial Standards and Responsibility Accounting

In an era of retrenchment in the hospital industry, professional nurses will be asked to reduce waste. While they will be expected to maintain high standards of care, they will also be expected to compare treatment expenses with clinical benefits. This will mean making objective, economic choices in use of supplies, equipment, and services. One way nurses can do this is through a system of responsibility accounting.

According to McCullers and Schroeder, a responsibility accounting system for making efficient decisions has these characteristics:

1. Decision usefulness. Information must be relevant and reliable.
2. Timeliness. The information can become available to the decision maker before it loses its capacity to economize expenditures.
3. Favorable cost/benefit ratio. The benefit desired from the information must exceed the cost of collecting, maintaining, and processing it.

4. Understandability. Information content must be intelligible to those who must handle it and be presented in a form they can grasp.
5. Relevance. The information collected must actually make a difference in decisions to be made.
6. Reliability. Information should faithfully represent what it purports to represent.
7. Verifiability. Agreement among independent measures using the same measurement methods can demonstrate content validity to referents.
8. Materiality. Information magnitude has a significant impact on the resources of the unit or the organization as a whole. However, magnitude by itself is not sufficient for a decision. The nature of the item and the circumstances in which the decision is made must also be considered.
9. Comparability and consistency. Current information can be compared with similar information about the same unit for another time period.
10. Neutrality. Accounting methods should be free from bias towards a predetermined result.
11. Predictive value and feedback value. The information should be able to help predictor confirm expectations.[4]

Like all other characteristics of quality control, a system of responsibility accounting needs pertinent standards against which accurate amounts can be measured. The differences between standard and actual amounts are called variances. They can be used by professional nurses to make clinical decisions about patient care. Financial standards can be developed through use of historical cost data from the accounting division. These will include financial standards for staffing, medical supplies, equipment, and services. Nurse managers should be sure they obtain input for these standards from practicing nurses. Responsibility accounting can be a motivational factor in making clinical nursing decisions.

In giving financial accountability, nurses have a first duty to give full accountability to their patients, who have given them their trust. They should be accountable for their work to themselves, their professional peers, and their employers. The last item includes financial responsibility and, in publicly funded institutions, responsibility to taxpayers.

One way or another the patient pays the costs of health care. It may be through insurance premiums, taxes, or fringe benefits or from the pocket. Financial accountability means that nurses and others can account for the efficient spending of the money paid for health care.

Nurse managers need to have information on the costs of all services provided by their institutions and competing institutions. This knowledge will in turn be provided to clinical nurses, who should know what it costs to do their work. Cost-consciousness leads to reduction in waste and to cost management.

Some managers believe that overspending can be controlled by controlling nursing labor power and expenditures. This misconception can be rectified by holding nurses accountable for their budgets, both revenues and expenses.

Nurse managers have to justify the cost benefit of services provided and devise new methods to increase cost-effectiveness. They should use computers to their advantage. Increasingly, information processing technology is covered in nursing curricula. As continuing education becomes more important, a stronger linkage between academics and clinical practitioners should be formed.

The Cost of Nursing Care

To determine the cost of nursing care, several factors should be considered. Nursing charges should be quantifiable. A patient acuity system can be used for this purpose. The patient acuity system usually separates patients into four or five levels of nursing care. Charges are set by level and will be negotiated with third-party payers. Non-nursing tasks are reassigned to ensure that the charges for nursing care reflect the actual cost of providing such care.

Nursing care requirements for each level of patient acuity should be enumerated. The cost of these requirements can then be separated from the cost of non-nursing requirements, and charges can be made accordingly.

A second method of costing nursing is determining the share of total hospital costs attributable to nursing. This will vary by DRG. An industry-wide effort for each region could produce standards for nursing costs and charges. Otherwise a majority of the approximately 7,000 acute care hospitals in the

United States will need to undertake research to determine nursing costs and charges on a hospital-specific basis. Multihospital corporations, of course, can apply research studies across member institutions.

DEFINITIONS

Budget

According to *Webster's New Twentieth Century Dictionary,* second edition, a budget is "a plan or schedule adjusting expenses during a certain period to the estimated or fixed income for that period."

Herkimer has stated that "an effective budget is the systematic documentation of one or more carefully developed plans for all individually supervised activities, programs, or sections. . . . The budget is a tool which can aid decision makers in evaluating operating performance and projecting what future operations might produce."[5]

A budget is an operational management plan, stated in income and expense terms, covering all phases of activity for a future division of time. It is a financial document which expresses a plan of operation in action. In the division of nursing it sets the limits of financial support, thereby controlling the extent and quality of nursing programs. The budget will determine the number and kinds of personnel, material, and money resources available to care for patients and to achieve the stated nursing objectives. It is a financial statement of policy.

Unit of Service

The unit of service is a measure of output of hospital service consumed by the patient. In the operating units and recovery room, it will be minutes or hours; in the emergency room, it will be visits; and in the nursing unit, it will be category of acuity of patients and hours per day expressed in RVUs. Measures include procedures, patient days, patient visits, and cases.

Revenue

Revenue is the income from sale of products and services. Traditionally, nursing revenue has been included with room charges. It is increasingly being unbundled from the room rate as a separate charge per patient acuity category and per visit, day, or procedure.

Revenue can include assets such as accounts receivable and income-producing endowments. The latter can be restricted to specific purposes. Buildings, land, and other items can be assets if they produce income or are capable of producing income. Total income is frequently termed gross income, with the excess of revenues over expenses being known as net income.

Revenues also come from research grants, gift shops, donations, gifts, rentals of cots and televisions, parking fees, telephone charges, and vending machines, among other sources.

Revenue Budgeting

Revenue budgeting or rate setting is the process by which a hospital determines revenues required to cover anticipated economic costs and to establish prices sufficient to generate that revenue. Complicating the process is the fact that all patients (purchasers) don't pay an equal share of a hospital's economic costs.

To remain viable any business, including a hospital, must generate sufficient revenue to cover operating costs and profit. These include increases in working capital needs, capital replacement, and inflation adjustment. Nonprofit hospitals are identified as such for tax status only! Profits are used to improve plants and services and cannot go to stockholders or owners.

Fundamental to the rate-setting process are adequate statistical data, historical and projected, for implementing the rate-setting methodology to be employed. This includes, on a departmental basis, volume of services, current rate, allocated costs, and rate increase constraints. The goal is to obtain the greatest impact from a minimum cumulative rate increase in today's cost management environment. This is done by increasing rates in high-profit departments while instituting rate reductions in low-profit departments, so that they offset each other. An example of this would be pediatric or rehabilitational services paid by charges versus internal medicine services paid by DRG.

In today's reimbursement milieu revenues are

often budgeted before expenses. This is necessary to determine how much revenue will be available.

Expenses

Expenses are the costs of providing services to patients. They are frequently called overhead and include wages and salaries, fringe benefits, supplies, food service, utilities, and office and medical supplies. As part of the budget they are a collection or summary of forecasts for each cost center account.

Full costs include both direct and indirect expenses or costs. While direct costs such as nursing can be traced to the source, indirect costs such as utilities, telephones, or purchasing services are allocated to the source by a standard formula. Accountants use a process called *cost finding* to determine full cost by allocating indirect costs.

Expense Budgeting

Expense budgeting is the "process of forecasting, recording, and monitoring the manpower, material and supply, and monetary needs of an organization in such a manner that the operation of the various components of the organization can be controlled."[6] The components of expense budgeting are cost centers. Purposes of expense budgeting include:

- Prediction of labor hours, material and supplies, and cash flow needs for future time periods.
- Establishing procedures for making comparative studies.
- Providing a mechanism for determining when changes in procedures need to be made, providing gross information on the kinds of changes needed, and providing evidence that control has been established or reestablished.

Historical trends are the single best inexpensive indicator available to the institution. They are valid for predicting present and future trends most of the time.

Patient Days

Patient days are statistics used to project revenues. They are commonly used as units of service to compute staffing. Patient-day statistics are usually derived from census reports that are done daily at midnight and summarized monthly, for the year to date, and annually. A patient admitted on May 2 and discharged May 10 is charged for nine patient days. See Table 6–1 for an illustration of patient days per unit for one month (June and July 1989 columns).

Fiscal Year (FY)

The fiscal year is the budgetary or financial year. It may be the calendar year in some organizations, beginning on January 1 and ending on December 31. Many organizations use the period of October 1 to September 30 as the fiscal year. Some use the period of July 1 to June 30. This is done to coincide with budget decisions of state legislatures and the U.S. Congress. In the latter examples, the fiscal year obviously overlaps two calendar years.

Year to Date (YTD)

The term "year to date" is used to describe the accumulated units of service at a particular point in the fiscal year. If the fiscal year begins October 1, the year-to-date patient days for December 31 would be the summary for 92 days. See Table 6–1 for an illustration of year-to-date statistics (1988–1989 and 1987–1988 columns).

Average Daily Census (ADC)

The census is summarized for a specific number of days and divided by that number of days. As an example, the average daily census for the month of June would be the total patient days for June divided by 30. In Table 6–1, the number of patient days for June was 7436. When this is divided by 30, the average daily census is 248.

Hours of Care

From the nursing viewpoint, hours of care has traditionally been the number of hours of care allocated per patient per day (24 hours) on a unit. With the use of patient acuity rating systems, hours of care can be determined to the hour or even parts of an hour. Usually patients are determined to fall

TABLE 6–1. University of South Alabama Medical Center Statistics as of July 31, 1989 and 1988 Including June 1989

	July 1989	OCC %	June 1989	Total to Date 1988–1989	OCC %	1987–1988
Nursing Station						
3rd Floor	1,014	79.8%	833	9,792	78.6%	8,650
4th Floor	811	76.9%	718	7,834	75.8%	7,255
5th Floor North	526	65.3%	524	5,300	67.1%	4,838
5th Floor South	622	77.2%	592	5,587	70.7%	5,603
6th Floor	792	71.0%	866	8,730	79.8%	8,176
7th Floor	850	68.5%	895	9,086	74.7%	8,885
8th Floor	0	0.0%	0	0	0.0%	4,403
8th Floor North	376	60.6%	383	4,624	76.1%	2,393
8th Floor South	303	69.8%	274	3,253	76.4%	1,729
9th Floor	0	0.0%	0	0	0.0%	5,138
9th Floor North	526	84.8%	501	5,332	87.7%	2,690
9th Floor South	481	77.6%	506	5,118	84.2%	2,617
MINU	104	83.9%	89	1,041	85.6%	432
SINU	73	58.9%	84	964	79.3%	471
Burn Unit	173	79.7%	188	1,723	81.0%	1,912
Labor and Delivery	138	37.1%	99	1,228	33.7%	1,258
CCU	206	83.1%	148	1,848	76.0%	1,937
Clinical Research Unit	137	73.7%	132	1,342	73.6%	1,361
EAU	23	0.0%	7	390	0.0%	634
MICU	213	85.9%	191	2,099	86.3%	2,291
PICU	169	54.5%	112	1,612	53.0%	1,834
SICU	229	92.3%	207	2,175	89.4%	2,302
NTICU	209	84.3%	87	1,891	77.8%	2,277
Total	7,975	73.1%	7,436	80,969	75.7%	79,086
Nursery						
Newborn	832	103.2%	632	7,666	97.0%	7,307
Intermediate	577	103.4%	457	4,761	87.0%	3,991
Intensive Care	955	110.0%	716	8,526	100.2%	7,022
Total	2,364	105.9%	1,805	20,953	95.7%	18,320

SOURCE: Courtesy of the University of South Alabama Medical Center, Mobile, Alabama.

into one of four or five categories, each assigned a specific number of hours of care per patient day.

Care Giver

Each nurse who works with patients is labelled a care giver. In nursing there are three commonly used types of care givers: registered nurses, licensed practical nurses, and nurses' aides. Most personnel budgets have a ratio of registered nurses to other care givers. There is considerable research supporting an all–registered nurse care giver staff. The current nurse shortage will alter this goal.

Cost-to-Charge Ratios

Cost-to-charge ratios are convenient tools for computing the cost of providing a service. For example, if the charges to a patient for fiber optic laboratory services were $1,000 and the cost-to-charge ratio 0.815626, one would know that the cost to the hospital for these services was approximately $815.63 (see Table 6–2). This cost includes the expense of running the fiber optic laboratory and a portion of the hospital's overhead cost. In some instances the cost-to-charge ratios are greater than one, which means the cost of operating these cost centers is greater than the charges.

The hospital is made up of two types of cost centers. The first type is revenue-producing cost centers, such as the fiber optic laboratory, which bill patients for services provided. The second type is overhead cost centers, such as the accounting department, which exist to support the revenue-producing centers. The cost of the overhead cost centers are added to the revenue-producing centers by various statistical methods. For example, utility costs are allocated to the revenue departments based on their square footage. However, the accounting department cost is allocated based on the operating budget of each revenue cost center. The cost-to-charge ratio is computed by dividing the total cost of the cost center, including direct and overhead, by the total charges for the same department.

TABLE 6–2. University of South Alabama Medical Center Cost-to-Charge Ratios as of 9/30/89.

Cost Center	Cost-to-Charge Ratio
Operating room	1.072993
Recovery room	0.731813
Delivery room	0.920547
Radiology	0.846045
Laboratory	0.502010
Respiratory therapy	0.288370
Physical therapy	1.261435
EKG-EEG-CVL	0.698327
Fiberoptic lab	0.815626
Medical supplies	0.303416
Drugs	0.275234
Cast room	0.238285
Emergency room	1.131543
Routine inpatient	1.321196
Surgical ICU	1.044988
Coronary care	0.892522
Burn unit	2.054106
Pediatric ICU	1.153027
Medical ICU	1.038597
Nursery ICU	0.756198
Nursery	1.138131

SOURCE: The University of South Alabama Medical Center, Mobile, Alabama. Reprinted with permission.

Product Line

Hospitals are reorganizing on the basis of product lines. These can include outpatient or ambulatory surgery, home health care, a burn center, a comprehensive cancer center, or other products. As in business or industry, each functions as a profit center within the overall accounting system. Even one DRG can be a product. A product must pay for itself, be paid for through cost shifting, or be deleted.

Financial Management Triad

The financial management triad includes planning, budgeting, and evaluation. Planning is essential to development and to survival. It considers philosophy, type of hospital, type of patient, size of units, projected occupancy, physical plant, modality of nursing, availability of ancillary services, staffing, variable costs for office supplies, medical supplies, food, and repair and maintenance of equipment. Planning projects the institution of new programs and expenses as well as curtailment or discontinuance of old programs. Through the operating and capital budgeting process a price tag is put on plans. When they are implemented they are evaluated for effect and efficiency. People who are involved in the financial management triad will put forth an effort to make it work. For this reason broad participation is preferred over narrow participation by employees.

Cost/Benefit Analysis

Cost/benefit analysis is a planning technique. What are the costs of pursuing a goal, an objective or a program? How do they compare with the benefits?

Vertical Integration

Purchase or establishment of free-standing diagnostic centers, nursing homes, chronic care facilities, and other organizations by hospitals is termed "vertical integration." This technique is used to increase financial stability and profit. A hospital may move backward in vertical integration and buy or acquire a medical supply business. Thus the hospital sells products it previously bought, an entirely new service to the hospital. It may move forward and acquire a health maintenance organization. In horizontal integration, hospitals merge.

Flexible Budgeting

Flexible budgeting is a budget model designed to allow for evaluation of varying costs and demand, rather than evaluating variances from a predetermined fixed level of demand. The flexible budget is adjusted to reflect actual activity levels. It will show meaningful variance analysis.

Contribution Margin or Percentage

This a mathematical computation that relates charges to costs to show the break-even point. The break-even point is the point at which charges or revenues equal cost of production. As the charges or revenues increase or decrease, the contribution margin or percentage increases or decreases. The margin of safety is the point to which charges can be dropped without incurring losses.

Zero-Base Budgeting

Zero-base budgeting provides no incentive but is rather a method of budgeting that relates to cost control. It ignores the previous budget and the previous historical data base. Zero-base budgeting starts from zero and justifies everything. A previous activity can be included in the budget but funding for it must be justified by its relation to the organizational objectives. In theory, each and every function in a zero-base budget is isolated to stand on its own merits. The merit of each function is reviewed annually. All labor power and costs are recalculated and decisions are made as to whether to continue the function and at what levels.

In actual practice, zero-base budgeting seldom reviews all costs. Much of the previous budget is accepted; a complete analysis could cost more than it saves. With cost studies becoming more prevalent in nursing, the application of zero-base budgeting techniques will increase.

OPERATING OR CASH BUDGETS

The cash budget is the actual operating budget in detail, excluding the capital budget. A cash budget requirement is cash flow that must be adequate to meet debt obligations, including replacement and expansion of facilities, unanticipated requirements, the payroll, payment for supplies and services, and a prudent investment program. Cash receipts come from third-party payers, tuition, endowment fund earnings, and sales of food, gifts, and services.

The cash budget is the day-to-day budget and represents money coming in and going out. It is advisable to have cash reserves so that cash flow, the money coming in, will pay the bills. Otherwise revenues must be speeded up or payment of bills slowed down.

Negative Cash Flow

The major factors influencing negative cash flow are:

1. Time lag between delivery of services and collection of payments.
2. The difference in cycles between the timing of net income and flow of cash.

TABLE 6–3. University of South Alabama Medical Center 85/86 Budget Worksheet, Surgical-9th Floor, Account Number 60686

Sub Code	Description	ABR	Prior Year Expense	Original Budget	Annualized Expense	Budget Detail	Budget Pool
200	Pool-Med/Surg Supply	0	.00	10,975.00		$10,780	$ 8,985
211	Med & Surg Supplies	4	10,893.80	.00	8,790	$ 8,790	
213	Drugs	4	129.59	.00	195	$ 195	
Pool Total			11,023.39	10,975.00	8,985		
220	Pool-General Supply	0	.00	2,705.00			$ 2,848
232	Office Supplies	4	303.34	.00	672	$ 810	−320
234	Printing	4	37.75	.00	3	$ 3	
240	Housekeeping Supply	4	1,404.06	.00	1,482	$ 1,482	
270	Food Expense	4	913.73	.00	523	$ 523	
Pool Total			2,658.88	2,705.00	2,680		
300	Pool-Travel/Entertain	0	.00	110.00			$ 50
314	Local Travel	4	13.80	.00	18	$ 50	
Pool Total			13.80	110.00	18		
320	Pool-Other Expenses	0	.00	130.00			$ 660
336	Equip Maint & Repair	4	66.60	.00	123	$ 610	
372	Books & Subscription	4	25.00	.00		$ 50	
Pool Total			91.60	130.00	123		
501	Minor Equipment	0	.00	.00	72	−53	$ 465
Pool Total			.00	.00	72		
Acct Total			13,787.67	13,920.00	11,878		

Total	$14,968
−	373
	$14,595

SOURCE: Courtesy of the University of South Alabama Medical Center, Mobile, Alabama.

3. Lag created by the large up and down cycles of volume during the different seasons (cash deficit during a busy census cycle or surplus during a low census cycle).
4. Labor expense (60 to 70 percent of operating expense) paid out in salary and wages not cycling concurrently with collections.

To maintain solvency, cash flow must be managed carefully and cycles of cash shortage planned for appropriately. The cash budget should plan for the ability to borrow cash during shortfalls, investment of excess cash, and *strict* monitoring and reporting of lost charges and of the billing and collecting process. The cash budget is a part of the total budget and is apportioned to departments based on individual cost-center activity.

Developing the Operating Budget

Operating budget information supplied to the chief nurse executive, department heads, and cost-center managers include a budget worksheet and an adjustment explanation worksheet. The budget worksheet depicts information by cost-center account number and subcode. It lists prior year expense,

FIGURE 6–3. Adjustment Explanation, Calendar Year 1985–1986

DEPARTMENT NAME   9th floor

DEPARTMENT NUMBER   60686

Subcode Number	Subcode Description	Adjustment Amount	Adjustment Explanation
		$ 30.00	2 lg blue policy binders 15.00 ea
		6.00	1 sm blue policy binder
		32.00	2 large red 4″ (8½ × 11) 3-ring binders—normal wear and tear 2 yrs old
232	Office Supplies	$ 25.00	4 black 3-ring binders (MAR & Kardex)—normal wear & tear
		28.00	48″ × 36″ cork & wooden frame bulletin boards—↑ appearance ↓ clutter
		17.00	25″ × 25″ ¼″ thick Plexiglas—↑ appearance
		$138	
		$	
		$ 30.00	Tabers Medical Dictionary—ref. book needed to ↑ professionalism
372	Books	$ 20.00	Websters Ninth New Collegiate Dictionary—↑ learning
		$ 50.00	

SOURCE: Courtesy of the University of South Alabama Medical Center, Mobile, Alabama.

original budget, and annualized expense. Usually this form is provided during a fiscal year and the annualized expense is the projected total expense if current rates continue to the end of the fiscal year. The columns headed "Budget Detail" and "Budget Pool" are empty so the cost-center manager can fill in the budget expenses for the projected fiscal year. Note in Table 6–3 that the cost center manager had projected an increased budget of $10,780 for sub-code 211, medical and surgical supplies. This was reduced to an annualized projection of $8,790 at the budget council hearings as hospital administration had decided not to project inflation.

Also in Table 6–3, note that subcode 232, office supplies, was increased by $138. This was justified on the adjustment explanation; see Figure 6–3. However, information available to the administrator indicated that $320 had been budgeted and expended in the current year for new chart backs. Since this was a one-time expense it was backed out of the budget. A similar transaction for $53 was backed out of subcode 501, minor equipment. Increases were approved for subcodes 501, minor equipment, and 372, books. The supply and minor equipment budget for FY 1985–86 for this cost center was approved for $14,595.

In the budget formulation stage described here, the assistant administrator for finance distributes the worksheets to the other assistant administrators and department heads. They develop budgets with their cost-center managers and defend them before the budget council.

PERSONNEL BUDGET

Most nursing personnel budgets are based upon quantitative workload measurements. Nursing ser-

---

FIGURE 6–4. Nursing Personnel Budget

Nursing Budget

1. The attached 1984–85 budget for all nursing units is based on a patient acuity rating system purchased from Medicus Systems. The standard is:

Acuity	Nursing Hours Per Patient Needed During 24-hour Period
.5	0–2 hours
1.0	2–4 hours
2.5	4–10 hours
5.0	10–24 hours

2. The staffing formula is:

$$\frac{\text{Average Census} \times \text{Nursing Hours} \times 1.4 \times 1.14}{7.5}$$

3. The total nursing personnel needed includes ward clerks and units not using a patient acuity rating system:

Maternal Child

Unit	ADC	Acuity	NSG/HRS	RN	LPN	NA	Other	Total
3rd	31.8	0.9	4	14	9	4	5	32
Peds	22.0	1.3	4.5	16	5	0	4	25
PICU	4.4	3.4	12	11	0	0	2	13
ICN	21.7	2.9	12	41	7	6	4	58
Inter.	11.9	2.3	4.5	6	4	1	1	12
NBN	19.7	1.0	4	9	6	1	3	19
Del. Rm.	—	—	—	20	3	1	4	28
Play Rm.	—	—	—	—	—	—	1	1
Total				117	34	13	24	188

(continued)

FIGURE 6–4. Nursing Personnel Budget (*continued*)

Unit	ADC	Acuity	NSG/HRS	RN	LPN	NA	Other	Total
Medical								
5 No.	14.3	1.3	4.5	11	3	0	3	17
5 So.	22.1	1.3	4.5	12	5	4	3	24
CRU	3.6	—	4.5	6	—	1	1	8
8th	25.1	1.7	4.5	15	7	2	3	27
MICU	7.2	4.0	12	18	0	0	3.5	21.5
CCU	6.5	3.0	12	16	0	0	1	17
Telemetry	—	—	—	—	1	5	0	6
Total				78	16	12	14.5	120.5
Surgical								
9th	16.2	1.2	4.5	11	2	2	3	18
6 Surg.	26.5	1.6	4.5	16	6	3	3	28
6 Ortho.	23.5	1.5	4.5	15	4	4	3	26
SICU	6.4	3.8	12	17	0	0	2	19
B.U.	3.7	2.8	12	8	2	0	1	11
Ortho Tech	—	—	—	—	—	—	1	1
Total				67	14	9	13	103
Psychiatry								
7th	23.5	—	5.5	11	4	11	6	32
OR/RR/EAU/ED								
OR	—	—	—	21	13	4	2	40
RR/EAU	—	—	—	16	0	1	2	19
ED	—	—	—	25	0	7	8	40
Administration								
N/S Adm.	—	—	—	13	0	0	3.5	16.5
Staff Dev.	—	—	—	8.5	0	0	1	9.5
Health Nurse	—	—	—	1	—	—	—	1
CVICU								
Pool	—	—	—	4.5	12	18	2	36.5
Total				362	93	75	76	606

NOTE: The formulary budget is based on actual ADC for 12 months (July, 1983–June, 1984). All positions above formula calculations are placed in CVICU budgeted cost center and held vacant.

SOURCE: Courtesy of the University of South Alabama Medical Center, Mobile, Alabama.

FIGURE 6–5. Calculating the Nursing Personnel Budget

The staffing formula is

$$\frac{\text{Average Daily Census} \times \text{Nursing Hours} \times 1.4 \times 1.14}{7.5}$$

Example: 3rd Floor

Average daily census = 31.8

Nursing hours = 4 (per 24 hours)

1.4 is a constant representing 7 days in a week with a full time worker working 5 days in a week:

$7 \div 5 = 1.4$

1.14 is a constant representing an allowance of 0.14 FTE for vacation, illness, etc. for each 1.0 FTE

7.5 represents one work day

$$\frac{31.8 \times 4 \times 1.4 \times 1.14}{7.5} = 27 \text{ FTEs}$$

There are 14 RNs, 9 LPNs, and 4 NAs (27 FTEs) budgeted for 3rd Floor. The "others" column represents ward clerks or other non-nursing personnel not included in the formula. While quantitative measurements justify a full complement of nursing personnel, the budget committee can reduce this number. Note that ICN has been reduced from the formula calculation by 1.0 FTE.

vice should have a patient acuity system. It is usually a computer program that produces staffing requirements by shift and by day. It produces an acuity index for each patient and the formula indicates needed staff by category (R.N., L.P.N., nursing assistant) and by shift. It also compares actual staffing with that required and can be summarized by month and year. Each day at a given time a registered nurse enters each patient's acuity rating into a computer terminal. To promote objectivity of the ratings, R.N.s should be trained to use the same procedures when evaluating each patient. Quality assurance tests can be performed to compare trainer ratings with those done by registered nurses.

Figure 6–4 is a nursing budget that is based upon a patient acuity rating system. The average daily census (ADC) is obtained from records produced in the admissions office. It is the result of dividing the total patient days for a unit for one year by 365 days. Census reports are computer-generated on a daily, monthly, and annual basis.

Acuity is the result of the sum of all acuities for one year divided by 365 days. This figure is also computer-generated daily, monthly, and annually. The nursing hours are generated from the acuity standard listed in paragraph 1 of Figure 6–4. Application of a staffing formula for preparing the personnel budget for a specific unit is illustrated in Figure 6–5.

In planning the personnel budget, the nurse manager has quantitative information related to staffing and can accurately predict the number of FTEs needed for patient care. Other considerations must be weighed at the same time. Will there be a pay increase next year? If so, it must be calculated and budgeted for. Will fringe benefits increase or decrease? They must also be budgeted for. If new programs are being implemented, do they require

FIGURE 6–6.   New Position Questionnaire, 1989–9_ Budget Year

1. Department _____ Department number _____

2. Position class, title _____ Position FTE _____

3. Minimum starting salary _____ Expected starting date _____

4. Permanent _____ Temporary _____ If temporary, ending date _____

5. Describe briefly the new position responsibilities:

_____

_____

_____

_____

Need for new position:

6. New service _____ Increased volume _____
   If new service, complete question 7.
   If increased volume, complete question 8.

7. Describe the new service to be provided and estimated new revenues.

_____

_____

_____

_____

_____

8. Document increased volume and provide staffing analysis for your department.

_____

_____

_____

_____

(Attach additional pages if necessary)

_____

SOURCE: The University of South Alabama Medical Center, Mobile, Alabama. Reprinted with permission.

additional labor power? Will this labor power come from cutbacks in other programs or from added FTEs? See Figure 6–6 for adding new positions to the budget.

Careful planning ensures that the nurse administrator will control the nursing budget. It will also ensure that the nurse administrator has a handle on the total dollar amount that will be expended on personnel and that personnel will generate income.

In the budgeting process, personnel account for the largest portion of the nursing budget. When one is preparing budgets for clinics, emergency departments, recovery rooms, operating rooms, and delivery rooms, it is important to have quantitative data. These include number of visits, procedures, deliveries, and the like. Samples of lengths of time required for each activity can be taken by using management engineering techniques in which visits, procedures, or other activities are charted over a period of time.

Data should be collected over a representative period to show the actual hours worked by shift and by day. These data will indicate fluctuations in the workload by shift and by day of the week. Use of a second data sheet is suggested to determine the total number of patients in the emergency room area at any one time, including those patients in a holding status. Conversion of these data into graphs provides information to compare staffing with workload. These data will provide the following information:

1. The current nursing hours available per patient visit.
2. Fluctuation in available hours by shift and day.
3. Fluctuation in workload by time of day.
4. Fluctuation in ratio of staffing levels to patient load.[7]

Piper indicates that the basic staffing of an emergency room should be calculated to handle a "critical mass," the staffing level required to handle an unexpected emergency. In addition to quantitative data, the nurse administrator should collect qualitative data from the staff to assist in containing stress, determining mix of staff, and in improving support services. Data can be compared with those from other institutions. The result will then be translated into personnel dollars.

In the process of budgeting, the nurse manager knows how much each decision will cost, whether it involves numbers and kinds of personnel or amounts and kinds of supplies and equipment. Few nurse managers will have the luxury of a budget that provides all of the resources that can be used. Hard decisions have to be made. They are easier to substantiate when workloads are quantified. In the personnel area, if the patient dependency or acuity system is reliable and valid and has quality checks on the raters, it will provide data that justifies the personnel budget. When the number of highest acuity level adult patients increases from 24 to 32 per shift and day, the budget must be adjusted. Comparisons must be made to determine whether other levels have decreased. Estimates must be made as to whether the increases and decreases are permanent or temporary. Then the budget decisions are made.

To provide for fluctuations in personnel costs, a personnel pool can be established. This can consist of permanent or temporary FTEs; full-time or part-time workers; persons who work flexible hours; a mixture of R.N.s, L.P.N.s, nursing assistants, and clerks; and provision for all shifts and days of the week. An effective PRN pool must be well managed by one line manager or staffing director. Its personnel require staff development programs and concern for managing them as a unique workforce of human beings. The nurse manager or administrator determines the level of service and then expresses it in financial terms to produce a budget.

SUPPLIES AND EQUIPMENT BUDGET

The supplies and equipment budget is part of the operating or cash budget. It includes all supplies and equipment used in provision of services except capital equipment and supplies charged directly to patients as revenues. Examples of supplies to be budgeted include office supplies, medical/surgical supplies, pharmacy supplies, and others. Refer to Table 6–3 and Figure 6–3.

Minor equipment includes such items as sphygmomanometers, otoscopes, ophthalmoscopes, and the like. It is equipment costing less than the base set for capital equipment. If the base is $500, all equip-

TABLE 6–4. University of South Alabama Medical Center Capital Budget 1986–1987 Status as of June 30, 1989

Department	Dept. No.	Item Description	Budget	Paid 06-30-89	Encumbrances	Total Committed	Budget Balance
Nursing Services							
Nursing Services—Admin	60601	Software License	$0.00	$18,135.00	$2,000.00	$0.00	$0.00
		External Modem		527.12			
		Electric & Manual Beds—6		31,704.72			
		Cardio System Special Care Beds		13,725.00			
		Telemetry Monitoring System		113,080.12			
		COMPAQ Computer		9,842.70			
		Department Total	189,014.66	187,014.66	2,000.00	189,014.66	0.00
Private U. 6th Floor	60609	Lifepack 7 Defibrillator		5,500.00			
		Facsimile Machine		1,600.00			
		Lifepack 7 Defibrillator		5,208.00			
		Department Total	12,308.00	12,308.00	0.00	12,308.00	0.00
Coronary Care	60615	Lifepack 6 Defibrillator		7,621.32			
		Department Total	7,621.32	7,621.32	0.00	7,621.32	0.00
5th Fl—Shared Supplies	60619	Facsimile Machine		1,550.00			
		Department Total	1,550.00	1,550.00	0.00	1,550.00	0.00
Fifth Floor—North	60622	Lifepack 7 Defibrillator		5,500.00			
		Department Total	5,500.00	5,500.00	0.00	5,500.00	0.00
CCU	60626	Telemetry Transmitters		3,300.00			
		Department Total	3,300.00	3,300.00	0.00	3,300.00	0.00
Pediatric Unit	60630	Lifepack 7 Defibrillator		5,500.00			
		Facsimile Machine		1,550.00			
		Department Total	7,050.00	7,050.00	0.00	7,050.00	0.00

SOURCE: The University of South Alabama Medical Center, Mobile, Al. Reprinted with permission.

TABLE 6–5. University of South Alabama Medical Center Investment in Plant Assets for the Ten Months Ended July 31, 1989

Plant assets consisting of land, buildings, and equipment are stated at cost or, if contributed, at fair market value at date of gift. No provision is made in the accounts for depreciation of plant assets. Investment in Plant is reduced for disposal of plant assets.

All Hospital equipment purchases are funded by the Renewals and Replacements Fund. The Hospital also uses plant assets purchased by the University. These assets are not presented in the Hospital's Financial Statements.

Depreciation expense is included in Medicare, Medicaid, and Blue Cross cost reports. This information is presented below.

	Cost	Deprn Expense 07-31-89	Accum. Deprn. 07-31-89	Net Book Value 07-31-89
Hospital-Designated Funds				
Land	$ 186,096	$ 0	$ 0	$ 186,096
Buildings	8,070,647	184,063	3,942,812	4,127,835
Fixed Equipment	10,386,318	605,671	5,878,008	4,508,310
Major Movable Equipment	15,079,892	1,235,052	8,971,493	6,108,399
Minor Equipment	186,757	0	186,757	0
Construction in Progress	762,874	0	0	762,874
Total	34,672,584	2,024,786	18,979,070	15,693,514
University-Designated Funds				
Buildings	1,544,927	39,481	581,958	962,969
Fixed Equipment	2,564,683	158,533	1,914,366	650,317
Major Movable Equipment	5,315,499	0	5,315,499	0
Total	9,425,109	198,014	7,811,823	1,613,286
Total equipment used for patient care	$44,097,693	$2,222,800	$26,790,893	$17,306,800

SOURCE: Courtesy of the University of South Alabama Medical Center, Mobile, Alabama.

ment under $500 is budgeted under the supplies and equipment budget as minor equipment.

Generally, the director of materials management furnishes information on the total cost of supplies and equipment per cost center to the accounting office. The accounting office generates a cost per patient day for supplies and equipment for each cost center. This is used for budgeting purposes, increases for inflation being a decision of top management. Based on projected patient days and revenues, decisions can be made to increase or decrease the supplies and equipment budget.

Costs can be decreased by controlling the amounts of supplies and equipment kept in inven-

tory. Nurse administrators should look at any inventories they control and reduce them according to usage.

CAPITAL BUDGET

A capital budget is usually separate from the operating budget; see Table 6–4. Each item of a capital budget is defined in terms of dollar value and is an item of equipment that is reused over a period of time. It projects the costs of major purchases. The budget provides for depreciation of each capital

TABLE 6–6. University of South Alabama Medical Center Statement of Changes in Fund Balance-Renewals and Replacements Fund for the Ten Months Ended July 31, 1989

Account Number	Description	Balances 10/01/88	Funded Depreciation	Other Additions Deductions	Expended for Plant Facilities	Intrafund Transfers	Balances 07/31/89
79008	Unallocated—USAMC	9,915,392.38	2,222,800.29	78,134.71	.00	159,538.18—	12,056,789.20
79030	Defects—Joint Commis	65,818.19	.00	.00	.00	65,818.19—	.00
79039	Information System	92,709.68	.00	.00	.00	.00	92,709.68
79050	Helicopter—USAMC	712,120.33	.00	127,667.94	.00	.00	839,788.27
79057	USAMC Emer Generator	48,562.09	.00	.00	.00	.00	48,562.09
79063	Donated Eq—Others	2,313.49	.00	153.00	1,928.70—	384.79—	153.00
79064	USAMC Aux Purch Eq	.00	.00	688.08—	538.08	150.00	.00
79068	Hosp Adm Purch Eq	.00	.00	33,809.52	33,809.52—	.00	.00
79075	HVAC System—Surgery	74,475.00	.00	.00	.00	74,475.00—	.00
79077	Labor Deliv Unit 3FL	291,990.72	.00	.00	.00	.00	291,990.72
79083	H.A.S. Telephone Sym	13,007.00	.00	.00	.00	13,007.00—	.00
79092	Capital Budget 86-87	364,110.78	.00	5,208.00—	334,654.47—	.00	24,248.31
79093	Xray Silver Recovery	49,944.03	.00	12,678.45	.00	.00	62,622.48
79095	Capital Exp <$10,000	75,414.38	.00	.00	146,864.18—	150,000.00	78,550.20
79097	Linear Accelerator	.00	.00	.00	45,994.26	45,994.26—	.00
79098	Mini Van	1,606.48	.00	2,847.51	.00	.00	4,453.99
79099	O/P Surg Cap Equip	161,720.27	.00	.00	225,718.54—	64,324.93	326.66
79101	O/P Surg Renov	37,425.00	.00	.00	1,316.60—	.00	36,108.40
79102	Angiograph Lab Eqmnt	1,000,000.00	.00	.00	189,259.00—	.00	810,741.00
79103	Nuclear Medical Eqmnt	284,000.00	.00	.00	246,035.68—	.00	37,964.32
79104	Telethon Purch Equip	.00	.00	40,185.00	40,185.00—	.00	.00
79105	Medical Rec Dict Sys	.00	.00	.00	.00	86,288.00	86,288.00
79106	Renal Transplant Prg	.00	.00	.00	.00	96,000.00	96,000.00
79110	ELENA-USAMC Damage	31,916.36	.00	5,629.15	.00	37,545.51—	.00
	Final Totals	13,222,526.18	2,222,800.29	295,209.20	1,173,239.35—	.00	14,567,296.32

Source: The University of South Alabama Medical Center, Mobile, Alabama. Reprinted with permission.

FIGURE 6–7. University of South Alabama Medical Center Capital Requests
1989–1990

DEPT. NAME: Operating Room (Orth.)

DEPT. NO.: 660

RETURN TO STEVE SIMMONS BY 2/10/89

1. LAYMAN'S DESCRIPTION OF EQUIPMENT: Wolf 70 degree Arthroscope and Attachments. Scope used to look in the knee at a different angle

2. EXPECTED USE:
    2 times per week

3. TOTAL PRICE:
    $3,600.00

4. INSTALLATION & RENOVATION COSTS:
    none

5. SHIPPING COST:

6. TRAINING COST:

7. STAFFING (INCREASE OR DECREASE)

8. EXPECTED USEFUL LIFE:
    15 years

QUESTIONS 9. & 10. ASSUMES BUDGET APPROVED 3/1/89:

9. EXPECTED ARRIVAL DATE:
    April, 1989

10. EXPECTED DATE OF FIRST PATIENT USE:
    April, 1989

11. TRADE IN VALUE OF REPLACED EQUIPMENT:

12. PROCEDURE CHARGE:
    $100.50

13. EXPECTED ANNUAL PROCEDURES:
    104 per year

14. COST OF SUPPLIES PER PROCEDURE:

(continued)

FIGURE 6–7. University of South Alabama Medical Center Capital Requests 1989–1990 (*continued*)

15. PROFESSIONAL FEES:

16. JUSTIFY PRIORITY: The 70 degree scope is needed to look in the posterior aspect of the knee behind the femoral condyles and this cannot be done with the 30 degree scopes that we own at the present time. With the increasing importance of arthroscopy and the expertise now supplied by Dr. Dondren being on the part-time faculty, this scope is badly needed to update our equipment.

SIGNATURES: DEPARTMENT HEAD   ASSISTANT ADMINISTRATOR

SOURCE: Courtesy of South Alabama Medical Center, Mobile, Alabama.

budget item, sets aside the amount of this depreciation in an escrow account, and uses this account to finance new capital budgets; see Table 6–5. In addition department heads are required to justify and set priorities on capital budget items. See Figure 6–7.

Capital budgets also deal with maintenance, renovations, remodeling, improvements, expansion, land acquisition, and new buildings; see Table 6–6. The financial manager for nursing is the nurse manager, who should evaluate past decisions and advise the nurse administrator on whether they were good or bad.

All proposals for capital equipment need to be fully evaluated for amount of use, payment methodology, safety, replacement, and duplication of service, and every conceivable angle including the need for space, personnel, and renovation. The needs and desires of the medical staff should be included. Their involvement in planning will help to ensure wise purchases of capital equipment.

The capital budget must address increased forms of competition, dwindling financial resources, and regulatory contraints. Its manager should provide conditions under which effective planning and capital budgeting increase the hospital's chance of long-term survival. Capital budgeting is a part of the overall budget planning process for the organization and not an entity unto itself.

When the capital budget list has been analyzed and reduced to the amount available, it is again tabulated. It is now ready to present to the board of directors; see Table 6–4. With their approval, the list is distributed to cost-center managers who prepare requisitions for purchase. The purchasing department prepares bid specifications, with input from cost-center managers. Purchases are finalized on the basis of results of bids submitted by vendors who meet the required specifications. Purchases are finally entered into the depreciation budget schedule. The latter is obtained from the American Hospital Association and is considered the standard for the industry; see Figure 6–8.

REVENUES

What are the sources for nursing revenue or for securing a financial base for nursing? They include grants, continuing education, private practice, community visibility, health care for students and staff, health maintenance organizations, city health departments, industries, unions, third-party payments, professional corporations, and nurse-managed centers.

Operating room nursing is an example of a cost center that can be billed as a source of revenue. This can be done by determining the level of care needed for different procedures and the room charges based on use of supplies and equipment, then bill-

FIGURE 6–8. Excerpt From Depreciation Schedule

Item	Years to Depreciate
Land improvements	
Heated pavement	10
Signs	12
Buildings	
Masonry, wood frame	20–25
Boiler house	15–25
Major movable equipment	7–12
Minor movable equipment	2–5

SOURCE: American Hospital Association, *Estimated Useful Lives of Depreciable Hospital Assets,* (Chicago: American Hospital Publishing, 1988), 1–2.

ing the services separately. In computing the nursing charges, the cost of nursing personnel per case can be determined from the records. To this can be added cost for preparation time for assembling supplies and equipment and setting up the room, visiting the patient preoperatively and postoperatively, nursing administration, and staff development. Room costs would include environmental services and maintenance.[8]

Maryland and Maine have passed legislation requiring hospitals to list nursing as a separate item on patients' bills. As the hospital bill is unbundled, all nursing cost centers will become major revenue-producing centers. Then all payers will be paying for nursing services based on business procedures. This will include allocated return on equity (profit) and proportionate losses due to bad debts.[9]

Using product line strategy, nursing divisions can sell staff development programs, consultation services, home health care, wellness programs, computer software, and many other product lines.

Many items and services have been used to generate revenues for hospitals. These include drugs, supplies, respiratory therapy, physical therapy, and others. In most instances the charges have been excessive and there have been areas where cost

shifting accounted for revenues (and profits) to cover services delivered and charged at a price below costs. As the hospital bill is unbundled, charges will eventually reduce to costs at a 1:1 ratio. Not-for-profit hospitals are not allowed a return on equity or credit for bad debts as a cost of doing business.

Budgeting is a competency of nursing managers indicating responsibility and accountability. A well-prepared unit budget indicates that the best head nurse has been delegated and has accepted the responsibility for this facet of the job. Management of the budget to keep expenditures and revenues in balance indicates the nurse manager accepts responsibility for it. Within the budgetary plan the nurse manager should be allowed some flexibility in making decisions about the mix of expenditures. This would mean that monies for staff, supplies, education, and other budgeted expenses could be interchanged so long as revenues are not exceeded and the objectives of the unit are being met.

A concept related to budgeting is "value for money." Is the unit or the organization getting full value for the money expended? This question relates to such areas as turnover of personnel, waste of supplies, ineffective use of clinical skills, and inaccurate staffing standards.[10]

RELATIONSHIPS OF PATIENT ACUITY RATING SYSTEMS TO BUDGETING

Historically, nursing staffing has been based on subjective formulas; the nurse administrator with the most persuasive list of personnel needs was most successful in obtaining greater allocations. Such a list might include formulas based on research, standards of professional and government agencies, and a number of facts and statements related to average daily census, number of admissions and discharges, number of operations, and complaints of stress by nurses and about nurses by physicians and nurse managers. All budgeted positions are seldom filled and requests for increased staffing do not usually affect the bottom line—costs. A CEO can respond positively to personnel requests that will probably not be filled.

During the 1980s we have seen the disappearance and reemergence of nurse shortages, the advent of prospective payment, and a more scientific quantitative approach to nurse staffing and personnel budgeting, the Patient Classification System (PCS). A PCS is actually mandated by the Joint Commission on Accreditation of Healthcare Organizations.

Among the benefits of such a system is the reduction of nursing staff tensions. Management predicts budgetary needs for personnel using objective data. Staffing based upon needs becomes predictable to management and subsequently to the staff.

Some hospitals are using the PCS to bill for actual nursing services. They are using patient classification billing systems composed of:

1. An accurate patient classification system.
2. Staffing based on patient classification.
3. Patients rated by nurses.
4. Defined units of care.
5. Rate per unit.

The advantages of this system include elimination of inequities of flat rate billing systems that shift costs from patients requiring few units of nursing care to subsidize the nursing care of those requiring many units of nursing care. Such a system also ensures adequate reimbursement for nursing expenses. Professional nurses see value placed upon their work and their morale is boosted.

The following are early examples of patient classification billing systems:

1. St. Luke's Hospital Medical Center, Phoenix (1974): points were assigned per nursing task based on time and skills; points per support or education of patient's family or friends; five categories for general units and two for intensive care; 24-hour billing rates.

2. Montana Deaconess Medical Center (1971): patients rated twice daily by nurses by types of service provided; hourly charge; four categories for general units, four for intensive care, three for the intensive care nursery, and five for critical care.

3. Massachusetts Eye and Ear Infirmary, Boston (1975): clinical care units; dollar rate per unit;

applied to specific diagnosis; bills varied by length of stay; one-time administrative charge; room and board fee daily.

Herzog attributes 50 percent of the total hospital expense budget to nursing. Since nursing costs are buried within other categories of financial data including room rates, laboratory charges, radiology charges, and so on, the true costs of nursing must be identified. The patient classification system is one important source for identifying hours of care per category of care given per patient. Nursing research can test nursing treatment modes. These would include selection of a procedure, selection of supplies, selection of category of personnel to perform it, and comparison of outcomes.[11]

While in business and industry, technology is used to reduce costs by increasing output, the opposite has been encouraged in the health-care industry by cost-based reimbursement schemes. Increases in equipment costs and types and numbers of procedures were paid for by third-party payers. That has changed with Prospective Payment System. With control of reimbursement, less expense is best. The old revenue producers such as drugs, respiratory therapies, laboratory tests, x-rays, and others are being reimbursed at their true costs. Nursing care is the source of revenue for the future. Nurses should identify the relative value units (RVUs) of care by which they will be reimbursed. They will learn to use information systems to process data. They will select and use the supply item that does the best job for the least money. They will standardize procedures and practices and they will review and revise jobs.

Fixed costs require that a hospital maintain high productivity. If productivity declines, costs must be decreased. This is done by decreasing staff and use of supplies and making other reductions in use of resources.

THE CONTROLLING PROCESS

Now that the nursing budget has been viewed from its planning and directing aspects, it will be looked at from its controlling or evaluating aspects. The budget establishes financial standards for the division of nursing and through its cost center for each nursing unit. Feedback on a daily, weekly, monthly, and quarterly basis will supply information needed to compare managerial performance with the established standards. The results are used to make adjustments. What kind of feedback is needed by nurse managers relative to their budgets and cost control? They need information to tell whether their goals are being met. Are they exceeding the budget? Is the excess both for cost and revenues? Are the supplies and expenses of the quantity and quality planned? Is the equipment being purchased and installed as scheduled? Are employees being recruited and utilized effectively to produce the needed quality and quantity of nursing services? Is employee morale good? What adjustments need to be made? Where are the problem areas and who is responsible for them?

Budget processes should be flexible, to allow for increased and decreased volume of business. The business office provides cost-center managers with needed biometric information to make adjustments in staffing and in use of supplies.

A planning-programming-budgeting system (PPBS), developed by the Rand Corporation for the Department of Defense in the 1960s, has found application in health-care management. Using this concept the nurse administrator would prepare a total budgetary package containing:

1. Defining the objectives (planning)
2. Analyzing the contributions the proposal will make toward accomplishing organizational objectives, including all pertinent costs and benefits that are part of the proposed program (programming),
3. Budgeting all resources including all future costs and benefits
4. Completing authorized programs
5. The analysis that was employed in evaluating alternative approaches for reaching the same goals.[12]

The last criterion (5) is considered to be a key one. Again, having specific, current, practical, written objectives for the division of nursing and each of its units is imperative to planning, budgeting, and effective cost control.

It should be remembered that a budget is a plan based on the best estimates of the costs of running an organization. It cannot be inflexible, but it also cannot hide waste and inefficiency.

The nurse administrator should be sure that nurse managers will not be penalized when budgetary objectives are not met due to events beyond their control. They are working within the confines of an organizational environment that is affected by both internal and external constraints. One of the external constraints facing them is federally mandated cost control or cost containment, which is seen by some administrators as reimbursement control.

DECENTRALIZATION OF THE BUDGET

Cost-center managers, usually head nurses and supervisors of wards or units, are capable of planning and controlling their own budgets. The nurse administrator, assisted by financial managers, should prepare them to do so. Through decentralized budgeting, cost-center managers propose innovative objectives. They gather data to defend their objectives and operating plans. The unit budget becomes their responsibility and they guard its integrity with zeal. They sense when adaptations have to be made because of increased costs or decreased revenues. In these instances they make or recommend immediate remedies. Decentralized budgeting provides for internal controls.

MONITORING THE BUDGET

While various techniques have been described and defined for monitoring the budget, all budget objectives should contain procedures for quality review. These techniques include identification of a team to perform such a review. If a program is not successful—is not meeting objectives or is running above predicted costs and below predicted revenues—a decision should be made to cancel it. This is very difficult but is essential to good control. The technique of cancelling budgeted programs is sometimes referred to as "sunsetting." A nurse manager should accept the responsibility for sunsetting programs that are costly and unprofitable.

In developing the nursing budget it is necessary that the unit structures for nursing administration are comparable. This can be ensured by developing

TABLE 6–7. University of South Alabama Accounting System Report

Account statement in whole dollars for 07/31/89

Computer Date 08/03/89 — Report Page 6722
Time of Day 06:47:57 — User ID 44.2
PGM=AM090-B1 — FAS1029
Acct: 4-60680 — To: Britten Sandy
Dept: 60680 — USAMC-NRS SVC Admin

83% of fiscal year elapsed
Distribution code = 700
Medical Intensive Care Unit—8th Floor—Expense

Sub Code	Description	Budgets		Actual		Open Encumbrances	Balance Available	Perc Used
		Original	Revised	Current Month	Fiscal Year			
100	Pool—Salary & Wages	948,742	901,053				901,053	0
130	Professional Salry			72,533	775,790		775,790—	***
135	Tech Salry & Wages			4,085	50,947		50,947—	***
140	Office Salaries			4,347	53,168		53,168—	***
155	Service Empl Wages			3,936	52,195		52,195—	***
160	Student Wages		14,898	1,518	14,898			100
166	Accrued Salaries		32,791	11,462	32,791			100
	Salaries	948,742	948,742	97,880	979,789		31,047—	103
170	Pool—Empl Benefits	254,683	55,722				55,722	0
182	Employers FICA		112		112			100
183	Group Life Ins		2,569	264	2,569			100
184	Disability Ins		4,869	526	4,869			100
185	Teachers Retirement		134		134			100
188	Group Health Ins		59,973	5,887	59,973			100
198	State Paid Retiremnt		62,158	5,591	62,158			100
199	State Paid FICA		69,146	6,313	69,146			100
	Employee Benefits	254,683	254,683	18,581	198,961		55,722	78
200	Pool—Med/Surg Supply	75,000	23,920				23,920	0
211	Med & Surg Supplies		128,235	14,846	128,235			100
213	Drugs		1,317	140	1,317			100
214	Solutions		36,091	4,389	36,091			100
	Med/Surg Supplies	75,000	189,563	19,375	165,643		23,920	87
220	Pool-General Supply	5,789	2,553—				2,553—	0

Account	Description	Original	Current Month	Liquidating Expenditures	Adjustments	Current Enc	%
232	Office Supplies	1,070	19	1,069		1	100
233	Copying & Binding	36	30	36			100
234	Printing	1,494	115	1,494			100
235	Printing Paper	633	83	633			100
240	Housekeeping Supply	1,880	323	1,880			100
243	Housekeeping Furnish	1,395		1,395			100
244	Linen Replacement	214		214			100
250	Maintenance Supplies	1,001		1,001			100
270	Food Expense	619	49	619			100
	General Supplies	5,789	620	8,341	1	2,553—	144
300	Pool—Travel/Entrtain	1,005				1,005	0
316	Workshop & Training	425		425			100
	Travel/Entertainment	1,430		425		1,005	30
320	Pool—Other Expenses	12,624				12,624	0
324	Contract Service	140,390	16,720	140,390			100
336	Equip Maint & Repair	3,700		2,950	750		100
372	Books & Subscription	286		286			100
	Other Expenses	157,000	16,720	143,626	750	12,624	92
501	Minor Equipment	4,000				4,000	0
	Total Expenses	1,561,207	153,176	1,496,785	751	63,671	96
	** Account Total **	1,561,207	153,176	1,496,785	751	63,671	96

Current month detail is shown on the Report of Transactions (AM091)
Questions: University call 460-6241, USAMC call 434-3535

Open Encumbrance Status

Account	P.O. Number	P.O. Date	Description	Original Enc	Adjustments	Liquidating Expenditures	Current Enc	Last Act Date
4-60680-232	H01764	10/06/88	Waller Brothers	.85			.85	10/18/88
4-60680-336	H07584	07/24/89	Scaletronix Inc	750.00			750.00	08/01/89
			*** Account Total **	750.85			750.85	

SOURCE: The University of South Alabama Medical Center, Mobile, Alabama. Reprinted with permission.

and providing financial policies and guidelines. This approach is most successful when the top administration team works together with the budget monitor in developing such financial policies. The nurse administrator will be part of this team and will bring to its meetings standards of service that are defensible, such as data on workload including numbers and types of procedures, patients, surgical operations, and visits. These policies should reflect the long-range plans of the governing board.

Part of the information furnished to nurse administrators and managers is in the form of reports. These include statistical reports of revenues and expenditures for the current year. Table 6–7 illustrates financial information that is needed by the cost-center manager and the nursing service administrator.

It will be noted that the account number at the head of the table is 4-60680. The prefix "4" denotes that the account balance does *not* turn over at the end of the fiscal year. The cost center or department is 60680. Any financial transaction, including purchase orders for supplies and minor equipment as well as the payroll, will be identified with this cost-center number and will be charged by purchasing and accounting to this number and to the appropriate subcode, 100 through 501. Horizontal columns indicate the operational budget; the actual expenditures for the current month of July 1989 and FY 1989; any open encumbrances and the balance available. Since 83 percent of the fiscal year (beginning October 1) had elapsed, this has some relationship to the percent used column. Although 103 percent of the budgeted salary has been used, only 78 percent of employee benefits have been used, indicating a use of overtime plus part-time employees working less than the 0.5 FTE required to qualify for fringe benefits. Zero percent of the budgeted monies for minor equipment had been spent to date. The total budget expenses were 96 percent, indicating 13 percent overspending. While this report serves as a control for nurse managers, the expenditure of budgeted monies for any one subcode could cause the total expenses to date to be greater than the percent of fiscal year elapsed without creating an alarm. In this instance overspending should be related to increased census and revenues.

Table 6–8 informs the nurse managers of the specific financial transactions that took place during the month of July 1989. They can be checked against Table 6–7.

Information on revenues is reported similarly. Table 6–9 illustrates the inpatient revenue for the Medical Intensive Care Unit which includes nursing and hotel services. It is all credited to nursing.

The revenue account is 4-30815 while the cost center is the same as for expenses, 60680. The budgeted revenues for the year are listed as were the revenues for the month of July and for the fiscal year. It will be noted that while 83 percent of the fiscal year has elapsed, only 76 percent of the budget revenues have been charged. Also, Table 6–10 indicates that 76 percent of budgeted equipment revenues have been charged.

Since the amount charged is 76 percent, being less than the 83 percent of fiscal year elapsed, the nurse managers can note that revenues are behind expenses, a negative financial report that needs to be analyzed. The goal is to control this kind of financial management to the end of the fiscal year.

Additional financial information can be furnished to each nurse manager. This includes summary reports in whole dollars and for all cost centers supervised. This can be done by subcode (see Table 6–11), by subcode and cost center (see Table 6–12), and by any unit or department (see Tables 6–13 and 6–14).

"Rollover" funds, designated by prefix "3," are also included in the financial reports that can be provided to the chief nurse executive. Balances in these funds are carried over into the next fiscal year to be spent at any future date. An example of a rollover fund is account 3-64155, the maternal/child health education fund. Table 6–15 shows activities for this fund for the month of July 1989 and Table 6–16 shows how the debits were spent.

Rollover funds can be managed by the chief nurse executive, a department head, or a cost-center manager.

MOTIVATIONAL ASPECTS OF BUDGETING

Budgeting can be a motivating force for personnel—if current programs must increase in effectiveness and efficiency to remain in the budget; if decentralization and staff involvement provides an increased sense of responsibility and satisfaction; and if merit increases, promotions, and bonuses are tied to budgetary performance.

TABLE 6–8. University of South Alabama Accounting System Report

Computer Date 08/03/89
Time of Day 06:47:57
PGM=AM091

Report Page 6724
User ID 44.2
FAS1030

Distribution code = 700
Medical Intensive Care Unit—8th Floor—Expense

Acct: 4-60680
Dept: 60680

To: Britten Sandy
USAMC-NRS SVC Admin

Sub Code	Description	Date	EC	Ref.	2nd Ref.	J.E. Offset Account	Budget Entries	Current Rev/Exp	Encumbrances	Batch Ref.	Batch Date
130	Payroll Expense	07/07	64	900001		0-10080-118CR		35,017.03		PPS584	07/07
130	Payroll Expense	07/21	64	900001		0-10080-118CR		37,516.33		PPS588	07/21
130	CM Total Professional Salry							72,533.36			
135	Payroll Expense	07/07	64	900001		0-10080-118CR		1,630.89		PPS584	07/07
135	Payroll Expense	07/21	64	900001		0-10080-118CR		2,454.11		PPS588	07/21
135	CM Total Tech Salry & Wages							4,085.00			
140	Payroll Expense	07/07	64	900001		0-10080-118CR		2,082.44		PPS584	07/07
140	Payroll Expense	07/21	64	900001		0-10080-118CR		2,264.26		PPS588	07/21
140	CM Total Office Salaries							4,346.70			
155	Payroll Expense	07/07	64	900001		0-10080-118CR		1,884.26		PPS584	07/07
155	Payroll Expense	07/21	64	900001		0-10080-118CR		2,051.29		PPS588	07/21
155	CM Total Service Empl Wages							3,935.55			
160	Payroll Expense	07/07	64	900001		0-10080-118CR		494.83		PPS584	07/07
160	Payroll Expense	07/21	64	900001		0-10080-118CR		1,022.81		PPS588	07/21
160	CM Total Student Wages							1,517.64			
166	Susp Corr/Accr Sal	06/30	60		S01544	0-13000-160CR		65.00		HJV002	07/10
166	Susp Corr/Accr Sal	06/30	60		S01543	0-13000-160CR		45.00		HJV002	07/10
	RVS Accrd Sal & Wage	07/01	60		075101	0-15300-220DR		40,318.00—		HJV001	07/10
	RVS Accrd Sal & Wage	07/01	60		075101	0-15300-220DR		65.00—		HJV001	07/10
	RVS Accrd Sal & Wage	07/01	60		075101	0-15300-220DR		45.00—		HJV001	07/10
	Accrued Sal & Wages	07/31	60		075100	0-15300-220CR		51,780.00		HJV019	07/31
166	CM Total Accrued Salaries							11,462.00			

(continued)

167

TABLE 6–8. (Continued)

Computer Date 08/03/89
Time of Day 06:47:57
PGM=AM091

Report Page 6724
User ID 44.2
FAS1030

Report of transactions for 07/31/89

Distribution code = 700

Medical Intensive Care Unit—8th Floor—Expense

Acct: 4-60680
Dept: 60680

To: Britten Sandy
USAMC-NRS SVC Admin

Sub Code	Description	Date	EC	Ref.	2nd Ref.	J.E. Offset Account	Budget Entries	Current Rev/Exp	Encumbrances	Batch Ref.	Batch Date
183	Payroll Expense	07/21	64	900001		2-77000-180CR		264.04		PPS588	07/21
183	CM Total Group Life Ins							264.04			
184	Payroll Expense	07/21	64	900001		2-77000-180CR		526.48		PPS588	07/21
184	CM Total Disability Ins							526.48			
188	Payroll Expense	07/07	64	900001		2-77000-180CR		65.81		PPS584	07/07
188	Payroll Expense	07/21	64	900001		2-77000-180CR		5,821.12		PPS588	07/21
188	CM Total Group Health Ins							5,886.93			
198	Payroll Expense	07/07	64	900001		2-77000-180CR		2,659.96		PPS584	07/07
198	Payroll Expense	07/21	64	900001		2-77000-180CR		2,930.66		PPS588	07/21
198	CM Total State Paid Retiremnt							5,590.62			
199	Payroll Expense	07/07	64	900001		2-77000-180CR		3,019.55		PPS584	07/07
199	Payroll Expense	07/21	64	900001		2-77000-180CR		3,293.55		PPS588	07/21
199	CM Total State Paid FICA							6,313.10			
211	Inventory Exp Alloc	07/31	60		075264	0-12100-140CR		14,845.75		HJV027	07/31
211	CM Total Med & Surg Supplies							14,845.75			
213	Pharmacy Distrib—Jul	07/31	60		075006	4-60730-213CR		140.34		HJV033	07/31
213	CM Total Drugs							140.34			

214	Inventory Exp Alloc	07/31	60		075264	0-12100-140CR	4,389.27		HJV027	07/31
214	CM Total Solutions						4,389.27			
232	Inventory Exp Alloc	07/31	60		075264	0-12100-140CR	19.49		HJV027	07/31
232	CM Total Office Supplies						19.49			
233	Xerox Expense-J/J 89	07/31	60		075008	4-60960-965CR	30.21		HJV026	07/31
233	CM Total Copying & Binding						30.21			
234	Print Shop Chrgs—Jul	07/26	60		075011	4-60960-960CR	115.20		HJV013	07/27
234	CM Total Printing						115.20			
235	Inventory Exp Alloc	07/31	60		075264	0-12100-140CR	82.69		HJV027	07/31
235	CM Total Printing Paper						82.69			
240	Inventory Exp Alloc	07/31	60		075264	0-12100-140CR	323.42		HJV027	07/31
240	CM Total Housekeeping Supply						323.42			
270	Inventory Exp Alloc	07/31	60		075264	0-12100-140CR	48.61		HJV027	07/31
270	CM Total Food Expense						48.61			
324	Nephrology Applicati	07/26	68		563631	0-15030-211CR	3,520.00		HPD850	07/26
324	Accure Jly	07/31	60		075259	0-15030-210CR	13,200.00		HJV024	07/31
324	CM Total Contract Service						16,720.00			
336	Scaletronix Inc	07/24	50	H07584				750.00	HEN010	07/31
336	CM Total Equip Maint & Repair							750.00		
	*** Account Total ***						153,176.40	750.00		

Source: The University of South Alabama Medical Center, Mobile, Alabama. Reprinted with permission.

TABLE 6–9. University of South Alabama Accounting System Report

Account statement in whole dollars for 07/31/89

Computer Date 08/03/89
Time of Day 06:47:57
PGM=AM090-B1

83% of fiscal year elapsed
Distribution code = 700
Medical Intensive Care Unit—8th Floor—Revenue

Report Page 6557
User ID 44.2
FAS1029

Acct: 4-30815
Dept: 60680

To: Asst Admin—Nursing
USAMC-NRS SVC Admin

Tab Code	Description	Budgets		Actual		Open Encumbrances	Balance Available	Perc Used
		Original	Revised	Current Month	Fiscal Year			
040								
0/0	Inpatient Revenue	1,511,400—	1,511,400—	115,500—	1,146,600—		364,800—	76
	Total Revenues	1,511,400—	1,511,400—	115,500—	1,146,600—		364,800—	76
	** Account Total **	1,511,400—	1,511,400—	115,500—	1,146,600—		364,800—	76

Current month detail is shown on the Report of Transactions (AM091)
Questions: University call 460-6241, USAMC call 434-3535

Source: The University of South Alabama Medical Center, Mobile, Alabama. Reprinted with permission.

TABLE 6–10. University of South Alabama Accounting System Report

Account statement in whole dollars for 07/31/89

Computer Date 08/03/89	Report Page 6559
Time of Day 06:47:57	User ID 44.2
PGM=AM090-B1	FAS1029

83% of fiscal year elapsed
Distribution code = 700
Medical Intensive Care Unit—SP&D—Revenue 8TH FLR

Acct: 4-30818
Dept: 60680

To: Asst Admin—Nursing
USAMC-NRS SVC Admin

Sub Code	Description	Budgets		Actual		Open Encumbrances	Balance Available	Perc Used
		Original	Revised	Current Month	Fiscal Year			
040	Inpatient Revenue		1,080,088—	101,637—	818,031—		262,057—	76
	Total Revenues		1,080,088—	101,637—	818,031—		262,057—	76
	** Account Total **		1,080,088—	101,637—	818,031—		262,057—	76

Current month detail is shown on the Report of Transactions (AM091)
Questions: University call 460-6241, USAMC call 434-3535.

Source: The University of South Alabama Medical Center, Mobile, Alabama. Reprinted with permission.

171

TABLE 6–11. University of South Alabama Accounting System Report

Summary report in whole dollars for 07/31/89

Distribution code = 750

Report Page 106
User ID 44.2
FAS1033

Sub Code	Description	Budgets		Actual			Open Commitments	Balance Available	Perc Used
		Original	Revised	Current Month	Fiscal Year	Project Year			
001	Prior Year Balance		302,976					302,978	0
002	Transfers								0
010	Income	16,419,272–	16,419,272–	1,342,529–	13,782,618–	13,782,618–		2,636,654–	84
020	Income			13,078–	127,981–	127,981–		127,981	0
023	Interest Income			1,353–	11,022–	11,022–		11,022	0
025	Original Budget 86/87	600,000–	600,000–	77,740–	1,236,565–	1,236,565–		636,565	206
026				191–	210–	210–		210	0
028	Bad Debt Recovery				169,932	169,932		169,932–	0
030									0
040	Inpatient Revenue			1,852–	29,682–	29,682–		29,682	0
041	Outpatient RF								0
042	Outpatient ED								0
050	Ded/Gross Revenue	75,009,000	75,009,000	8,904,127	72,586,402	72,586,402		2,422,598	97
099	State Paid Benefits								0
	Total Revenues	57,989,728	58,292,706	7,467,383	57,568,256	57,568,256		724,450	99

100	Pool—Salary & Wages	1,416,748	82,157				82,157	0
110	Exec & Adm Salaries		170,518	23,443	170,518	170,518		100
120	Instruction Salaries							0
130	Professional Salary		210,392	15,839	210,592	210,592	200—	100
131	Interns Salaries							0
135	Tech Salary & Wages		11,906	1,195	11,906	11,906		100
140	Office Salaries		840,893	79,028	840,893	843,866	2,973—	100
150	Craft/Trade Wages				143	808	808—	0
155	Service Empl Wages					154	154—	0
159	Temp Craft/Trade Wge					2,431	2,431—	0
160	Student Wages		20,975	2,678	20,975	20,975		100
164								0
166	Accrued Salaries		41,158	10,264	41,158	41,158		100
167								0
168	Tuition Reimbursemnt		6,971	2,756	6,971	6,971		100
169	Budget Correction							0
	Salaries	1,416,748	1,384,969	135,202	1,303,156	1,309,378	75,591	95
170	Pool—Empl Benefits	340,007	116,982				116,982	0
180	Employee Benefits	187,747	205,413	3,318	421,300	421,300	215,888—	205
181	Unemployment Ins	41,307	41,307	7,722	22,717	22,717	18,590	55
182	Employers FICA	266	266	54	266	1,871	1,605—	703
183	Group Life Ins	91,969—	91,969—	435	91,969—	91,967—	3—	100
184	Disability Ins	9,090	9,090	1,015	9,106	9,110	20—	100
185	Teachers Retirement	4	4		4	4		100
186	Meal Books							0
187	TIAA-CREF Retirement	2,068	2,068	259	2,068	2,068		100
188	Group Health Ins	96,262	96,262	12,650	116,322	116,342	20,080—	121
190	Tuition Reimbursemnt	56,911	56,911	7,955	49,916	49,916	6,996	88

SOURCE: The University of South Alabama Medical Center, Mobile, Alabama. Reprinted with permission.

TABLE 6–12. University of South Alabama Accounting System Report

Subcode summary audit report for 07/31/89

Computer Date 08/03/89   Distribution code = 750   Report Page 111
Time of Day 05:06:11   User ID 44.2
PGM=AM095-B1   BUS1033

Sub Code	Subcode Description	Original Budget	Revised Budget	Current Month	Year to Date	Project to Date	Open Commitments	Balance Available
001								
364100	General Hospital Fnd	0.00	30,653.57	0.00	0.00	0.00	0.00	30,653.57
364105	Burn Unit	0.00	22,495,81	0.00	0.00	0.00	0.00	22,495.81
364110	Intensv Care Nursery	0.00	4,438,37	0.00	0.00	0.00	0.00	4,438.37
364120	J Erwin Ped Surgery	0.00	942.96−	0.00	0.00	0.00	0.00	942.96−
364127	Heart Statn—Holters	0.00	14,205.00	0.00	0.00	0.00	0.00	14,205.00
364173	Helping Hands/3&4 Fl	0.00	3,618.70	0.00	0.00	0.00	0.00	3,618.70
364174	Telethon—C&W USAMC	0.00	32,797.51	0.00	0.00	0.00	0.00	32,797.51
364175	Heart Fund Donations	0.00	864.10	0.00	0.00	0.00	0.00	864.10
364176	Telethon—C&W 1987	0.00	71,327.96	0.00	0.00	0.00	0.00	71,827.96
364178	WOCD/Palmer Mem Fund	0.00	1,403.81	0.00	0.00	0.00	0.00	1,403.81
364179	Telethon—C&W 1988	0.00	122,923.92	0.00	0.00	0.00	0.00	122,923.92
364197	Payroll Inserter	0.00	1,308.00−	0.00	0.00	0.00	0.00	1,308.00−
	Subcode Total	0.00	302,977.79	0.00	0.00	0.00	0.00	302,977.79

SOURCE: The University of South Alabama Medical Center, Mobile, Alabama. Reprinted with permission.

Budgeting facilitates communication within interdependent departments, thus increasing knowledge and understanding of other areas. It provides needed learning opportunities for future nurse managers.

The budget can be dysfunctional and fail to facilitate attainment of organizational objectives when it is viewed as an end rather than a means. This happens:

- If it is inflexible and permits no deviation from the established plan.
- If it is viewed as being externally imposed by administrators who do not understand patient care.
- If health-care providers feel left out of budget decisions.
- If there is an overemphasis on staying within the budget, leading to a decrease in interdepartmental communication and cooperation.
- If managers are held accountable without being given authority.[13]

Using the Budget for Innovation

In many hospitals head nurses manage from twenty-five to thirty full-time and part-time staff members, with operating budgets exceeding a million dollars. This is as much as other major department heads manage, and more than some. The nurse executive encourages and supports head nurses to develop simulated budgets for proposed expansion and changes in utilization of facilities or modification of unit schedules. Well-qualified head nurses do not need to be overseen by directors of nursing so closely that their creativity is stifled. When such excessive oversight occurs the head nurses often spend time doing the work of directors rather than their own. In a decentralized organization the head nurses are department heads who develop their

TABLE 6–13. University of South Alabama Accounting System Report

Responsibility roll-up report as of 07/31/89

Revenue—Britten

Time of Day 05:09:39
PGM=AM047-H1

Cost-Center 9-82301
Reports to: 9-81000
Ledgers: 4

To: Britten Sandy

	Budgets		Actual			Open Commitments	Balance Available	Perc Used
	Original	Revised A	Current Month	Fiscal Year	Project Year B	C	A-B-C	(B+C)/A
Responsibility Units								
Cardiovas Rehab	790—	790—		869—	869—		79	110
Revenue-Enter Thpy	3,968—	3,968—	2,960—	39,582—	39,582—		35,614	997
Chemothrapy-O/P Revn	90,729—	90,729—	15,107—	110,452—	110,452—		19,723	121
Clinical Research Un	268,800—	482,051—	34,340—	346,521—	346,521—		135,530—	71
Cardiac ICU	1,524,600—	3,254,816—	252,996—	2,426,084—	2,426,084—		828,732—	74
Orthopedic Cast Room	108,459—	108,459—	8,128—	91,765—	91,765—		16,696—	84
5th Floor North/Reve	31,592—	31,592—	4,013—	39,076—	39,076—		7,484	123
5th Floor South/Reve	2,054,000—	2,977,320—	236,359—	2,331,656—	2,331,656—		645,664—	78
Psychiatric Unit/Rev	1,701,300—	1,725,507—	137,906—	1,463,792—	1,463,792—		261,715—	84
8th Flr Medical/Reve	2,315,220—	2,959,584—	216,324—	2,456,181—	2,456,181—		503,403—	82
Medical ICU/Revenue	1,773,840—	2,853,928—	244,778—	2,232,035—	2,232,035—		621,893—	78
Coronary Care/Revenu	2,148,888—	2,148,888—	167,130—	1,801,879—	1,801,879—		347,010—	83
6th Flr Surgical/Rev	1,787,100—	2,409,563—	172,079—	1,930,916—	1,930,916—		478,648—	80
Burn Center/Revenue	1,254,000—	3,090,809—	193,436—	2,155,646—	2,155,646—		935,163—	69
9th Flr Surgical/Rev	2,029,260—	3,122,028—	230,728—	2,446,790—	2,446,790—		675,238—	78
Neuro/Trauma ICU/Rev	1,504,800—	1,504,800—	111,100—	1,035,650—	1,035,650—		469,150—	68
Newborn Nursery/Reve	804,600—	896,817—	87,603—	794,535—	794,535—		102,282—	88
Premature Nursy/Reve	615,672—	615,672—	71,803—	596,432—	596,432—		19,240—	96
Neonatal Nursy/Reven	4,692,600—	5,468,373—	580,112—	5,178,067—	5,178,067—		290,306—	94
Obstetric Unit/Reven	1,930,440—	2,379,997—	217,489—	2,091,217—	2,091,217—		288,781—	87
Pediatric Unit/Reven	1,438,080—	2,013,282—	171,673—	1,658,513—	1,658,513—		354,769—	82
Pediatric ICU/Revenu	1,141,800—	1,915,268—	115,489—	1,208,778—	1,208,778—		706,490—	63

(continued)

175

TABLE 6–13. (Continued)

Responsibility roll-up report as of 07/31/89

Revenue—Britten

Time of Day 05:09:39
PGM=AM047-H1

Report Page 11
User ID XX.1
Page 1

Cost-Center 9-82301
Reports to: 9-81000
Ledgers: 4

To: Britten Sandy

| | Budgets | | Actual | | | Open Commitments | Balance Available | Perc Used |
	Original	Revised A	Current Month	Fiscal Year	Project Year B	C	A-B-C	(B+C)/A
Delivery Room/Reven	3,396,552—	3,396,552—	410,192—	3,553,291—	3,553,291—		156,738	104
Emergency Room	4,922,867—	4,922,867—	446,310—	4,716,353—	4,716,353—		206,514—	95
Total	37,539,957—	48,373,660—	4,128,055—	40,706,080—	40,706,080—		7,667,586—	84
Rev/Exp by Fund								
Operating Revenues	37,539,957—	48,373,660—	4,128,055—	40,706,080—	40,706,080—		7,667,586—	84
Total	37,539,957—	48,373,660—	4,128,055—	40,706,080—	40,706,080—		7,667,586—	84
Rev/Exp by Type								
Revenues	37,539,957	48,373,660	4,128,055	40,706,080	40,706,080		7,667,586	84
Expenses								
Salaries								
Employee Benefits								
Med/Sur Supply								
Office/Other Suply								
Travel/Entertain								
Other Expenses								
Minor Equipment								
Cost Offsets								
Total Expenses								

SOURCE: The University of South Alabama Medical Center, Mobile, Alabama. Reprinted with permission.

176

TABLE 6–14. University of South Alabama Accounting System Report

Computer Date 08/03/89
Time of Day 05:09:39
PGM=AM047-H1

Report Page 9
User ID XX.1
Page 1

Responsibility roll-up report as of 07/31/89

Expense—Britten

Cost-Center 9-82300
Reports to: 9-81000
Ledgers: 4

To: Britten Sandy

| | Budgets | | Actual | | | Open | Balance | Perc |
	Original	Revised A	Current Month	Fiscal Year	Project Year B	Commitments C	Available A–B–C	Used (B+C)/A
Responsibility Units								
Medical Nursing	1,446,644	1,561,207	153,176	1,496,785	1,496,785	751	63,671	95
Psychiatric Nursing	659,186	661,552	63,520	590,664	590,664	566	70,323	89
Staff Development	274,449	274,748	17,680	295,828	295,828	2	21,082—	107
Nursing Svcs-Admin	869,036	880,078	91,347	779,791	779,791	6,242	94,044	89
Clinical Resch Unit	211,846	222,854	17,962	250,545	250,545	16	27,707—	112
Cardiac ICU	429,808	429,807	3,424	53,440	53,440		376,367	12
Float Nurses Pool			110	2,589	2,589		2,589—	
Orthopedic Cast Room	27,195	27,196		12,461	12,461	1,172	13,563	50
Employee Health Nurs	155,423	155,423	18,779	149,601	149,601	5	5,817	96
9th Floor-North	527,221	527,222	46,442	496,133	496,133	98	30,991	94
9th Floor-South	521,411	521,412	40,785	461,240	461,240	2	60,170	88
8th Floor-Medical	810,508	894,965	109,696	1,131,504	1,131,504	1,557	238,095—	126
5th Floor-Shrd Supp	66,529	157,455	25,770	185,295	185,295	862	28,702—	118
Burn Center	546,449	940,030	77,567	836,022	836,022	3,353	100,656	89
6th Floor-Surgical	1,222,187	1,363,087	117,908	1,278,709	1,278,709	2,101	82,276	93
Surgical ICU	1,074,332	1,332,394	138,564	1,309,157	1,309,157	338	22,899	98
7th Floor-Shrd Supp	626,522	696,032	72,802	833,026	833,026	787	137,781—	119
Newborn Nursery	667,925	939,910	81,197	892,992	892,992	868	46,051	95

(continued)

177

TABLE 6–14. (*Continued*)

Computer Date 08/03/89
Time of Day 05:09:39
PGM=AM047-H1

Cost-Center 9-82300
Reports to: 9-81000
Ledgers: 4

Responsibility roll-up report as of 07/31/89

Expense—Britten

Report Page 9
User ID XX.1
Page 1

To: Britten Sandy

	Budgets		Actual			Open Commitments	Balance Available	Perc Used
	Original	Revised A	Current Month	Fiscal Year	Project Year B	C	A-B-C	(B+C)/A
Intermediate Nursery	236,612							
Intensive Care Nursy	1,810,927	1,944,960	202,179	1,749,864	1,749,864	1,241	193,856	90
Obstetric Unit	628,047	668,254	64,748	632,055	632,055	226	35,974	94
Pediatric Unit	923,577	998,643	91,105	895,375	895,375	263	103,005	89
Pediatric ICU	560,288	645,410	48,874	568,314	568,314	50	77,045	88
Delivery Room	1,113,286	1,208,604	134,770	1,107,944	1,107,944	20,154	80,506	93
Emergency Room	1,613,253	1,691,149	160,935	1,524,713	1,524,713	13,885	152,550	90
Patient Transport	220,377	220,377	18,889	186,146	186,146	40	34,191	84
Total	17,243,038	18,962,769	1,798,229	17,720,193	17,720,193	54,579	1,187,999	93
Rev/Exp by Fund								
Nursing Division	17,060,420	18,750,317	1,771,862	17,527,171	17,527,171	53,402	1,169,746	93
Professional Division	27,195	57,029	7,588	43,421	43,421	1,172	12,436	78
Administrative Divis	155,423	155,423	18,779	149,601	149,601	5	5,817	96
Total	17,243,038	18,962,769	1,798,229	17,720,193	17,720,193	54,579	1,187,999	93

Rev/Exp by Type

Revenues

Expenses

Salaries	12,382,495	12,461,654	1,256,095	12,391,869	12,391,869		69,785	99
Employee Benefits	3,031,241	3,033,250	239,363	2,487,863	2,487,863		545,387	82
Med/Sur Supply	1,502,492	3,020,154	262,420	2,447,985	2,447,985	30,781	541,387	82
Office/Other Suply		109,306	9,788	107,656	107,656	1,652		100
Travel/Entertain	43,989	45,788	2,209	27,555	27,555		18,233	60
Other Expenses	212,976	211,676	19,555	196,765	196,765	4,019	10,891	94
Minor Equipment	55,585	66,681	7,590	21,443	21,443	18,127	27,113	59
Cost Offsets	14,060	14,060	1,209	39,057	39,057		24,797—	273
Total Expenses	17,243,038	18,962,769	1,798,229	17,720,193	17,720,193	54,579	1,187,999	93
Net Revenue/Expense	17,243,038	18,962,769	1,798,229	17,720,193	17,720,193	54,579	1,187,999	93
Total	17,243,038	18,962,769	1,798,229	17,720,193	17,720,193	54,579	1,187,999	93

Source: The University of South Alabama Medical Center, Mobile, Alabama. Reprinted with permission.

179

TABLE 6–15. University of South Alabama Accounting System Report

Account statement in whole dollars for 07/31/89

Computer Date 08/03/89	83% of fiscal year elapsed
Time of Day 06:47:57	Distribution code = 700
PGM=AM090-B1	Maternal Child Health Education Fund

Report Page 6544
User ID 44.2
FAS1029

Acct: 3-64155
Dept: 64155

To: Mair Betty
USAMC—Nursing Svc

Sub Code	Description	Budgets		Actual		Open Encumbrances	Balance Available	Perc Used
		Original	Revised	Current Month	Fiscal Year			
001	Prior Year Balance		3,624				3,624	0
020	Income				5,285−		5,285	***
021	Refunds				55		55−	***
	Total Revenues		3,624		5,230−		8,854	144−
224	Recreation Supplies				60		60−	***
231	Postage				60		60−	***
234	Printing				257		257−	***
	General Supplies				377		377−	***
311	Travel			459	1,463		1,463−	***
314	Local Travel				27		27−	***
316	Workshop & Training			3,338	3,498	2,500	5,998−	***
	Travel/Entertainment			3,796	4,989	2,500	7,489−	***
422	Honorarium				425		425−	***
450	Expense Offset				1,000−		1,000	***
	Total Expenses			3,796	4,790	2,500	7,290−	***
	** Account Total **		3,624	3,796	440−	2,500	1,563	57

Current month detail is shown on the report of transactions (AM091)
Questions: University call 460-6241, USAMC call 434-3535

Open Encumbrance Status

Account	P.O. Number	P.O. Date	Description	Original Enc	Liquidating Expenditures	Adjustments	Current Enc	Last Act Date
3-64155-316	H04118	01/26/89	Perdido Hilton Hotel	2,500.00			2,500.00	03/22/89
			*** Account Total ***	2,500.00			2,500.00	

TABLE 6–16. University of South Alabama Accounting System Report

Computer Date 08/03/89　　　　Report of transactions for 07/31/89　　　　Report Page 6545
Time of Day 06:47:57　　　　　　　　Distribution code = 700　　　　　　　　　User ID 44.2
PGM=AM090　　　　　　　　　Maternal Child Health Education Fund　　　　　FAS1030

Acct: 3-64155　　　　　　　　　　　　　　　　　　　　　　　To: Mair Betty
Dept: 64155　　　　　　　　　　　　　　　　　　　　　　　　USAMC—Nursing Svc

Sub Code	Description	Date	EC	Ref.	2nd Ref.	J.E. Offset Account	Budget Entries	Current Rev/Exp	Encumbrances	Batch Ref.	Batch Date
311	Dorothy May	07/11	48		218418			458.65		HPC804	07/11
311	CM Total Travel							458.65			
316	Perdido Beach Hilton	07/19	48		220893			3,337.73		HPC832	07/19
316	CM Total Workshop & Training							3,337.73			
	*** Account Total ***							3,796.38			

SOURCE: The University of South Alabama Medical Center, Mobile, Alabama. Reprinted with permission.

181

FIGURE 6–9. New Programs

1. Expand the intensive care bed capacity.
2. Establish a helicopter aeromedical evacuation service.
3. Replace monitoring equipment in MICU.
4. Update defibrillators.
5. Expand clinical ladder levels II and III.
6. Reorganize nursing administration.

own objectives, programs, and budgets. They are assisted by staff experts in such tasks as staffing and scheduling.

Proposals originated in this way present a variety of options and are subject to cost/benefit analysis, a process with which the head nurses thus become familiar. They are provided with staff service in this area by the chief nurse executive or a staff expert.

New Programs

Complete management plans should be made if new programs are to be implemented. The plans should include objectives; actions that identify procedures, supplies, equipment, and personnel; target dates for implementing each action; and accomplishments noted as they occur. Figure 6–9 illustrates a list of programs that would require such management plans.

CUTTING THE BUDGET

When the budget has to be cut, planning is a vital aspect of the process. This is happening today as hospital admissions and stays decrease and reimbursement takes on a new character. The form and the process of nursing management can determine the course of events when the budget has to be cut.

A nursing administration that delegates decision making to the lowest level and encourages participative management is an effective administration. When clinical nurses are informed at the unit level and invited to give their input, they will help with suggestions for cutting costs. They will

later implement and support the activities they view as resulting partly from their input. A nursing organization that promotes self-direction at the clinical nurse level, head nurse level, clinical consultant level, and executive nurse level will support direction to reduce cost and to increase productivity and profit. As an example, when a hospital CEO discovered that self-pay patient care was the only category not reviewed for use of resources, a review process was established by a clinical nurse. This process was supported by physicians and other health care professionals.

Nursing budgets are enormous, with budgets for a single unit running into hundreds of thousands of dollars a year. Pay awards or increases have to be met by budget cuts (personnel cutbacks), use of cheaper supplies and techniques, or increased productivity. The latter requires more paying patients, shorter stays, and increased sales of all paying services. When personnel cuts are to be made, numbers make nursing vulnerable. Some cuts can come from all services but nursing has greater numbers. The nurse manager who controls these numbers daily, weekly, and yearly will have greater credibility. Many sources indicate that turnover is costly. The cost of turnover of personnel low on the salary scale is sometimes weighed against the higher cost of employees who are at the top of the salary scale. An assumption is made that long-term employees are better satisfied with their jobs and do better work, an assumption that needs to be validated through research.

As workload data indicates shifts from one unit to another, resources must be shifted. This can be done by asking for volunteers, moving vacated positions, and using PRN pools. There is a shift today from inpatient procedures in hospitals to outpatient procedures, either in hospitals or ambulatory surgery centers. Also, many more diagnostic procedures are done on an outpatient basis. As a result, inpatients are often a sicker group.

Because nurse administrators control multimillion dollar budgets they are powerful people. They are also vulnerable for personnel cuts. Much of this vulnerability stems from external controls imposed by the state and federal governments and health insurance companies. Power comes from the ability of nurse administrators to use knowledge and skills in defending their budgets and in directing and controlling them. They learn to hold the line on staffing, on overtime, and on appropriate use for items of supply and equipment.

Development of an Operating Room Budget

Prior to 1982, prices in hospitals were developed to maximize reimbursement. Inflated prices were charged for ancillary services such as pharmacy, radiology, and respiratory therapy. The semiofficial base for determining costs and setting prices or charges has been the Medicare Cost Report. It is used by other third-party payers and although some financial people indicate there could be better ways of determining health care costs, either none have been developed or they have not been used.

The data in Table 6–17 have been extracted from the Medicare Cost Report of the University of South Alabama Medical Center. They are for FY 1987–88.

The charges are greater than the costs, indicating no adjustments should be made. However, in previous years costs exceeded charges in the operating room while in other services the charges greatly exceeded the costs. These inequities in the costing and pricing of health-care services are gradually being addressed as services become more competitive and as reimbursement mechanisms change with prospective payment.

The Operating Room Committee

In the past, many nursing managers did not deal with their own budget, leaving it to financial managers. In select areas of a hospital, the budget is still not based upon good quantitative data. The surgical suite or operating room is one of these. The budget here needs to be developed based on policies laid down by the operating room committee. The committee should include the nursing manager and a representative of hospital administration. Policy will be developed that answers the following questions:

1. What are the total hours needed for delivery of service?
2. How will these hours be distributed?
3. How will emergencies be staffed?

4. What will be included in the costs of running an operating room?

Total Hours

The total hours needed for delivery of service can be based on historical data. A decision will be made as to what time is counted. It can be from the call for the patient to delivery to the recovery room. These data can be kept on a computer. Coordination with the chair of the department of surgery will elicit information on expansion of services, since this individual will usually know of new services coming into the area that will increase the need for personnel, equipment, and supplies.

Once an estimate is made of the total hours of service expected, staffing can be estimated. Productive hours per FTE can be established by subtracting nonproductive time, including meal breaks, staff development, and other time, from 40 hours per week. If productive time is determined to be 36 hours per week and each FTE is estimated to work 48 weeks per year after vacation and illness, then each FTE produces 1728 hours of work per year. Two nurses or one R.N. and 1 L.P.N. are required per team.

If operating hours are estimated to be:

Day shift (8 rooms × 8 hours × 260 days)   16,640

Emergencies   2,400

The number of FTEs needed to staff will be:

Day shift: 16,640 ÷ 1728 × 2 = 38.52 = 39 FTE

Emergencies: 2,400 ÷ 1728 × 2 = 2.78 = 3 FTE.

If it is decided to staff weekends, evenings, and nights, emergencies can be covered in this manner.

Distribution of Hours

Distribution of hours of operating room services needs to be based on policy agreed upon by the surgical committee. The following can be an example:

1. Eight rooms, 5 days a week.
2. One room, 2 days a week for weekend emergencies.

TABLE 6–17. The Operating Room Budget (Expenses)

Operating Room
  Direct expenses (directly assigned)
  Salaries
  Other (employee benefits, personnel services, supplies, etc.)

Total	$3,039,624

Indirect Expenses Apportioned to O.R., Capital Buildings & Fixtures

(square feet—percentage to total depreciated over 30 year period)	$ 29,882
Capital Equipment, Movable (Dollar value. Each item has useful life)	127,318
Employee Benefits (Workmen's Compensation, Life Insurance, etc.)	21,968
Communications (number of instruments)	8,353
Data Processing (units of service)	29,414
Purchasing (supply expense)	51,441
Admitting (gross inpatient revenue)	54,359
Patient Accounts (total revenue)	142,070
General Administration (accumulative costs)	127,406
Plant Operations (square footage)	164,804
Biomedical (labor hours)	19,901
Laundry (pounds)	–0–
Housekeeping (man hours)	78,269
Nursing Administration (FTEs)	95,191
Patient Transport (survey 2 weeks)	141
Preparation (time study 2 weeks)	677,103
Central Supply (costed requisitions)	28,276
Pharmacy (costed requisitions)	4,380
College of Nursing (cost allocated in on FTEs)	79,392
Interns and residents (surgical residents) and others	1,575,480
Total Costs	6,354,772
Total Charges	8,774,102
Cost-to-charge ratio	0.724265

SOURCE: The University of South Alabama Medical Center, Mobile, Alabama. Reprinted with permission.

3. One room, 7 evenings a week for emergencies.
4. One room, 7 nights a week for emergencies.

Policies will cover elective schedules for evening, night and weekend shifts, and call teams.

The total FTEs needed to run the staffing of these rooms will be:

1. Day shift	39 FTE
2. Day shift weekends	1 FTE
3. Evening shift	3 FTE
4. Night shift	3 FTE
5. Management	2 FTE
6. Clerical	3 FTE
7. Housekeeping and transport	5 FTE
Total	56 FTE

A budget can now be prepared for the operating room using the format shown in Figure 6–10.

FIGURE 6–10. Operating Room Budget (Hours)

Estimated Operating Hours 19,040

Personnel		Budget
RNs	25 × average hourly rate × 2080 hours	$ _____ . _____
LPNs	23 × average hourly rate × 2080 hours	_____ . _____
Clerks	3 × average hourly rate × 2080 hours	_____ . _____
Housekeeping and transport	5 × average hourly rate × 2080 hours	_____ . _____
Total for 56 FTEs		_____ . _____
Fringe benefits @ _____ percent of total		_____ . _____
Overtime @ _____ percent of total		_____ . _____
Call @ _____ percent of total		_____ . _____
Staff development		_____ . _____
Total personnel budget		_____ . _____
Supplies (previous cost per hour plus any allowance for inflation × 19,040)		_____ . _____
Indirect costs apportioned		
Building depreciation (square feet × rate)		$ _____ . _____
Equipment depreciation (amount of inventory × rate)		_____ . _____
Administration (square feet × rate including nursing administration, hospital administration)		_____ . _____
Operation of plant (square feet × rate)		_____ . _____
Laundry and linen		_____ . _____
Housekeeping in excess of personnel budget (square feet × rate)		_____ . _____
Central sterile supply		_____ . _____
Intern-Resident Service (FTEs × hourly rate × 2080 hours)		_____ . _____
Employee benefits		_____ . _____
Communications		_____ . _____
Data processing		_____ . _____
Purchasing		_____ . _____
Admitting		_____ . _____
Patient accounts		_____ . _____
Biomedical		_____ . _____

(continued)

FIGURE 6–10. Operating Room Budget (Hours) *(continued)*

Preparation	_____ . _____
Pharmacy	_____ . _____
College of Nursing	_____ . _____
Total indirect	_____ . _____
Working capital (accounts receivable and inventories)	_____ . _____
Capital (land, buildings and equipment to be bought)	_____ . _____
Profit or return on equity (If allowed)	_____ . _____
Deductions from patient revenues or bad debts (If allowed)	_____ . _____
Total Costs (Expenses)	_____ . _____
Charges per hour (total expenses ÷ estimated operating hours of 19,040)	_____ . _____

Legitimate Budget Activities

It is the contention of the author that hospitals should be managed like other businesses. Charges should be determined from costs and should include allowance for profits or return on equity and for bad debts. The practice of cost shifting to make certain services revenue producers should be stopped.

Oszustowizc suggests a seven-step system by which total financial requirements eventually determine the gross patient revenue equal to meet the financial needs of a department. These seven steps are:

1. Detail demand for nursing services and equipment needs.
2. Detail direct expenses.
3. Detail indirect expenses.
4. Detail working capital requirements.
5. Detail capital requirements.
6. Detail earnings (profit) requirements.
7. Detail deductions from patient revenues.[14]

SUMMARY

It is important for nurse managers to have a working knowledge of the objectives of a cost-accounting system and of such components as cost factors, fixed costs, variable costs, direct costs, indirect costs, service units, costing standards, charts of accounts, inventories, cost transfers, and performance reporting. Every activity that takes place in a hospital costs money. There must be a standard for assigning costs to user departments. The nursing department should pay its user share and no more. Knowledge of the cost-accounting system will provide accurate information for budgeting and for cost management.

Budgeting operations for the nursing manager include those for personnel, supplies and equipment, and capital budgets. The nursing personnel budget for today's hospital is based on accurately quantified data from a patient acuity rating system. Nurse managers thus need to develop a staffing philosophy and plans that will expand and contract staffing to provide for fluctuation. This can be partially done with part-time personnel, float pools, and the use of historical census data.

Nursing personnel budgets will be ultimately regarded as revenue budgets as laws and regulations change to allow for direct reimbursement for nursing care. Efficient nurse managers will use a budget calendar that covers formulation, review and enactment, and execution stages of the total budget process.

Evaluation is an administrative aspect of budgeting that in itself serves as a controlling process. Decentralization vests control at the lowest competent level of decision making. Good budget feedback information is essential for use of the budget as an effective controlling process. This includes information about revenues and expenses and internal comparisons of projected and actual budgets. The budget can be used to motivate professional nurses and to facilitate their development of innovations.

This chapter has detailed development of an operating room budget that identifies costs and charges from the *Hospital and Hospital Health Care Complex Cost Report Certification and Statement Summary,* commonly known as the Medicare Cost Report. It provides a format that can be adapted to develop the operating room budget.

The belief of nurse managers that budgets are beyond comprehension can effectively sabotage their effectiveness in a managerial position. Spiraling health-care costs, hospital cost-containment efforts, and increasing accountability from individual cost responsibility centers should serve as an impetus to learn at least the fundamentals of budgets and the budget process. To assume the responsibility of budget work increases the nurse manager's potential realm of planning, predicting, and reviewing programs within his or her jurisdiction.

Similar to a nursing care plan, the budget is an activity guidance tool. It is a plan expressed in monetary terms, carried out within a time frame. To be effective as a caregiver the nurse knows how to develop and use a nursing care plan; similarly, to be most effective the nurse manager knows how to develop and use a budget.

NOTES

1. J. N. Althaus, N. M. Hardyck, P. B. Pierce, and M. S. Rodgers, *Nursing Decentralization: The El Camino Experience* (Rockville, MD: Aspen, 1981). Reprinted as abridged by permission. © 1981 Nursing Resources, available from Aspen Systems Corporation, 1600 Research Blvd., Rockville, MD 20850.
2. B. Nordberg and L. King, "Third-Party Payment for Patient Education," *American Journal of Nursing,* Aug. 1976, 1269–1271.
3. B. Huttman, "Taking Charge: Selling Your Budget," *RN,* Apr. 1964, 25–26.
4. L. D. McCullers and R. G. Schroeder, *Accounting Theory Text and Readings* (New York: John Wiley & Sons, 1982), 18–23.
5. A. G. Herkimer, Jr., *Understanding Hospital Financial Management* (Rockville, MD: Aspen, 1978), 132.
6. R. P. Covert, "Expense Budgeting," *Handbook of Health Care Accounting and Finance,* William O. Cleverly, Ed. (Rockville, MD: Aspen, 1982), 261–278.
7. L. R. Piper, "Basic Budgeting for ED Nursing Personnel," *Journal of Emergency Nursing,* Nov./Dec. 1982, 285–287.
8. P. N. Palmer, "Why Hide the Revenue Produced by Perioperative Nursing Care?," *AORN Journal,* June 1984, 1122–1123.
9. In business and industry bad debts are considered an expense of doing business. In hospitals bad debt is subtracted from revenue, so it becomes a reduction of revenue rather than a cost of doing business. Profit or return on equity is not allowed by Medicare or Medicaid except in for-profit hospitals. A few third-party payers allow a return on equity.
10. C. Hancock, "Value for Money," *Nursing Focus,* Sept. 1981, 447–449.
11. T. P. Herzog, "Productivity: Fighting the Battle of the Budget," *Nursing Management,* Jan. 1985, 30–34.
12. R. M. Hodgetts, *Management: Theory, Process, and Practice,* (Philadelphia: W. B. Saunders, 1975), 208–209. L. C. Megginson, D. C. Mosley and P. H. Piehri, Jr., Management: Concepts and Applications, (2d. ed., New York: Harper and Row, 1986), 522–523.
13. A. E. Hillestad, "Budgeting: Functional or Dysfunctional?" *Nursing Economics,* Nov./Dec. 1983, 199–201.
14. R. J. Oszustowizc, "Financial Management of Department of Nursing Services," NLN Publ. 20-1798, National League for Nursing, 1979, 1–10.

REFERENCES

American Hospital Association, *Chart of Accounts for Hospitals* (Chicago: American Hospital Publishing, 1976).

American Hospital Association, *Managerial Cost Accounting for Hospitals* (Chicago: American Hospital Publishing, 1980).

Cochran, Sr. Jeanette, "Refining a Patient-Acuity System Over Four Years," *Hospital Progress,* Feb. 1979, 56–60.

Esmond, T. H., Jr., *Budgeting Procedures for Hospitals, 1982 Edition.* (Chicago: American Hospital Publishing, 1982).

Goetz, J. F., and H. L. Smith, "Zero-Base Budgeting for Nursing Services: An Opportunity for Cost Containment," *Nursing Forum,* Feb. 1980, 122–137.

Hallows, D. A., "Budget Processes and Budgeting in the New Authorities," *Nursing Times,* Aug. 4, 1982, 1309–1311.

Hancock, C., "The Nursing Budget," *Nursing Mirror,* Oct. 20, 1982, 47–48.

Hicks, L. L. and K. E. Boles, "Why Health Economics?," *Nursing Economics,* May-June 1984, 175–180.

Hutton, J. and D. Moss, "Budgetary Control—The Role of the Director of Nursing Services and Treasurers," *Nursing Times,* Aug. 11, 1982, 1364–1365.

Johnson, K. P., "Revenue Budgeting/Rate Setting," in *Handbook of Health Care Accounting and Finance,* W. O. Cleverly, Ed. (Rockville, MD: Aspen, 1982), 279–311.

La Violette, S., "Classification Systems Remedy Billing Inequity," *Modern Healthcare,* Sept. 1979, 32–33.

Lyne, M., "Grasping the Challenge," *Nursing Times,* Nov. 23, 1983, 11–12.

Marriner, A., "Budgetary Management," *The Journal of Continuing Education in Nursing,* Nov./Dec. 1980, 11–14.

McCarty, P., "Nursing Administrators Control Millions," *The American Nurse,* Sept. 20, 1979, 1, 8, 19.

Orem, D. E., *Nursing Concepts of Practice,* 3d. ed. (New York: McGraw-Hill, 1985).

Rowsell, G., "Economics of Health Care," *AARN Newsletter 37,* No. 7, July/Aug. 1981, 6–8.

Ruskowski, U. "A Budget Orientation Tool for Nurse Managers," *Dimensions in Health Service,* Dec. 1980, 30–31.

Sonberg, V., and K. E. Vestal, "Nursing as a Business," *Nursing Clinics of North America,* 18, No. 3, Sept. 1983, 491–98.

Suver, J. D., "Zero-Base Budgeting," in *Handbook of Health Care Accounting and Finance,* William O. Cleverly, Ed. (Rockville, MD: Aspen, 1982), 353–376.

Swansburg, R. C. and P. W. Swansburg, *The Nurse Manager's Guide to Financial Management* (Rockville, MD: Aspen, 1988).

Trofino, J., "Managing the Budget Crunch," *Nursing Management,* Oct. 1984, 42–47.

Vracin, R. A., "Capital Budgeting," in *Handbook of Health Care Accounting and Finance,* William O. Cleverly, Ed., (Rockville, MD: Aspen, 1982), 323–351.

Managing a Clinical Practice Discipline

7

INTRODUCTION

Nursing is a clinical practice discipline. Effective nurse managers realize this and treat its practitioners accordingly. This means that nurse managers will facilitate the work of clinical nurses, a difficult goal for supervisor-employee relationships in bureaucratic organizations. Professional nurses want autonomy in their own practice. They want to apply their nursing knowledge and skills without interference from nurse managers, physicians, or persons in other disciplines. This is best done by nurse managers who establish professional peer relationships with practicing professional nurses. Such a relationship does not abrogate the supervisor-employee relationship. Nurse managers develop a relationship that embodies trust. The nurse manager trusts the professional nurse to apply knowledge and skills correctly in caring for a group of patients. In turn, the clinical nurse trusts the nurse manager to coordinate supplies, equipment, and support systems with personnel of other departments.

Nurse managers ask clinical nurses for input on implementation of policies and procedures. Clinical nurses come to respect a human relations management process in which they participate rather than one in which they have rules and regulations imposed upon them. They use the body of nursing knowledge (theory) gained in nursing school and maintained through continuing education and staff development to practice nursing as they determine it should be practiced. In doing so they adhere to management policies regarding such things as documentation or quality assurance because these requirements are also part of clinical nursing practice.

USE OF NURSING THEORIES

In developing nursing as a scientific discipline, nursing educators and researchers have developed theoretical frameworks for the clinical practice of nursing. These theoretical frameworks are used by clinical nurses as models for testing and validating applications of nursing knowledge and skills. Their results are added to the body of knowledge now commonly called the theory of nursing. Theory gives practicing nurses a professional identity. It is based on scientific inquiry: nursing research. Each result of nursing research adds tested facts to nursing theory that can be learned by nursing students and active practitioners.

Models and Examples

Models are frequently used in the development of nursing theory. A model usually communicates in graphic format an abstract entity, structure, or process that cannot be directly observed. Models depict behavioral processes that exist in reality but cannot be directly observed except as indirect behaviors of those engaged in the process. They order, clarify, and systematize selected components of the phenomenon they serve to depict. Models illustrate and clarify theories. Because nursing theories have not been widely applied they are frequently described as models.[1]

Theories of Orem and Kinlein.   Dickson and Lee-Villasenor report testing of Orem's self-care nursing theory as modified by Kinlein. As independent generalist nurses they did their research in a private nursing practice setting. They used grounded theory methodology to systematically obtain data from clients and analyze them. As the clients spoke, they recorded, identifying self-care assets, self-care demand, and self-care measures with their clients.

In performing a content analysis, Dickson and Lee-Villasenor classified events as expression of need, self-care assets, self-care demand, and self-care measures. They catalogued events by numbers of expressions of need: a perception of self, an action taken, a want, a wish, or a question; and by perception of self according to mind-body combination. Events were also catalogued according to evidence of patterns of self-care actions that contributed positively to the client's state of health and number of self-care assets: action, motivation, knowledge, and potential.[2]

This model can be duplicated by clinical nursing research in hospital settings, home health-care settings, and other areas in which nurses practice.

The results will add to the body of nursing theory. Nurse managers will facilitate the practice of clinical nursing by supporting acquisition of new knowledge. This can be done through staff development by having unit programs, providing periodicals or journal clubs, or offering release time for library use.

Theory of Roy.   Roy advocates adaptation level theory to nursing intervention. She notes that a person adapts to the environment through four modes: physiologic, self-concept, role mastery, and interdependence.[3] Just as the individual patient adapts to changes in the environment, so does the nursing worker.

According to Roy the goal of nursing is to assist the patient to adapt to illness so as to be able to respond to other stimuli. The patient is assessed for positive or negative behavior in the four adaptive modes. Once the assessment is made at the necessary (first or second) level, intervention is established by a nursing care plan of goals and approaches. The approach is selected to match the goal.[4] Roy's adaptive modes can be applied to develop a theory for nursing management.

According to Mastal and Hammond, Roy's views are "that the developing body of nursing knowledge now contains verifiable theories and general laws related to: (1) persons as holistic beings and (2) the role of nursing in promoting the person's maximum potential health and harmonious interaction with the environment."[5]

While Roy's theory is directed toward the care of patients as persons, the model has the potential of being adapted to management of the practitioner. Nurse managers then have two options: (1) implementing Roy's theory at the clinical practice level or (2) constructing a management model adapting Roy's theory. The latter may appear as a conceptual model; see Figure 7–1.

A nurse manager could support a clinical nurse in her or his adaptation by substituting "practicing nurse" for "client" in Roy's outline of a six-step nursing process:

1. Assess the client's behaviors in each of the modes and determine whether they are adaptive or inefficient.
2. Assess the stimuli that influence those behaviors and classify them as to whether they are focal, contextual, or residual. All stimuli (both

Figure 7–1.   Adaptation of Roy's Theoretical Concepts to Nursing Management

Roy's Concept	Adapted to Management
1. Person is an adaptive system or biopsychosocial being who functions as a totality in constant interaction with a changing internal or external environment. The cognator adaptive mechanism "identifies, stores, and relates environmental stimuli to effect symbolic responses. It acts consciously by thought and decision, and unconsciously through defense mechanisms." (p. 73) The regulator adaptive mechanism responds through the autonomic nervous system with reflex action by approach, attack, or flight.	1. The clinical nurse is the focus of nursing management and is affected by the actions of the nurse manager. These management actions can affect the internal or external environment of the clinical nurse. The cognator mechanism of the clinical nurse responds consciously or unconsciously to stimuli from the nurse manager. A nurse manager who creates an autocratic environment may cause clinical nurse responses varying on a continuum from awareness to resignation from the job and that include suppressed anger, nausea, expressed anger, absenteeism, and so on.
2. Environment provides the stimuli that provoke adaptation. Stimuli are stressors.	2. The nurse manager can invoke stressors that impede or facilitate goal achievement by clinical nurses.
3. Adaptation is both a process and an end state. It is a person's response to environmental stimuli to promote that person's goals of survival, growth, reproduction, and self-actualization.	3. A clinical nurse may feel so harassed by a nurse manager as to go on a permanent shift to survive. If a clinical nurse cannot achieve career goals, this person may transfer, change jobs, or adapt his or her work schedule.
4. Health-illness is a dimension of a person's life that occurs on a continuum: 4.1 peak wellness. 4.2 high-level wellness. 4.3 good health. 4.4 normal health. 4.5 poor health. 4.6 extreme poor health. 4.7 death.	4. The health-illness concept applies to all persons but nurse managers need an awareness of its impact on the performance of the clinical nurse.

Source: Adapted from M. F. Mastal and H. Hammond, "Analysis and Expansion of the Roy Adaptation Model: A Contribution to Holistic Nursing," *Advances in Nursing Science*, July 1980, 71–81; S. C. Roy, *Introduction to Nursing: An Adaptation Model* (Englewood Cliffs, NJ: Prentice-Hall, 1976).

positive and negative) must be considered if a valid situational assessment is to be achieved.

3. Identify and state the adaptation problem.
4. Establish goals in terms of desired behaviors.
5. Manipulate those stimuli that will promote adaptation. Manipulation refers to removing, changing, increasing, or decreasing the stimuli so that adaptive behaviors are reinforced and inefficient ones are modified.
6. Evaluate the person's response to nursing intervention in terms of meeting the established goals.[6]

Theory of Newman.   Engle tested Newman's conceptual framework of health in a sample of older women. She indicates that Newman uses Rogers's concept of the life process and the relationship of the individual within the environment. In this model aging is considered a natural process, the person's individual state being a fusion of health and disease. Movement is a correlation of health measured by a basic time factor or tempo.[7]

Engle indicates tempo to be the characteristic rate of performing a task. Time is the second correlation of health. Tempo and time occur in a succession of events, rhythmic patterns of temperatures and movement, and patterns within the environment. Time perception and tempo are hypothesized to be altered by age and illness. The patient does self-assessment of his or her health as a criterion measure. Self-assessment and physician assessment of health have been shown to correlate. Self-assessment of health is altered by ability to perform everyday activities, by age self-concept, and by movement and time.[8]

In her study Engle measured personal tempo, time perception, and self-assessment of health by using the Cantril Ladder in 114 females aged 60 or older. She found no age effect for time perception in this study, nor did Newman and Tompkins in similar studies. Nor was there any age effect for personal tempo.[9]

There was a significant relationship between time perception and personal tempo that could have significance for the patient and the clinical nurse. The patient or nurse with a physical or mental condition that alters personal tempo may have an altered perception of time. This could be true in older nurses in whom physical and mental states are more often altered. Further research in this area is needed, particularly as the population ages.

Theory of Levine.   Levine indicates that nursing practice has mirrored prevailing theories of health and disease. Nursing has created an environment for healing: cleanliness, safety, and physical and emotional comfort. Nursing enhances the reparative process. Nursing became "disease-oriented" when diseases, not patients, were the focus of treatment. As nurses became concerned with the multiple factors affecting the course of disease, they developed the "total patient care" concept.[10]

People respond to illness in individual ways. Nursing intervention should match the individual response, which is identified from observation and data analysis. Assessment reveals unique needs requiring unique nursing measures. Nursing supports repair and maintenance of a person's integrated self—homeostasis and equilibrium. Equilibrium is maintained by adaptation. The nurse intervenes to support successful adaptation, to achieve a therapeutic or supportive role.[11]

Levine's theory could be applied to nursing management within an organization. The nurse manager wants to maintain the equilibrium of a unit, service, department, or division. When this equilibrium is upset because of staff turnover, nurse managers need to act in concert with clinical nurses to adapt to working with fewer professional nurses. Data are collected and analyzed to make adjustments that can include increased productivity and increased efficiency as well as changes to decrease turnover.

Theory of Johnson.   The Johnson Behavioral Systems Model is a theory of nursing practice. Johnson incorporated the nursing process (assessment, planning-diagnosis, intervention, and evaluation) into a general systems model. Rawls applied it to care of a patient for the purpose of testing, evaluating, and determining its utility for predicting the effect of nursing care on a patient. Rawls indicates the model has disadvantages but is a tool that can be used "to accurately predict the results of nursing interventions prior to care, formulate standards of care, and most importantly administer truly holistic empathic nursing care."[12]

The Johnson Behavioral Systems Model could be applied to nursing management. It could be tested as a predictor of the effect of nursing management on clinical nurses.

Theory of Peplau.   While Peplau's theory that nursing "is a significant, therapeutic, interpersonal process" has been applied to clinical nursing, there is merit to its application to nursing management. The nurse manager uses the interpersonal process in relationships with personnel, patients, families, visitors, and other individuals and groups. As a manager of clinical nurses, the nurse manager could use the interpersonal process in assisting employees to manage life situations that cause anxiety, depression, or insecurity.

Peplau's theory involves communication techniques, assessment, definition of problems and goals, direction, role clarification, and other concepts relevant to human resource management. The nurse manager adept in the theory could assist personnel in meeting their needs, thereby preventing or reducing anxiety. Room exists for research in application of Peplau's theory to nursing management. This would include identification of principles that apply.[13]

Theory of Orlando.   Orlando's theory of nursing develops three basic concepts:

1. Professional nursing has as its function the identification and meeting of patients' immediate needs for help.
2. Professional nursing has as its outcome or product both verbal and nonverbal improvement in the patient's behavior.
3. Regardless of its form, the patient's presenting or initial behavior may be a plea for help.

Orlando's theory has been implemented in a department of nursing under the leadership of a director of nursing. Thus nursing theory is used by nurse managers to promote clinical nursing.

Schmieding applied Orlando's theory to solving problems in managing the behavior of clinical nurses. She recommends that the work of one theorist be used as the practice model within a given organization. This application of Orlando's model has helped nurses apply common concepts and a framework for nursing. The model could be adapted if the nursing staff synthesized the concepts of several theories.[14]

Applications to Nursing Management

Nurse managers use management skills to motivate clinical nurses. Their work rests on a theoretical understanding of communication, motivation, and leadership (directing activities), as well as of planning, organizing, and evaluating. The adaptive aspects of the nurse manager's behavior are multidimensional in their response to management problems, just as is clinical nursing behavior in response to the problems of sick patients.

Just as modern clinical nurses have access to theory, so do nurse managers. Scientific management knowledge is as essential to the nurse manager as scientific biological, physical, and social knowledge is to the clinical nurse. The nurse manager is responsible for maintaining the wholeness, integration, and equilibrium of the clinical nurse.

Cleland points to a methodology for research in nursing management. She suggests starting with a nursing problem of interest and of empirical significance. One would work directly from empirical data, expressing concepts from relative formulations, and deductively from theoretical formulations, with frequent close interaction between data and conceptualization.[15]

To illustrate her points, Cleland described research to predict the career patterns of inactive registered nurses. She referred to the Barnard Simon theory of organizational equilibrium to examine the decision to participate in an organization. She also referred to Herzberg's motivation and hygiene factors theory. Reference group theory would be used to examine role conflicts between married nurses and their spouses, relating norms of socioeconomic class. Cleland developed hypotheses from general management theory, indicating how nursing management theory can be used to solve problems. The problems can be solved through applied or basic research, a lesson for nurse managers.[16]

According to Goldstein the tendency to actualize oneself is the only motive by which human activity is set going. If this theory is applied to the nurse manager it has two possible directions: promotion of self-actualization in clinical nurses by nurse managers and development of the self-actualization motive within nurse managers.[17]

Clinical nurses learn theories of nursing in preservice programs. They learn to synthesize knowledge and skills and apply them in clinical practice. Through staff development and personal endeavors they add to their body of nursing theory knowledge as the knowledge is tested and disseminated.

Nurse managers facilitate the process by encouraging learning, research, and excellence of performance. They pursue research in nursing management and draw upon the theory of business, management, human relations, and related disciplines as well as the theory of nursing.

Clinical practitioners in any field need to apply some management theory to their work. Structure is always an essential element. Work needs to be planned, goals set, outcome criteria set, organization designed, budget and resources identified, controlling techniques established, and the decision-making process determined. Nurse managers assist and support applications of management theory in their relationships with clinical nurses. They provide the work processing tasks that include procedures, tools, techniques, harmonious work relationships, problem solving, budget and schedule preparation, communication, and working.

Nurse managers thus facilitate clinical nurses to:

1. Utilize the nursing process.
2. Perform nursing diagnosis and treatment.

3. Accept accountability for nursing activities of other nursing personnel.
4. Accept accountability for nursing outcomes.
5. Control the nursing practice environment.[18]

Participation in the management process by clinical nurses can be fostered by nurse managers in at least five ways:

1. Upward participation—Professional nurses become involved in the manager's work. Nurse managers accustomed to autocratic management may not support such a process if they have difficulty giving up control. When they involve the nurses in the structuring process, it is more likely to be successful. Nurse managers should teach employees the skills of upward participation.

2. Downward participation—Nursing work is structured by nurse managers who may become involved in it. This can be positive or negative in its effect on employees. If there is mutual agreement that defines the reason for and the scope of the manager's involvement, the result will be positive. Participation can be from the division, department, or service level to any lower level or levels, including the unit level.

3. Lateral participation—Collaboration among nursing units requires skills in group processes and in managing individual and group differences. Usually the unit or departments will be within a nursing service or the nursing division.

4. Organizational participation—Collaboration across divisions or departments corrects isolationism and separation, requiring strong managerial and clinical leadership to breach territorial imperatives. Nurses sometimes want to participate with other professionals and in other departments, but they do not always welcome reciprocal participation.

5. Personal participation—The individual uses personal mental and physical capabilities in doing work. Nurse managers should remove barriers to autonomy of practice. Personal participation enhances self-esteem and feelings of professional and personal worth in nurses.[19]

Many other applications and suggested applications of nursing theory to nursing administration theory, practice, and research have been made. These include cultural care theory (Leininger); systems theory (King); humanity-living-health theory (Parse); and unitary human beings theory (Rogers).[20]

MODALITIES OF NURSING PRACTICE

Several modalities or methods of nursing practice have evolved during the past 35 years. These include functional nursing, team nursing, primary nursing, case method, joint practice, and case management. All are practiced in various forms in health-care institutions in the United States. While nurse managers frequently decide the method of nursing practice to be used in their organizations, it is best to involve practicing clinical nurses in making this decision. The latter are the ones who will do it; if the choice is theirs they will make it work. Clinical nurses should be provided with sufficient information about the modality and how the institution will support it so they can provide input for a workable decision.

Once the decision is made an ad hoc committee can develop policies and procedures for implementing the modality. There should be adequate resources, including appropriate categories of nursing personnel, to make the modality work. Personnel need to be adequately prepared through staff development programs. These can be supported by staff development instructors in large organizations. Small organizations may need assistance from a consultant, usually available within the larger organizations of the nearest urban area.

Functional Nursing

This is the oldest nursing practice modality. It can best be described as a task-oriented method in which a particular nursing function is assigned to each staff member. One registered nurse is responsible for administering medications, one for treatments, one for managing intravenous administration; one licensed practical nurse is assigned admissions and discharges, another gives bed baths; a nurses aide makes beds, passes meal trays, and so on. No nurse is responsible for total care of any patient. The method divides the tasks to be done, with each person being responsible to the nurse manager. It is efficient and may be the best system when confronted with a large patient load and a shortage of professional nurses.

The advantage of functional nursing is that it accomplishes the most work in the shortest amount of time.

Disadvantages of functional nursing are that:

- It fragments nursing care.
- It decreases the nurse's accountability and responsibility.
- It makes the nurse-client relationship difficult to establish, if it is ever achieved.
- It gives professional nursing low status in terms of responsibility for patient care.

Functional nursing was largely a development of the World War II era, when large numbers of nurses entered military service and ancillary personnel were trained to staff many nursing functions of hospitals. It is still alive and well in many institutions.[21]

Team Nursing

Team nursing developed in the early 1950s, when various nursing leaders decided that a team approach could unify the different categories of nursing workers. Under the leadership of a professional nurse, a group of nurses would work together to fulfill the functions of professional nurses. Assignment of patients is made to a team consisting of a registered nurse as a team leader, and other staff R.N.s, L.P.N.s, and aides as team members.

The team leader has the responsibility for coordinating the total care of a block of patients and is the leadership figure. Team nursing is practiced in many institutions.[22]

The intent of team nursing is to provide patient-centered care. The patient's nursing care needs are identified and met through nursing diagnosis and prescription. Ward clerks and unit managers perform the non-nursing functions of the unit. The process requires planning to meet the objective of taking nursing personnel to the bedside so that they can focus upon nursing care of patients.

Implementing team nursing requires study of the literature on the team plan, development of a philosophy of team nursing, planning for appropriate utilization of all categories of nursing workers, and planning for team conferences, nursing care plans, and development of team leadership. Figure 7–2 depicts an original schema for a team nursing organization. It would be somewhat modified today to depict a less bureaucratic structure, with team members performing different roles.

The following is a summary of the team plan as advocated by Newcomb and Swansburg:

The team plan gives priorities to the development of leadership potential—leadership in the practice of nursing—leadership that is creative and that encourages improvement of communications among team members, patients, and leaders. It gives priority to emphasis on democratic leadership, the nurturing of cooperative effort, and free expression of ideas of all team members. It gives

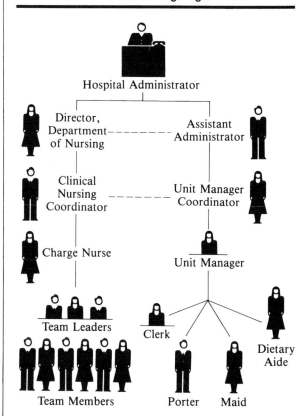

FIGURE 7–2. Team Nursing Organization

SOURCE: D. P. Newcomb and R. C. Swansburg, *The Team Plan* (New York: G. P. Putnam's Sons, 1953, 1971).

priority to motivation of people to grow to this self-approved or maximum level of performance. Through the team plan the contributions of all team members in improving patient care are recognized. Priority is given to the strengthening of their weaknesses.

Patient-centered care employs effective supervision and recognizes that personnel are the media by which the objectives are met in a cooperative effort between team leaders and team members. Through supervision the team leader identifies nursing care goals; identifies team members' needs; focuses on fulfilling goals and needs; motivates team members to grow as workers and citizens; guides team members to help set and meet high standards of patient care and job performance—all of them supporting the priority of *practicing nursing.*[23]

The advantages of team nursing are:

- It involves all team members in planning patients' nursing care, through use of team conferences and writing nursing care plans.
- It provides the best care at the lowest cost, according to some advocates.

Disadvantages of team nursing include:

- It can lead to fragmentation of care if the concept is not implemented totally.
- It can be difficult to find time for team conferences and care plans.
- It allows the R.N. who is the team leader to have the only significant responsibility and authority.[24]

The disadvantages of team nursing can be overcome by educating competent team leaders in the principles of nursing management.

Primary Nursing

The most touted method of assignment and practice today is that of primary nursing. It is an extension of the principle of decentralization of authority, the primary authority for all decisions about the nursing process being centered in the person of the professional nurse. The primary nurse is assigned to care for the patient's total needs for the duration of the hospital stay.

Responsibility covers a 24-hour period, with associate nurses providing care when the primary nurse is not there. The care given is planned and prescribed totally by the primary nurse.[25]

Marram, Schlegel, and Bevis state "Primary nursing . . . is the distribution of nursing so that the total care of an individual is the responsibility of one nurse, not many nurses."[26] They indicate autonomy to be the key to the development of professional nursing. Characteristics of the primary nursing modality are:

1. The primary nurse has responsibility for the nursing care of the patient 24 hours a day, from admission through discharge.
2. Assessment of nursing care needs, collaboration with patient and other health professionals, and formulation of the plan of care are all in the hands of the primary nurse.
3. Execution of the nursing care plan is delegated by the primary nurse to a secondary nurse during other shifts.
4. The primary nurse consults with head nurses and supervisors.
5. Authority, accountability, and autonomy rest with the primary nurse.[27]

Primary nursing parallels decentralized patient education because the nurse becomes the primary provider. In comprehensive patient care the primary nurse is responsible and accountable for patient education.[28]

Since 1974 primary nursing has been implemented in many hospitals and has undergone numerous modifications. Primary nurses frequently do the hands-on nursing care of the patient. Sometimes they direct other care givers while retaining the functions of decision makers.

Fagin states that research studies on primary nursing indicate it reduced hospital stays and complications of renal transplant patients at the University of Michigan Medical Center in Ann Arbor. They saved $51,000 in one year. Primary nursing at Evanston Hospital in Illinois resulted in fewer nursing hours and less salary expense per patient during a 5-year period. Nurses aides had 27 percent unoccupied time per day while R.N.s had 8 percent at Rush Presbyterian. Also, turnover was decreased in the operating room with an increased R.N. to operating room technician ratio. Other studies indicate that primary nursing saves money; increases job satisfaction, group adhesion, and patient satisfaction; and decreases costs of overtime, sick time, and compensatory time.[29]

Studies support primary nursing as enhancing patient satisfaction, nurse satisfaction, and cost-effectiveness. They also suggest that "individual differences in nurses and nurse competencies may have a greater impact on the quality of care than does the primary nursing structure." It should be noted, however, that when educational backgrounds of nurses were matched, differences in quality of care between team and primary nursing disappeared. The structure for primary nursing is generally a better system for organizing care. Effectiveness of primary nursing differs for types of nurses, patients, hospitals, and even nursing units within a single hospital.[30]

Both primary and team nursing need efficient nursing support systems: communication, distribution, transportation, and unit management. Shukla proposes the contingency theory that primary nursing is more effective when support systems are efficient and patients' dependence on nurses is high. Primary nursing is not better than team nursing for all hospitals, all nursing units within a hospital, or all types of patients.

Decentralized support systems such as those for moving supplies, linens, and drugs to patients' rooms are more efficient and improve the benefit of primary nursing over team nursing. When primary nurses have to go to centralized areas for such items, they are impeded in providing direct care. Also, modular nursing or modified primary nursing alternatives require performance of more indirect and routine nursing and non-nursing tasks. Patients requiring extensive care benefit more from primary nursing than those capable of self care. Primary nursing is best for intensive care.[31]

Rosenman and Jenkins report a pilot project to change from a functional modality to a patient-oriented one. The outcomes included fewer patient complaints, more letters of praise of nursing staff, more communication and collegiality with physicians, a higher census, and nurses wanting to give their own reports. Primary nursing promoted esprit de corps, with nurses identifying with patients, patients with nurses, and physicians with nurses. High levels of staff satisfaction resulted and attendance and punctuality increased.[32]

Ingersoll reports implementation of primary nursing in a surgical outpatient department using change theory. One primary nurse was assigned over two specified surgical clinics with an L.P.N. as associate nurse. Individualized care plans were placed on the charts, indicating problems to date, course of action, evaluation, information from patients and families, the name of the primary nurse, and the phone number of the surgical outpatient department. The outpatient primary nurse visited the patients as inpatients before they were discharged to the surgical clinic. Results included improved patient care (documented), increased responsibility and satisfaction of nurses, and communication to allay patients' anxieties.[33]

The Information for Legislators prepared by the Nevada Nurses Association stated sixteen instances in which professional nurses practicing primary nursing advanced cost effective care. A fact sheet promotes primary nursing care of inpatients and primary care services by advanced practitioners of nursing care of outpatients.[34]

Watson reports the results of a project to have patients evaluate a primary nursing project. The hypothesis tested was that patients would perceive primary nursing as more personalized than other modalities. Results show that patients perceived that fewer nurses cared for them in primary care and the nurses were friendly and prepared to sit down and talk. They perceived that nurses were concerned about their families. Patients in all situations said it was much easier to approach nurses rather than doctors for information. Communication with patients and between doctors and nurses was perceived by patients to be better in primary units. Patients on primary units stated they were better prepared for discharge. Patients made comments that indicated that primary nurses gave them comfort and security.[35]

Advantages of primary nursing are the following:

- It provides for increased autonomy on the part of the nurse, thus increasing motivation, responsibility, and accountability.
- It assures more continuity of care as the primary nurse gives or directs care throughout hospitalization.
- It makes available increased knowledge of the patient's psychosocial and physical needs, because the primary nurse does the history and physical assessment, develops the care plan, and

acts as liaison between the patient and other health workers.

■ It leads to increased rapport and trust between nurse and patient that will allow formation of a therapeutic relationship.

■ It improves communication of information to physicians.

■ It eliminates nurses aides from the administration of direct patient care.

■ It frees the charge nurse to assume the role of operational manager: to deal with staff problems and assignments and to motivate and support the staff.

The main disadvantage of primary nursing is that it is said to require the entire staff to be R.N.s, which increases staffing costs. However, this has been disputed in cost studies. For example, money is saved when non-nursing duties are performed by other categories of personnel and are not taken over by R.N.s.[36]

Case Method

The case method of nursing provides for a one-to-one R.N.-to-client ratio and the provision of constant care for a specified period of time. Examples are private duty, intensive care, and community health nurses. This method is similar to that of primary nursing except that relief nurses on other shifts are not associate R.N.s.[37]

Joint Practice

Joint practice is more than a modality. It entails nurses and physicians collaborating as colleagues to provide patient care. They work together to define their roles within the joint practice setting, such goals being reciprocal and complementary rather than mutually exclusive. They may use mutually agreed-upon protocols to manage care within a primary setting.[38]

The primary nursing modality is preferred for joint practice or collaborative practice. There must be adequate professional nurses freed of non-nursing tasks. Nurse managers facilitate the growth of individual professional nurses. Decision making is decentralized and in-service education and certification are used to upgrade the nurse's scope of practice. Compensation is increased to match increased responsibility and accountability.

Physicians are required to accept responsibility for their part in joint collaborative practice. Administration includes joint practice nurses on every committee within the hospital. It may take as long as a year to establish true functional relationships. Both physicians and nurses have to modify their behaviors.

The elements needed to establish successful joint practice in a hospital setting are:

1. A committee of physicians and nurses with equal representation and equal voice in establishing the objectives and ground rules of operation.
2. An integrated patient record.
3. Primary nursing and case management.
4. Collaborative practice with honest communication and encouragement of clinical decision making by nurses.
5. Joint education of physicians and nurses.
6. Joint nurse-physician evaluation of patient care.
7. Trust.

Results of a joint practice demonstration project at four hospitals concluded that:

■ Patients receive better nursing care and are highly satisfied with their care.

■ Doctor-nurse communications are better and there is increased mutual respect and trust between nurses and physicians.

■ Both doctors' and nurses' job satisfaction is increased.[39]

Case Management

Case management is also more than a modality of nursing. It has been described as:

> a system of patient care delivery that focuses on the achievement of outcomes within effective and appropriate time frames and resources. Case management focuses on an entire episode of illness, crossing all settings in which the patient receives care. Care is directed by a case manager who ideally is involved in a group practice. Case management incorporates the principles of managed care.[40]

Case management involves collaborative practice that in turn involves groups of professional nurses who collaborate to move the patient through the system. It is episode-based rather than unit-based. Nurses of various units collaborate to move the patient on a critical path through the hospital stay.[41]

Group practice is:

a formal structure for case-based nursing care delivery and management throughout an episode of illness. Membership includes pre-identified primary nurses from serial units (and agencies) who work in partnership with (1) the key physicians for that case type and (2) the patients and their families to facilitate care that meets specific clinical standards within appropriate resource obligation.[42]

Collaborative practice is group practice that includes physicians. At the New England Medical Center group practice is mainly composed of nurses. Joint practice, like collaborative practice, implies a joint effort by M.D.s and R.N.s. The aims of these practice modalities appear to be similar.

Managed Care

Managed care in its broadest sense goes beyond the health maintenance organization and preferred provider organization or hospital plans. In this book, managed care is case management by nurses as developed by Zander and others and adopted as a system by many hospital nursing organizations.

Managed care is:

unit-based care that is organized to achieve specific patient outcomes within fiscally responsible time frames (length of stay) utilizing resources that are appropriate in amounts and sequence to the specific case type and to the individual patient. Care is structured by case management plans and critical paths which are based on knowledge by case type regarding usual length of stay, critical events and their timing, anticipated outcomes, and resource allocation.[43]

Managed care can employ any modality of nursing, including team nursing, primary nursing, functional nursing, or case management. Tools for managed care include case-management plans and critical paths; see Figures 7–3 and 7–4.

At the New England Medical Center critical paths have been developed for approximately one hundred fifty diagnostic-related groups (DRGs) and case management plans for approximately 50 DRGs as of early 1988.

In addition to being cost-effective, managed care meets established quality control indicators. It is outcome-based and identifies the business of nursing. A professional nurse who practices managed care may be doing primary care nursing, a solo act of case management, or collaborative practice with nurses in other units such as the operating suite or emergency department—or all at the same time.

Managed care develops management skills that include variance identification and analysis, negotiation, consulting, clinical assessment, time management, problem solving, and priority setting. Management development of staff nurses is a factor in managed care.[44]

NURSING ASSESSMENT: SKILLS AND TECHNIQUES

The Washington State Board of Nursing has a legal definition of nursing practice that includes "the observation, assessment, diagnosis, care or counsel, and health teaching of the ill, injured, or infirm, or . . . the maintenance of health or prevention of illness of others" and "performance of such additional acts . . . recognized jointly by the medical and nursing professions as proper to be performed by nurses licensed under this chapter and which shall be authorized by the board of nursing through its rules and regulations."

The law opens the door to nurses' legally performing minor surgery and prescribing: "This chapter shall not be construed as . . . (15) permitting the performance of major surgery, except such minor surgery as the board may have specifically authorized by rule or regulation duly adopted . . . [or] (16) permitting the prescribing of controlled substances as defined in schedules I through IV of the Uniform Controlled Substances Act." In short, nurses in the state of Washington can neither perform major surgery nor prescribe controlled substances, but they may perform minor surgery and prescribe other substances.

This advanced law says the nurse is "directly accountable to the individual consumer for the quality of nursing care rendered."[45]

FIGURE 7-3. New England Medical Center Hospitals Department of Nursing Case Management Plan

DIAGNOSIS: Transurethral Resection of Prostate Benign UNIT: Proger 5 North

DRG: 337 MDC: 12 LENGTH OF STAY: 5.8 days USUAL OR DAY (from admission day = 1):

Health Outcomes

Diagnosis	Outcome (The patient . . .)	DAY VST	Intermediate Goal (The patient . . .)	DAY VST	Process (The nurse . . .)	DAY VST	Process (The physician . . .)
Alteration in urinary elimination patterns related to indwelling catheter	* Is draining urine freely through the catheter system. * Has no fever, chills, or foul smelling urine. * Has no ureteral discharge or tissue inflammation.	2-3	* Informs nurse of any problems with foley catheter, i.e.:: clots abdominal distention muscle spasms fever or chills.	2-3	* Assesses foley catheter drainage for color, clots, and volume glh for 8 hrs, then g4h for 24 hrs.	2-3	
					* Provides an explanation of catheter function and corrects any misconceptions the patient might have.	2-3	
					* Teaches the patient to recognize problems with the catheter.	2-3	
					* Irrigates blood clots from the bladder and tubing as necessary to prevent distention.	2-3	
					* Monitors VS q4h.	2-3	
					* Keeps catheter anchored to prevent dislodging.	2-3	
					* Forces fluids. * Gives appropriate care of catheter equipment and charts on the treatment sheet. * Maintains strict I/O.	2-3	

Nursing Diagnosis		Patient Outcomes		Nursing Interventions
Alteration in elimination following removal of indwelling catheter.	4–5	* Resumes a normal voiding pattern. * Experiences minimal discomfort secondary to dysuria/frequency and urgency.	4–5	* Records the time and volume of each void for 48–72 hours. * Measures and records strict I/O. * Notes character of urine for:
		* States that there may be some discomfort, burning, frequency, or lack of control while voiding for the first 24–72 hours.		

		* States that he should drink at least eight 8 oz glasses of fluid daily, preferably before 6 P.M.	3
			4
			5
				punch colored urine
				   dark tea colored
				   light tea to amber.

		* States the importance of sphincter exercises.	2–3	* Reassures patient regarding transient frequency urgency, etc. * Checks for bladder distention and discomfort. * Instructs patient to do sphincter exercises.
Alteration in comfort related to pain.	2–5	* Discomfort is controlled, enabling the patient to mobilize and complete ADLs.		* Informs nurse of any abdominal distention, burning, spasms, or pain in penis or scrotom
			*2–5	* Assesses etiology of pain. Offers analgesics as ordered. Administers antispasmodics as ordered. * Applies scrotal support and changes prn. * Applies ice to scrotom if necessary. * Encourages ambulation. * Notifies MD of any pain not relieved after comfort measures.

SOURCE: Sally Barney and Barbara Toland. Reprinted with permission of K. Zander, K. Bower, and M. Etheridge, The Center for Nursing Care Management, New England Medical Center, Boston, MA.

FIGURE 7–4. New England Medical Center Hospitals Department of Nursing, TURP Critical Path

Patient _____			Case Type _____TURP_____	
MD _____			DRG _____336_____	
Case Manager _____			Expected LOS _4 Days_	
Date Critical Path			Pratt 4	
Reviewed by MD _____				

Date	_____	_____	_____	_____
Outpatient	Day 1	Day 2	Day 3	Day 4
>-------- OR-P4 --				
Consults	Admit after OR			
Tests Pre-Op				
Work-Up		HCT		
		LBC		
Activity	Spinal Anesthesia	OOB -------------------------->		
	Bedrest 6–8 Hr,			
	then OOB w/Assist			
Treatments	IV -------------------->	D/C IV		
	Pulmonary Toilet -->			
	Foley Care -->D/C Foley			
	Foley Irrigation -->			
Meds	IV Antibiotic × 1	Begin --> (Total 10 Days)		
	Pre-Op	Oral		
	Post-Op Gentamycin	Antibiotics		
	× 2 Doses, then			
	D/C Parenteral			
	Narcotics --------------> P.O. Narcotics -->			
	Stool Softeners --> D/C if voiding			
				w/o difficulty
				and BM × 1
Discharge	Preop Phone Call	Contact Social	If VNA indicated	Discharge
Planning	and Social Assess-	Service, PRN, i.e.	write & call in.	
	ment Reinforce	Homemaker	Assess transpor-	
	4 Day LOS	Services	tation needs.	
Teaching		Med Teaching		Reassess compre-
		Activity Restriction		hension and rein-
		TURP Teaching		force necessary
		Plan		content.

Admission Date _____   Discharge date _____   Discharge Time _____

Days in ICU _____   Variations from standard (record on back) Days in Routine Bed _____

SOURCE: Copyright New England Medical Center Hospitals 1987, Department of Nursing. Reprinted with permission.

Since its passage, other states have revised their nursing practice laws to give nurses the legal right to use such terms as "diagnosis," "prescribe," and "counsel."

Nursing Process

Miller described the components of skilled nursing care as follows:

1. Nursing diagnosis.
2. Nursing pharmacology.
3. Nursing psychology and psychiatry.
4. Family counseling.
5. Specific nursing techniques.
   a. Bathing, dressing, feeding.
   b. Bladder and bowel management.
   c. Ostomy care.
   d. Inhalation therapy.
   e. Intravenous management of water, electrolytes, and medications.
   f. Nasogastric tube feedings.
   g. Decubitus prevention and management.
6. Restorative nursing care.
7. In-service training.
8. Nursing research.
9. Administrative nursing.[46]

Certainly the skills of nursing assessment can be related to any or all of these components of skilled nursing care. A nursing diagnosis will result from the taking of the nursing history and doing a physical assessment. It will be based on the history taker's scientific and technical knowledge. It will be learned through continuing education and staff development. Nursing research will contribute to its refinement, and the total process will be managed through administrative nursing.

Today's nurses are educated to extend the assessment process throughout the patient's illness. In addition to the initial observations and nursing diagnosis, they identify changing patient conditions related to changing medical and nursing entities and the onset of changing pathological and psychological patterns of behavior. They identify this altered status in the home as well as in institutions.

A nursing history and physical assessment provide the means by which information can be accurately and completely obtained, thus providing the professional nurse with the basis to assess the patient's problems. It does not matter who gathers information so long as it is complete. Some technicians can be taught to gather portions of this information accurately and completely. The important point to be made here is that they must be taught, since someone has to systematically gather sufficient information to allow a professional nurse to make a nursing diagnosis, categorize the patient's problems, and organize them into a meaningful list of problems to be addressed in a nursing care plan. Categorization of the problems requires the depth of knowledge that only a professional nurse has. This is also true of the nursing prescription or plan of what care will be given to solve the problems. The direction of its application, how that nursing care will be given, is also the exclusive province of the professional nurse. Technicians may again be taught the skills used in application of the nursing care, under professional direction. During this time observations indicate the effectiveness of the nursing skills applied and give the professional nurse feedback whereby she or he can evaluate and judge whether problems are being resolved or needs met. Evaluation may result in modification of the nursing prescription. Resources need to be pooled so that a professional nurse directs the delivery of sound, economical care to patients.[47]

Consider the reasons for doing a nursing assessment and a nursing care plan. The Joint Commission on Accreditation of Healthcare Organizations (JCAHO) states, in standard NR5, "individualized goal-directed nursing care is provided to patients through the use of the nursing process."[48] This standard cannot be implemented unless the patients' problems are diagnosed through the assessment process—the nursing history and physical assessment.

Other authoritative sources include the statements of mission, philosophy, and objectives of the institution, division, department, or units; job descriptions and performance standards; operating or management plans and instructions; the American Nurses Association *Standards for Organized Nursing Services and Responsibilities of Nurse Administrators Across All Settings* and *Standards of Nursing Practice;* and numerous others. The patient deserves that problems be assessed and care be given to meet them.

Nurse managers manage the clinical practice discipline of nursing. To do this efficiently and effectively they should establish consultation with the practicing clinical nurses. Together they will use such management processes as management by objectives, participatory management and others. The global goals are to meet professional and legal standards; to meet patients' needs both in terms of the nursing care process and its outcomes; and to provide for the economic and professional well-being of nurses.

Stevens states that despite all the reasons for writing nursing care plans, they receive only token support from registered nurses. They state that they do not have time to do them and that nursing care plans serve no real purpose. Stevens goes on to state that the nurse is educated as a scientist and to plan her clinical care on scientific principles. In practice she makes judgments that do not always produce the planned outcomes. The result is that she does not want to commit plans to paper for all to see when they may result in failure. A possible solution to the problem is to assign responsibility for each care plan to one individual. Stevens states:

> Thus the care plan needs to be under the direction of one nurse over a sustained period of time if nursing strategies are to be consistent. A strategy that changes every day is no strategy at all. Certainly, lines of communication should be developed to permit recommendations from other staff members, and procedures should be established for instituting emergency changes as needed. The head nurse or other selected authority should be responsible for evaluating plans and guiding the assigned nurses in their care plan formulation.[49]

Stevens says that the nurse leader should follow these principles to promote use of nursing care plans:

1. Evaluate each care plan on its inherent worth as well as on patient outcomes.
2. Be supportive of nursing care plans that are thoughtfully and logically developed by the responsible nurses, even if you would personally have selected other strategies. (Adherence to the approved care plan should be required of all staff; the care plan cannot be treated as an optional guide).
3. Provide some means for the nurse to explain and communicate the reasoning behind her nursing plans to other staff members.
4. Assign responsibility for a care plan to one particular nurse over a sustained period of time.

5. Derive a system for staff input to the planning nurse.
6. Provide a system for review of care plans and of guidance to the planning nurse by a selected nursing expert.[50]

Use of a systems approach may facilitate the development and use of nursing care plans within the conceptual framework of primary nursing. Such an approach would include information gathering, nursing diagnosis, nursing prescription, and planned nursing care.

Ryan defines a system as a "a set of elements or units in interaction to achieve a specific goal" or an "orderly, logical arrangement of interdependent parts into an interrelated whole to accomplish a given purpose. . . . A system operates to convert or process energy, information, or materials into a planned outcome, a product, or information."[51] Characteristics of a system are as follows:

1. Input—the part that receives, stores, or takes energy in the form of information or material such as time, money, people, equipment, effort, or information.
2. Throughput—the processor, converter, or assimilating means of changing the energy received.
3. Output—the outcome, result, or product.
4. Feedback—the regulating mechanism that functions as a monitor, evaluator, or control to ensure that the planned goals are obtained. Output should be reintroduced to input at proper phases.

An open system continuously gathers and receives information about the environment and behavioral reactions to events occurring within and between component relationships, using this information as the means of signaling directions or adaptations toward the goals of the system.

The nursing care plan is such a system:

> A nursing care plan is an information receiving, processing, sending, and evaluating center initiated by the professional nurse through the use of specialized assessment, diagnostic, communication, and judgmental skills and compiled as a guide for directing nursing activities toward the fulfillment of health needs of the patient and the achievement of related nursing goals. . . . The

nursing care plan is expected to (1) bring a broad area of information to bear on the health problems of an individual patient and (2) control the operations or performance of the nursing care team in the coordinated manner of a single mind.[52]

These are principles to follow in developing nursing care plans:

1. The system receives input information from numerous sources, including the patient, the family, and records, and by systematic assessment through a history taking, a physical examination, and observational process.
2. The input is analyzed to identify problems and provide the throughput of a nursing diagnosis that is entered into a nursing care plan.
3. The output is a set of nursing orders or prescriptions that are entered into the plan and applied to the patient for the purpose of achieving goals or objectives.
4. The patient's responses are evaluated and the resulting information is given as feedback into the input phase of this system.

A standard format for nursing care plans improves their use and the documentation of care while retaining individualization.[53] The format for such plans can be coordinated with that for nursing history and assessments.

ETHICAL CONCERNS

There are many ethical issues directly related to the provision of patient care services. These have become more important during the past decade because of the increased sophistication of medical science and technology, concern about practical limits on financial resources for health care, changes in society, and growing emphasis on the autonomy of the individual.[54]

Nurse managers implement the employer's policy concerning the moral responsibilities for health care. Nurse managers have responsibility for supervision and review of patient care, meeting quality standards, making certain that decisions about patients are based on sound ethical principles, developing policies and mechanisms that address questions of human values, and responding to social problems and dilemmas that affect the need for health-care services.[55]

To fulfill this responsibility the nurse manager supports nurses confronted with ethical dilemmas and helps them think through situations by open dialogue. Nurse managers establish the climate for this. Davis recommends ethics rounds as a means of discussing ethical dilemmas. Such discussions can focus on hypothetical cases, case histories, or a current patient. Ethical reasoning requires participation by a knowledgeable person. Davis describes four ethical principles:

1. *Autonomy.* Personal freedom of action is an ethical principle to be applied by nurse managers toward professional nurses, who in turn apply the principle in the care of the patients. The professional nurse is given autonomy to deliberate about nursing actions and has the capacity to take nursing actions based on this deliberation.

Hospitalized or ambulatory patients may have diminished autonomy and the professional nurse becomes an advocate or autonomous agent for their rights. The patient is responsible for making decisions about care. The family may be involved with the patient's consent.

2. *Nonmaleficience.* Avoidance of intentional harm or the risk of inflicting harm on someone is termed "nonmaleficience." The use of restraints is an area that pits the principles of autonomy and self-determination against that of nonmaleficience. When risks outweigh costs, one must protect the patient. Side-rails, safety vests, tranquilizers, and wrist restraints all have the potential for abuse.

Discharge planning can prevent negative outcomes and potential errors. When errors occur, the nurse acknowledges them to the patient or a surrogate with full and immediate disclosure to the physician and institution's administration.

Nurses can protect patients from incompetent practitioners but protect their own rights at the same time.

3. *Beneficience.* Nurses view persons as autonomous and do not harm them, contributing to their health and welfare.

4. *Justice.* Nurses give patients what is due or owed, deserved or legitimately claimed.[56]

There are many ethical issues that relate to nursing and health care. One of these is the issue of the right to health care. We do not have a law that says society is obliged to provide health care. Other ethical issues are:

1. The rights of individuals and their surrogates versus the rights of the state or society. This issue creates confrontations among consumers and practitioners. As an example, cancer cases frequently lose money under reimbursement mechanisms. This may lead to management efforts to cut costs by cutting services (staff) or closing treatment centers. A survey of the Association of Community Cancer Centers indicated that 84 percent of them staff oncology units higher than other medical/surgical units.[57]
2. The rights of patients unable to make their own decisions versus the rights of their family versus the rights of institutions.
3. The right of patients to forego treatment versus the rights of society.
4. Issues related to:
   4.1 Reproductive technology, preselection of desired physical characteristics of children, genetic screening.
   4.2 Organ harvesting and transplants.
   4.3 Research subjects.
   4.4 Confidentiality.
   4.5 Restraints.
   4.6 Continuity of care.
   4.7 Disclosure.
   4.8 Informed consent.
   4.9 Patient incapacity.
   4.10 Court intervention.

The American Nurses Association (ANA) Committee on Ethics has published several position statements and guidelines which seek to assist nurses in making ethical decisions in their practice. These guidelines are based on ethical theory and the ANA Code for Nurses, which is an expression of "nursing's moral concerns, goals, and values." They are designed to provide nurses with guidance on a range of ethical issues, including the withdrawing or withholding of food and fluid; risk versus responsibility in providing care; safeguarding client health and safety from illegal, incompetent, or unethical practices; nurses' participation in capital punishment; and nurses' participation and leadership in ethical review practices.[58]

Nurse managers need to know the legal framework for their actions. They should help clinical nurses to balance teaching, research, clinical investigation, and patient care. All should work for social justice to ensure a quality of life and health-care services that is desirable. Nurses may promote compassion and sensitivity through protest of public policies that reduce quality or access to health care for the poor. They pursue human values, wholeness, and health values.[59] This does not mean that nurses must subsidize health care by working for lower salaries; rather they should work to have the cost shared by all of society.

Lee indicates that all organizations should develop a policy on ethics. Business ethics help people find the best way to satisfy the demands of competing interests. Ethics is part of corporate culture. Ethical organizations try to satisfy all of their stockholders, are dedicated to a high purpose, are committed to learning, and try to be the best at whatever they do.[60]

Leaders of ethical organizations have the moral courage to change direction, hire brilliant subordinates, encourage innovation, stick to values, and persist over time. Polaroid established internal conferences on ethics in 1983 and 1984. These included philosophers, ethicists, and business professors who looked at the language and concepts of ethics. They broadened the conferences to include leadership and dilemma workshops to apply the knowledge to company cases.[61]

Nurse managers can explore similar modes of studying ethics. They can do so with clinical nursing staff. This will include looking at how business is done versus how it should be done. It will set the organizational climate for ethical decision making. Ethics can be built into orientation, management development, participative management, and policies and procedures.

According to Beckstrand, "the aims of practice can be achieved using the knowledge of science and ethics alone." To apply her theory to nursing management, nurse managers would apply their knowledge of change to the nursing work environment to realize a greater good where and when needed.[62]

Education in management knowledge and practice changes the behavior of managers. Changes in management practice that reflect appropriate goals will result in meeting the needs of practicing clinical nurses. The ultimate outcome will be improved nursing care by persons satisfied with their nursing roles.

Current dilemmas in nursing are partly due to limitations in nursing management knowledge. Changes are needed that address values and goals. There could be a hierarchy of values in managing practice. Nurse managers need to determine how much decision-making power clinical nurses want and how much they can delegate. A theory of ethics should be meshed with a theory of nursing management. Nurse managers need a theory of ethical conduct that is congruent with one for clinical nurses.

Both clinical nurses and managers use scientific knowledge to determine whether conditions support change. The intrinsic value of the management actions should be given careful thought and should be debated by nurse managers who consciously attempt to practice management that realizes the highest good. The manager is more apt to be successful if scientific management knowledge is applied.

Ethics in management was the topic in an interview with Kenneth Blanchard. His comments are applicable to nurse managers; translated into nursing theory, they can be summed up as follows:

1. Nurse managers can influence the ethical behavior of nursing personnel by treating them ethically.
2. Nurse managers have a code of ethics that peers have agreed upon (see Appendix 7–1). They enter into ethical dilemmas when they go against that code.
3. Nurse managers fall into moral dilemmas when they go against their internal values.
4. While ethical and moral dilemmas differ, an ethical nurse manager is a moral nurse manager.
5. Ethical functions can be confronted by three questions:
   5.1 "Is it legal?" Resolves some dilemmas but not nonsensical laws and policies.
   5.2 "Is it balanced?" The nurse manager should aim for a win-win solution.
   5.3 "How will it make me feel about myself?" The nurse manager should consider the impact of each action on her/his self-respect.
6. Nurse managers with high self-esteem usually have the internal strength to make the ethical decision.
7. An ethical leader is an effective leader.

8. Nurse managers should apply six principles of ethical power:

   8.1 The chief nurse executive promotes and ensures pursuit of the stated mission or purpose of the nursing division, since this statement reflects the vision of its practicing nurses. While the mission should be reviewed periodically, goals or objectives are set for yearly achievement.
   8.2 Nurse managers should build an organization to win, thereby building self-esteem of employees through pride in their organization.
   8.3 Nurse managers should work to sustain patience and continuity through a long-term effect on the organization.
   8.4 Nurse managers should plan for persistence by spending more time following up on education and activities that build commitment of personnel.
   8.5 Nurse managers should promote perspective by giving their staff time to think. They should practice good management for the long term.
   8.6 Nursing service managers should consider developing an organization-specific code of ethics expressed in observable and measurable behaviors.[63]

Ethics should be ingrained in employees to create a strong sense of professionalism. A code of ethics can be developed to do this. Such a code should be the basis of a planned approach to all management functions of planning, organizing, directing, and controlling.

Nursing employees can help develop the code of ethics, can help implement it, and can help determine the rewards and punishment associated with it. A code of ethics should be read and signed by employees. It should be reviewed and revised on a regular schedule.

Contents of a code of ethics include definition of ethical and unethical practices, expected ethical behavior, enforcement of ethical practices, and rewards and punishments. To be objective a code of ethics specifies rules of conduct. It should be applied to all persons to be effective.[64]

Two centers exist to help organizations, including nursing, to establish standards for ethics programs:

Ethics Resource Center. Located in Washington, DC, the Ethics Resource Center is involved with "research on ethics and advising associations, businesses, educational institutions, and government agencies in the development of ethics programs."

Center for the Study of Ethics in the Professions. Located at the Illinois Institute of Technology in Chicago, this organization has concentrated on engineering and science, including nursing.[65]

SUMMARY

Nurse managers work with staff who are clinical practitioners. Educated in nursing management, they can assist these practitioners to guide their work according to the models of such theorists as Orem, Kinlein, Roy, Newman, Levine, Johnson, Peplau, Orlando, and others.

Several modalities of nursing have evolved during the past 40 years. In the 1940s, functional nursing was predominant because many professional nurses were in the armed forces during World War II and hospitals where thus staffed with auxiliary personnel.

Later, team nursing became the modality of choice for many hospital nursing services. Under the leadership of a professional nurse, a group of nurses work together to provide patient care. Team nursing rests on theoretical knowledge related to philosophy, planning, leadership, interpersonal relationships, and nursing process.

During the past two decades the modality of total patient care through primary nursing has evolved. With primary nursing the total care of a patient and a case load is the responsibility of one primary nurse.

Joint or collaborative practice by a physician-nurse team has developed as a modality of nursing in a very few hospitals. The latest development is case management, a method of practicing nursing that incorporates any modality but in which the knowledgeable nurse becomes the case manager, making or facilitating all clinical nursing decisions about a case load of patients during an entire episode of illness.

Clinical skills in nursing include history taking, making a nursing diagnosis, prescribing nursing care, carrying out nursing care, evaluating the results, and making needed changes. Nurse managers establish the climate for meeting all requirements for professional nursing. They do so with abilities that provide satisfaction to professional nurses, enhance the productivity of nurses, and make nursing care profitable and of high quality.

NOTES

1. H. A. Bush, "Models for Nursing," *Advances in Nursing Science,* Jan. 1979, 13–21.
2. G. L. Dickson and H. Lee-Villasenor, "Nursing Theory and Practice: A Self-Care Approach," *Advances in Nursing Science,* Oct. 1982, 29–40.
3. S. C. Roy, "Adaptation: A Basis for Nursing Practice," *Nursing Outlook,* Apr. 1971, 254–257.
4. Ibid.
5. M. F. Mastel and H. Hammond, "Analysis and Expansion of the Roy Adaptation Model: A Contribution to Holistic Nursing," *Advances in Nursing Science,* July 1980, 71–81.
6. Ibid.
7. V. F. Engle, "Newman's Conceptual Framework and the Measurement of Older Adults' Health," *Advances in Nursing Science,* Oct. 1984, 24–36.
8. Ibid.
9. Ibid.
10. M. E. Levine, "Adaptation and Assessment: A Rationale for Nursing Intervention," *American Journal of Nursing,* Nov. 1966, 2450–2453.
11. Ibid.
12. A. C. Rawls, "Evaluation of the Johnson Behavioral System Model in Clinical Practice," *Image,* 1980, 12–16.
13. L. Thompson, "Peplau's Theory: An Application to Short-Term Individual Therapy," *Journal of Psychosocial Nursing,*" Aug. 1986, 26–31.
14. N. J. Schmieding, "Putting Orlando's Theory into Practice," *American Journal of Nursing,* June 1984, 759–761; I. J. Orlando, *The Discipline and Teaching of Nursing Process: An Evaluative Study* (New York: G. P. Putnam's Sons, 1972); I. J. Orlando, *Nurse-Patient Relationship: Function, Process, Principles* (New York: G. P. Putnam's Sons, 1961).
15. V. S. Cleland, "Research—How Will Nursing Define It?," *Nursing Research,* Spring 1967, 118–121.
16. Ibid.
17. S. Fredette, "The Art of Applying Theory to Practice," *American Journal of Nursing,* May 1974, 856–859; K. Goldstein, *Human Nature Is the Light of Psychopathology* (New York: Schocken, 1963), 201.
18. "Accountability in Nursing Practice," *Nursing Management,* November 1984, 72.
19. S. R. Hinckley, Jr., "A Closer Look at Participation," *Organizational Dynamics,* Winter 1985, 57–67.
20. B. Henry, C. Arndt, M. DiVincenti, and A. Marriner-Tomey, Eds., *Dimensions of Nursing Administration: Theory, Research, Education, Practice* (Boston: Blackwell, 1989).
21. R. C. Swansburg and P. W. Swansburg, *Strategic Career Planning and Development for Nurses* (Rockville, MD: Aspen Publishers, 1984), 26–27.

22. Ibid., 27; D. P. Newcomb and R. C. Swansburg, *The Team Plan* (New York: G. P. Putnam's Sons, 1953, 1971); R. C. Swansburg, *Team Nursing: A Programmed Learning Experience,* 4 vols. (New York: G. P. Putnam's Sons, 1968).

23. D. P. Newcomb and R. C. Swansburg, op. cit., 56.

24. R. C. Swansburg and P. W. Swansburg, op. cit., 27.

25. Ibid.

26. G. D. Marram, M. W. Schlegel, and E. O. Bevis, *Primary Nursing: A Model for Individualized Care* (Saint Louis: Mosby, 1974), 1.

27. Ibid., 16–17.

28. S. Malkin and P. Lauteri, "A Community Hospital's Approach—Decentralized Patient Education," *Nursing Administration Quarterly,* Winter 1980, 101–106.

29. C. M. Fagin, "The Economic Value of Nursing Research," *American Journal of Nursing,* Dec. 1982, 1844–1849.

30. R. K. Shukla, "Primary or Team Nursing? Two Conditions Determine the Choice," *The Journal of Nursing Administration,* Nov. 1982, 12–15.

31. Ibid.

32. R. Rosenman and M. Jenkins, "A Nursing Staff Designs Its Own System," *Nursing Management,* Feb. 1986, 32–34.

33. G. L. Ingersoll, "Implementing Primary Nursing in a Surgical Outpatient Department," *Nursing Management,* May 1984, 32–33, 36–38.

34. Nevada Nurses' Association, *Nevada RNformation,* March 1985, 1.

35. J. Watson, "Patient Evaluation of a Primary Nursing Project," *The Australian Nurses' Journal,* Nov. 1978, 30–33, 49.

36. R. C. Swansburg and P. W. Swansburg, op. cit., 27–28.

37. Ibid., 28.

38. The National Joint Practice Commission, *Guidelines for Establishing Joint or Collaborative Practice in Hospitals* (Chicago, IL: Neely Printing, 1981).

39. Ibid.

40. E. Comeau, K. Zander, K. Bower, M. L. Etheredge, and J. G. Somerville, "Glossary," New England Medical Center Hospital, Department of Nursing, 1987.

41. K. A. Bower and J. G. Somerville, "Managed Care and Case Management Outcome-Based Practice: Creating the Environment," unpublished presentation at Sheraton Grand Hotel, Tampa, FL, Feb. 15–16, 1988.

42. E. Comeau, et al., op. cit.

43. Ibid.

44. Ibid.

45. "Diagnosing, Prescribing Included in Washington's Definition of Nursing," *American Journal of Nursing,* November 1973, 1962. *The Law Relating to Registered Nurses,* 18.88RCUW, (Olympia, WA: State of Washington Department of Licensing, July 1987).

46. M. B. Miller, "A Physician Views Skilled Nursing Care," *Journal of Nursing Administration,* Jan.-Feb. 1973, 20–29.

47. R. C. Swansburg, *Management of Patient Care Services* (St. Louis: Mosby, 1976): 172–173.

48. *Accreditation Manual for Hospitals, 1989* (Chicago: Joint Commission on Accreditation of Healthcare Organizations, 1989), 138.

49. B. J. Stevens, "Why Won't Nurses Write Nursing Care Plans?" *Journal of Nursing Administration,* Nov.-Dec. 1972, 67, 91–92.

50. Ibid.

51. B. J. Ryan, "Nursing Care Plans: A Systems Approach to Developing Criteria for Planning and Evaluation, *Journal of Nursing Administration,* May-June 1973, 50–58.

52. Ibid.

53. C. W. Sanborn and M. Blount, "Standard Plans: For Care and Discharge," *American Journal of Nursing,* Nov. 1984, 1394–1396.

54. Report of the Special Committee on Biomedical Ethics, *Values in Conflict: Resolving Ethical Issues in Hospital Care* (Chicago: American Hospital Association, 1985).

55. Ibid.

56. A. J. Davis, "Helping Your Staff Address Ethical Dilemmas," *The Journal of Nursing Administration,* Feb. 1982, 9–13.

57. L. E. Mortenson, "Are Oncology Nurses Too Expensive?," *Oncology Nursing Forum,* Jan./Feb. 1984, 14–15.

58. Committee on Ethics, American Nurses' Association, *Ethics in Nursing: Position Statements and Guidelines* (Kansas City, MO: American Nurses' Association, 1988).

59. J. E. Sauer, "Ethical Problems Facing the Healthcare Industry," *Hospital & Health Services Administration,* Sept./Oct. 1985, 44–53.

60. C. Lee, "Ethics Training: Facing the Tough Questions," *Training,* March 1986, 30–33, 38–41.

61. Ibid.

62. J. Beckstrand, "The Need for a Practice Theory as Indicated by the Knowledge Used in the Conduct of Practice," *Research in Nursing and Health,* Dec. 1978, 175–179.

63. K. C. Fernicola, "Take the High Road . . . to Ethical Management: An Interview with Kenneth Blanchard," *Association Management,* May 1988, 60–66.

64. M. Mizock, "Ethics—The Guiding Light of Professionalism," *Data Management,* Aug. 1986, 16–18, 29.

65. "Ethics Programs: More Than Lofty Phrases," *Association Management,* May 1988, 66–67.

REFERENCES

American Academy of Nursing, *Primary Care by Nurses: Sphere of Responsibility and Accountability* (Kansas City, MO: The Academy, 1977).

Berger, K. and Fields, *Pocket Guide to Health Assessment* (Reston, VA: Reston Publishing, 1980).

Chinn, P. L. and M. K. Jacobs, *Theory and Nursing: A Systematic Approach* (St. Louis: Mosby, 1987).

Ciske, K. I., Response to Zander's "Primary Nursing Won't Work . . . Unless the Head Nurse Lets It," *Journal of Nursing Administration,* Jan. 1978, 26, 43, 50.

Felton, G., "Increasing the Quality of Nursing Care by Introducing the Concept of Primary Nursing: A Model Project," *Nursing Research,* Jan.-Feb. 1975, 27–32.

Little, D. E. and D. L. Carnevali, *Nursing Care Planning,* 2d ed., (Philadelphia: Lippincott, 1976).

Mulligan, H. A., "Scruples Not Just Name of a Game," *The Augusta Chronicle, Augusta Herald,* Apr. 23, 1989, 1D, 4D.

Rotkovitch, R. "ICON: A Model of Nursing Practice for the Future," *Nursing Management,* June 1986, 54–56.

Roy, S. C., "Relating Nursing Theory to Education: A New Era." *Nurse Educator*, Mar.-Apr. 1971, 16–21.

Sherman, J. L. Jr. and S. K. Fields, *Guide to Patient Evaluation*, 3d ed. (Garden City, NY: Medical Examination Publishing, 1978).

Shukla, R. K., "Structure Versus People in Primary Nursing: An Inquiry," *Nursing Research*, July-Aug. 1981, 236–241.

Williams, L. B. and D. W. Cancian, "A Clinical Nurse Specialist in a Line Management Position," *The Journal of Nursing Administration*, Jan. 1985, 20–26.

Zander, K. S. "Primary Nursing Won't Work . . . Unless the Head Nurse Lets It," *Journal of Nursing Administration*, Oct. 1977, 19–23.

Zander, K., "Nursing Case Management: A Classic," *Definition*, Spring 1987.

APPENDIX 7–1.   ASNSA Code of Ethics

Preamble. This code of ethics is intended to give direction to and facilitate accomplishment of the goals of nursing service administration through the integrity and expertise of practitioners in the field of nursing service administration. Effective executive functioning demands that nursing service administrators affirm and accept the responsibility to practice their profession according to the highest professional nursing and management standards.*

Nursing service administrators believe in the worth and dignity of man. Nursing service administrators share responsibility for the multifaceted delivery of health care and are committed to maintain standards of excellence in facilitating an environment for the provision of nursing care. Nursing service administrators are prepared to undertake a valid and consistent approach to the solution of patient care problems.

This code of ethics is applicable to professional individuals having responsibility as nursing service administrators in any health care setting and complies with existing policies of the American Hospital Association.

Accountability. Nursing service administrators must meet four primary accountabilities: to the consumer; to themselves in accomplishing their responsibilities as nursing service administrators and for and to the staffs for whom they are responsible; to the chief executive officer or chief operating officer of the health care agency; and to the American Society for Nursing Service Administrators.

Nursing service administrators are expected to adhere to the *Guidelines of Ethical Conduct and Relationships for Health Care Institutions* formulated by the American Hospital Association. They are expected to utilize the standards of nursing practice as determined by professional nursing. Therefore, the nursing service administrator shall:

1. Maintain and support interpersonal relationships within the organization that will assure an environment conducive to humane and appropriate care of those served
2. Continually strive to merit the confidence and respect of patients, staff, and community through quality and scope of nursing services

3. Cooperate with other disciplines engaged in or supportive of health services
4. Develop, implement, and periodically review nursing service organization and management, professional policies, practices, standards of performance, and activities for quality assurance

In matters of professional and personal ethics, the nursing service administrator has a duty to:

1. Observe at all times the existing local, state, and federal laws as a minimum guide for fulfillment of responsibilities
2. Conduct activities on behalf of and within the health care agency in a manner that is honest and ethical

The Governing Body and Chief Executive/ Operating Officer. Effectiveness in nursing service administrative performance depends on mutual respect and harmonious relationships between the nursing service administrator, the chief executive/operating officer, and the governing authority. Such accord can be maintained best when functions and prerogatives of each are carefully defined, understood, and followed.

In the fulfillment of defined functions the nursing service administrator shall:

1. Exercise authority required to conduct nursing service activities of the organization in accordance with nursing and health care agency policies adopted by the governing body
2. Demonstrate personal integrity and professional competence with capable leadership that merits confidence and respect
3. Consider as a major factor the corporate interest in all matters affecting the nursing service administrator's role and responsibility

Medical Staff. The nursing service administrator shall promote effective channels for exchange of thinking and decision making between the medical staff and nursing service administration.

To effect the above, the nursing service administrator shall:

1. Promote coordination, supportive mechanisms, and understanding through colleagueship with the medical staff to carry out responsibilities and activities with respect to quality of nursing care provided patients
2. Enhance, through appropriate channels, the policies established for the rights and responsibilities of patients

Nursing Staff. The nursing service administrator shall strive to enhance the knowledge and expertise of nursing service personnel to assure the highest level of care to the patient.

To effect the above, the nursing service administrator shall:

1. Establish and implement appropriate philosophy, objectives, policies, and standards for nursing care of patients in concert with corporate policies and resources
2. Provide and implement a departmental plan of administrative authority clearly delineating accountability and responsibility for all categories of nursing personnel
3. Establish staffing requirements for nursing services and recommend and implement policies and procedures to assure an appropriate and competent nursing staff
4. Estimate needs for supplies, facilities, and equipment and implement an effective evaluation and control system
5. Initiate, utilize, and participate in studies and research projects designed for the improvement of patient care and health care agency services
6. Provide and implement a program of continuing education for all nursing personnel
7. Facilitate an environment for professional nursing practice that enables staff to continue to learn and students to have clinical experience in nursing
8. Assume responsibility for preparation and management of both operating and capital equipment budgets for nursing services

Interdepartmental Relationships. The nursing service administrator shall foster an effective interdepartmental relationship between nursing service and all other departments existing in the health care setting. The nursing service administrator coordinates the needs of nursing service with those of supporting departments and, together with general administration and department heads, plans solutions to problems related to the welfare of the patient and staff.

Agency Relationships. Nursing service administrators shall maintain a spirit of cooperation with representatives of other health care organizations where there is a sharing of common objectives. They assist other nursing service administrators and their organizations through participation in activities and services that will improve the quality of patient care programs. They cooperate with education and planning organizations that contribute to the advancement of health care.

Conflict of Interest. Nursing service administrators shall conduct their personal and professional relationships in such a way as to assure themselves, their organizations, and the public that decisions they make are in the best interest of the patient and the organization. Exercise of judgment is required to determine whether a potential conflict of interest exists. A conflict of interest exists when a nursing service administrator is in a position, apart from the remuneration received from employment, to profit directly or indirectly through the application of personal or administrative authority. The nursing service administrator shall endeavor to avoid conflict of interest by providing full disclosure to the chief executive/operating officer and the governing body of any potential conflict of interest.

Systems Conflict. Because of the need to coordinate and participate in the operation of the larger health care system, nursing service administrators are often elected and appointed to the governing bodies of health-related organizations, such as planning bodies, state and national hospital associations, and other health care organizations. Inherent in such positions is a potential conflict of interest because of the duality of interest of the nursing service administrator. Such duality of interest is acceptable only when there is no conflict of interest.

Confidential Information. Confidential information belongs to the health care agency. Use of it by nursing service administrators, their business associates, friends, or relatives for their own gain is a violation of the code of ethics.

P332-500-10/1/78

*A committee to administer this code of ethics will provide a clarifying and supportive function to nursing service administrators.

Nursing Service Policies and Procedures 8

INTRODUCTION

Policies, procedures, rules, and regulations are the standing plans of the nursing organization. Standing plans are fixed in both nature and content. They apply until reviewed and modified or abandoned.[1] While hospitals and other employers of nurses seldom use the terms "rules" or "regulations," they frequently develop and maintain policies and procedures that incorporate the rules and regulations imposed by such government agencies as the Health Care Financing Administration, which administers Medicare and Medicaid.

NURSING SERVICE POLICIES

Nursing service policies exist for standardization and as a source of guidance of the nursing staff. As guidelines they give the nurse manager input into nursing activities of each unit, ward, and clinic in which nursing personnel practice. Generally policies fall into three main categories: those which apply to patients, those which apply to personnel, and those which apply to the environment in which patients are cared for and in which personnel work. A fourth category could be that of relationships with other disciplines or departments. Nursing management also gives input into institutional policies and policies of other departments sharing in the care of patients. Major administrative policies of the division of nursing are best developed by the chief nurse executive in consultation with representatives of all groups concerned in their implementation, including clinical nurses. Such a process of participatory management assumes that employees will follow and support policies they have helped to develop.

Policy making is a part of the planning function of top nursing management. All policies of lower levels of management supplement and support those of top management. Although any supervisor may set a policy, it cannot conflict with one enforced by a higher authority; policy may be made by a manager only for the area over which that manager has authority.

Meggison, Mosley, and Pietri define policies as "broad general statements of expected actions that serve as guides to managerial decision making or to supervising the actions of subordinates."[2] Figure 8–1 offers an example. The first and last paragraphs fit the definition of a *policy* while the guidelines more properly fit the *procedures* category.

Policies are usually developed by a policy committee. At the organizational level the committee will be representative of departments and top management. At the nursing division level the committee will be representative of nursing specialties and top nursing management. The policy development process includes the following steps:

1. Determination that a policy is needed.
2. Assignment of the development of each policy to a committee member or members.

3. Development of policy from appropriate sources of information, such as those for the policy on "no code."[3] Sources for developing such policies can be found through computer searches or by using references from published sources.
4. Review of the draft policy by the committee.
5. Circulation of the draft to appropriate clinical committees of physicians who will write orders and nurses who will carry them out. A "no code" policy, for example, would go to these groups, while other policies would go to other appropriate groups.
6. Review of returned comments.
7. Referral to the organization's attorney for approval when indicated (such as "no code" policy).
8. Final approval by committee and signature of the organization's chief executive officer.
9. Distribution with appropriate communication. In the case of a "no code" policy, all personnel who would respond to a cardiac arrest need to be informed.

FIGURE 8–1.　Subject: "No Code"

A decision not to resuscitate a patient is the responsibility of the attending physician. An order must be written on the physician's order sheet by the attending physician or delegated to a house officer. [Such orders cannot] be accepted verbally.

The following guidelines will be adhered to by the physician when writing "no code" orders and documented in the progress notes.

1. Assess for: Viability of the patient, quality of life of the patient, and competency of the patient.
2. Discuss with the patient and/or family the results of this assessment and the writing of a "no code" order by this physician.
3. This order for "no code" will be reviewed by the physician daily and updated weekly. Changes will then be made as needed.

The hospital nursing procedure for "code 1" will be immediately implemented on all patients without a "no code" order.

SOURCE: Courtesy of the University of South Alabama Medical Center, Mobile, Alabama.

A policy is a mechanism that establishes constraints or boundaries for administrative action and sets a course to be followed. Within those boundaries, nursing personnel still have latitude for independent action. A clinical nurse working alone can refer to policies to make decisions.

Policies are closely related to departmental and unit mission, philosophy, objectives, and operating plans. Objectives may be expressed through policies, and policies may be used to help achieve objectives.

Policies will not always be written down, since a consistent pattern of administrative decisions and actions related to specific problems also indicates policy. An example of unwritten policy in an organization is that an employee who is within two years of retirement is not promoted, even though her record may be better than employees with less service. Such covert policies are sometimes precedent-setting policies. Employees make decisions and act on their own without comment or action by supervisors. Thus they set a precedent for other clinical nurses. Also, supervisors sometimes act in such a way as to imply policy. Policies established by precedent or implied action are the covert or unwritten policies of nursing.

Policies are formal or informal, written or covert. Formal policies are those that apply to:

1. Organizations as a whole.
2. A functional entity such as a division or department.
3. A basic unit such as a ward, floor, special care unit, or clinic.

Policies impact nursing at each of these levels.

Policies that define an organization's philosophy or position on philosophical issues such as ethics or religion are apt to be developed at top management level. Those that enforce legal rules or government regulations are the responsibility of top management. Policies must be in harmony with legal aspects of organizational operations.

Policies have value because of their effect in promoting consistency of action and stability. They provide guidance from top management to lower levels, and in so doing they transfer and thus speed up some decision making. Absence of policy creates situations in which similar problems are addressed over and over again, sometimes within several sections at one time, without establishing a management position. Policies conserve time by setting standards, discipline problems being an example. If there are no policies one manager can terminate an employee for the same act for which another manager gives counsel, written warning, or suspension. Uniformity of policies prevents conflict and promotes fairness.

Too much imposition of policies is frequently perceived by professionals as authoritarian and bureaucratic. Administrative directives in any form, including policies, could be kept to a minimum. They should be pertinent, concise, and comprehensive and should state their underlying reasons. When policies are written for every eventuality, they stifle independent thought and action.

How Is Policy Made and Used?

Formulation of Policy.   Before a policy is instituted, relevant information should be gathered and analyzed. Other departments may need to be consulted. A tentative draft can be prepared and circulated asking for comments on potential effects. A nurse manager should remember that published policy represents the official position of the organization.

Communication of Policy.   People who are going to be affected by policies need to know about them, particularly if they must apply them and conform to them. Written policies have advantages of being a source for future reference, especially for new personnel, part-time personnel, and those on relief duty in areas in which they are not regularly assigned. Written policies also are not garbled by verbal transmission.

Policies need to be written in simple, easy-to-understand language. They can be communicated by supervisors verbally or by letters, bulletin board announcements, newspaper accounts, handbooks, or policy manuals. Training conferences are valuable forums for explaining and discussing the use of existing policies. In these sessions the purposes and events leading to their development can be questioned and discussed. A good practice that will help make new policies known to nursing personnel is to place two copies in each unit, one in the policy book and the other on the bulletin board to be read and initialed by employees. To be effective, new policies should be discussed with personnel, who will be told the reasons for change. This will prevent irritation and annoyance. A system should be developed for handling policies so that they will not be posted on disorganized and crowded bulletin boards or in a format that will be disregarded by nursing personnel. Their relative value will be indicated by the manner in which they are distributed and made known.

Application of Policy.   Administrative judgment is essential to application of policy. Application should be consistent and fair; then the policy will be valued. Flexibility can be written into policy when needed. An example would be policy that describes management actions for discipline: when to counsel, reprimand, suspend, or terminate employees. Policy that is not applied is of little value and can indicate unfair practices or irrelevance.

Review and Appraisal.   A schedule for review of policies will keep them from becoming outmoded. Some organizations have a system for annual review on a suspense file data basis. Files can be maintained in a nursing management information system. As objectives change, related policies need to be reviewed and updated. Effective management is partly the result of successful policy changes.

FIGURE 8–2. Excerpt from a Table of Contents of Hospital-wide Policies

---

Organization of the Policy and Procedure Manual

Purpose

Exceptions

Distribution of Manual

Responsibility for Policy Implementation

Types of Policy Change

Policy Change

Policy/Procedure Committees

Hospital

Organizational Chart

Hospital Mission Statement

Philosophy of the University of South Alabama Medical Center

Functional Plan of Organization of the University of South Alabama Medical Center Mission Statements Administrative Responsibility (Weekend, Night, and Holiday)

Admission, Deposit Requirements for Inpatients, Noninsured

Admitting Services

Adoption

Adverse Drug Reaction Report

Anesthesiology

Audit Policy, Hospital

Authority of Intervention

Battered Child Syndrome

Beds, Moving of

Bomb Threats

Brain Death Protocol

Building Modifications

Business Office

   Purpose

   Organization

   Hours of Operation

   Business Services

Cardiovascular Laboratory

Chaplain Services

Check Cashing

Circulation Technology

Code One (1)

Code Five (5)—Security Announcements

Communicable Disease, Exposure

SOURCE: Courtesy of the University of South Alabama Medical Center, Mobile, Alabama.

Policy-Making Responsibility

Part of the responsibility for policy making results from external forces such as applicable laws, accreditation standards, and standards of professional associations. Government regulation of health-care services is expanding. Organized labor influences the establishment of organizational policy, particularly in the area of personnel policies. Although employees may not have direct input into policy making, their position and views are often considered.

Because the nurse administrator has overall responsibility for divisional direction, that person must have control of key policy decisions. Such policies will usually be broad and related to divisional objectives. Organizational structure will influence policy making, since it describes relationships among departments and among units within departments. This structure describes the responsibilities of each department and will define how policy making is delegated.

Personnel are usually experts in specific areas and can help develop many of the departmental policies. As examples in nursing, policies for intensive care units, coronary care units, and other specialized areas should be developed and reviewed by the appropriate nurse manager. Clinical nurses know laws, practices, and other up-to-date information about the specialties.

Lower-level managers adopt the broad policies of top management. Management plans will include provision for input into policy making from all levels. This input may be accepted or rejected by the nurse administrator. Figure 8–2 is an excerpt from a table of contents of hospital policies. Figure 8–3 is an excerpt from a table of contents of nursing division policies.

FIGURE 8–3. Excerpt from Table of Contents for Nursing Division Policies

SOURCE: Courtesy of the University of South Alabama Medical Center, Mobile, Alabama.

Personnel Policies

Personnel policies will usually be developed by the personnel section or department, depending on the size of the institution. They should be developed with input from the division of nursing. Their purpose will be to attract and retain nursing personnel who will make an effective contribution to achieving the objectives of the nursing services. Personnel policies should be consistent with overall organizational policies and policies recommended by the American Nurses Association. They should provide for an employee health program and a grievance procedure, cover the benefits and conditions of work, including salary, and promote job satisfaction and stability of staff. They should exist in written form and should be given to and discussed with each applicant for a position.

Policies frequently cover selection and placement of personnel in an area in which they are interested and for which they have been prepared through education and experience. Policies should promote a work environment in which all nursing staff participate in planning, implementing, and evaluating nursing care. Policies will include assignments of personnel to allow them to devote most of their duty time to the primary functions of nursing so as to provide continuity as well as satisfaction to them, to patients, and to families. See Appendix 4–1.

Scheduling should be covered by firm yet fair personnel policies. Coverage will include:

- Minimum requirements per shift.
- Weekends off.
- Work stretch policies.
- Holiday, days off, vacation by request.
- Equitable rotation.
- Modifications.
- Part-time personnel.
- Staff preferences.
- Equity.[4]

It is also a good plan to include processes for effective communication between nursing staff and management personnel in departmental policy. Nurse managers know the organization's personnel policies and procedures. These are usually provided in an updated version by the personnel or human resources department. In many organizations the important policies are summarized in an employee handbook.

In many instances, management of employees is governed by major federal legislation. It is important for nurse managers to refer to the organization's personnel manual and to confer with personnel of the human resources department. A summary of major federal antidiscrimination laws is listed in Figure 8–4.

Human resources departments also stay up to date on state laws that affect personnel policies and procedures. A nursing department's policies and procedures that pertain to personnel management should be coordinated with organizational personnel policies and procedures, manuals, and handbooks.

Personnel manuals are a form of communication with employees. Figure 8–5 shows an excerpt from the table of contents of a personnel manual.

1. Philosophy.
2. Objectives.
3. Organizational plan.
4. Recognition of patient's cultural, economic, and social differences and their value systems.
5. Collaborative planning with patients, their families, and the interdisciplinary team.
6. Fiscal resource management.
7. Staffing.
8. Assignments.
9. Clinical nursing privileges.
10. Advancement in clinical practice.
11. Quality assurance.
12. Support services.
13. Orientation.
14. Education.
15. Ethics.
16. Research.

Standards

Some written policies are required by the Joint Commission on Accreditation of Healthcare Organizations (JCAHO). Implementation of standards implies that policies will be developed for carrying them out. Many will affect administrative areas; these should be reviewed by the nurse administrator, who provides recommendations for policy development, revision, and implementation as it relates to the care of patients and the activities of nursing personnel. Policies will need to include standards applicable to the practicing nurse, particularly with regard to clinical privileges and standards of professional ethical practices. These clinical privileges will be covered by the state nursing practice act and will be based on education, experience, and demonstrated competence and judgment. They will include policies related to assignments; diagnostic and therapeutic orders of medical staff members; medication administration; confidentiality of information and the role of the nursing staff in discharge planning and in patient and family education; the maintenance of required records, reports, and statistical information; cardiopulmonary resuscitation; patient, employee, and visitor safety; and the scope of activity of volunteers or paid attendants.[5]

The American Nurses' Association's (ANA) *Standards for Organized Nursing Services and Responsibilities of Nurse Administrators Across All Settings* imply nursing policies related to:

In addition, ANA standards state that nurses should be involved in policy making.[6]

Specific written hospital policies are required for management of patient care services. Since nursing personnel are frequently responsible for implementing these policies, the nurse administrator should be involved in their development and revision. It has been the experience of many nurse administrators that these policies have to be totally developed, revised, and implemented by the nursing staff. Other areas related to JCAHO standards for which nurse managers will have to assist in developing, revising, or implementing policies are diagnostic radiology services, hospital-based home care services, hospital-sponsored ambulatory care services, pharmaceutical services, anesthesia services, dietetic services, emergency services, infection control, medical record services, nuclear medicine services, plant technology and safety management, professional library services, quality assurance, radiology oncology services, rehabilitation services, respiratory care services, social work services, and special care units.

Specific policies and procedures for ambulatory care services and special care units are of particular import to nursing personnel. In the standards for special care units it is required that each special care unit have specific written policies and procedures that supplement the basic hospital policies and procedures. An administrator or manager of a division of nursing knows the standards of the JCAHO

FIGURE 8–4. Major Federal Discrimination Laws

The following summary of the major federal legislation and requirements under which questions of prohibited discrimination most commonly arise is not all-inclusive. A number of other federal laws also exist and, in addition, requirements enacted by the various state and/or local governments also must be ascertained.

Source of Regulation	Employer Coverage	Discrimination Prohibited	Enforcing Agency
I. Employers Generally			
U.S. Constitution	Public employers and private employers acting "under color of state law"	Race, religion, national origin; sex questionable	None specified
Title VII of the Civil Rights Act of 1964	Public and private employers with 15 or more employees for at least 20 weeks in the year	Race, color, religion, sex, national origin	EEOC
Civil Rights Act of 1866 (§1981)	Private, state, and local governments	Race; perhaps national origin	None
Civil Rights Act of 1871 (§1983)	State and local governments and private persons acting "under color of state law"	Rights protected by federal constitution and laws (e.g., race, national origin, sex)	None
Equal Pay Act of 1963	Private and public employers	Unequal pay for equal work by males and females	EEOC
Age Discrimination in Employment Act (ADEA)	All private employers with 20 or more employees for at least 20 weeks in the current year, state and local governments	Age (40–70)	EEOC
Veterans Reemployment Act	All public and private employers	Returning veterans, employees on military leave, employees who leave to go into the military, reservists	Department of Labor (DOL) Office of Veterans' Reemployment Rights (OVRR)
Apprenticeship Act	Sponsors of apprenticeship programs	Race, color, religion, national origin, sex	DOL
II. Federal Contractors			
Executive Order No. 11,246	Employers who are party to a contract with the federal government (1) in excess of $10,000 per year (2) in excess of $50,000 per year plus 50 employees	Race, color, religion, sex, national origin In addition, employers must adopt written affirmative action plan	Office of Federal Contracts Compliance Programs (OFCCP)

FIGURE 8–4. Major Federal Discrimination Laws (*continued*)

The following summary of the major federal legislation and requirements under which questions of prohibited discrimination most commonly arise is not all-inclusive. A number of other federal laws also exist and, in addition, requirements enacted by the various state and/or local governments also must be ascertained.

Source of Regulation	Employer Coverage	Discrimination Prohibited	Enforcing Agency
Executive Order No. 11,141	Employers who contract with federal government	Age	Federal agency entering into contract
Veterans Readjustment Act	Employers who are party to a contract with the federal government in excess of $10,000 per year	Disabled veterans, the Vietnam era veterans	OFCCP
Section 503 of the Rehabilitation Act	Employers who are party to a contract with the federal government in excess of $2,500 per year	Handicap	OFCCP

III. Federally Assisted Programs

Title VI of the Civil Rights Act of 1964	Employers with programs or activities receiving federal financial assistance*	Beneficiaries of programs/ activities due to race, color, national origin; employment regulated if primary objective of federal assistance is to provide employment	Federal department/ agencies providing assistance
Section 504 of the Rehabilitation Act	Same as Title VI	Handicap; extends to beneficiaries and employees/applicants†	Office of Civil Rights
Age Discrimination Act of 1975	Same as Title VI	Age (employer not covered unless CETA funded)	Various CETA funds

*The federal regulations designate Medicare and Medicaid as federal financial assistance, 45 C.F.R. Part 80, app. A, pts. 1 and 2; 45 C.F.R. Part 84, app. A, subpt. A, 1–2. Also, see United States v. Baylor University Medical Center, _____ F.2d _____, No. 83-1398 (5th Cir. July 19, 1984).
†Consolidated Rail Corp. v. Darrone, 104 S. Ct 1248 (1984).

SOURCE: K. H. Henry, *The Health Care Supervisor's Legal Guide,* Appendix 6-A, (Rockville, MD: Aspen Publishers, © 1984), 162–164. Reprinted with permission.

and develops policies and procedures for all areas in which nursing personnel perform services. A practical way of doing this is to make a checklist of these standards and involve appropriate nurse managers and clinical nurses in developing policies that will be workable and helpful to all who have need to refer to them.

Continuing education has become a condition of employment written into some personnel policies. It is required by the employer for clinical advancement and may or may not be a fringe benefit. Policies also cover the organization of committees, including purposes, membership, and operating procedures. Other areas frequently covered by policies include:

1. Personnel policies reflecting goals of an affirmative action program to maintain equal employment practices while maintaining an efficient, productive work force.
2. Moving and travel costs.
3. Sabbaticals.
4. Pay.
5. Programs to recognize outstanding performances and achievements.
6. Suggestion programs.
7. Orientation programs that foster creativity.
8. Provisions that make jobs meaningful.
9. Four-day workweeks.
10. Flexible hours in workweek.
11. Drug and alcohol abuse.
12. Handicapped employees.
13. Performance appraisal.
14. Management by objectives.

Most of these fourteen areas would be covered by organizational policies. In large organizations entire staff positions may be devoted to policy and procedure writing.

These policies will usually be written and available as manuals and used by appropriate personnel. There will be provision for their periodic review and revision. For this reason it is practical to have them in a loose-leaf notebook.

Policies may be combined with procedures, with policy stated first. Policies may stand alone or require many procedures to be implemented.

FIGURE 8–5. Excerpt from Table of Contents of Personnel Policies Manual

1.0 Introduction
2.0 Major Employment Policy Statements
    2.1 Equal Opportunity and Affirmative Action
    2.2 Rights of Management
3.0 Employment
    3.1 Eligibility Guidelines
        3.1.1 Minimum Requirements
        3.1.2 Age
        3.1.3 Employment of Relatives
        3.1.4 Aliens
        3.1.5 Former Employees
        3.1.6 Hospital Employees
    3.2 Employment Status
        3.2.1 Definition of Status
        3.2.2 Probationary Period
        3.2.3 Dual Employment
        3.2.4 Outside Employment
        3.2.5 Service Periods
    3.3 Change in Status
        3.3.1 Promotion
        3.3.2 Transfer
        3.3.3 Demotion
        3.3.4 Resignation
        3.3.5 Retirement
    3.4 Personnel Record
        3.4.1 Confidentiality
        3.4.2 Reporting Changes
4.0 Attendance and Leave
    4.1 Work Schedules
        4.1.1 Hours, Rest Periods, and Lunch Periods
        4.1.2 Emergency Closings
        4.1.3 Overtime
    4.2 Time Sheets and Time Cards
    4.3 Sick Leave

SOURCE: Courtesy of the University of South Alabama Medical Center, Mobile, Alabama.

NURSING SERVICE PROCEDURES

In addition to policies, a written and current nursing procedures manual should be available to all nursing personnel. Procedures outline a standard technique or method for performing duties and serve as a guide for action. Procedures are detailed plans for nursing skills that include steps in proper sequence; see Figure 8–6.

Purposes

Procedures are used for communication, understanding, standardization, and coordination. They are referred to for review when an employee has not done a procedure for some time. They are used to teach and evaluate students and new employees, to orient new employees to distinguishing characteristics of an institution's procedures, and to update employees in developing technologies.

FIGURE 8–6. Nursing Policy on Patient Care Assignments

I. Policy Statement. Patient care assignments for nursing personnel will be made by a qualified professional registered nurse/charge nurse according to the University of South Alabama Medical Center standards of care.

II. Purpose. To guarantee the best possible nursing care for the patient, based on the patient's care needs and the staff competencies.

III. General Information. Patient assignments will be made at the beginning of each shift. Each patient's care will be directed by a written management plan. Patient care will be supervised by an R.N.

IV. Equipment.

Management plan

Patient Kardex

Assignment sheets

V. Procedures

Nursing Action	Basis for Nursing Intervention
1. Have written assignment for staff members.	1. Allows staff to see duties required on that shift.
2. Receive a verbal report on the patients.	2. Allows nurse to communicate any changes in plans of care or patient status.
3. Take orders from management plan and doctors' orders.	3. Allows for review of management plan and current physician orders.
4. Review patient assignment with staff members.	4. Allows R.N. to direct other staff members and clarify care orders.

VI. Documentation Write assignments on assignment sheet and update as needed. Include patient acuity on assignment sheet.

SOURCE: Courtesy of the University of South Alabama Medical Center, Mobile, Alabama.

Patient care procedures should inform, teach, and reduce errors. They should relate new and changing equipment to patient care practices. They should tell where to order, call, or send for something, how to perform tasks, and why. Procedures are updated by a committee of professional nurses representing those who use them, relate to them, and contribute theoretical insights. The following is a recommended sequence of events to follow in developing a new procedure:

1. A task or title is stated.
2. A need is identified (purpose stated).
3. A draft is made by a user (an outline on paper of all possible steps and substeps).
4. References and experts, including manufacturers, are consulted.
5. The committee member responsible for development of the specific procedure drafts it in standard format, including related policies, equipment needed, line drawings, location of equipment, and ordering procedure. The draft provides step-by-step instructions in performance, brief theory statements, and supporting documents.
6. The draft is edited.

FIGURE 8–7.   Excerpt from Table of Contents, Procedure Manual

	Revised/Reviewed				
	1986	1987	1988	1989	1990
A					
Abbreviations					
Absenteeism and Tardiness					
Accidents					
Admission of Patients					
Air Mattress					
Allergies					
AMBU Bag, Use of					
Assignments					
Educational Programs					
B					
Bedside Rails					
Blood Collection by Registered Nurses					
Blood Glucose Monitoring					
Blood Transfusions, Outpatients					
Bottle Feeding					
Breast Feeding					
C					
Cardiac Monitoring System					
Cardio Pulmonary Resuscitation					
Cardiac Rehabilitation					
Catheter, Insertion of					
Catheter, Irrigation of					
Catheter, Medication Instillation of					
Cervical Traction, Application of					
Cesium, Therapy					

FIGURE 8–7. Excerpt from Table of Contents, Procedure Manual (*continued*)

	Revised/Reviewed				
	1986	1987	1988	1989	1990
C					
Chaplain Services					
Charting					
Chest Tube Clamping					
Circumcision, Assisting with					
Clinitron Therapy, Initiation and Maintenance of					
Code I Team					
Code I Pediatric Alert					
Color Code for Charts					

SOURCE: Courtesy of University of South Alabama Medical Center, Mobile, Alabama.

7. An index code number is assigned.
8. The procedure is typed and distributed to reviewers (labelled "draft") with a deadline for feedback.
9. Returned drafts are used to revise the procedure.
10. The revised manuscript is submitted to approval authorities.
11. When approved, the procedure is printed and distributed.
12. In-service training on the procedure is given to all appropriate personnel.[7]

Policies and procedures are reviewed, revised as necessary, and dated to indicate the time of the most recent review. They must be abandoned when obsolete. Figure 8–7 is an excerpt from a table of contents for a procedure manual.

Advantages

Six major advantages of procedures are that they:

1. Conserve management effort.
2. Facilitate delegation of authority.
3. Lead to more efficient methods of operation.
4. Permit significant economizing in personnel.
5. Facilitate control.
6. Aid in coordination of activities.[8]

Disadvantages

Policies and procedures do not always encourage participatory management. They provide a "party line," thereby limiting individual discretion and decision making. For this reason their review should include such questions as, "is this policy (or procedure) really needed?" and "can this policy (or procedure) be modified to give more leeway to clinical and managerial decision making throughout the division?"[9]

Nurse administrators can review commercially produced nursing skills books with the object in mind of adopting one that meets most needs. It can be supplemented with only those procedures absolutely necessary for organizational fit. Nurses are thus saved untold hours of procedure meetings.

Rules and Regulations

Most rules and regulations are included in policy and procedures manuals. They describe what can or cannot be done under specified circumstances. They permit no variations. As previously stated, flexibility should be written into the document itself. Figure 8–8 shows how rules are spelled out in hospital policy.

OTHER MANUALS

Policy and procedure manuals are only two of the possible manuals developed for use in hospitals or other health-care institutions. Depending upon the size of the institution there may be manuals on safety, disaster preparedness, nutrition and food service, pharmacy, and others.

Grubb recommends the following process for developing manuals:

1. Initiating.
2. Proposing.
3. Gathering data.
4. Analyzing data.
5. Setting content priorities.
6. Delegating responsibilities.
7. Selecting format.
8. Organizing materials.
9. Outlining topics.
10. Writing.
11. Checking facts.
12. Reviewing rough draft.
13. Rewriting.
14. Evaluating.
15. Typing final draft.
16. Proofreading.
17. Numbering pages.
18. Indexing.
19. Printing.
20. Binding.
21. Distributing.
22. Utilizing.
23. Maintaining.
24. Revising.

These steps can be applied to procedures also.

This process is more likely to be followed if one person is responsible for it. That person will advise the committee and implement its work. Bylaws of a policy and procedure committee are presented in the chapter on committees, as is an example of policy and procedure minutes.

Manuals may be used in many ways, including conferences, meetings, and procedure demonstration days or through exercises and games, demonstrations, videotapes, case studies, and group learning sessions. A predetermined and coded distribution list should be a part of each policy.

FIGURE 8–8.   University of South Alabama Medical Center Hospital Body Substance Precautions

Policy.   Body substance precautions will be used by all departments in this institution and are to be used for *any* contact with *all* patient blood or body secretions.

Purpose.   The purpose of these guidelines is to prevent the transmission of infectious diseases within this institution.

General Information.   Use body substance precautions on all patients and for all patient care at *all times*.

Some of the steps to be taken for *all* contact with patient substance and/or fluids are:

1. Wash your hands for at least 15 seconds both before and after any patient contact.
2. Wear gloves when touching *any* body substance or mucous membrane.
3. Wear gowns when clothing or uniform is likely to be soiled.
4. Place soiled linen in a laundry bag.
5. Place used needles or sharps in needle disposal containers. *Do not recap needles!!*
6. Inform Infection Control Nurse if patient has an infectious disease for appropriate isolation.
7. Wear goggles when splashing of body fluids is possible.

Remember: Gloves should be worn for all contact with mucous membranes, nonintact skin, and moist body substances, for *all patients at all times*.

Note: Direct all inquiries to the Infection Control Department.

SOURCE: Courtesy of the University of South Alabama Medical Center, Mobile, Alabama.

SUMMARY

In developing a theory of nursing management, nursing service policies and procedures are conceptual plans translated into physical entities, usually called manuals. Both should be developed with input from clinical nurses who will be led to view them as one source of nursing standards.

Lower-level policies support upper-level ones. All are developed from appropriate sources of information and are updated periodically. It is important for nurses to note that policies and procedures set standards and hold the profession to meeting them.

Although many policies come from external sources and are mandated, nurse managers should work with clinical nurses to determine the necessity for each policy.

All policies and procedures are communicated to users, making it essential that nurse managers have such a communication plan and exercise it periodically.

Some policies and procedures cover topics so extensively as to be developed into separate manuals. These include disaster plans and safety manuals. Including representatives of all categories of professional nurses on policy and procedure committees helps them to accept responsibility for activities in which they participate.

NOTES

1. L. C. Megginson, D. C. Mosley, and P. H. Pietri, Jr., *Management: Concepts and Applications*, 2d ed. (New York: Harper & Row, 1986), 129–131.

2. Ibid., 130

3. M. Cushing, " 'No Code' Orders: Current Developments and the Nursing Director's Role," *Journal of Nursing Administration*, Apr. 1981, 22–29.

4. R. C. Jellinek, T. K. Zinn, and J. R. Brya, "Tell the Computer How Sick the Patients Are and It Will Tell How Many Nurses They Need," *Modern Hospital*, Dec. 1973, 81–85.

5. JCAHO, *Accreditation Manual for Hospitals 1989* (Chicago: American Hospital Association, 1987), 133–143.

6. ANA Task Force on Standards for Organized Nursing Services and Responsibilities of Nurse Administrators, *Standards for Organized Nursing Services and Responsibilities of Nurse Administrators Across All Settings* (Kansas City, MO: ANA, 1988).

7. M. A. Grindol, "A Manager's Guide to Procedure Manuals," *Nursing Management*, Jan. 1984, 12–14; J. Griffith and D. Ignatavicius, "Procedure Development: A Simplified Approach," *Journal of Nursing Administration*, Sept. 1984, 27–31.

8. L. C. Megginson, D. C. Mosley, and P. J. Pietri, Jr., op. cit., 132–134.

9. C. W. Clegg and T. D. Wall, "The Lateral Dimension of Employee Participation," *Journal of Management Studies*, Oct. 1984, 429–442.

10. R. D. Grubb, *Hospital Manuals: A Guide to Development and Maintenance* (Rockville, MD: Aspen, 1981).

REFERENCES

Rowland, H. S. and B. L. Rowland, Eds., *Hospital Administration Handbook* (Rockville, MD: Aspen, 1984).

Swansburg, R. C., *Management of Patient Care Services* (Saint Louis, MO: Mosby, 1976).

Decision Making and Problem Solving

9

CLAUDETTE T. COLEMAN Ed.D., R.N.
Assistant Professor, School of Nursing
Auburn University at Montgomery
Montgomery, Alabama

INTRODUCTION

Decision making is essential to problem solving. It is doubtful that anyone would argue with that statement. Nurses already know how to do this, don't they? Nurses have been making decisions since they were small children. Certainly these decisions were not always made after careful deliberation, by consciously following specified steps in a process. Nurses may not have known how they did it; they just did. Thus a nurse might be thinking, "I wouldn't be where I am professionally if I didn't know how to do this—so I'll go to the next chapter."

Wait! How often have nurses made bad decisions? Why were they bad? How do they prevent making similar errors in future decisions? How do they deal with indecision?

The answers to these questions are explored in this chapter. Complex decision making is a part of any level of nursing management. To function successfully the nurse manager must consistently demonstrate problem-solving skills in rapidly changing and uncertain situations in which indecisiveness or poor decisions are costly. Ability to foster organizational decision making and problem solving are personal skills essential to the nurse manager. This chapter will deal with models and strategies which can be used by the nurse manager to strengthen personal skills successfully and further develop the decision-making and problem-solving abilities of staff members.

The theory of decision making is an essential component of the nursing process and the management process. It is a required competency for all professional nurses.

THE DECISION-MAKING PROCESS

Definition

Since everyone is involved at some time in making decisions, it may be assumed that innate abilities,

226

past experience, and intuition form the basis for successful decisions. Decisions are often made by choosing among known alternatives. But what about unknown alternatives? Making a choice is not the only element of decision making. The process involves a systematic approach of sequenced steps and it should be adaptable to the environment in which it is used. Lancaster and Lancaster defined decision making as a systematic, sequential process of choosing among alternatives and putting the choice into action. This definition does not eliminate natural and learned abilities, while providing orderliness and continuity to the process of decision making.[1]

Models

A review of the literature yields a number of models of decision making. Three models are covered in this chapter.

The Normative Model. This model is at least 200 years old. It is assumed to maximize satisfaction and fulfills the "perfect knowledge assumption" that "in any given situation calling for a decision, all possible choices and the consequences and potential outcome of each are known."[2] Seven steps are identified in this analytically precise model:

1. Define and analyze the problem.
2. Identify all available alternatives.
3. Evaluate the pros and cons of each alternative.
4. Rank the alternatives.
5. Select the alternative that maximizes satisfaction.
6. Implement.
7. Follow up.

The normative model for decision making is unrealistic because of its assumption of clear-cut choices among identified alternatives.

The Decision Tree Model. Various adaptations of decision tree analysis are found in the literature; the essential elements described in the 1960s are standard. All factors considered important to a decision can be represented on a decision tree. Vroom used answers to seven diagnostic questions in the form of a decision tree to identify types of leadership style used in management decision-making models. The questions focus on protecting the quality and acceptance of the decision and deal with adequacy of information, goal congruence, structure of the problem, acceptance by subordinates, conflict, fairness, and priority for implementation.[3] Magee and Brown depict decision trees as starting with a basic problem and making "event forks" and "action forks" represented as branches. The number of branches at each fork correspond to the number of identified alternatives. Every path through the tree equates to a possible sequence of actions and events, each with its own separate consequences. Probabilities of both positive and negative consequences of each action and event are estimated and recorded on the appropriate branch. Additional options (for example, delaying the decision) and consequences of each action–event sequence can be depicted on the decision tree. Computer simulations of decision trees are now available and are adaptable to a limited or highly complex number of "branches" involved in the decision making process. Normal analysis of the tree is conducted by computing predicted consequences of all event forks (the right hand edge of the tree), substituting that value for the actual event fork and its consequences, and selecting the action fork with the optimum expected consequences. Both the optimum strategy and its expected consequences will be determined. Quantitative analysis in the form of decision trees can be used for any type problem but may be unncessary in simple problems involving limited consequences.[4]

Descriptive Model. Simon developed the descriptive model based on the assumption that the decision maker is a rational person looking for acceptable solutions based on known information. This model allows for the fact that many decisions are made with incomplete information because of time, money, or people limitations and the fact that people do not always make the best choices. Simon wrote that few decisions would ever be made if we always sought optimal solutions. Instead, he contended, we identify acceptable alternatives. Steps in the descriptive model (Figure 9–1) include:

1. Establish acceptable goal.
2. Define subjective perceptions of the problem.
3. Identify acceptable alternatives.
4. Evaluate each alternative.
5. Select alternative.
6. Implement decision.
7. Follow up.[5]

FIGURE 9–1.   The Decision-Making Process

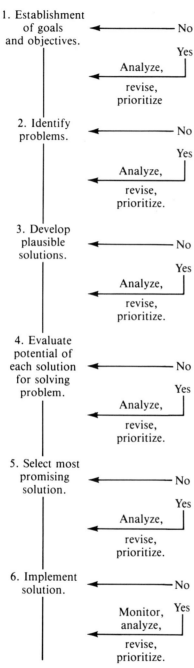

1. Establishment of goals and objectives. ← No

Yes

Analyze, revise, prioritize

2. Identify problems. ← No

Yes

Analyze, revise, prioritize.

3. Develop plausible solutions. ← No

Yes

Analyze, revise, prioritize.

4. Evaluate potential of each solution for solving problem. ← No

Yes

Analyze, revise, prioritize.

5. Select most promising solution. ← No

Yes

Analyze, revise, prioritize.

6. Implement solution. ← No

Yes

Monitor, analyze, revise, prioritize.

The establishment of goals and objectives requires that decisions be made as to how they will be achieved. A first decision may be the priority in which they will be carried out. Decisions do not relate only to problems. They relate to development of plans and programs to accomplish nursing goals and objectives. A best alternative that does not work requires making a decision whether to start over from Step 1 if other alternatives have less chance of success.

This descriptive model may lend itself well to nurse managers faced with daily decision making that must be completed rapidly and with significant consequences. Steps in the model are not unlike those in the familiar nursing process, although sequencing is different. Readers may readily identify conditions in their own environments similar to those described by Simon and see immediate applicability.[6] Lancaster and Lancaster illustrated use of this model for nursing administrators.[7]

Steps in the Process

From these and other models of decision making, five general steps of the process are identified.

First the problem must be identified. While this step may seem simple, recognizing and defining the problem is complex because of the diversity of individual perceptions. Since all individuals affected by the problem should be involved in discussing it, authority for decision making should be delegated to individuals at the level of impact. When this is impossible, representatives of various affected groups may provide input. Each may have a different perspective as to what the outcome should be. Nurse managers should make certain that the identified problem is one that requires their attention and cannot be handled alone by those involved. Collecting factual information in addition to subjective perceptions is essential. Logical and systematic fact finding includes questioning all sources for divergent opinions and objective data. When the difference between desired and present situations or outcomes is significant, problem recognition may occur.

Once the problem has been identified, the nurse manager must then evaluate the potential for a solution and determine the priority of the problem. Reitz suggests three approaches to prioritizing problems:

1. Deal with problems in the order in which they appear.
2. Solve the easiest problems first.
3. Solve crisis problems before all others. A decision will depend on the time and energy that can be devoted at that time. When a high-priority problem is identified with limited potential for resolution, the decision maker may be forced to give it lower priority until more information is collected and acceptable alternatives can be found. The fact that needed information is missing may

help define the real problem underlying the perceived one.[8]

The second step in decision making is gathering and analyzing information related to the solution. This step involves defining the specifications to be met by the solution through a series of activities. A thorough information search may be essential for validating the correct identification of a problem. This search should include knowledge of organizational policy, prior personal experience or training, or experiences of others. Externally, the nurse manager begins to identify alternatives comparing the potential alternatives with the desired outcome and the desired outcome with available resources. In organizational settings, data base information systems may provide this information quickly. Establishing goals with measurable objectives for attainment helps focus the search for alternatives. Certainly to be considered while comparing potential alternatives is the cost involved for implementation, time required and available, and the capabilities of those who will be involved in implementing a decision. Once again it is essential to involve in discussions of alternatives those individuals who are or will be affected by the choice. Irrelevant, insignificant, and extraneous factors must be eliminated from consideration. Gaining a commitment to implement a decision before the choice is made supports the process. It is possible to reach a point of information overload when the searcher has received information too quickly to process or in too great a quantity. Research indicates that the quantity of information sought has a direct positive correlation with the degree of anticipated risk in the decision to be made. Personal confidence of the decision maker also affects the amount of information required for support of choices in decision making. Less searching is required by the manager who recognizes patterns or similarities to previously encountered problems and confidently makes a choice of alternatives.

The third step in decision making is evaluating all alternatives and selecting one for implementation. In the evaluation of alternatives, possible positive and negative consequences of each choice are identified with probability of each estimated. A common approach involves identifying the best and worst possible outcomes to an alternative and then the outcomes that fall between the two extremes. As each alternative is evaluated, additional options may become apparent. Disagreement may stimulate

the imagination and produce better solutions. The effects of taking no decision must be weighed against the effects of each proposed solution. Each alternative must be systematically evaluated for its efficiency and effectiveness in accomplishing the desired outcome as well as the likelihood of achievement with available or obtainable resources. The advantages and disadvantages of each alternative are identified to determine risk factors in possible outcomes. Identifying the solution which best satisfies specifications should receive attention before any compromises, concessions, or revisions are made between involved parties. An alternative which provides the greatest probability of an acceptable desired outcome using available resources is most likely to be selected.

A fourth step in the decision-making process is to act on or implement the selected alternative. Knowledge and skills of the decision maker transform the alternative into action by completing any necessary plans involving sequencing of necessary steps and preparing individuals to implement the solution, effectively communicating the process with all involved.

Orton suggests asking oneself seven questions to increase the success of one's decision choice:

1. Does the quality of the decision really make a difference?
2. Do I have all the information I need to make the decision alone?
3. Do I know what I'm missing? Do I know where to find the information? Will I know what to do with the information I'm given?
4. Do I need anybody's commitment to make sure this succeeds?
5. Can I gain commitments without offering participation in the decision?
6. Do those involved in the decision share the organization's goals?
7. Is there likely to be conflict about the available alternatives?[9]

A final step in the process of decision making is to monitor the implementation and evaluate outcomes. The nursing manager compares actual results with anticipated outcomes and makes modifications as needed to accomplish the desired outcome. Evaluation criteria obtained from measurable objectives provide feedback for testing the validity and effectiveness of the decision against the actual sequence of events in the process. Determination of flaws or gaps in the process may assist the decision maker to monitor the process more closely in the future and prevent the reoccurrence of such problems. The effective decision maker consciously follows these five steps in a logical sequence.

PITFALLS OF DECISION MAKING

While information technology is increasing its effect on decision making, pitfalls in the process stem more from the individual than from computers. Individual managers still are resistant to change involving risk and new ideas, often lacking trust in others who will test new areas. Such attitudes stifle not only individuals but groups. When nurse managers find themselves resisting needed change they should analyze their behavior toward the goal of becoming more imaginative and creative managers. It is important to move away from being authoritarian, controlling managers. If the manager chooses to control decision making and omit those affected by the decision from the process, less commitment to implementing the decision is a natural result. When feasible, the nurse manager may use a team approach to decision making, as in a matrix organization. Group decision making usually produces greater commitment to putting the selected alternative into action and working for success.

Other pitfalls of decision making include:

■ Inadequate fact finding. Decisions should be based on accurate information. For this reason, information should be obtained from wide and varied sources who are authorities on the subject. They do not have to be contacted personally; instead their publications can be reviewed.

■ Time constraints. Collection and analysis of facts, opinions, assumptions, and feelings of those directly involved should be completed in a timely fashion. Pressures of time, resources, and priorities render the decision-making process more complex. It is not always possible to obtain all the necessary facts. This produces a degree of uncertainty, especially when multiple alternatives are identified.

■ Poor communication. Communicating the decision to appropriate individuals is as essential as following up to determine if results are as expected.

■ Failing to systematically follow the steps of the decision-making process will likely result in unanticipated results.

IMPROVING DECISION MAKING

Basic precepts are identified in the literature for improved decision making. In addition to those already mentioned they include: educating people so they know how to make decisions; securing support of top management for decision making at the lowest possible level; establishing decision-making checkpoints with appropriate time limits; keeping informed of progress by ensuring access to firsthand information; using statistical analysis when possible to pinpoint problems for solution;[10] and staying open to use of new ideas or technologies in analyzing problems and identifying alternatives. Numerous strategies and tools are available to improve our decision-making abilities.

A successful manager is one who stays informed about decisions being made at different levels of the organization after appropriately delegating these responsibilities, deals only with those decisions requiring his/her level of expertise, supports implementation of decisions, and credits the decision maker. McKenzie states that managers who make all decisions themselves convey a lack of trust in the ability or loyalty of their subordinates. Delegation of decision making on a selective basis gains the support of the staff and raises their self-esteem. They gain a sense of belonging and develop loyalty. Delegation leads to leadership. Leaders share authority and power rather than impose it. This is not to say that leaders do not ever make decisions without input from subordinates. This may be necessary on occasion and is acceptable to subordinates who know they participate in decisions that rely on their level of knowledge and experience.[11] Wrapp wrote that good managers don't make policy decisions. Instead they concentrate on a limited number of significant issues, identify areas where they can make a difference, judge how hard to force an issue, give a sense of direction to the organization through open-ended objectives, and spot opportunities that permit others to "own" their ideas and plans for implementation. Wrapp's description of the successful manager portrays a motivator who is knowledgeable and skilled in both decision making and problem solving and serves as a role model for others.[12]

PLACE OF INTUITION IN THE DECISION-MAKING PROCESS

There is a place in the decision-making process for intuitive reasoning abilities. Intuition is a powerful tool guiding executive decision making. So-called left-brain activities such as analytical and logical thinking, mathematics, and sequential information processing are essential in decision making and problem solving. But right-brain functions allow us simultaneously to process information, conceive and use contradictory ideas, fantasize, and perceive intuitively. Intuition is defined as a power of apprehending the possibilities inherent in a situation. It is a subspecies of logical thinking and integrates information from both sides of the brain—facts and feeling cues.[13] Nurse managers with an ability to think intuitively have a sense of vision, generating new ideas and ingenious solutions to old problems. Agor reported research involving 2000 managers using a Myers-Briggs Type Indicator for measuring intuitive ability. Initial findings showed intuitive ability varying by managerial level, with higher ability in top-level managers than in middle or lower-level managers.

Factors cited by middle and lower managers that impeded the use of intuition included lack of confidence, time constraints, stress factors, and projection mechanisms such as dishonesty and attachment. Follow-up of the 200 top executives scoring in the top 10 percent of the first study revealed all but one using intuitive ability as one tool in guiding decisions. These managers stated their intuitive ability stemmed from years of knowledge and experience. From this research, eight conditions were identified in which intuitive ability seems to function best:

1. When a high level of uncertainty exists.
2. When little previous precedent exists.
3. When variables are less scientifically predictable.
4. When "facts" are limited.
5. When facts don't clearly point the way to go.
6. When analytical data are of little use.
7. When several plausible alternative solutions exist to choose from, with good arguments for each.

8. When time is limited and there is pressure to come up with the right decision.[14]

Nurse managers can certainly identify with each of these decision-making situations. It should be gratifying to know that research has supported the use of intuition in decision making. However, it is stressed that there are appropriate times for use of intuition as an "adjunct" to the logical steps of decision making—*not* where objective data are complete. Because basic nursing education stresses the need for assessment of facts and avoidance of personal opinions, it may be difficult for some nurse managers to activate intuition for decision making. Techniques and exercises used by executives to activate and expand their intuitive decision-making abilities have been identified by Agor, including relaxation and mental/analytical techniques. A full account of Agor's research is beyond the scope of this chapter; the reader is referred to Agor's extensive writings on the subject of intuitive decision making.[15]

ORGANIZATIONAL VERSUS PERSONAL DECISIONS

Various models for decision making have been identified and specific steps involved in the process including the role of intuition have been described. Now the question must be raised of when to make organizational versus personal decision.

When are organizational decisions necessary? It would be easy to say we deal with professionals who are capable of making decisions related to their practice. No effective manager would make decisions others can make. However, incapacity of subordinates, uncertain instructions, novel conditions, conflicts, or failure of authority to make effective decisions or to make decisions at all may cause decisions to be appealed to a higher authority. Effective organizational decisions require collaboration and consultation with those having specialized knowledge. Organizational decisions relate to organizational purpose; constant refinement of organizational purpose is required as the organizational environment changes. This process would provide opportunities for participative management styles to be functional, thereby giving subordinates the prerogative and responsibility of professional decision making.[16]

From an organizational standpoint, decisions may be analyzed on the basis of futurity, impact, qualitative or value factors, and recurrent, rare, or unique decisions. Futurity is defined as the amount of time the decision will affect the organization in the future and the time required to reverse its impact. Impact refers to the number of individuals or departments affected as a determinant of the level at which the decision is made. When philosophy or ethics are involved, decisions must be made at a higher level. The last characteristic refers to the uniqueness of the decision; recurrent decisions are made following a rule or principle already established.[17]

But what about institutional policy? Historically, decision making in nursing has been authoritarian, with minimal input from nursing staff, particularly in institutional policy. Nurses have also been limited in their professional autonomy. Literature on the sociology of professions has indicated that a professional person has an ultimate or independent decision-making authority granted by society on the basis of unique knowledge and skill. This viewpoint gave physicians control over nurses. The traditional definition of autonomy no longer applies, as patients demand more input in decision making and increasing patient care technology requires nurses to make independent life-and-death decisions. McKay redefined professional autonomy as "both independent and interdependent practice-related decision making based on a complex body of knowledge and skill."[18] Primary nursing promotes nurse accountability, intraprofessional and interprofessional consultation, and an assertive synthesis of nursing and medical care plans. Interdependent decision making promotes professional autonomy.

Since nurse care givers are functioning with increasing professional autonomy, nurse managers are moving into more executive positions in health-care administration. Nurse managers recognize advantages of nurses being involved in strategic institutional decisions such as major programs, policies, promotions, personnel, and budgets. In addition to enhancing professional autonomy, the involvement of nurses in decision making has resulted in higher job satisfaction, better morale, lower turnover, improved communication, improved professional relationships with peers and colleagues from other disciplines, and higher productivity.[19] The nurse administrator can maximize the opportunity for staff nurses to be involved in interdependent decision making by involving them at all levels of patient care decision making, especially on interdisciplinary institution-wide committees. Strategies which have proven successful in involving nurses in institutional decision making and policy development include:

1. Decentralization to the unit level. This requires educated nurse managers and clinical nurses to make managerial and clinical decisions. While the middle manager cannot effect this change for the institution, the practice can be used at the unit level to involve all clinical nurse staff in decision making.

2. Committee systems. Opportunity is provided for nurse participation on interdepartmental, interdisciplinary, and institution-wide committees with knowledge that collectively made decisions are more apt to be collectively implemented and supported.

3. Governance systems. While usually discussed in terms of the entire nursing division within the context of the institution, self-governance concepts are adaptable to the middle nurse manager. A set of bylaws, developed by the unit professionals, governs internal affairs of the unit. The theory of participative management could be operationalized as management by committees instead of by nurse managers. Each committee has coordination responsibilities for specific management tasks. This system requires voluntary support and respect for the clinical management role of peers and places control of nursing practice in the hands of professional nurses.[20]

Since nurses are involved in making critical decisions affecting individuals as well as institutions, emphasis needs to be placed on improving their decision-making skills. This can be done by involving them in institutional governance, by structuring the nursing organization for maximum decision making by clinical nurses, and by preparing them for these roles through staff development programs. These areas are covered in other chapters of this book.

THE PROBLEM-SOLVING PROCESS

At this point one may be wondering about the relationship between decision making and problem solving. The first step in decision making was to identify the problem. But problem solving may involve multiple incidents of decision making. The best way to define their relationship is to define the steps of problem solving.

Steps in the Process

In reality, the steps of the problem-solving process are the same as the steps of the nursing process: assess and analyze, plan, implement, and evaluate. Assessment includes systematic collection, organization, and analysis of data into related information which may be associated with a specific problem or need. It involves logical fact-finding, questioning all sources, and differentiating between objective facts and subjective feelings, opinions, and assumptions. Knowledge and experience guide in data collection and analysis. Assessments should also determine whether a commitment exists to implement a decision/action before the process goes any further.[21] Making certain there is no readily apparent solution is also a time saver in consideration of the number of people who may become involved in problem solving. Once a problem is identified, it must be determined if it requires other than routine handling; that is, whether it is a rare or unique situation, not a recurrent one. This will lead into the second step of problem solving: planning.

Planning involves several phases. In nursing terms we determine priorities, set goals and measurable objectives, and plan interventions. Management literature essentially says the same: break the problem down into components and establish priorities, develop alternative courses of action, determine probable outcomes for each alternative; decide which course is best in relation to resources, goals, risks, and the like, and decide on a plan of action with a timetable for implementation.[22]

Nurse managers should relate the problem to the corporate mission when determining priorities. Decisions involve a selection among alternative courses of action. Decisions must have an acceptable effect on those directly involved, other areas affected, and the entire organization. Plans should include when and how to alter a course of action when undesired results occur.

The third step is implementation of the plan. The manager should keep informed of the status of the process, since it is unlikely she or he will be directly involved. This is the one step in the process most likely to be delegated to subordinates. Imple-

mentation requires knowledge and skills appropriate to specific selected alternatives. Evaluation, the final step in problem solving, includes determining how closely goals and objectives were met, the success or failure of actions taken in resolving the problem, and whether the plan should be terminated because the problem is resolved or continued, with or without modification.

Group Problem Solving

While each step of the problem-solving process can be approached by the individual, input from all affected individuals or areas promotes the probability of more complete data collection, creative planning, successful implementation, and evaluation indicating problem resolution. Managerial problem-solving groups are often formed in organizations with the expectation that the group's effect will prove to be greater than the sum of its parts. Brightman and Verhoeven state that a

> team of problem solvers has greater potential resources than an individual, can have a higher motivation to complete the job, can force members to examine their own beliefs more carefully, and can develop creative solutions.[23]

Two types of group techniques which may prove successful in problem solving have been identified, Delphi and nominal group techniques. In the Delphi group technique, only the group leader knows the identity of members. Questionnaires are completed by each member, consolidated, and recirculated until a consensus emerges. The Delphi technique is especially useful when group members are experts physically separated from each other. Electronic mail has eliminated the primary limitation of this technique by reducing the amount of time required for sending and tabulating the questionnaires.

The nominal group technique avoids development of a self-proclaimed expert by combining independent activity with interacting group structures at specific points in the problem-solving process. Individuals first generate solutions for a problem independently, then present and defend the alternatives individually. Each person may be questioned for clarification but not criticized. The group leader collects the written ideas; after group members interact to reach agreement, each member ranks each option silently and independently. Group size of five to ten members is suggested. Delphi and nominal group techniques are more fully discussed in another chapter.

Scharf suggests a problem-solving team of five to ten persons plus a facilitator to be most effective because each is assigned a specific responsibility. His effective team has a person who has a real interest in the problem, one who will be implementing the selected alternative, one who will receive output from the alternative, a decision maker with sufficient power to implement, a needed technical expert, a resource controller, an "integrator," or uninvolved party, and a trained workshop team facilitator. Perhaps the success of such a group lies in individual autonomy for a specific task and a facilitator who motivates and monitors the group function.[24]

If group problem solving has so many advantages, why would the failure rate be high? Brightman and Verhoeven cite a number of reasons for failure of managerial problem-solving groups. Among them are the group leader's ineffective leadership skills and lack of a game plan, a homogeneous group using similar styles of problem solving, use of improper group structure (for example, interacting), and developing counterproductive norms such as "groupthink," in which consensus is sought at the expense of critical thinking and realistic consideration of alternative ideas.[25]

Effective groups need varied perspectives and values. That means members are needed who use their senses to evaluate hard facts as well as members who use intuition to imagine. People are needed who use their feelings as well as people who think logically and analytically. Effective group leaders comprehend group dynamics and use appropriate intragroup intervention skills and techniques to promote open sharing, constructive conflict, minority opinion, and clarification of all ideas and feelings.

Whether functioning essentially as an individual or participating with a group, the nurse manager must daily make decisions related to problems encountered by and with individual patients, their families, nursing staff, and the organization in which they function. Systematic use of the decision-making and problem-solving processes described in this chapter should enhance professional growth and consistency in making sound decisions and resolving problems.

SUMMARY

Decision making and problem solving occur concurrently with all major functions of nursing management. Three models of the cognitive thinking skills involved in decision making are presented: the normative model, the decision tree model, and the descriptive model.

Decision making involves having an objective, gathering data pertaining to the objective, analyzing the data, identifying and evaluating alternative courses of action that will achieve the objective, selecting an alternative (the decision), implementing it, and evaluating the results. Nurse managers make the best decisions through knowledge and use of the theory of decision making combined with intuitive ability developed over years of experience.

While problem solving is not the exact equivalent of decision making, it employs a similar thinking process. Decision making is different from problem solving in that the objective does not have to pertain to a problem. It can be an objective that relates to change, to progress, to research, and to implementation of any operational or management plan.

NOTES

1. W. Lancaster and J. Lancaster, "Rational Decision Making: Managing Uncertainty," *Journal of Nursing Administration,* Sept. 1982, 23–28.
2. Ibid., 23.
3. V. H. Vroom, "A New Look at Managerial Decision Making, Organizational Decision Making," *Organizational Dynamics,* Spring 1973, 66–80.
4. R. V. Brown, "Do Managers Find Decision Theory Useful?," *Harvard Business Review,* May-June 1970, 78–89; J. Magee, "Decision Trees for Decision Making," *Harvard Business Review,* July-Aug. 1964, 126; J. Magee, "How to Use Decision Trees in Capital Investment," *Harvard Business Review,* Sept.-Oct. 1964, 79.
5. H. A. Simon, *Administrative Behavior,* 3d ed. (New York: The Free Press, 1976).
6. Ibid.
7. W. Lancaster and J. Lancaster, op. cit.
8. J. H. Reitz, *Behavior in Organizations* (Homewood, IL: Richard D. Irwin, 1977), 154–199.
9. A. Orton, "Leadership: New Thoughts on an Old Problem," *Training,* June 1984, 28, 31–33.
10. D. Graham and D. Reese, "There's Power in Numbers," *Nursing Management,* Sept. 1984, 48–51.
11. M. E. McKenzie, "Decisions: How You Reach Them Makes a Difference," *Nursing Management,* June 1985, 48–49.

12. H. E. Wrapp, "Good Managers Don't Make Policy Decisions," *Harvard Business Review*, Sep./Oct. 1967, 91–99.
13. W. H. Agor, "The Logic of Intuition: How Top Executives Make Important Decisions," *Organizational Dynamics*, Winter 1986, 5–18.
14. Ibid., 9.
15. Ibid., 5–18.
16. C. Barnard and M. Beyers, "The Environment of Decision," *The Journal of Nursing Administration*, March 1982, 25–29.
17. R. C. Swansburg, *Management of Patient Care Services* (Saint Louis: C.V. Mosby, 1976), 149–170.
18. P. S. McKay, "Interdependent Decision Making: Redefining Professional Autonomy," *Nursing Administration Quarterly*, Summer 1983, 21–30.
19. American Hospital Association, *Strategies: Nurse Involvement in Decision Making and Policy Development*, 1984, 1–10.
20. Ibid.
21. A. Scharf, "Secrets of Problem Solving," *Industrial Management*, Sept.-Oct. 1985, 7–11.
22. B. Blai, Jr., "Eight Steps to Successful Problem Solving," *Supervisory Management*, Jan. 1986, 7–9.
23. H. J. Brightman and P. Verhoeven, "Why Managerial Problem Solving Groups Fail," *Business*, Jan.-Mar. 1986, 24–29.
24. A. Scharf, op. cit.
25. H. J. Brightman and P. Verhoeven, op. cit.

REFERENCES

Argyris, C., "How Tomorrow's Executives Will Make Decisions," reprint from *Think Magazine*, IBM, 1967.

Argyris, C., *Reasoning, Learning and Action* (San Francisco: Jossey-Bass, 1982), 87, 102.

Denton, D. K., "Problem Solving by Keeping in Touch," *Business*, July-Sept. 1986, 40–42.

Galbraith, J. K., *The New Industrial State* (Boston: Houghton Mifflin, 1967).

Goldstein, M., D. Scholthaver, and B. B. Kleiner, "Management on the Right Side of the Brain," *Personnel Journal*, Nov. 1985, 40–45.

Grandori, A., "Prescriptive Contingency View of Organizational Decision Making," *Administrative Science Quarterly*, June 1984, 192–209.

Greiner, L. E., D. P. Leitch, and D. P. Barnes, "Putting Judgment Back into Decisions," *Harvard Business Review*, Mar.-Apr. 1970, 59–67.

Holland, H. K., "Decision-Making and Personality," *Personnel Administration*, May-June 1968, 24–29.

Kersey, J. H. Jr. "Responsibility Accounting: Making Decisions Efficiently," *Nursing Management*, May 1985, 14, 16–17.

Leo, M., "Avoiding the Pitfalls of ManagemenThink," *Business Horizons*, May-June 1984, 44–47.

Locke, E. A., D. M. Schweiger, and G. P. Latham, "Participation in Decision Making: When Should It Be Used?," *Organizational Dynamics*, Winter 1986, 65–79.

Miller, M., "Putting More Power into Management Decisions," *Management Review*, Sept. 1984, 12–16.

Southern Council on Collegiate Education for Nursing, *Preparing Nurses for Decision Making in Clinical Practice: A White Paper* (Atlanta: SCCEN, 1985).

Suding, M. J., "Decision Making Controlling the Computer Input," *Nursing Management*, July 1984, 44, 46, 48–52.

Implementing Planned Change   10

INTRODUCTION

As a catalyst, the nurse manager causes or accelerates changes by using knowledge and skills that are *not* permanently affected by the reaction. In essence, the nurse manager may be considered a change agent. Let us first consider the philosophy embodied in theories of human resource management, theories based on adequate assumptions about human nature and motivation. Has the nurse manager organized money, materials, equipment, and personnel in the interests of providing quality services to patients and thereby giving them their money's worth? Have nursing employees had experiences of supervision that have made them passive and resistant to organizational needs? Or do nursing employees work under conditions that inspire them to develop their potential, assume increased responsibility, and work to achieve their personal goals as well as those of the organization? Are clinical nurses able to direct their own efforts?

Nurse managers should start looking for ways to inspire nursing personnel to utilize their capabilities, to encourage them to accept responsibility, and to encourage them to be active and to seek real meaning in their work. Autonomy and self-direction are traits that people desire. They are traits that when freed satisfy people's ego needs. Nurse managers can show nurses how to achieve these goals by gaining knowledge and skills that will satisfy their desire to control their own destinies.[1]

Machiavelli said, "There is nothing more difficult to take in hand, more perilous to conduct, or more uncertain in its success, than to take the lead in the introduction of a new order of things."[2] With a few notable exceptions (such as the weather), most of the change that takes place in our society is planned change. This means that nurse managers can plan with clinical nurses to implement change. It must first be decided that a new skill or technique using a new apparatus or technology is needed to improve patient care and ability to deliver that care. Then nurse managers and clinical nurses can plan and carry out the changes they want to make.

Spradley defines planned change as "a purpose-ful, designed effort to bring about improvements in a system, with the assistance of a change agent."[3] Change occurs whether one wants it to or not. New technology is developed; new treatments result, causing personnel and organizational adjustments. These changes need to be controlled or managed. Hence we refer to the process as "planned change."

THE NEED FOR CHANGE

Four general reasons for designing orderly change have been defined by Williams:

1. To improve the means of satisfying somebody's economic wants.
2. To increase profitability.
3. To promote human work for human beings.
4. To contribute to individual satisfaction and social well-being.[4]

The basic motivation for a change could be that orderly change needs to be designed to improve patient care while lowering costs and increasing nursing's economic status. It could be that the organization should profit by being able to do more for less or at the same cost or by improving its reputation for quality care. The goal could be making the work situation or environment better for the employees. Or it could be improvement of individual satisfaction and social well-being for both patients and staff members.

Implementation of planned change will alter the status quo. New programs of patient care will modify existing relationships among nursing personnel and between them and other members of the health-care team.

Change can help achieve organizational objectives as well as individual ones. Individual nurses and the institution of nursing will grow and prosper if they change with improved technology, especially if that technology will cure disease, save infant lives, prolong life without increasing suffering, and in general promote social improvement.

What are the common types of change with which nurses must deal? One obvious type is technological. A few years ago a 200-watt-per-second defibrillator was considered satisfactory. Now 400 watts per second is desirable. Changes also occur in methods and procedures related to machinery and equipment, electronic thermometers and ventila-tory equipment being two examples. Changing work standards delineate up-to-date competencies for both nurse managers and clinical nurses.

Other changes include personnel and organizational adjustments, for example constant turnover of personnel or changes in organizational structure. Nurses are certainly aware of their changing relationships with those who hold authority and power, changes in responsibility and status, and changes in organizational, departmental, and unit objectives. Some employees resist change, but others welcome it as an opportunity to make adjustments in existing work situations, alter their relationships with their associates, and achieve personal goals.

During the past 25 years there have been significant changes in the nature of health-care organizations, the demands placed on nurse managers, and the needs and motivations of nursing personnel. Successful nurse managers have learned to manage change and have publicly related the role of nursing as being an involved and concerned element of society. They recognize the growing complexity of the health-care organization, particularly today's division of nursing, and they recognize the changing values of nurses within the profession. Nurses want opportunities for advancement or promotion, recognition for their work, and more help from their peers and supervisors to improve their job skills. One dramatic change has been the impetus of nurses to develop their professional standards to higher levels to which they must raise their credentials, particularly with regard to education. They have also recognized the need for continuing education to deliver up-to-date services. A glance at a nursing journal shows nurses' awareness of society's current problems and their increasing involvement in them. These include problems of health, environmental pollution, poverty, social equality, education, civil rights, religion, and many others. Nurse managers see themselves as agents of change functioning within a profession that draws its basic support from society.

Evidence suggests that technological innovation can cause scientists' and engineers' knowledge to become obsolete in 10 years if they do not pursue further education. Parallel evidence could be developed to support the same conclusion about nursing. Today's nurses are more committed to task, job, and profession than they are loyal to an organization. They look at the kind of services provided (short-term versus critical versus chronic), management's philosophy (participative versus authoritarian), experimental outlook, and physical and geographical location. Nurses want control over their work environment and are dissatisfied otherwise. For these reasons nursing management philosophies and assumptions are changing. Nurse managers are changing their management styles, policies, procedures, relationships with subordinates, and employment and compensation practices. Hospital managers are looking at the kinds of health services they offer. Nurse managers are seeking knowledge of community, state, and national affairs, government trends, individual needs, and group motivations. They are learning to function in a computerized world of business systems.

No longer is the nursing worker bound down by threat and ritual. Nurses are still in great demand in the job market and are highly mobile. The professional nurse looks forward to moving and frequently has the next move planned while still at the present job. This nurse is willing to work but desires an environment where there is humor and opportunity to use imagination. Nurse managers have to change their behavior to suit the changing profile of this new breed of worker. Nurse managers need to learn how to provide avenues for need satisfaction of clinical nurses. They need to look at their own style of management and how it affects others and learn to be more flexible and individualized in dealing with their employees. They learn to be candid and to confront conflict so that each can express feelings, thoughts, and reactions to others. The change in management in nursing aims to promote ideas of all people, to encourage attentive listening, and to reward people for becoming personally involved and committed to their work.

Adaptation to change has always been a job requirement for nursing. Nursing personnel work for numerous bosses, including individual patients, physicians, the head nurse, and a different charge nurse each change of shift. Nursing practitioners will find their roles changed many times in a day, sometimes being a manager, sometimes a clinical nurse, sometimes a consultant, and always in multiple roles.

Among the reasons for change is evidence that something needs changing. The nurse manager needs to recognize the symptoms. They can be glaring or subtle. An example of the subtle would be offhand comments of float personnel such as "I'd rather work anywhere than ward 3F" or "Could you send me someplace else?"

The health-care system is constantly changing. Changes include a labor force that wants wages comparable to other professions, hours of work that fit their personal needs, and the power to make their own professional decisions about patient care. Many times the change focuses on technology without consideration for human relationships and political sensitivities. A case in point is the American Medical Association's 1988 push to solve the nursing shortage by proposing a new health-care technician.

Nurse managers require extensive knowledge of community affairs, government trends and constraints, world affairs, international practices and procedures, the changing nature of individual needs, and group motivation. Even the supply and demand of nurses relates to these many areas. Within nursing, needs change with new systems of computers, planning, business, accounting, control, and marketing.[5]

Younger nurses, like other younger professionals, are mobile and have salable skills. They want to use all of their skills and to be collaborative and democratic.[6]

Change is the key to progress and to the future.

CHANGE THEORY

Reddin has developed a planned change model that can be used by nurse managers. Maximum information is important to the success of change. At least four announcements should be made by management:

1. That a change will be made.
2. What the decision is and why it was made.
3. How the decision will be implemented.
4. How implementation is progressing.[7]

Widely used theories of change are those of Reddin, Lewin, Rogers, Havelock, and Lippitt.

Reddin's Theory

Reddin has suggested seven techniques by which change can be accomplished:

1. Diagnosis.
2. Mutual setting of objectives.
3. Group emphasis.

4. Maximum information.
5. Discussion of implementation.
6. Use of ceremony and ritual.
7. Resistance interpretation.

The first three techniques are designed to give those who will be affected by the change an opportunity to influence its direction, nature, rate, and method of introduction. They are then able to have some control over it, to become involved in it, to express their ideas more directly, and to propose useful modifications.

Diagnosis is scientific problem solving. Those affected by the change meet and identify problems and the probable outcomes. Perhaps other team members can be involved in diagnosing the problem by having them gather some of the needed information.

Mutual objective setting is like practicing management by objectives. The goals of both groups, those instituting the change and those affected by it, are brought in line. It may be necessary to bargain and compromise.

Group emphasis is sometimes referred to as team emphasis. Change is more successful when supported by a team rather than a single person. To have group emphasis there must be a group; a manager should not have already made a decision. Groups are influential in reducing resistance to change, since they take the focus off the individual. "Groups develop powerful standards for conformity and the means of enforcing them."[8]

Lewin's Theory

One of the most widely used change theories is that of Kurt Lewin. Lewin's theory involves three stages:

1. *The unfreezing stage.* The nurse manager or other change agent is motivated to create change. Affected nurses are made aware of this need. The problem is identified or diagnosed and the best solution is selected. Three possible mechanisms giving inputs to the initial change are: Individual expectations are not being met (lack of confirmation); the individual feels uncomfortable about some action or lack of action (guilt-anxiety); or a former obstacle to change no longer exists (psychologic safety). The unfreezing stage occurs when disequilibrium is introduced into the system, creating a need for change.[9]

2. *The moving stage.* The nurse manager gathers information. A knowledgeable, respected, or powerful person influences the change agent in solving the problems (identification). This person can be an influential nurse manager, peer, or superior. A variety of sources give a variety of solutions (scanning) and a detailed plan is made. People examine, accept, and try out the innovation.[10]

3. *The refreezing stage.* Changes are integrated and stabilized as part of the value system. Forces are at work to facilitate the change (driving forces). Other forces are at work to impede change (restraining forces). The change agent identifies and deals with these forces, and change is established with homeostasis and equilibrium.[11]

Roger's Theory

Everett Rogers modified Lewin's change theory. Antecedents included the background of the change agent involved and the change environment. There are five phases. Phase 1, awareness, corresponds to the unfreezing phase of Lewin. Phases 2, interest, 3, evaluation and 4, trial, correspond to his moving phase. Phase 5, adoption, corresponds to Lewin's refreezing phase. In the adoption phase the change is accepted or rejected. If accepted it requires interest and commitment.[12]

Roger's theory depends upon five factors for success:

1. The change must have the relative advantage of being better than existing methods.
2. It must be compatible with existing values.
3. Complexity—more complex ideas persist even though simple ones are implemented more easily.
4. Divisibility—change is introduced on a small scale.
5. Communicability—the easier the change is to describe, the more likely it is to spread.[13]

Havelock's Theory

Havelock's theory is another modification of Lewin's, expanded to six elements. The first three correspond to unfreezing, the next two to moving, and the sixth to refreezing. Havelock's phases are:

1. Building a relationship.
2. Diagnosing the problem.
3. Acquiring the relevant resources.
4. Choosing the solution.
5. Gaining acceptance.
6. Stabilization and self-renewal.

Havelock's theory emphasizes the planning stage as being where the significant change occurs.[14]

Lippitt's Theory

Lippitt added a seventh phase to Lewin's original theory. The seven phases of his theory of the change process are as follows.

Phase 1: Diagnosing the Problem. During this phase the nurse manager as change agent looks at all possible ramifications and who will be affected. People who will be affected are involved in the change process. The nurse manager holds group meetings to involve others and win their commitment. The change agent also involves key people in top management and policy-making roles to ensure success.

Phase 2: Assessment of the Motivation and Capacity for Change. Possible solutions are determined and the pros and cons of each are forecast. Consideration is given to implementation methods, roadblocks, factors motivating people, driving forces, and facility forces.

Assessment considers financial aspects, organizational aspects, structure, rules and regulations, organizational culture, personalities, power, authority, and the nature of the organization. During this phase the change agent would coordinate activities among a number of small groups.

Phase 3: Assessment of the Change Agent's Motivation and Resources. The change agent can be external or internal to the organization or division. An external change agent may have fewer bases but must have expert credentials. An internal change agent, on the other hand, knows the people. There may be both. The change agent needs a genuine desire to improve the situation, a knowledge of interpersonal and organizational approaches, experience, dedication, and a personality to suit the

situation. The change agent should be objective, flexible, and accepted by all.

Phase 4: Selecting Progressive Change Objectives. The change process is defined, a detailed plan is made, time tables and deadlines are set, and responsibility is assigned. The change is implemented for a trial period and evaluated.

Phase 5: Choosing the Appropriate Role for the Change Agent. The change agent will be active in the change process, particularly in handling personnel and facilitating the change. Conflict and confrontation will be dealt with by the change agent.

Phase 6: Maintenance of the Change. During this phase emphasis is on communication, with feedback on progress. The change is extended in time. A large change may require a new power structure.

Phase 7: Termination of the Helping Relationship. The change agent withdraws at a specified date after setting a written procedure or policy for perpetuation. The agent remains available for advice and reinforcement.[15] Figure 10–1 offers a comparison of these theories.

It should be noted that all five theories are similar to the problem-solving process, indicating that the latter could be used to implement planned change. The nurse manager should select the theory she or he feels most comfortable with after identifying the change to be made. A management plan is then made to cover the phases of making the change. The planning phase requires gathering data to support a decision for change. The nurse manager would work with the nursing staff who will be affected by the change to set objectives. Thus the entire group becomes aware of the need for change and interested in it. A relationship is built between the nurse manager and nursing employees. The plan can then be made cooperatively, implemented by an enthusiastic group, and evaluated and maintained by the group.

Spradley's Model

Spradley has developed an eight-step model based on Lewin's theory. She indicates that planned change must be constantly monitored to develop a fruitful relationship between the change agent and

FIGURE 10–1. Comparison of Change Theories

Reddin	Lewin	Roger	Havelock	Lippitt
1. Diagnosis 2. Mutual objective setting	1. Unfreezing	1. Awareness	1. Building a relationship 2. Diagnosing the problem 3. Acquiring the relevant resources	1. Diagnosing the problem 2. Assessment of the motivation and capacity for change 3. Assessment of the change agent's motivation and resources
3. Group emphasis 4. Maximum information 5. Discussion of implementation 6. Use of ceremony and ritual	2. Moving	2. Interest 3. Evaluation 4. Trial	4. Choosing the solution 5. Gaining acceptance	4. Selecting progressive change objective 5. Choosing the appropriate role of the change agent
7. Resistance interpretation	3. Refreezing	5. Adoption	6. Stabilization and self-renewal	6. Maintenance of the change 7. Termination of the helping relationship

the change system. The eight basic steps of the Spradley model are:

1. *Recognize the symptoms.* There is evidence that something needs changing.
2. *Diagnose the problem.* Gather and analyze data to discuss the cause. Consult with the staff. Read appropriate materials.
3. *Analyze alternative solutions.* Brainstorm. Assess the risks and the benefits. Set a time, plan resources, and look for obstacles.
4. *Select the change.* Choose the option most likely to succeed that can be afforded. Identify the driving and opposing forces, using challenges that include assimilation of the opposition.
5. *Plan the change.* This will include specific measurable objectives, actions, a timetable, resources, budget, an evaluation method Performance Evaluation Review Technique (PERT), a plan for resistance management, and stabilization.
6. *Implement the change.* Plot the strategy. Prepare, involve, train, assist, and support those involved.
7. *Evaluate the change.* Analyze achievement of objectives and audit.
8. *Stabilize the change.* Refreeze; monitor until stable.[16]

Figure 10–2 provides an illustration of this model.

The Change Agent

As one reads change theory one notes that the applications tend to mimic the problem-solving process. The nurse manager operating as a change agent uses change theory to identify and solve problems. This nurse manager learns to anticipate impending change, including that from interdependent systems, responds to change, and takes action to direct its course.

FIGURE 10–2. Planned Change Model

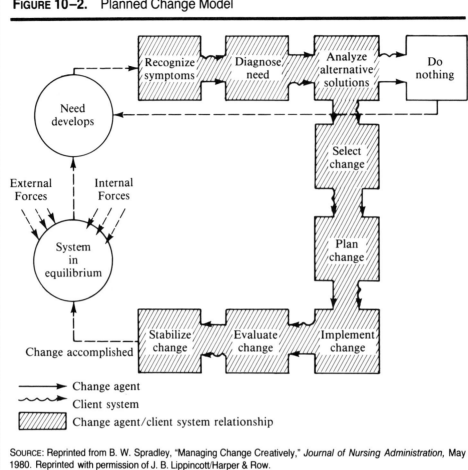

SOURCE: Reprinted from B. W. Spradley, "Managing Change Creatively," *Journal of Nursing Administration,* May 1980. Reprinted with permission of J. B. Lippincott/Harper & Row.

Nurses can compete successfully in the world of health care by doing things a new way. Nursing executives are expected to have the vision to change things, to be change agents.[17] Outsiders are resisted as change agents.

Nurse managers can plan change by establishing procedures to evaluate obsolescence and estimate the best time for replacement of equipment and procedures, which in turn engenders a need for updating the cognitive, affective, and psychomotor skills of practicing nurses. Hunt and Rigby recommend modification of change theory with a more open-minded model: unfreezing-changing-unfreezing rather than unfreezing-changing-refreezing.[18]

Beyers recommends development of scenarios for the future of nursing services. Scenarios could be written to describe various future environments for nurse managers. They could be presented through role playing at management development programs. They would be used to make change decisions.[19]

Examples of the Application of Change Theory

Retrenchments involving layoffs do not always use appropriate change theory. As a consequence there are considerable unnecessary pressures on nurse managers, including unfavorable publicity. The organizational climate becomes tense and disruptive and gives personnel a sense of loss of security. The nurse executives feel tired and drained. They need a sense of organizational atmosphere, of performance levels, and of physical and emotional responses. Some verbal harassment from employees can occur.

Causes of these problems include policies and plans being developed after the fact, with few policies developed to deal with employees remaining with the organization. The media can be used to inform the public of changes in the health-care system that necessitated the layoff.

Among the positive responses that will minimize resistance to the change of retrenchment are:

1. Having a strong orientation toward reality, preparedness, knowledge of human behavior, stress management, and openness and honesty in dealing with employees.
2. Developing organization-wide retrenchment plans and policies with the advice of the personnel/human resource management department and legal counsel.
3. Considering use of consultants.
4. Evaluating the criteria for layoffs: seniority, performance appraisal, and job categories. The principle of "last hired, first fired" should be a strong consideration.
5. Having the public relations department (or a consultant) handle publicity.
6. Dealing with rumors positively by newsletters, informal discussions, and open meetings.
7. Reassure remaining employees by being visible and available. Make frequent rounds.
8. Do team building with chaplains, psychiatric specialists, and human resource specialists.
9. Form a nurse manager support group and include families, friends, colleagues, and non-nursing professional peers.
10. Be fair and honest and handle people with dignity and care.[20]

In one hospital faced with the need to respond to changes of a contracting marketplace, competition, and changing reimbursement, the administration formed a task force of *all* involved parties. They brainstormed to plan for these changes; their efforts led to value improvement, cost reduction, and quality enhancements simultaneously. The results:

1. By looking at factors affecting length of stay, therapies were able to be started earlier, leading to earlier discharges.
2. Prosthetic devices were standardized, leading to reduced inventory levels and saving time, carrying charges, space, and paperwork.
3. Operating room procedures were standardized,

reducing core time, anesthesia, and loss of blood and leading to improved recovery.
4. One million dollars were saved and there was improved quality of care with a synergy of costs, comparisons, involvement, and implementation.[21]

RESISTANCE TO CHANGE

Resistance to change, or attempting to maintain the status quo when efforts are being made to alter it, is a common response to change. Change evokes stress that in turn evokes resistance.

Resistance to change is often based on a threat to the security of the individual, since it upsets an established pattern of behavior. Questions that should be answered if the problem-solving approach is used will fall under the area of workability of the solution. They include the following: Will the change affect the work standard and subsequent employment, promotion, and raises? Will it mean an increased workload at an accelerated pace? Do employees visualize how they will fit into the picture if this change occurs? In-service education is part of the answer; continuing education may also help meet the goal.

Factors that stimulate resistance to change include habits, complacency, fear of disorganization, set patterns of response to change, conservatism, perceived loss of power, ego involvement, insecurity, perceived loss of current or meaningful personal relationships, and perceived lack of rewards.[22]

People are afraid of change because of lack of knowledge, prejudices resulting from a lifetime of personal experience and exposure to others, and fear of the need for greater effort or of a higher degree of difficulty.

People have developed fears, biases, and social inhibitions from the cultural environment in which they live. They cannot be employed devoid of these cultural barriers, so it is necessary to find ways of managing them within a system.

Barriers to change include a perception of implied criticism: "You are changing the system because you don't like the way I do it." Employees perceive machines and systems replacing them or making their jobs less interesting. As an example, a programmed system could be developed for patients to take their own nursing histories.

Change may necessitate the investment of a

great deal of time and effort in relearning. If nurses are to be independent practitioners, what happens to those who are not prepared? "Probably the greatest single personal barrier is that individuals do not understand or refuse to accept the reasons for the change or the need for it. Unfortunately, it is not always easy to equate the reasons and the needs and to communicate them in meaningful and compelling language."[23]

People are members of a social system in a community and will resist change if it affects that social system. Social changes that threaten social customs, values, self-esteem, and security are resisted more than technical changes. One member of the social system may influence others even if they are unaffected by the change.

Values and Beliefs

Cognitive frameworks are based on values and beliefs about effective means of achieving these values. Nurse managers who value the chain of command, policies, and procedures and who believe their management experience does not need input from clinical nurses may not look for problems needing change. So long as they are successful they are strengthened by success that builds their self-respect. This success fosters resistance to change that threatens the integrity of the framework. People resist discarding their own ideas. Accepting another's idea reduces their self-esteem. They may consider a good idea a unique event to be preserved. Ideas should have life cycles. They shine and then dim and need to be replaced. Ideas should be put on a depreciable basis.[24]

Change is affected by the crucial differences among geographical regions. Some regions are more open to fast change while others accept slow change. Cultural changes are affected by religious or political beliefs. People hold fast to meaningful beliefs.[25]

Other Causes of Resistance to Change

Success leads to imprinting and resistance to change. Remember the saying "if it works, don't fix it?" Units within a division of nursing change at different paces, but in a complex organization many problems require their interaction. The nurse manager as effective change agent must orchestrate this interaction. Time perspectives differ among nursing units. When personnel transfer they have to adjust to the changed pace. Different generations of nurses also have different rates of change.

Sometimes nurse managers want to change things at too fast a pace. Excessive changes make a nurse manager and the organizers unpredictable and distrusted.

Gillen claims that change stimulates increased levels of energy. It is called "hyper-energy" and is *not* stress. Hyper-energy is the heightened drive a person feels in response to a perceived challenge or threat. If not managed, hyper-energy is used by employees to think of surreptitious ways of preventing change. Hyper-energy can be pooled for collective resistance to change. It distracts employees, causing errors and accidents.[26] Skilled nurse managers bring employees into the change process so the latter do not view it as a threat. Employees' hyper-energy is then channelled into involvement in the change process.

An Example

Niland describes the failure of change in an attempt to convert an acute care unit into a swing unit of patients awaiting transfer to a nursing home. The reasons given for the failure illustrate the importance of change theory:

1. The unit's goals were not made known to the staff or clinical manager.
2. The workload was too demanding.
3. There was poor communication and planning.
4. The managers were not aware of these staff perceptions:
   4.1 They were being used as workhorses.
   4.2 The unit was a waiting area for patient placement.
   4.3 The reason was fiscal.
   4.4 There was no nursing home bed shortage.
   4.5 The unit had become a geriatric unit in which they did not choose to work.
   4.6 They were doing the work of nurses aids.

These problems could have been avoided through careful planning using change theory.[27]

It should be remembered that both individuals and organizations need continuity in policies and procedures so that recurring needs can be dealt with routinely and problems do not have to be resolved anew each time they appear. Hierarchical, bureaucratic frameworks with rules achieve stability, one reason for resistance to change.

The major symptoms of resistance to change are refusal; confrontation; covert resistance such as nonpreparation for meetings or misunderstandings of the place or time; incomplete reports; refusal to accept responsibility; uncooperative employees; passive aggressiveness; absenteeism; and tardiness.[28]

STRATEGIES FOR OVERCOMING OBSTACLES TO CHANGE

Managed Change

Change can be managed, with nurse managers acting as change agents. One of the strategies a nurse manager can use is to request the services of a consultant to make the managerial diagnosis and recommend programs that will improve the productivity of nursing personnel while giving them job satisfaction. Such measures can include educational programs to improve those areas where there are problems.

There is ample evidence that modified forms of management by objectives are an effective strategy for change. The nurse administrators will be the change agents for its success.

Effective managed change leads to improvement of patient care services, raised morale, increased productivity, and meeting of patient and staff needs. Change is an art, the mastery of which can be exhilarating, refreshing, challenging, and exciting, because change represents opportunity. Change is facilitated when nursing employees are matched to demands for adaptability to jobs.

Collection and Development of Data

Nurse managers need to gather data about their work that can be discussed, analyzed, and used to effect change when indicated. Personnel, particularly managers, can be educated to make and manage change. They will learn about labor power planning and utilization rather than considering this to be the specialized area of the human resources department. They will learn about financial management rather than depending upon the accounting office to take care of them. These are areas in which effective strategies can be developed for

external cooperative efforts among chief nurse executives of similar institutions within a community. Such concepts can be expanded to clinical services. If a division of nursing cannot afford to use such specialists as a full-time mental health nurse practitioner, several organizations can collectively contract for the services of one. Thus change becomes a cooperative venture.

Integration of computers and automated equipment is essential to the change process. This is particularly true when managers are competing for professional nurses as well as for health-care dollars. Within this domain nurse managers can elicit the advice and skills of nursing management information system personnel as impartial third-party critics of the change being effected. Thus these personnel will give nurse managers effective feedback while providing management information support systems.

Preparation or Planning

Preplanning will help to overcome many of the obstacles to change. Planning will keep interpersonal relationships from being disrupted if persons with common frames of reference are brought together. The planner can assist people to meet their goals while minimizing fear and anxiety. Fear is stimulated by the external threat of change. Anxiety is internally stimulated; it is self-induced dread. Planning will help people accept the change without fear or anxiety.

In making changes nurse managers should plan to have people unlearn the old (unfreeze) and use the new (refreeze). Implementation of nursing management information systems can refine much unfreezing and refreezing. Often nurse mangaers help their staff learn the new without having them unlearn the old. This is a major problem in nursing today because of how the role of nurses is changing. As an example, nurse managers are not helping nurses unlearn the non-nursing routines. This is a big challenge for nurse managers and staff development personnel.

To prepare a plan carefully, share information and decision making, work for common perception and understanding, and support and reinforce the nursing staff's effort to effect change. Clear statements of philosophy, goals, and objectives are needed in preparation for change. The chapter on mission, philosophy, objectives, and management plans offers guidelines for evaluation.

Beyers recommends that nursing executives be involved in the following elements of strategic planning:

1. Product/market planning.
2. Business unit planning.
3. Shared resource planning.
4. Shared concern planning.
5. Corporate level planning.[29]

Nursing in all areas, both clinical and managerial, must consider competition. The patient will go where there is higher-quality nursing care. High-quality nursing care results from effectively planned and managed change. Nurse managers should perform market surveys to determine the nursing products and services wanted by consumers.[30] This activity itself will constitute change and will also result in changes.

In preparation for change, nurse managers should envision the future so as to create better systems. They should develop a long-range view of nursing as a basis for strategic planning. As an additional preparation for change, nurse managers can voluntarily rotate their own assignments among units and departments to develop their capacity for dealing with a fast pace of change. In this way they can expand their managerial experience and perceptions.

Plans should list everyone on whom the change depends and their level of involvement. Who will oppose and who will support the change? The dominant coalition in the organization and the forces that will stimulate change should be identified and their support enlisted. Appropriate current events should be noted through reading and through meetings, highlighting those that will enhance the mission of the organization and for which the clinical nurses will claim or share ownership.[31] This activity brings new ideas and new knowledge to stimulate and justify the need for change.

Planning will also require thinking in multiple time frames: changes to be effected in 6 months, 1 year, and so on. Identify the trade-offs between nursing and other departments, between clinical and management staffs, and within the change process itself. List ways to enlist support.[32]

Be careful not to overplan. Leave some room for the people who will implement the change to exercise intelligent initiative. Be sure the rewards or benefits to individuals and to the group are carefully communicated. If people want a change to work, they will make it happen.

Training and Education

Many factors play a part in new learning, including attracting people's attention and stimulating their desire to learn. The staff development instructor and the nurse manager have to find the cues that trigger the desired behavior. This may necessitate working backward from desired behavior to cues. Next they must determine the values that will personally satisfy the learner. When a match is made that satisfies both individual and employer, a new system can be implemented.

The frequency of training and education should match the frequency of change. Nursing personnel will require constant staff development programs to keep from depreciating in knowledge and competence. From initial hiring and orientation, change should be portrayed as an integral part of nurses' jobs.[33]

Rewards

Rewards for old behavior patterns should be removed after the individuals have been helped to see the reasons for the proposed change. They need to see the necessity for the new behaviors, and real incentives, financial or nonfinancial, should be provided. Here is where job standards come in. The job standards should incorporate the new methods or skills and phase out the old ones. To provide an incentive, performance appraisals can be based on the new standards. Time must be allowed and opportunity provided for retraining.

Employees affected by change should receive sympathetic understanding from the nurse manager. Also, compensation programs need to be changed for the benefit of more people in the division of nursing rather than being concentrated on the top level. Some effective programs have rewarded outstanding performance with special certificates and ceremonies that cited the behavior earning the award. Rewards should be increased legitimately and should be consistent throughout the organization. There should be a fair arrangement for employees who stand to lose from change.

Other forms of nonfinancial rewards include enriching jobs and encouraging self-development. These activities can provide satisfaction of individual needs.

Using Groups as Change Agents

Groups in themselves are often effective change agents. When the group appears to work in harmony and to have well-understood goals, it may be used to institute the change. If the idea can be planned in the group, it will be implemented more successfully. A group is more willing to assume risks than most individuals. Planning should make clear the need for change and provide an environment in which group members identify with such needs. Objectives should be stated in clear, concise, and qualitative terms. Administrative policy should contain broad guidelines for achieving the objectives. They should be communicated to the group. The procedures they contain also need to be understood.

As agents of change, nurse managers need to utilize the talents of their staff through use of temporary work teams to solve specific problems and effect change. They need to participate on interdisciplinary task forces. They need to prepare people for job mobility through planned experiences that will facilitate it. Third-party critics may help diagnose and solve problems.

The informal group can promote and support change. It can be formed by enlisting the help of a strong leader and by forming a strong group that will communicate their perception of needed change to nurse managers.[34]

Nurse managers assume multiple managerial roles in matrix organizations. They perform for several bosses and perform several tasks at a time. Improving group teamwork is essential to managed change. In the new work of nursing management no social group or set dominates.

Communications

Too often change is announced by rumor when it should be clearly introduced. Announcements should be factual and comprehensive and should state the objectives, nature, methods, benefits, and drawbacks of the change. If the announcement can be face-to-face, it will be better received.

Discussion of implementation should give people maximum information. The discussion should cover the rate and method of implementation, including the first steps that will be taken and the rate, sequence, and people involved in each element.

Ceremonies may be effective in various aspects of the change. They are useful for retirements; promotions; introduction of a new coworker, superior, or subordinate; a move to a new job; start of a new system; and reorganization. When used well, ceremonies focus on the importance of the ongoing institution and underline the importance of individual loyalty to that institution and its positions. They convey that the organization and the employees are both needed.

The nurse manager as change agent discusses reasons for resisting change with people. When people understand their real reasons for it, they are not as resistant. They should be encouraged to sound off.

Planned change needs to be successfully communicated to all employees even if they are not directly or immediately involved. Verbal announcements can be followed up with written ones and progress reports. Change occurs smoothly in direct proportion to the positive and democratic behavior that demonstrates management's philosophy and practice at all levels from the top down.

The Organizational Environment

Nurse managers could be more successful if they paid attention to the organizational environment into which change is introduced and the manner in which this is done. Managers need to be committed to a change and to support it by their actions, which express their attitudes. When the nurse administrator attempts to impose change on people in an authoritarian manner, they often resist it.

Managers can establish an environment for change when they:

1. Stress relationships with and between groups.
2. Bring out mutual trust and confidence.
3. Emphasize interdependence and shared responsibility.
4. Contain group membership and responsibility by limiting individuals from belonging to too many groups and ensuring the same responsibilities are not given to several groups.

5. Have a wide sharing of control and responsibility.
6. Resolve conflict through bargaining or problem-solving discussions.[35]

Concern for employees is as important as concern for patients.

In assessing the environment the nurse manager identifies prestige factors, leaders, and the communication network. They seek out and introduce change in the unit where success is best ensured.[36]

Other aspects of the organizational environment that support change include:

1. Permitting job movement to facilitate careers.
2. Anticipating and rewarding change, thus institutionalizing it.[37]
3. Modifying the nursing organizational structure to accommodate changes that provide growth and development.
4. Promoting a "can-do" attitude.

When the organizational climate changes, employees change behaviors. A desired organizational climate fosters high-quality patient care.[38]

Anticipating Potential Failures

While preparation is the key to successful change, it should include anticipation of potential failure. Three questions need to be answered before actions for change begin. First, nurse managers should determine what the risks are and how much they are willing to expect in terms of resources. Second, they should decide who will do the work. Third, they should have a flexible agenda and plan what will be done when it goes wrong.

Mistakes will happen. The importance of the change will determine how much risk the nurse manager is prepared to take. For example, one might risk a great deal and reorganize an entire unit to achieve the goal of having professional nurses perform as case managers. Changes can be introduced in one unit, evaluated, and modified before being extended to other units.

Change should be evaluated by people who the manager knows will work to make them successful. Evaluators should be equal to the size and nature of the problem. As problems emerge from the experiment with change, they can be addressed and

solved. Plans should include the action to be taken when anticipated problems occur. It is necessary for the manager, the change agent, to have the will to change, particularly because instituting change means stirring up problems.

The positive aspect of resistance to change is that it pushes the change agent to plan more carefully, listen with sympathetic understanding, and reexamine goals, functions, priorities, and values. When properly addressed, resistance uses less of people's energy. Other effective responses to resistance are respect for honest questions and differences of opinion, altering of strategy and tactics, altering of composition of groups, and proceeding in an objective, firm, assertive, and nonjudgmental manner.[39]

CREATIVITY AND INNOVATION

Creativity Defined

One would be remiss to neglect to define what is meant by creativity or innovation, the latter term being used interchangeably today in many articles exploring the subject. Creativity is defined in *Webster's Dictionary* as "artistic or intellectual inventiveness." Innovation is defined as "the introduction of something new." From these definitions, it would appear that we can use these two terms interchangeably. A person could say that creativity is the mental work or action involved in bringing something new into existence, while innovation is the function of that effort.[40] Creativity is a way of using the mind.[41] Research indicates that creativity is *not* intelligence.[42] If one wishes to differentiate, a nurse can create or invent a new nursing product, process, or procedure (creativity) or can effect change by putting a new product process or procedure into use (innovation).

Creativity has also been defined as an attitude brought to the job by workers. It behooves nurse managers, then, to determine whether workers have brought this attitude of creativity to the job. A nurse manager might well determine if clinical nurses come to their jobs with attitudes that indicate belief in progress. Do they believe there are goals to be accomplished? That changes are inevitable? Or do they simply come to the job because it is a way of earning a living by application of old practices? Creativity is needed because change is constant.

Nurse managers create the environment that fosters and encourages new ideas.[43]

Creativity is original thought and action. It is the human expression of reaction to a challenge, usually a challenge to the intellect of a person. Some would call it "ability to generate new ideas" or the "basic human facility for solving problems."[44] It certainly involves new thoughts about old problems; in short, it involves ideas.

Creativity has been defined in terms of these elements:

1. Creativity is a mental activity.
2. It is triggered by specific problems.
3. It results in novel solutions.
4. These solutions usually have implications or applications beyond their immediate uses.[45]

While there seems to be no lack of creativity in nursing, there does seem to be a lack of ability to put new ideas into operation. Such innovation requires not only money and time, but also executive leadership. Either the leadership must be endowed with ability to make ideas work, or they must be able to identify the nurses who can. In the process, all must be willing to overcome problems that arise during the process of innovation.

Confusion should not be mistaken for creativity. Innovation will be accomplished by following a plan or blueprint that makes allowances for variation in approaches. The change itself will be disturbing enough.

Why Creativity?

Business leaders would argue that creativity yields profits. With creativity, new products can be developed and a company can compete. Not just products but new methods are also fruits of creativity. For many years nurses have tended to think of selling their services like a product as being mercenary or unethical. This thinking has changed as nurses have acquired more education and become more autonomous. More professional nurses have become entrepreneurs in establishing independent business enterprises. This development was predicted by Sister Reinkemeyer when she wrote that "university programs try to produce independent personalities and thinkers capable of facing some of the modern scientific and psychosocial changes in nursing."[46]

A constant flow of new ideas is needed to procure new products, services, processes, procedures, and strategies for dealing with the changes occurring in every sphere of endeavor: technology, social systems, government, and everyday living. Health care is big business.

Drucker advocates a reporting system that calls attention both to things that go wrong and to those that go better than expected, forecast, or budgeted. Following his advice, nurses would be entrepreneurs if the organization would not penalize them. He also states that entrepreneurship should neither be mixed with operations and rewards nor put on the bottom of the organization to be killed. Instead good people should be put to work in the new enterprise with a full-time person in charge. Even if the organization is middle-sized it can have some people working in a new service. While innovation needs order, it does not need excess policy. It requires reception and a market to be successful.[47]

Establishing a Climate for Creativity

For creativity to prosper, the organization should provide a warm intellectual environment that gives employees recognition, prestige, and an opportunity to participate. They will be involved in planning their work and making decisions that give them a sense of ownership and commitment. The manager who practices management by objectives supports creativity.

Nurse managers promote creativity through sensitivity that gives people the individual attention they want and treats them as having individual differences. Professionally competent managers inspire creativity through taking risks as well as through showing confidence, praise, and support, being nourishing, using tact, and having patience.[48]

Metamanagement.   Metamanagement is a term describing a cooperative effort of entrepreneurial or creative managers, strategic planners, and top management. It is:

> a planning framework that cuts across organizational boundaries and facilitates strategic decision making about current practices and future directions; a flexible and creative planning process that stimulates in-house entrepreneurial thinking and behavior; and a consistent and accepted value system that reinforces management's commit-

ment to the organization's strategy and stresses teamwork, organizational flexibility, open communication, innovation, risk taking, high morale, and trust.[49]

Nurse managers practicing metamanagement will organize the organization's structure, dynamics, nature, and position. They will demonstrate an innovative, committed, enlightened, disciplined, and courageous management willing and able to restructure thinking and organizations and generate and execute successful plans for a profitable nursing business. They will stimulate the input of their clinical nurses, thereby generating direction for the nursing organization and occupation.

The External Environment.　The external environment includes all aspects of the larger system, such as a hospital, that determine how conducive to creativity a group of clinical nurses perceives its climate to be. Such aspects include management controls, communications, reward systems, attitudes, feedback, information, energy, supplies, and values. The following task-related actions by nurse managers will help to develop and maintain a creative climate:

1. Providing freedom to experiment without fear of reprimand.
2. Maintaining a moderate amount of work pressure.
3. Providing challenging yet realistic work goals.
4. Emphasizing a low level of supervision in performance tasks.
5. Delegating responsibilities.
6. Encouraging participation in decision making and goal setting.
7. Encouraging use of a creative problem-solving process to solve unstructured problems.
8. Providing immediate and timely feedback on task performance.
9. Providing the resources and support needed to get the job done.[50]

Creative Problem Solving.　Creative problem solving starts with vague or ill-defined problems as challenges. Problems can be attacked intuitively to generate as many ideas as possible. Solutions may create new challenges and new cycles of creative problem solving. Gordon and Zemke support using creative thinking when the logical approach does

not work. Ideas are no good if no action results. These authors argue that the left brain–right brain model of creative problem solving is not working.[51]

There are several theories of creative problem solving. Lattimer and Winitsky suggest the following:

1. *Thinking.* Identify the factors to be used in solving issue or developing a strategic plan. The choice is between a risk-free alternative and a risky one.

2. *Decomposing.* Break down the situation into components—alternatives, uncertainties, outcomes, consequences; work with each and combine the results for a decision.

3. *Simplifying.* Determine the important components and concentrate on them. What are the most crucial factors and most essential relationships? Then make intuitive judgements.

4. *Specifying.* Establish the value of key factors, the probabilities for the uncertainties, and preferences for the outcomes.

5. *Rethinking.* Was the original analysis sensible regarding omissions, inclusions, order, and emphasis?[52]

Godfrey recommends an alternative theory of creativity that has five steps, as follows:

1. *Perception.* Realizing there is a problem.
2. *Preparation.* Research, data collection, and arrangement of information to define the problem.
3. *Ideation.* Analysis and structure of a variety of formats that stimulate analogies and images; brainstorming.
4. *Incubation.* Withdraw and relax when the flow of ideas ends. The unconscious takes over and forms images of possible solutions.
5. *Validation.* Test a solution.[53]

Drucker's Strategies for Innovation.　Drucker indicates that every corporation needs a strategy for innovation. He suggests four, as follows:

1. *The first with the mostest.* Be first in the market and the first to improve a product or cut its price. This discourages prospective competitors.

2. *The second with the mostest.* Let someone else establish the market. Satisfy markets with narrow needs and specific capabilities. Provide excellent products for big purchasers with narrow needs. Offer few features. This strategy is evident in the competitive health-care market, where certain corporations have specialized in psychiatric services, rehabilitation services, or drug dependency services.

3. *The Niche Strategy.* Corner a finite market, making it unprofitable for others. When the niche becomes a mass market, change the strategy to remain profitable.

4. *Making the Product Your Carrier.* One product carries another. This has been done by medical supply companies whose electronic thermometers sell disposable covers and intravenous pumps sell fluid administration sets.[54]

Creativity Training.   Training can help people to be creative. It can teach them to develop creative thinking skills and logical techniques that can lead to successful results. General Electric established creativity training for its engineers in 1937. Many other companies also provide creativity training. Before developing creativity training, nurse managers should establish some general concepts of what they want employees to bring into existence that is new (products, techniques, markets, etc.).

Creativity training aims to increase the creative capacity or creative behavior of individuals or groups. The techniques of creativity training can include brainstorming, synectics, morphological analysis, forced fit, forced relationships, brainwriting, visualization, cueing, lateral thinking, and divergent thinking,[55] as illustrated in Figure 10–3.

Other Approaches to Creativity.   Avoid the "six rules for stifling innovation" identified by Kanter:

1. Regard any new idea from below with suspicion—because it is new, and because it is from below.
2. Insist that people who need your approval to act go through several other levels of management to obtain their signatures first.
3. Express your criticisms freely and withhold your praise. (That keeps people on their toes.) Let them know they could be fired at any time.

4. Make decisions to reorganize or to change policies in secret, and spring them on people unexpectedly. (That also keeps people on their toes.)
5. Control everything carefully. Make sure people count anything that can be counted, frequently.
6. Never forget that you, the higher-ups, already know everything important about this business.

To stimulate innovation, just do the reverse.[56]

Nurses will be motivated to be creative when nurse managers encourage them to express their ideas openly and accept divergent ideas and points of view. Other motivators of creativity by nurses include providing assistance to develop new ideas, encouraging risk taking while buffering resisting forces, providing time for individual effort, providing opportunities for professional growth and development, encouraging interaction with others outside the group, promoting constructive intragroup and intergroup competition, recognizing the value of worthy ideas, and exhibiting confidence in workers.[57]

Research studies indicate that creative behavior is inherent in human nature and can be developed. Elements or pieces necessary for creating something new exist and must be arranged in new and useful combinations. Excessive motivation, caused by high rewards for performance or anxiety over failure possibilities, has been proved to have inhibited creativity. It causes people to pursue ideas down blind alleys.

The actions for producing original, goal-oriented ideas are the following:

1. Assemble the separate elements needed and that will be creatively combined to produce a product or a new process. The problem must be identified in terms of usefulness of this product or process. If a known element is missing, what is available to replace it?
2. Use the available and assembled elements in combinations that produce original ideas.
3. Remove inhibitions to creativity such as excess motivation, anxiety, fear of taking risks, dependence on authority, or habitual modes of thinking and talking about things. Creativity is not confined to a small, exclusive set of gifted people. Language contains the potential for creative thought so all of us have the potential.
4. Study techniques of creativity so that the elements can be used.[58]

FIGURE 10–3. The Creativity Jargon Jungle

Here is a list of the ten techniques and terms we heard most often while researching the wonderful world of creativity training. Our thumbnail definitions are in no way USDA-approved. And remember that terms sometimes mean anything a particular speaker wants them to mean.

Creativity Training. According to the *Encyclopedia of Management* (Van Nostrand Reinhold, 1982), General Electric established in 1937 a two-year work/study program for engineers "showing creative promise during the first months of employment." This first recorded creativity training program focused on nurturing that promise through work assignments and educational experiences.

Today the term is used to cover a multitude of processes and means neither more nor less than the speaker wants it to mean. As used in this story, it refers to training that aims to increase the creative capacity or creative behavior of individuals or groups; it does not refer to efforts to foster a creative "climate" in an organization.

Brainstorming. A group-based idea-generating technique developed by Alex Osborn in 1938 and popularized in his book *Applied Imagination* (Scribner, 1953). Brainstorming is not a room full of people madly shouting out whatever comes into their heads. It is a structured, moderated process. The group is led by a chairman who controls time, presents the problem to be worked out, and controls the progress of the storm. Brainstorming usually starts with a warm-up wherein the participants review the rules ("no critiquing others' ideas, piggybacking is good, be far out, etc."), and loosen up with practice exercises ("How many uses can you think of for a sick cat?").

Then the real problem is presented and participants call out as many ideas as they can dream up. Someone records every idea. The idea-generation phase typically lasts an hour to 90 minutes. Participants then cluster and categorize the ideas, evaluate their potential, and recommend the most promising ones to the problem owner.

Brainstorming groups have been convened to find new uses for an old product, to name a new product, and to develop slogans for campaigns from sales to safety. Proponents see the technique's uses as vritually unlimited. Brainstorming is the longest running act in the idea-generating business; there are probably as many variations as there are people who hold creativity sessions.

Synectics. A group-based problem-solving technique that stresses control over the creative environment and reasoning by analogy. In 1944 W. J. J. Gordon set out to study creativity through the psychoanalysis of inventors.

George Price joined Gordon, popularized his findings, added to them and translated them into practical procedures. In 1960 they founded Synectics, Inc., which sells training in the method. The firm is credited with coining the expression, "making the familiar strange and the strange familiar." Synectics comes from the Greek *synetikos,* meaning "the joining together of apparently irrelevant elements." A short description of synectics is just about impossible. The major stages are: 1) problem as given, 2) short analysis of the problem as given, 3) purge (the problem as given is clarified and simplified), 4) problem as understood (the problem is reinterpreted in analogy or metaphor), 5) excursion (the group leaves the problem and "plays" with analogies), 6) fantasy force fit (a metaphor is forced onto the original problem), 7) viewpoint (the problem is redefined in a "new light").

Morphological Analysis. Developed in the late 1940s by a mathematician named Frank Zwicky, and refined later by Myron Allen, morphological analysis is a system of breaking an idea or problem into its components for study. It's seen as falling toward the logical end of the creative problem-solving spectrum.

You specify the attributes of the problem and then make a grid or cube of them. For instance, you're trying to come up with a new method of transportation. You choose "energy" as a minor dimension, and list under that heading all the ways that a thing can be powered (wind, gas, steam, etc.). That list forms one side of a morphological grid. Acorss the other axis you write "surfaces" and list ground, air, water, etc. This gives you a series of "boxes" where each factor listed under one of your major headings intersects with each factor listed under the other. Where "wind" and "water" intersect, we think of a sailboat. Ah, but what about "wind" and "ground"? Add a third major dimension and you can create a three-dimensional cube instead of a grid.

Force Fit/Forced Relationships. A basic idea in creative problem solving and in the creativity literature as a whole is that if you rub two old ideas together you sometimes come up with a new one. But ideas don't necessarily stick to one another easily: sometimes they have to be forced together and examined for fit. Force fitting refers to going back to a list of interesting, outrageous, preposter-

FIGURE 10–3. The Creativity Jargon Jungle (*continued*)

ous—as well as sensible—ideas and twisting and squeezing them until they become a reasonable or at least a possible solution to the problem. Sometimes ideas are jammed together with objects, sights, sounds, etc. Smell, particularly, is considered a powerful sensory trigger.

The terms direct force fit and get-fired technique also show up in connection with this process. In "get-fired" the challenge to the group is to come up with solutions that would work, but that would lead to the sponsor getting fired. Once such a solution is determined, the task becomes to scale or tone it down so that the problem gets solved but the sponsor saves his or her job. Force-Fit Game is a team competition in idea generating developed by Helmut Schlicksupp of the Battelle Institute in Frankfurt, Germany.

Brainwriting. This is an idea-generating technique for groups that aren't exactly groups, much like the Nominal Group Technique, Crawford Slip Method, and Collective Notebook. All are methods that encourage free association and the recording of ideas in writing, without verbal interaction with other people but with their "assistance." In brainwriting, originally developed by Bernd Rohrback, the technique is simple. Participants are given a set of forms, consisting mostly of lines and white space. They listen to an explanation of the problem and are asked to write four ideas (solutions, suggestions, thoughts, etc.) about the problem on the form. The teams are then exchanged. Reading others' ideas is supposed to stimulate more ideas, which are then written on the form. The process continues until no one can think of something else to write.

Visualization. Most of us have little movie projectors in our heads that we can use to review the past, speculate about the future or create "pictures" of impossibilities. For some time, psychologists have tapped into this ability to help people overcome phobias and fears in a process called *systematic desensitization.*

People like T. H. Carl Krueger of Encina Corp., Las Cruces, N. Mex. have conducted several studies in high technology settings that suggest that it is possible to control and harness this natural skill 85% of us share (15% of the adult population cannot spontaneously visualize) and to fine-tune it for problem solving. A wide range of creativity consultants have been claiming that for years. Excursion, the generation of a fantasy scenario having no apparent relation to the problem being solved, is a form of visualization used in the synectics process and in many other courses.

Lists. There are a lot of them: Osborn's List, Arnold's list, the Davis and Houtman List, Polya's Checklist and more. They tend to be sets of specific questions to ask in specific problem-solving situations. For instance, if you are trying to make a change in a product, a checklist might ask, "Can you make it smaller? Larger? A different color?" The items on the checklists are intended to act as cues to new ways of considering the problem.

Attribute listing is a specific technique. The characteristics of a product or problem are spelled out. The group—or an individual—then speculates on ways of modifying the characteristics or obtaining the same characteristic in another way: "What can we substitute that has the same characteristics?" Walter Mettal uses the example of running out of packing material the evening before the moving trucks arrive. Packing material is "light, shock-absorbent, available, etc." These characteristics lead to a creative solution: "Go into the kitchen and pop a bushel or two of popcorn. Use the popcorn as packing material."

Lateral Thinking. A term coined by Edward de Bono to represent the need to escape from conventional ways of looking at problems to solve them. In his 1970 book, *Lateral Thinking* (Penguin Books), he divided problems into three types: those whose solutions require the processing of information, those where the "problem" is one of accepting what cannot be changed, and those that can only be solved by reorganizing information and assumptions about the problem. To solve the third type, you have to be illogical or "think laterally." Training in this area primarily involves learning to challenge assumptions and developing the awareness that methods other than straight logical reasoning can solve problems.

Divergent Thinking. A term that refers to expanding one's view of a problem. In divergent thinking, we roll the problem over in our minds and think about it in different ways without necessarily trying to solve it—just to "get a handle on it." Convergent thinking is just the opposite: the problem is cut into smaller and smaller pieces to obtain a manageable size and perspective. The key is to know when to do which. Predominantly, divergent thinkers are referred to as impractical, woolgatherers, perhaps scatterbrained. Insistently convergent thinkers are accused of jumping to solutions and being narrow-minded. Divergent thinking is most often stressed, but both skills are useful in creative problem solving.

Characteristics of a Creative Person

Creative people, including nurses, have a broad background of knowledge. They have the mental skills of curiosity, openness, sensitivity to problems, flexibility, ability to think in images, analysis, and synthesis.[59]

Creative nurses use their knowledge to stimulate their sensory perceptions. In addition to solving problems they create new problems to solve by formulating questions about the "whys" and "hows" of established practices. To foster their independence and creative talents nurse managers will assume that creative nurses are not odd or eccentric. As a consequence, barriers will not be erected among peer groups. Nurse managers will communicate and cooperate with clinical nurses to set new goals or new practices for achieving goals.[60]

Creative people have been thought of as being different from other people. This difference has been described by one writer thus: "The public would have him nearsighted but far-seeing, brilliantly innovative but absentminded, widely acclaimed but impervious to applause, capable of highly involved abstract thinking but naive and eccentric in his everyday reasoning."[61] The truth of the matter is that the creative person *is* different but is *not* a monster "strangely mysterious and incomprehensible."[62] An individual may appear to have been gifted with a brilliant intellect. During childhood this individual may have been the curious type who searched for books to read and tasks to do that satisfied his or her curiosity. Searching for the approval and encouragement of parents, friends, or teachers but not receiving it, a person may have become somewhat of a loner.

Creative individuals value the work and association of other creative individuals. They stimulate each other to think and perhaps even to be competitively creative. Creative people can tolerate ambiguity; they have self-confidence, the ability to toy with ideas, and persistence.[63]

While the creative nurse may not always invent or discover something entirely new, she may find an idea in almost any professional publication, or even in popular magazines. One team leader questioned why the job description of the department of nursing still reflected head nurse and staff nurse. As a result of her questioning a committee was established to investigate the possibility of changing the job titles as well as the listed duties and responsibil-

ities. The result was new job descriptions for clinical nursing coordinators (formerly called head or charge nurses).

A clinical nursing coordinator has set up her own cancer clinic. She convinced the physicians of her ability to perform the functions and of its benefit to them and to the patients. Patients now make direct appointments to this clinic, which has expanded to become a health screening clinic for women. In addition to coming for a Pap test and breast examination, clients have a history taken by the nurse practitioner. They are referred to the physician only when there is evidence of pathology. Many patients now come for personal health counselling. Future clinics to be established by clinical nursing coordinators include those in which patients with medical and surgical problems will be screened, referred to physicians as necessary, and referred back to the nurse for nursing care.

In another instance an assistant to the director of nursing questioned the time-honored practice of nurses counting narcotics and controlled drugs three times a day. With the advice of legal counsel it was decided that this was only being done because it had become common practice. Policy has been changed so that the narcotics and controlled drugs are inventoried by the pharmacist when he orders the medications each morning and by the unit manager before he leaves at the end of his shift. Discrepancies are reported to the head nurse. Thus nurses lost another non-nursing function.

A creative nurse manager could pursue a goal of developing a partnership of nurses and physicians in private practice on a contractual basis. It could be done to provide better health care to the American public, particularly if self-care theory were pursued. It could keep people out of hospitals and diminish the cost of medical expenses while keeping some individuals in the productive performance of their jobs. The physicians would practice medicine and the nurses would practice nursing without finely drawn lines between the two.

Managing Creativity

The nurse manager can encourage creativity through interpersonal relationships that establish trust. This requires acceptance of differing behaviors and ideas and a willingness to listen. It requires friendliness and a spirit of cooperation. It will also require respect for the feelings of others and a lack of defensiveness.[64]

Creative nurses produce a lot. They are unconventional and individualistic. Their critical skills are problem awareness and specification, skills that lead to problem resolution.[65]

Nurse managers can plan to nourish creativity in nursing personnel by:

1. Noting creative abilities of those persons who develop new methods and techniques.
2. Providing time and opportunity for people to do creative work. This can be planned during the performance appraisal process.
3. Recognizing that those who are masters or experts in nursing work in clinical practice, teaching, research, and management.
4. Encouraging nursing personnel to become involved in new nursing endeavors at work, in the community, in professional organizations, as well as undertaking other activities that increase knowledge and skills.
5. Encouraging risk-taking and acceptance of personal responsibility.

THE RELATIONSHIP OF NURSING RESEARCH TO CHANGE

The Need for Nursing Research

While there are many predictions of the future directions of health care, it will probably be different from all of them. Nursing research is essential to preparation for the future and for competition within the health-care system. Nurse managers must have good information to keep nursing competitive with other care givers in providing patient care. They must also have the knowledge to be competitive among employers and in a global economy. This requires the development and employment of nursing scientists who are researchers. Employment of these nursing researchers will commit nurse managers to developing research in managing human beings to their full potential. It is an investment that keeps people, the future human capital, from depreciating.[66]

Nursing research improves practice. A profession grounds practice in scholarly inquiry. Nurse managers will improve the quality of nursing practice when they promote nursing research and the application of the findings of nursing research. Nursing administration research will validate the discipline of nursing administration.[67]

Nurse managers, clinical nurses, instructors, and others are often eager to effect change. They like to try something new, to apply the latest technologies; they can do so through the nursing research process. There are two kinds of research activities, those in which nurses are the subjects and those in which they develop their own nursing research program. Real research requires preparation and time.

Nursing Research in the Service Setting

It follows, then, if there is to be research in nursing, and if it is to be part of the organizational goals, there must be planning. Plans incorporate a budget, a staff, and defined problems for research. Staff nurses working in clinical jobs and management personnel usually do not have time for this kind of research. They can use the results of such research and apply it to their situation so as to build better health-care delivery systems.[68]

A nursing management position filled by a scholar will enhance the chances of a nursing research program being successful. A scholar will have the knowledge to increase nursing administration research of a high intellectual and professional caliber. A nursing researcher can promote the reunification model of nursing education and nursing service through joint appointments and joint research endeavors, supporting cooperation between service and education. Nursing faculty tend to disengage from practice because of the numerous demands of their teaching roles. One reason that faculty focus on wellness may be their disengagement from practice. Since nursing faculty are often well-prepared scientists, nursing managers should find ways to budget for released time for practice and arrange to pay the school for their work. A coalition will benefit all nurses since faculty will be recognized for research activities that keep them up to date and managers will benefit from improved patient care.[69]

Nursing administration scholars will allow clinicians adequate time to develop their projects. They will provide a resource link to help clinicians find research partners with whom they can practice relevant nursing research.[70]

The Nursing Research Process

The nursing research process includes both scientific and technical steps. The format for writing up research is a problem-solving one and includes:

1. *Introduction*—includes an overview of the problem and tells why the research is being done.

2. *Statement of the problem*—an explicit and precise expression of the research question.

3. *Purpose of the study*—answers the question: what is the long-range goal of the research, the ultimate purpose that will be achieved by the findings? The statement also relates to current nursing concerns and the motivation for the study. If readers of a study cannot determine its purpose, they should read no further.

4. *Review of the literature*—a summary of the studies done and their results and a statement indicating what this study will add. The review should present a conceptual framework for the study; concepts and theories documented in previous studies; and evidence to support the approach. It should also indicate how the proposed study goes beyond what has already been achieved. The dependent variables to be measured and the independent variables to be manipulated should be identified.

5. *Hypothesis*—a formal statement of the research question, of what relationships are being tested and how they are measured. The variables are specifically defined.

6. *Methodology or design*—describes the setting, the subjects, how the subjects are chosen, procedures, analysis, and data collection. Measurement techniques used will be those appropriate to the hypothesis.

7. *Results*—answers the research question objectively. The presentation of results stays within the parameters of the designed study.

8. *Analysis*—a statistical test that measures the effect of the independent variable.

9. *Discussion*—includes any unexpected results as well as the conclusions reached.[71]

This format can be used to evaluate research reports; steps 1 through 5 indicate how to develop a research proposal. Plans for steps 6 through 9 should be included in the proposal.

The Research Question. The research question comes from many intensive hours of thought, literature review, and reflection. It avoids value judgments and opinions. The research question needs more than one variable. It may be a question or a statement. The researcher begins by getting thoughts down on paper, by writing an annotated statement of the question without concern for grammar and refining it later. A literature search is undertaken to find out what is known about the subject including facts, relationships, and level of confidence.

Written abstracts are made by the researcher, including types of studies and categories of variables. The researcher also defines the independent and dependent variables and has peers critique them. Questions answered include: Are these variables related so that change in one is apt to produce change in the other? What variables other than the one to be tested could influence the variable(s) to be measured?[72] A sample research question is given in Figure 10–4. According to Lindeman and Schantz, a good research question will meet the following criteria:

1. It can be answered by collecting observable evidence or empirical data.
2. It contains reference to the relationship between two or more variables.
3. It follows logically and consistently from what is already known about the topic.[73]

They state that experimental studies should not be done if no descriptive ones exist.[74]

The Research Design. The research design is the blueprint created to answer the research question. It follows development of the research question, the literature search, and statement of the hypothesis. Six elements of a good research design are:

1. *Setting*—the place where research will be done. There must be enough cases or variables specific to

FIGURE 10–4. Sample Research Question

Research Question. What is the difference in attendance between continuing education (CE) programs that are based on a needs survery and those that are not? (This question is researchable, while "Should a CE needs survey be done?" is not.)

Test	Other Factors	Measure
Independent variable: The variable being tested, examined, or manipulated. Provides measurement of the dependent variable	Extraneous variables: Conditions, behaviors, or characteristics known to exist but not considered of primary importance to the research. The research design may or may not control for these.	Dependent variables: The variables being measured, studied, or investigated to evaluate the impact of the first variable. The outcome or criterion: what will result from the study?
Needs survey	*Cognitive mapping, rewards, threats, personal needs*	*Attendance at CE programs*

SOURCE: Adapted from C. A. Lindeman and D. Schantz, "The Research Question, "*Journal of Nursing Administration*, Jan. 1982, 6–10. Reprinted with permission of Lippincott/Harper and Row.

the intent of the research, thereby strengthening internal and external validity and the ability to generalize.

2. *Subjects*—should be profiled and limited to those most useful in answering the research question. Their human rights will be protected.

3. *Sampling*—the method for choosing the sample size or number of subjects. Increasing the size of a sample adds strength, power, and meaningfulness.

4. *Treatment*—subjects of the sample are assigned to groups at random: experimental versus control. They are manipulated to increase the difference between the groups.

5. *Measurement*—statistical tests are selected to measure the differences between the groups. A reliable instrument produces consistent results. A valid instrument measures what it claims to measure.

6. *Communicating the results*—data are analyzed and results reported to others. Findings related to the research question are given first, then surprise data.[75]

Research Strategies

Nursing Research in a Health-Care Agency. Utilization of nursing research findings is poor in all spheres of nursing. This is improving as nurse administrators establish nursing research programs within their organizations. Two efforts to introduce research findings into practice and to evaluate the results have been conducted by the Western Interstate Commission for Higher Education in Nursing and the Regional Program for Nursing Research Development.[76]

Once the nurse administrator, with input from practicing nurses, defines the objectives of a nursing research program, a decision can be made regarding the organizational design for it. If resources are so scarce that additional budgeted personnel cannot be hired, a standing research committee can be established. A standing committee will promote stability by maintaining effective protocols and standards. The chair should have research expertise.

Since program resources are a determinant of the scope of the research program, the nurse administrator will need to establish a budget related to the objectives. This may include reallocation of money, generation of external funding, or revenue-generating activities by the professional nursing staff.

Budget permitting, the nurse administrator may hire a research specialist full- or part-time. Sometimes a budgeted position is shared by another nurse specialist. It could be a joint appointment with the college of nursing faculty.[77]

A research consortium can be established as a cooperative venture with other organizations within the community. This can include hospitals, home health-care agencies, nursing homes, and others.

Given a larger budget the nurse executive can establish a research department as a separate cost center. Such a department will have direct account-ability and clearly structured authority. It can even be a self-supporting department. Success will reflect strong commitment and will give increased visibil-ity. Figure 10–5 shows examples of nursing re-search studies from one institution.

The ultimate purpose of service-based nursing research is to improve patient care. Nursing man-agement research will answer questions related to the management of resources used in providing patient care. As practicing nurses become aware of the availability of competent nurse researchers they will refer research questions to them.

Four phases occur in the application of research findings to practice:

1. Evaluation of the strength of the research de-sign.
2. Evaluation of the feasibility and desirability of making the change in practice.
3. Planning the introduction and implementation of the change.
4. Using a pretest and post-test to evaluate the effect of the proposed change on practice.[78]

Milieu. A University of Michigan study of the conduct and utilization of research in nursing (CURN) included participating hospitals with mi-lieus that supported research. These milieus were found to include an active clinical faculty for under-graduate and graduate students, existing research programs, influential nurse administrators, librari-ans, and other resources. Each facility had ex-perienced, degree-prepared nurses with flexible, autonomous roles who facilitated research. They perceived nursing research to have increased the status and visibility of nursing on both sides, educa-tion and practice.[79]

Organizational Considerations. Once nurse ad-ministrators decide that nursing research will be a component of the nursing organization, they must plan the program design within the organizational structure. The mission, philosophy, and objectives will give direction to a nursing research program design. Input can be obtained from interested pro-

FIGURE 10–5. Nursing Research Studies Completed at Northeast Georgia Medical Center, 1986–1988

"A Comparison Study of Three Self-Monitoring Blood Glu-cose Meters," Shannon Garner, R.N., Debbie Cleland, R.N., and Susan Stone, R.N.

"The Recruitment and Retention of Registered Nurses in a Hospital Setting," Susan Stone, R.N., and Dan Walter, M.B.A.

"A Comparison Study of Heparinized Saline and Normal Saline in Maintaining INT Catheter Patency," Susan Stone, R.N., NGMC IV team.

"The Perceived Personal Needs of Families of Acute Brain-Injured and Spinal Cord–Injured Patients," Tracy Car-lisle, R.N., and NGMC neuroscience nursing staff.

"ICU Mortality Prediction Model," Susan Stone, R.N., Ruth Kunkle, R.N., NGMC ICU Nursing Staff.

"Nurses' Attitudes Towards Alcohol-Dependent Clients," Joan Burnham, R.N., North Georgia College.

"The Effects of Music Therapy on Critically Ill Patients in an ICU Setting," Sonja Chaffin, R.N., Angela Chambers, R.N., Fran Rusk, R.N., and Susan Stone, R.N., NGMC ICU Nursing Staff.

"Nurse Retention: Staff Nurse Perspectives," D. Patricia Gray, R.N., Susan Stone, R.N., NGMC neuroscience nursing staff.

"The Effects of Nocturnal Bottle-Feeding Patterns on Infant Weight and Maternal Satisfaction," Gay Mortimer, R.N., and Susan Stone, R.N., NGMC newborn nursery staff.

SOURCE: Reprinted with permission of Northeast Georgia Medical Center, 743 Spring Street, Gainesville, GA 30501-3899. The author visited this hospital and noted that while administration provided seed money, nursing research was expected to pay for itself through improved practice and cost savings.

fessional nurses at the planning stage. This can be done through an ad hoc committee that defines clear objectives for both clinical and administrative research activities. These objectives can include those for research conducted to satisfy departmental, personal, and interdisciplinary needs of the institution, graduate students, staff, faculty, and others. Other ad hoc committees can be formed to conduct research studies or to evaluate and implement research findings. Their composition will be determined by their objectives and by the interests and expertise of participating nurses.

Research Strategies. Protocols can be developed to benefit the entire institution. A hospital-wide research department or committee can include nurses. Such a committee can standardize procedures for approval, evaluation, and implementation of all research.

Staff development programs can support interest in the nursing research program. Instructors can communicate to the nursing staff the relevance of nursing research studies and teach nursing staff their roles. The nursing staff can be provided with rewards of nursing research in the form of money, improved care, and prestige. This will be supplemented with consistent communication in memoranda, study abstracts, literature, references, presentations, seminars, and conferences.[80]

Figure 10–6 presents details of an actual nursing research study.

Areas for Nursing Management Research

A Delphi study done in 1985 indicated these twelve research questions as having the highest mean score priority:

1. What are the cost-effective components of clinical nursing care that yield high patient satisfaction, decrease the number of complications, and shorten hospital stay for identified groups and patients?
2. How can nursing research in the practice setting be used to decrease cost, improve the quality of care, and increase patient and nurse satisfaction?
3. What is the relationship of patient acuity to cost of care, nursing resource needs, and nursing judgment of acuity?

FIGURE 10–6. ICU Mortality Prediction Model

Purpose. As health-care resources become limited and the cost of intensive care increases, reliable methods are needed to predict patient outcomes in the critical care setting. Determination of those patients who are most likely to benefit from the intensive care unit (ICU) could be useful to evaluate the need for admission and to estimate resources required for the ICU.

Northeast Georgia Medical Center (NGMC) was invited to participate in a national study funded by the National Center for Health Service Research Grant HS 04833. The purpose of this study was to describe the severity of illness of patients admitted to ICU and to predict the mortality of ICU patients based on clinical variables assessed on admission.

Study Design. A sample of 100 consecutive patient admissions was drawn from the ten-bed NGMC ICU. Each ICU nurse was instructed on the use of the ICU mortality prediction model (MPM) admission and discharge forms. Each MPM admission form was completed by an ICU nurse within four hours of the patient's admission to the ICU. Following patient discharge, the MPM discharge forms were completed and each was reviewed by the clinical nursing researcher. Confidentiality and anonymity were assured. Logistic regression and analysis were used to interpret the data.

Results. One hundred patients participated in the study. The mean patient age was 53 years. Fifty-eight percent were admitted to surgical service; 26 percent to medical service; 16 percent to neurological service. Average patient acuity according to the Medicus Patient Classification System was 3.91. Two of the patients were categorized as "do not resuscitate" by the physician.

The *actual* ICU mortality rate was 7 percent. The *predicted* ICU mortality rate, according to the ICU Mortality Prediction Model, was 16.5 percent. Among the other sixteen hospitals included in the study, the average predicted mortality rate was 17 percent. The predicted mortality range was 10 to 31 percent.

The average probability of dying among the living was 0.138 for NGMC. The average probability of dying among the dead was 0.519 for NGMC. Ninety-one of the 100 patients were correctly classified by the MPM. There were no patients who died who were predicted to live. For the ten highest calculated probabilities, 6.59 patients were expected to die and four actually died.

SOURCE: Reprinted with permission Northeast Georgia Medical Center, 743 Spring Street, Gainesville, GA 30501-3899.

4. How is nursing productivity measured in units of service or nursing care hours? How does it compare with the quality of care patients received?
5. What are the actual direct and indirect costs of providing nursing services?
6. What are the alternative approaches to measuring nursing intensity and patient need for nursing services?
7. How are intensity of nursing care, selected patient characteristics, and the cost of nursing services related?
8. How can nursing costs be effectively and efficiently estimated?
9. What education and skill mix of nurses provide the highest quality care and are the most cost-effective in health-care agencies of varying size, purpose, organization, and location?
10. What is the revenue-producing capability of nursing services?
11. What are the effects of cost containment on the planning, delivery, and evaluation of nursing services?
12. What are the effects of diagnostic-related groups on relative intensity measures of nursing care and on the quality of in-hospital nursing care?[81]

SUMMARY

Ability to manage planned change is a necessary competency for all nurse managers, since it represents viability of the nursing organization. Since planned change is a necessity, nurse managers create the climate for its reception by nursing personnel. Change, the key to innovation and the future, has its basis in change theory.

Lewin's change theory is widely used by managers and involves three stages: unfreezing, moving, and refreezing. In the unfreezing stage, employees are made aware of needed changes. A plan for change is made and tested in the moving stage. During the refreezing stage the change becomes a part of the system, establishing homeostasis and equilibrium.

Rogers, Havelock, and Lippett each modified Lewin's original change theory. Reddin's theory has many similarities and all have common elements of problem solving and decision making.

Resistance to change is evoked by stress from threatened security of affected employees. It can be overcome by planning that involves those to be affected, particularly if they can see a benefit. Established values and beliefs, imprinting, time perspectives, and hyper-energy all stiffen resistance to change.

The nurse manager as change agent is the manager of change and thus requires knowledge of the theory of change. Education and training are necessary for nursing personnel who will be affected. Intrinsic and extrinsic rewards are another management tool. Using groups to effect change will help absorb the risks of change, since risks are part of the process.

Creativity and innovation are important aspects of nursing management. They lead to better practice as new knowledge and skills are applied. The result is change that leads to maintenance of a competitive share of the health-care market, thus assuring the position of nursing.

Nursing managers can promote change through nursing research, thus committing nursing to a clinical practice based on scholarly inquiry. Promotion of nursing research effects change through application of research findings. Nursing research can be income-producing when it produces more effective and efficient nursing prescriptions.

Change involves nurse managers in many functions of nursing. It requires planning. The organization is adapted to accommodate the changes. The nurse manager uses communication, leadership, and motivation theory to overcome resistance and gain support in making the change work. The implemented change is continually evaluated to keep it working and effective.

NOTES

1. D. McGregor, *Leadership and Motivation* (Cambridge, MA: MIT Press, 1966), 15–16.
2. W. J. Reddin, "How to Change Things," *Executive*, June 1969, 22–26.
3. B. W. Spradley, "Managing Change Creatively," *The Journal of Nursing Administration*, May 1980, 32–37.
4. E. G. Williams, "Changing Systems and Behavior," *Business Horizons*, Aug. 1969, 53–58.
5. R. D. Brynildsen and T. A. Wickes, "Agents of Changes," *Automation*, Oct. 1970.
6. Ibid.

7. W. J. Reddin, op. cit.
8. Ibid.
9. B. W. Spradley, op. cit.; L. B. Welch, "Planned Change in Nursing: The Theory," *Nursing Clinics of North America,* June 1979, 307–321.
10. Ibid.
11. Ibid.
12. L. B. Welch, op. cit.
13. Ibid.
14. Ibid.
15. Ibid.
16. B. W. Spradley, op. cit.
17. J. V. Roach, "U.S. Business: Time to Seize the Day," *Newsweek,* April 4 1988, 10; M. Beyers, "Getting on Top of Organizational Change: Part 1, Process and Development," *Journal of Nursing Administration,* Oct. 1984, 32–39.
18. R. E. Hunt and M. K. Rigby, "Easing The Pain of Change," *Management Review,* Sept. 1984, 41–45.
19. M. Beyers, op. cit.
20. J. Feldman and D. Daly-Gawenda, "Retrenchment: How Nurse Executives Cope," *Journal of Nursing Administration,* June 1985, 31–37.
21. "Managing to Improve Value," *Managing Change* (Travenol Management Services), Spring 1985.
22. E. G. Williams, op. cit.
23. M. J. Ward and S. G. Moran, "Resistance to Change: Recognize, Respond, Overcome," *Nursing Management,* Jan. 1984, 30–33.
24. R. E. Hunt and M. K. Rigby, op. cit.
25. Ibid.
26. D. J. Gillen, "Harvesting the Energy from Change Anxiety," *Supervisory Management,* Mar. 1986, 40–43.
27. D. Niland, "Managing Change: Same Staff, Same Unit—New Role," *Nursing Management,* Dec. 1985, 31–32.
28. M. J. Ward and S. G. Moran, op. cit.
29. M. Beyers, op. cit.
30. Ibid.
31. Ibid.; D. J. Gillan, op. cit.
32. D. J. Gillen, op. cit.
33. R. E. Hunt and M. K. Rigby, op. cit.
34. M. J. Ward and S. G. Moran, op. cit.
35. R. E. Endres, "Successful Management of Change," *Notes & Quotes,* Nov. 1972, 3.
36. W. J. Ward and S. G. Moran, op. cit.
37. R. E. Hunt and M. K. Rigby, op. cit.
38. M. Beyers, op. cit.
39. W. J. Ward and S. G. Moran, op. cit.
40. D. P. Newcomb and R. C. Swansburg, *The Team Plan: A Manual for Nursing Service Administrators,* 2d. ed. (New York: G. P. Putnam's Sons, 1971), 136–172.
41. R. L. Lattimer and M. L. Winitsky, "Unleashing Creativity," *Management World,* Apr. 1984, 22–24.
42. J. Gordon and R. Zemke, "Making Them More Creative," *Training,* May 1986, 30ff.
43. Ibid.
44. T. Comella, "Understanding Creativity," *Notes & Quotes;* reprint from Apr. 1966 *Automation* (Hartford: Connecticut General Life Insurance Company), Sept. 1966, 1.
45. Ibid.
46. Sr. M. H. Reinkemeyer, "A Nursing Paradox," *Nursing Research,* Jan.-Feb. 1968, 8.

47. A. J. Rutigliano, "An Interview with Peter Drucker: Managing the New," *Management Review,* Jan. 1986, 38–41; A. J. Rutigliano, "Peter Drucker—On Managing The New," *Newsweek,* October 1988, S6–S7.
48. R. R. Godfrey, "Tapping Employees' Creativity," *Supervisory Management,* Feb. 1986, 16–20.
49. R. L. Lattimer and M. L. Winitsky, op. cit.
50. A. G. Van Gundy, "How to Establish a Creative Climate in the Work Group," *Management Review,* Aug. 1984, 24–25, 28, 37–38.
51. J. Gordon and R. Zemke, op. cit.
52. R. L. Lattimer and M. L. Winitsky, op. cit.
53. R. R. Godfrey, op. cit.
54. P. F. Drucker, "Creating Strategies of Innovation," *Planning Review,* Nov. 1985, 8–11, 45.
55. J. Gordon and R. Zemke. op. cit.
56. R. M. Kanter, *The Change Masters* (New York: Simon & Schuster, 1983). Material from workshop presented by Dr. Kanter.
57. A. G. Van Gundy, op. cit.
58. S. Glucksberg, "Some Ways to Turn on New Ideas," *Think* (IBM), Mar.-Apr. 1968, 24–28.
59. R. R. Godfrey, op. cit.
60. D. P. Newcomb and R. C. Swansburg, op. cit.
61. H. Levinson, "What An Executive Should Know About Scientists," *Notes & Quotes* (Hartford: Connecticut General Life Insurance Company), Nov. 1965, 1.
62. Ibid.
63. R. R. Godfrey, op. cit.
64. A. G. Van Gundy, op. cit.
65. J. Gordon and R. Zemke, op. cit.
66. T. R. Horton, "Poised for Tomorrow," *Newsweek,* October 5 1987, S-4.
67. M. L. McClure, "Promoting Practice-Based Research: A Critical Need," *Journal of Nursing Administration,* Nov.-Dec. 1981, 66–70; American Hospital Association, *Strategies: Integration of Nursing Research into the Practice Setting* (Chicago: AHA Nurse Executive Management Strategies, 1985).
68. R. C. Swansburg, *Management of Patient Care Services* (Saint Louis: Mosby, 1968), 334.
69. M. L. McClure, op. cit.
70. K. P. Krone and M. E. Loomis, "Developing Practice-Relevant Research: A Model That Worked," *Journal of Nursing Administration,* Apr. 1982, 38–41.
71. C. A. Lindeman and D. Schantz, "The Research Question," *Journal of Nursing Administration,* Jan. 1982, 6–10; D. Schantz and C. A. Lindeman, "Reading a Research Article," *Journal of Nursing Administration,* Mar. 1982, 30–33.
72. C. A. Lindeman and D. Schantz, op. cit.
73. Ibid.
74. Ibid.
75. D. Schantz and C. A. Lindeman, "The Research Design," *Journal of Nursing Administration,* Feb. 1982, 35–38.
76. E. A. Hefferin, J. A. Horsley, and M. R. Ventura, "Promoting Research-Based Nursing: The Nurse Administrator's Role," *Journal of Nursing Administration,* May 1982, 34–41.
77. American Hospital Association, op. cit.
78. E. A. Hefferin, J. A. Horsley, and M. R. Ventura, op. cit.
79. K. P. Krone and M. E. Loomis, op. cit.
80. American Hospital Association, op. cit.

81. B. M. Henry, L. E. Moody, J. O'Donnell, J. Pendergust, and S. Hutchinson, *National Nursing Administration Research Priorities Study,* Division of Nursing, Bureau of Health Professionals, Health Resources and Services Administration, US PHS (R01 NU 01085), Oct. 30, 1985, 19.

REFERENCE

Beyers, M., "Getting on Top of Organizational Change: Part 2. Trends in Nursing Service," *Journal of Nursing Administration,* Nov. 1984, 31–37.

Organizing Nursing Services

11

ORGANIZATIONAL THEORY

Once plans are made, the mission, purpose, or business for which the organization exists has been established, the philosophy has been developed and adopted, and the objectives have been formulated, resources are organized to sustain the philosophy and to accomplish the mission and objectives. Organizations develop as goals become too complex for the individual and have to be divided into units that individuals can manage.[1]

Fayol referred to the organizing element of management as the form of the body corporate and stated that the organization takes on form when the number of workers rises to the level requiring a supervisor. It is necessary to group people, distribute duties, and adapt the organic whole to requirements by putting essential employees where they will be most useful. An intermediate executive is the generator of power and ideas.[2] The body corporate of the nursing organization includes executive management and its staff, departmental managers (middle managers), technical managers (first line managers), and practicing professional and technical nursing personnel. Professional nursing personnel manage the performance of technical nursing personnel. In a theory of nursing management, nurse managers have as their object the development of a nursing organization that facilitates the work of clinical nurses.

Definitions of Organizing

Urwick referred to organizing as the process of designing the machine. It should allow for personal adjustments, but these will be minimal if a design is followed. It should show the part each person will play in the general social pattern, as well as the responsibilities, relationships, and standards of performance. Jobs should be put together along the lines of functional specializations to facilitate the training of replacements. The organizational struc-

263

ture must be based on sound principles, including that of continuity, to provide for the future.[3]

Organizing is the grouping of activities for the purpose of achieving objectives, the assignment of such groupings to a manager with authority for supervising each group, and the defined means of coordinating appropriate activities with other units, horizontally and vertically, which are responsible for accomplishing organizational objectives. Organizing involves the process of deciding the necessary levels of organization needed to accomplish the objectives of a nursing division, department or service, or unit. For the unit it would involve the type of work to be accomplished in terms of direct patient care, the kinds of nursing personnel needed to accomplish this work, and the span of management or supervision needed.

Principles of Organizing

The Principles of Chain of Command. The chain-of-command principle states that to be satisfying to members, economically effective, and successful in achieving its goals, organizations are established with hierarchical relationships within which authority flows from top to bottom. This principle supports a mechanistic structure with a centralized authority that aligns authority and responsibility. Communication flows through the chain of command and tends to be one-way—downward. In a modern nursing organization the chain of command is flat, with line managers and a technical and clerical staff that support the clinical nursing staff.

The Principle of Unity of Command. The unity-of-command principle states that an employee has one supervisor and there is one leader and one plan for a group of activities with the same objective. This principle is still followed in most nursing organizations but is increasingly modified by emerging organizational theory. Primary nursing and case management support the principle of unity of command, as does joint practice.

The Principle of Span of Control. The span-of-control principle states that a person should be a supervisor of a group that he or she can effectively supervise in terms of numbers, functions, and geography. This original principle has become an elastic one—the more highly trained the employee, the less supervision is needed. Employees in training need

more supervision to prevent blunders. When different levels of nursing employees are used, the nurse manager must coordinate more.

The Principle of Specialization. The principle of specialization is that each person should perform a single leading function. Thus there is a division of labor: a differentiation among kinds of duties. Specialization is thought by many to be the best way to use individuals and groups. The chain of command joins groups by specialty, leading to functional departmentalization.

The hierarchy or scalar chain is a natural result of these principles of organizing. It is the order of rank, from top to bottom in an organization. These principles of organizing are interdependent and dynamic when used by nurse managers to create a stimulating environment in which to practice clinical nursing.

Bureaucracy

Bureaucracy evolved from the early principles of administration, including those of organizing. It is a term coined by Max Weber. Bureaucracy is highly structured and usually includes no participation by the governed. The principles of chain of command, unity of command, span of control, and specialization support bureaucratic structures. These structures do not work in their pure form and have been greatly adapted in today's organizations.

Among the historical strong points of bureaucratic organizations is their ability to produce employees who are competent and responsible. They perform by uniform rules and conventions, are accountable to one manager who is an authority, maintain social distance with supervisors and clients, thereby reducing favoritism and promoting impersonality, and receive rewards based on technical qualifications, seniority, and achievement.

The characteristics of bureaucracy include formality, low autonomy, a climate of rules and conventionality, division of labor, specialization, standardized procedures, written specifications, memos and minutes, centralization, controls, and emphasis on a high level of efficiency and production. These characteristics frequently lead to complaints about red tape and to procedural delays and general frustration.[4]

Using the bureaucratic model as a reference, Hall studied ten organizations using these six dimensions: division of labor, hierarchy of authority, employee rules, work procedures, impersonality, and technical competence. He found these dimensions each varying in degree. An organization could be highly bureaucratized in one dimension while not in others. Highly bureaucratic structures would have a high degree of bureaucracy in each of the six dimensions. Bureaucracy is a matter of degree among organizations. Similar organizations may have similar degrees of bureaucracy.[5]

Hall also found that age and size of organization do not relate to its degree of bureaucratization. The "technical qualifications" dimension did not appear to correlate with the other five dimensions. It is the rational aspect of bureaucracy. A high degree of impersonality develops in organizations that deal with large numbers of customers or clients.[6]

This study has significance for nursing administration. The scale can be used for testing in health-care organizations and in nursing divisions. It can be used to measure and compare the six dimensions of bureaucracy.

Professionalism and Bureaucracy. Hall also studied the relationship between professionalization and bureaucratization. He surveyed 542 persons in eleven occupations and twenty-seven organizations, including nurses employed in a university student health service and in a general hospital. For a study using both structural aspects and attitudinal attributes of a profession, his findings were as follows:

1. Attitudes are strongly associated with behavior: professional organizations, certification.
2. Nurses are high in professionalism in terms of belief in service to the public, belief in self-regulation, and sense of calling to the field, but low in feelings of autonomy and using the professional organization as a reference point.
3. Nursing is high in bureaucratization, except for technical competence.
4. There is less hierarchy of authority in autonomous organizations. (Autonomous organizations are those that promote autonomy of professional practitioners.)
5. An organization's size does not affect hierarchy.
6. There is less division of labor in autonomous organizations.
7. There are fewer procedures in autonomous organizations.

8. There is an emphasis on technical competence in autonomous and heteronomous organizations. (These organizations promote differences in practice patterns among autonomous-practitioners of nursing.)
9. Professionalism increases with decreased division of labor, decreased procedures, decreased impersonality, and increased autonomy. Hierarchy is accepted if it serves coordination and communication functions.
10. Bureaucracy inhibits professionalism.[7]

The conclusion would be that the less bureaucratic the organization, the more nurses perceive themselves as professionals.

Role Theory. Role theory indicates that when employees face inconsistent expectations and lack of information they will experience role conflict, leading to stress, dissatisfaction, and ineffective performance. Role theory supports the chain-of-command and unity-of-command principles. Multiple lines of authority are disruptive, divide authority between profession and organization, and create stress. They force employees to make choices between formal authority and professional colleagues. The result is role conflict and dissatisfaction for employees and reduced efficiency and effectiveness for the organization. Role conflict reduces trust, personal liking, and esteem for the person in authority; reduces communication; and decreases employee effectiveness. Rizzo, House, and Lirtzman indicate that role conflict and ambiguity can be reduced by management that provides for:

1. Certainty about duties, authority, allocation of time, and relationship with others.
2. Guides, directives, policies, and the ability to predict sanctions as outcomes of behavior.
3. Increased need fulfillment.
4. Structure and standards.
5. Facilitation of teamwork.
6. Toleration of freedom.
7. Upward influence.
8. Consistency.
9. Prompt decisions.
10. Good, prompt communication and information.
11. Using the chain of command.
12. Personal development.
13. Formalization.

14. Planning.
15. Receptiveness to ideas by top management.
16. Coordinating work plans.
17. Adapting to change.
18. Adequacy of authority.

The implications for nurse managers are obvious. Role conflict and role ambiguity are separate dimensions, role conflict being more dysfunctional. Some employees find stress rewarding.[8]

Organizational Development

Organizational development (OD) deals with changing the work environment to make it more conducive to worker satisfaction and productivity. An underlying premise is that "people planning" is as important as technical and financial planning. OD allows managers to attend to the psychological as well as the physical aspects of organizations. Change is the terrain in which OD applies.

OD can sustain the favorable or desirable aspects of bureaucracy. Change can be employed to modify the undesirable aspects of bureaucracy. There is room for directive as well as nondirective leadership within organizations. Nurse managers have to be strong and tough in supporting the values of clinical nurses. They have to be proactive in planning, designing, and implementing new organizational structures and work environments. The object is to develop people, not to exploit them. OD emphasizes personal growth and interpersonal competence.[9]

Autonomy and Accountability.   Among the psychological and personality attributes of OD are autonomy and accountability, crucial elements of nursing professionalism. A professional nurse is obliged to answer for decisions and actions. According to Johnson and Luciano this would be achieved by using a management by results (MBR) approach. They developed a performance management program for unit supervisors that defined performance standards, incorporating acceptable behavior and results. It included tracking for progress, performance feedback, making adjustments, and personnel accountability.[10]

Characteristics of professional autonomy include self-definition, self-regulation, and self-governance. Professional nurses respond to demographic changes in society to define and reshape the content of nursing practice. They address society's needs, including the need for increased care for the elderly and the control of resources. Autonomy will be strengthened by unbundling the hospital bill and by direct reimbursement for nursing services by third-party payers.

Self-governance for nursing includes a nursing administrator hired or elected with input from nurses, self-employment for nurses, approval of nursing staff privileges by peer review with privileges revoked by the nursing staff organization, and case management.[11]

Argyris describes people as complex organizations who work for an organization for their own needs or gains. These needs exist at varying degrees or depths that must be understood by organizations. People seek out jobs to meet their needs. They develop and live on a continuum from infant to adult. This continuum is reflected throughout life in work and leisure.[12] Figure 11–1 shows the developmental continuum.

Ridderheim describes a hospital administrator's action to change a management style that was paternalistic, used downward communication, encouraged dependency, and inhibited management development. In an opinion survey, employees scored high on patient care and personal pride in their work but low in decision-making ability. Among the changes made by the administrator after organizational assessment and consultation were:

1. Decisions were turned back to operating managers, giving them freedom to act within broad policy guidelines.
2. Operating management was restructured into an executive operating committee (EOC) that included the administrator and assistants for medical staff affairs, operations, facilities, patient care, personnel, and finance. Each assistant had policy-making status.
3. A core group was established at lower levels of management to focus on the technical interests and objectives of the hospital.
4. Task forces were established for special projects.
5. A team was set up to monitor terminations, retirements, recruitments, advancements, and demotions.
6. Performance standards were developed for each manager.
7. Team-building seminars were held.

FIGURE 11-1. Developmental Continuum

Infant	Adult
Dependent	Independent
Submissive	Autonomous
Few abilities	Many abilities
Shallow abilities	Deep abilities
Short time perspective	Long time perspective
Frustrated by:	Motivated or inspired by:
Lack of self-control	Self-control
Being controlled	Self-direction
Directive (authoritarian) leadership	Job involvement
	Participative (democratic) leadership. (Electing own leaders.)
Lack of self-actualization	Self-actualization
Lack of opportunity to learn	Opportunity to learn
Lack of opportunity to advance	Opportunity to advance
Repetitive work	Variety in work
Dull work	Interesting work
Lack of equipment	Resources to do job
Lack of information	Feedback
Low pay	High pay
Powerlessness	Autonomy and responsibility
Fractionalized jobs	Job enlargement
Lack of education restricting job opportunity to lower levels	Education that increases job opportunity at higher levels
Structured jobs that inhibit individual growth	Opportunity for independent thought, action, growth, and feelings of accomplishment
Overstaffing	Understaffing (perform multiple roles)
Specialization of tasks	Generalization and wholeness of jobs
	Rewards for learning
	Self-governance
Routine work	Complex work
Responds by:	Responds by:
Fighting for redesign or control (union)	Allocating own tasks
Leaving (turnover)	Staying
Psychological apathy or indifference	Seeking out intrinsic rewards
Becoming oriented to payoffs of being market-oriented or instrumentally oriented	Increasing productivity
	Focusing on job content
Absenteeism	Attendance
Daydreaming	Being industrious and attentive
Aggression toward supervisors	Being innovative
	Cooperating
Aggression toward coworkers	Participation
Restricting output	
Making mistakes or errors	
Postponing difficult tasks or decisions	Accepting responsibility
Focusing on pay, fringe benefits, hours of work	Focusing on self-direction, self-expression, individual accomplishment, opportunity to use abilities or help people

(continued)

FIGURE 11–1. Developmental Continuum (*continued*)

Infant	Adult
Lack of interest in work	
Alienation	
Decreased job rating associated with:	Increased job rating associated with:
Reduced community participation	Increased community participation
Decreased leisure involvement	Increased leisure involvement
Decreased political activity	Increased political activity
Decreased participation in voluntary activities, culture,	Increased participation in voluntary activities
cerebral skills, group activities	
Being solitary	
Being withdrawn	

SOURCE: Adapted from C. Argyris, "Personality and Organizational Theory Revisited," *Administrative Science Quarterly*, V.18, 1973, 141–167.

8. After nine months, progress was critiqued at a retreat—first by the EOC, then by subordinate managers.
9. Achievement in relation to goals, individual growth, and teamwork was stressed over seniority.
10. Subsequent surveys showed improvements in job satisfaction, supervisory concern for employees, supervisory emphasis on goal achievement, work group emphasis on teamwork, decision-making practices, and motivational conditions.[13]

Culture. Organizational culture is the sum total of an organization's beliefs, norms, values, philosophies, traditions, and sacred cows. It is a social system that is a subsystem of the total organization. Organizational cultures have artifacts, perspectives, values, assumptions, symbols, language, and behaviors that have been effective.

Organizational cultures include communication networks, both formal and informal. They include a status/role structure that relates to characteristics of employees and customers or clients. Such structures also relate to management style—whether authoritarian or participatory. Management style impacts individual behavior greatly. In a health-care setting these structures promote either individuality or teamwork. They relate to classes of people and could be identified through demographic surveys of both employees and patients.

The basic mission of the organization is part of its culture: employment, service, learning, and research. There is a technical or *operational system* for getting the work done. Also, there is an *administrative system* of wages and salaries, of hiring, firing, and promoting, of report making and quality control, of fringe benefits, and of budgeting.

The artifacts of an organizational culture may be physical, behavioral (rituals), or verbal (language, stories, myths). Verbal artifacts result from shared values and beliefs. They include traditions, heroes, and the party line and result in ceremonies that embody rituals. They include ceremonies to reward years of service, the annual picnic, the Christmas party, and the wearing of badges and insignia.[14]

Metaphors are used to characterize personalities and work styles:

1. The military—language includes such terms as battle zone, tight ship, captain, troops, battles, campaigns, enemies, or stars. Award ceremonies also contain military metaphors.
2. Sports—terms such as teams, stars, or quarterback are used. Award ceremonies may also reflect the sports metaphor.
3. Anthropology—terms include family, novice, big daddy, big momma, elder, or prodigal son.
4. Television—terms include sitcom, soap opera, country club, playground, nursery, and jungles.

5. Mechanistic—terms such as factory, assembly line, or well-oiled machine are used.
6. The "zoo"—terms such as sly fox, chicken, or top dog appear.[15]

Perspectives are shared ideas and actions. They relate to decision-making methods. For example, social, technical, and managerial systems or subsystems will either support innovation or demand conformity.[16]

Dress, personal appearance, social decorum, and the physical environment are all part of the organizational culture. They will require strict compliance through written or implied rules.

Values are the general principles, ideals, standards, and sins of the organization. Basic assumptions are the core of the culture. They include the beliefs groups have about themselves, others, and the world.

Culture and the Manager. When output or productivity decreases in amount or kind, managers look at the social, technical, and managerial systems that are part of the organizational culture. They know that people behave in accordance with their understanding of the organization's norms and values. If they want to be successful they identify these norms and values and apply their efforts in conformity with them. They gather data on needs: market analysis, attitude surveys, management statements, directives, and climate surveys. Then they address the real needs. These will include a marketing campaign to build strong customer relations. They continually do self-criticism, looking at usefulness of projects, plans, programs, and products.[17]

A successful manager identifies and accepts the prevailing culture before making changes. It is more difficult to change a culture at the level of basic beliefs, values, and perspectives. It is easier to change technical and administrative systems.

Changing the culture uncovers the sacred cows and taboos. del Bueno and Vincent include diploma graduates, collective bargaining, mission, the competition, layoffs, converting positions, education, and clinical ladders among the sacred cows or taboos. Organizational culture focuses on work life. There is potential for conflict between a collection of differing personal norms of individuals and opposing cultural norms of the organization.[18]

Managers and personnel who survive in a culture learn how to support the values and norms of that culture. Their conformity impedes change and innovation. Dyer and Dyer suggest that the social, technical, and managerial systems are changed through organizational development. Organizational culture is far more difficult to change because it operates at the level of basic beliefs, values, and perspectives. Change in the organizational culture often involves revolution and conflict, so it is a tough issue. To change the organizational culture may require installing a new leader.[19] See Figures 11–2, 11–3, and 11–4.

Research indicates that a strong culture that encourages participation and involvement of employees in shared decision making affects an organization's performance positively. Such organizations outperform competitors two to one in return on investments and sales. The organizational culture can be influenced by the CEO.[20] See Figure 11–5.

Climate. The organizational climate is the emotional state shared by members of the system. It can be formal, relaxed, defensive, cautious, accepting, trusting, and so on. It is employees' subjective impression or perception of their organization. The employees of greatest concern to nurse managers are the practicing nurses. Practicing nurses create, or at the very least contribute to the creation of, the climate perceived by patients. The work climate set by nurse managers in turn determines the behavior of the practicing nurses in setting the work climate.

Practicing nurses want a climate that will give them job satisfaction. They achieve job satisfaction when they are challenged and their achievements recognized and appreciated by managers and patients. They achieve satisfaction from a climate of collegiality with managers and other health-care providers, in which they have input into decision making.

Practicing nurses want a climate that provides good working conditions, high salaries, and opportunities for professional growth through counseling and career development experiences that will enable them to determine and direct their professional futures. They want a climate of administrative support that includes adequate staffing and shift options. It has been known for years that the personnel shortage, frustration, failure, and conflict in nursing required sweeping changes in intrinsic and extrinsic rewards, including career development programs that increase the ability of professional

FIGURE 11–2.   OD Cycle: System Change

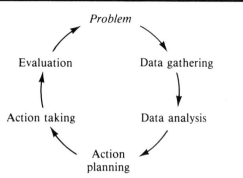

nurses to develop their self-esteem through self-actualization.

Many studies have been done to determine work climate, within business, industry, and healthcare organizations. One head nurse designed and implemented a project to motivate the nursing staff of a medical unit to better service and greater self-satisfaction. She designed an "employee of the month" motivational strategy that included measurable performance criteria. While the staff were initially uninterested, they eventually increased their interest and participation. Productivity also increased, as did emergence of talents. The strategy culminated in a recognition ceremony, a free lunch or dinner, and the employee's picture on the bulle-

---

FIGURE 11–3.   OD Cycle: Culture Change

1. A crisis calls into question the leader's assumptions. → 2. There is a breakdown of symbols, beliefs, and structure.

6. The new leadership establishes new symbols, beliefs, and structure to sustain the new culture.   3. New leadership emerges with a new set of assumptions.

5. If the crisis is solved and new leadership are given credit for the improvement, they become the new cultural elite. ← 4. Conflict occurs between the old and new cultures.

FIGURE 11–4.   Differences between System Change and Culture Change

System change	Culture change
1. Problem-oriented	1. Value-oriented
2. More easily controlled	2. Largely uncontrollable
3. Involves making incremental changes in systems	3. Involves transforming basic assumptions
4. Focuses on improving organization output/measurable outcomes	4. Focuses on the quality of life in an organization
5. Diagnosis involves discovering nonalignments between subsystems	5. Diagnosis involves examining dysfunctional effects of core assumptions
6. Leadership change is not essential	6. Leadership change is crucial

FIGURE 11–5.   The Effects of Management Style on Five Aspects of Corporate Life

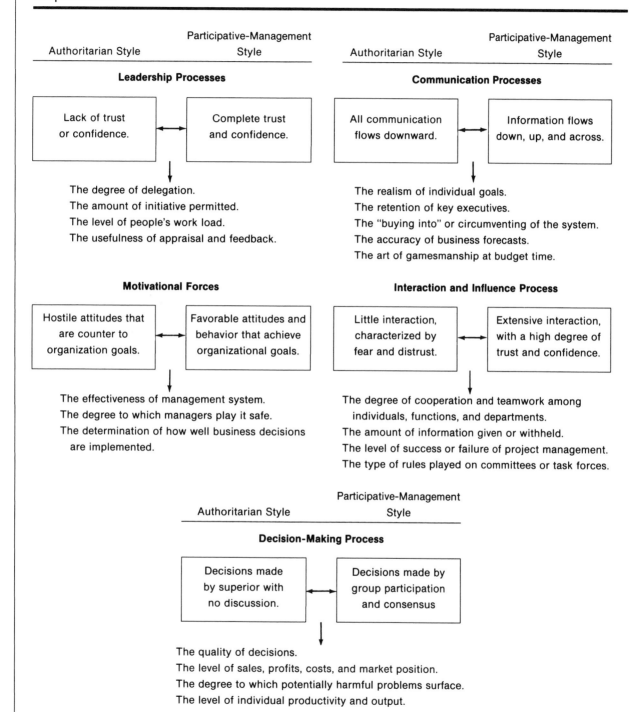

tin board. By the end of six months, twenty-five out of 144 employees had earned the title, their voluntary participation indicating that it met some of their needs.[21]

Guthrie, Mauer, Zawacki, and Conger reported use of the Health Professional Motivational Inventory (HPMI) to diagnose whether jobs motivated people. They measured forty-one female nurse managers and found them more satisfied than other managers previously reported. This, they speculated, was due to the increased variety of clinical and management skills required and the nurses' ability to see the results of their work. The nurse managers scored high on autonomy. The authors indicated that despite the widely held belief that nurse managers are constrained, their questionnaire indicated the opposite. The nurse managers were also satisfied with their pay.[22]

It is interesting to compare a similar study of practicing clinical nurses. Are they constrained by the nurse manager? One study of thirty-one nurses in a northwest Texas hospital indicated they were dissatisfied by physician-nurse conflict and lack of nursing management support, peer conflict, inadequate staffing, political conflicts between physicians and administration, lack of flexible scheduling, lack of patient care accomplishments, lack of overtime pay or payback, inflexible roles of leaders, lack of positive feedback from physicians, poor orientation, and lack of visitors following rules.

These same nurses reported obtaining satisfaction from patient and family care and education, the variety of work experiences, interaction with staff members, their paycheck, mental challenges, being needed, friendly staff and physicians, observed patient improvement, patients' compliments, knowledge of a job well done, exciting and unpredictable work, the ability to contribute, learn, and achieve, the availability of senior professionals to assist and teach, developing new staff, and having predictable work schedules.[23]

A study of five Midwest hospitals indicated that:

1. The behavior of professional nurses was positively affected by charge nurses who gave honest pep talks keying in on feelings, made fair and equitable assignments, handled orders efficiently, helped when the workload was great, listened to complaints and ideas and promoted cooperation, treated their staff as resource persons for clinical

expertise and valued their opinions, and were up to date in their knowledge and skills and taught others.

2. Behavior was negatively affected by charge nurses who were two-faced, phony, gossiped and took advantage, favored friends in making assignments, ignored questions and refused advice or help, did not help with patients when the need arose, did not communicate orders, did not follow suggestions they asked for, were disorganized, and did not know policies and procedures.

3. Staff nurses put high value on self-esteem and self-fulfillment, achievement, recognition, tasks assigned, advancement and responsibility.[24]

A survey of one hundred students enrolled in a hospital school of nursing indicated that practicing nursing met their self-esteem needs. Sources of job satisfaction included personal satisfaction (77.5 percent), collegial relationships (43.75 percent), security (12.5 percent), choice of work area (12.5 percent), and hours (11.25 percent).[25]

Desatnick indicates that management climate surveys measure clarity and understanding of an organization's goals, effectiveness of decision-making processes, integration, cooperation, vitality, leader effectiveness, openness and trust, job satisfaction, opportunities for growth and development, level of performance, orientation and accountability, effectiveness of teamwork and problem solving, and overall confidence in management. He suggests using surveys to make a diagnosis and to:

Establish new strategic directions.

Clarify an organization's mission, objectives, and goals.

Identify managers' and supervisors' training and development needs.

Reallocate resources.

Prepare a foundation for cultural change.

Revise hiring priorities using a patterned interview to "select in" those who share the same values.[26]

A study of customers' views of the organizational climate of a bank indicated these features important to them: convenience, short waiting time, personal friendly service, full-service banking, safety, and decoration. These features were evident in the caliber of employees who helped each other in serving customers, treated all customers equally, and appeared happy. These summary climate perceptions could be extended to nurses and thence to patients.[27]

Using the Hackman and Oldham *Job Diagnostic Survey (JDS)*, 160 registered nurses in a 350-bed Midwestern hospital were surveyed to determine the motivating potential score (MPS) of six nursing practice areas. In this study the ratings on the MPS were: (1) coronary care, (2) "other" nursing, (3) pediatrics, (4) obstetrics, (5) medical-surgical, and (6) psychiatry. These MPS results indicate medical-surgical and psychiatry have the greatest potential for problems with job satisfaction and would require the greatest attention to organizational climate by nurse managers.[28]

The nursing climate makes use of the individual practicing nurse's skills and motivational potential. Obsolete nursing organizational structures and communication can be changed. Nursing management practice can be brought in line with technological and environmental changes and the aspirational and value changes of practicing nurses. Rules, habits, and bureaucratic process can be modified to enable nurses to use their potential energy and creativity. New nursing management philosophies, styles, and structures can be developed to relate to nursing providers and consumers of nursing products and services. Communication, trust, and involvement can be established among nurse managers and practicing nurses. The organizational climate for educated nurses can provide for personal enrichment and involvement in decisions—a piece of the action. Practicing nurses who are given problems to solve will solve them. Otherwise nurses are oversupervised and underled!

Nurse managers should emphasize those management tasks or activities that stimulate motivation in nursing employees. They can then establish an organizational climate that supports such activities. This climate will include motivational characteristics or "satisfiers" to keep practicing nurses happy. Productivity will increase with fair compensation plus the intrinsic motivators of task identity or degree of completion of a whole piece of work with the visible outcome of patients who improve in health status, are maintained in comfort, or die

peacefully as a consequence of nursing action. In the ideal climate, nurses will be able to use a variety of skills and talents to achieve this impact, acting with autonomy while receiving adequate feedback.

Nurse managers should establish a management strategy to support new nurses and involve them in decision making. They should not merely plug them into vacant slots but match them to job choices and follow up to determine that all goes well.

Nurse managers should establish a climate in which discipline is applied fairly and uniformly. Nurses whose work is unsatisfactory should be discharged, following policies and procedures that protect their rights. The entire work climate should clearly promote employee rights. It should indicate that their ideas are being used. Nurse managers should promote competitive wages and fringe benefits by staying informed of the personnel policies of their competitors.

The nurse manager should work to establish an organizational climate that provides incentives for clinical nurses, that places them on committees, that is creative and equitable in all staffing matters, that emphasizes pride, promotes participation, rewards seniority and achievement, and reduces boredom and frustrations. This nurse manager will rate high in labor relations.[29]

Nurse managers should learn to use organizational climate surveys to find out the issues and concerns of practicing clinical nurses. They can then establish strategies that produce the climate that motivates their nurses to increased productivity.

Nurse managers who fail are no different from other managers. They fail when they go about business as usual, do not learn the business, apply their technical skills too quickly, ignore organizational problems, ignore strategic business needs, treat all responsibilities equally, take on too many conflicting priorities, promise without delivering, try to do the jobs of other line managers, do not respond adequately to higher concerns, represent selective interests, do not evaluate the anticipated impact of their actions on other people and projects, have poor timing, do not criticize themselves, do not market and merchandise their wares, are insensitive of internal client needs, and fail to understand the organization's culture.[30]

If nurse managers believe that trust is a key

element of recognition and that recognition and trust are desirable elements of the organizational climate, they will eliminate signs of distrust. Physical signs of distrust include time clocks and signs forbidding certain activities. The successful nurse manager hires practicing nurses who can be trusted and then trusts them. She or he supports subordinates without rescuing them or smothering them.

Nurse managers need management education and training. Such training should begin before nurses move into a management role and should continue to be provided by the organization and sought after by the individual. Management training is less expensive than turnover among practicing nurses. Educated nurse managers will foster an organizational climate of serenity, camaraderie, solidarity, and identification with the organization—a climate of excellence. Such a climate will stir up and excite nurses' energies by providing stimulating opportunities. Nurse managers and practicing nurses can work together to manage the work and the work environment so that energy is channeled into accomplishing personal and organizational goals.[31]

The job environment has become a major builder or destroyer of self-esteem and self-actualization. There are many sources of knowledge available for improving organizational climate. It remains for nurse managers to selectively learn and use them.

Job satisfaction is not a right of employees but a joint employer-employee responsibility. There are mutual benefits. Values and expectations must be rational. The employee must make a careful career choice and work to satisfy it. The employer must provide a supportive organizational climate. This will include matching employee and job through a realistic pre-employment interview, fostering job satisfaction, and being honest and truthful. There are no substitutes for either the nurse manager or the practicing nurse.

A study of organizational climate and its effect upon scientists indicated that they perceived structure as related to organizational climate. The research did not support this relationship as the structural data were poor. Flat organizations and large organizations tended to have scientists with more autonomy. Scientists perceived the climate as more competent, potent, responsible, practical, risk-oriented, and impulsive when performance reviews were tied to compensation programs. Scientists had greater autonomy over projects, assignments were general, and there were more informal research budgets. Risk-orientation decreased with increased performance reviews. These organizational climate factors improved performance and job satisfaction.[32]

Activities to Promote a Positive Organizational Climate

1. Develop the organization's mission, goals, and objectives with input from practicing nurses. Include their personal goals.
2. Establish trust and openness through communication that includes prompt and frequent feedback and stimulates motivation.
3. Provide opportunities for growth and development, including career development and continuing education programs.
4. Promote teamwork.
5. Ask practicing nurses to state their satisfactions and dissatisfactions during meetings and conferences and through surveys.
6. Market the nursing organization to the practicing nurses, other employees, and the public.
7. Follow through on all activities involving practicing nurses.
8. Analyze the compensation system for the entire nursing organization and structure it to reward competence, longevity, and productivity.
9. Promote self-esteem, autonomy, and self-fulfillment for practicing nurses, including feelings that their work experiences are of high quality.
10. Emphasize programs to recognize practicing nurses' contributions to the organization.
11. Assess unneeded threats and punishments and eliminate them.
12. Provide job security with an environment that enables free expression of ideas and exchange of opinions without threat of recrimination, which may occur as negative performance reports, negative counseling, confrontation, conflict, or job loss.
13. Be inclusive in all relationships with practicing nurses.
14. Help practicing nurses to overcome their shortcomings and develop their strengths.
15. Encourage and support loyalty, friendliness, and civic consciousness.

16. Develop strategic plans that include decentralization of decision making and participation by practicing nurses.
17. Be a role model of performance desired of practicing nurses.

Team Building. The commonly used terms related to the state of "feelings" of an organizational climate are "good morale" or "poor morale." Morale is a state of mind that refers to the zeal or enthusiasm with which someone works. A person who works courageously and confidently, with discipline and willingness to endure hardship would be manifesting high or good morale. Poor morale is evident in the person who is timid, cowardly, devious, fearful, diffident, disorderly, unruly, rebellious, turbulent, or indifferent as a result of job dissatisfaction and organizational milieu.

Morale is a motivation factor related to productivity and product or service quality outcomes. Firms want high morale among employees and use activities to promote it.

A team is a group of two or more workers striving for a common purpose or mission. They depend upon each other. The leader will emerge (if not appointed) as the person sustaining the confidence of the group. Confidence will be sustained by the leader's expertise in their purpose or mission and the enthusiasm expressed by the leader's verbal and nonverbal behavior. High enthusiasm by the leader will spark high enthusiasm within the group, thereby boosting group morale and stimulating *esprit de corps*, their spirit and sense of pride and honor.

One continually hears such remarks as "This organization does not care about the employees" or "This organization really cares about its employees." It goes without saying that nurse managers want to hear the positive statement. People who have low morale are not satisfied with their work. Dissatisfied workers will not contribute positively to *esprit de corps*.

Today's nurse managers will be effective if they are informed about nursing personnel's values. These include the following:

1. Work conflicts with family responsibilities and leisure activities, so some people want fewer or more flexible hours. The nurse manager determines how many hours each worker wants of work—per day, per week, per month, and per year. The result is matched with the givens.
   1.1 What are the legal givens?
   1.2 What are the organizational givens? Are they flexible? Can a person contract to work shorter than 8-hour shifts? Ten- and 12-hour shifts and even 16-hour shifts are commonplace. Under what conditions can a person work 4-hour shifts, 6-hour shifts, or some variation such as three 10-hour shifts and two 5-hour shifts? Can the beginning and ending times of shifts be set at other than 7:00 A.M., 3:00 P.M., 7:00 P.M., and 11:00 P.M.? Why not noon and midnight or other times?
   1.3 When child care services are provided, are they only available during the shift or can employees use them when they are off duty? Can use fees be waived, reduced, or purchased with vouchers given as awards for service?
2. The fast pace of the information age creates impatience. Everyone wants the rewards of being at the top. They want to live the lifestyle of the rich and famous depicted in television soap operas. This drive overrides any sense of loyalty.

   People know they cannot all reach the top so they want to be involved in decisions about their work. What can be done to involve them at the unit level, department level, division level, and organizational level?
3. People want inside knowledge about their organization. Some view this as a right. This desire can be accommodated by a solid communication plan that can be made to work by building quality assurance into the plan. This need should be addressed regularly, without fail, and actions under the plan should be made to meet their stated purposes of providing employees with information.

These values are consistent with those of people in other occupations in today's society.[33]

Nurse managers should create a humanistic environment for nursing employees, one that fosters trust and cooperation. Such an environment treats employees, rather than technology and buildings, as the most important asset. It is one in which minor rules are sometimes bent, complaints and ideas are heard, and self-worth and self-esteem are highlighted.

Nurses who have high self-esteem are energetic, confident, take pride in their work, have genuine respect and concern for patients, visitors, colleagues, and others. Their self-worth is evident in their behavior including their language. They are committed to excellence in patient care. These nurses have high morale. They work with *esprit de corps.*

The objective of team building is to establish an environment of cohesiveness among shift personnel and among different shifts in a unit. This is extended to other units, the department, and the division. The first step in team building is to find out why nursing employees are unhappy or dissatisfied. This can be accomplished through a questionnaire, although an open meeting is probably best. The meeting will be more productive if it is held away from the unit, to eliminate interruptions and the shadow of the organization.

The head nurse or another manager can assume the leadership or allow the group to select a leader. In any event the nurse manager will have to explain what the effort is all about and what the group is supposed to accomplish. Begin with identification of satisfactions if possible, to set a positive note.

Next, the leader must focus on identifying problems and prioritizing them for action. If the nurse manager can assume the role of facilitator rather than leader, the group will probably proceed at a faster pace.

Once problems or dissatisfactions are identified, a calendar should be established for addressing them. It is important to make a schedule of meetings and attendees for all phases of team-building activities. Meetings should be held at times most of the staff can be there. They should be short and focused on the problems, in priority sequence. It is best to make a brief management plan that includes the problem, objectives, actions the team can accomplish on its own authority, actions needing management support, persons assigned specific responsibilities, target dates, and a list of accomplishments.

As the plan is put into effect it should be communicated to the entire staff of the unit, department, or division. Evaluation should occur on a continuous basis to keep the momentum going. Each person can be encouraged to fulfill commitments, and everyone's accomplishments recognized. While each shift can work on their own plans, an occasional open forum of personnel on all three shifts is essential for intershift problems.

Figure 11–6 provides a worksheet for making management plans. Each problem and objective will use a similar format. Make provisions for wrap-ups of activities and for ensuring that problems remain solved. A similar approach was termed a communication model by Cohen and Ross. They used role negotiation and objectives for the team building process related to individual interface, cooperation and communication, intershift commitments, problem-solving mechanisms, and reinforcement by a head nurse as a 24-hour manager. The results included improved *esprit de corps,* improved unit cohesiveness among shifts, and the subjective belief that productivity increased.[34]

Jacobsen-Webb reported the use of the SELF Profile (Personal Dynamics, Inc., Minneapolis, MN) in a team-building exercise. Team members were given the SELF Profile to diagnose their behavioral patterns as *s*elf-reliant, *e*nthusiastic, *l*oyal, or *f*actual. Teams were formed based on the four behavioral types. The leadership position changed with the problem-solving task and the type of expert needed. A democratic and participatory climate was maintained by the team leader, who tapped the skills of team members and built commitment through effective group process. Progress was tracked through use of Program Evaluation Review Technique charts. When conflicts surfaced they were discussed and resolved through the team with input from each behavioral style. This process increased self-esteem and subsequent successful collaboration. It also increased skills of assertion, aggression, deference, interpersonal comfort, empathy, decision making, and effective communication.[35]

Recognition of the individual worth of the individual nurse is an important morale builder. It gives the individual self-esteem. Managers can stimulate self-esteem with praise that promotes a sense of competence, success, and worth. Nurse managers have to feel worthy before they can nurture that feeling in subordinates. Each nurtures the other. Managers who have self-esteem are not afraid to explore their personal feelings with colleagues or subordinates.

Professional nurses can think very highly of themselves while believing that others do not think highly of them. This tends to cause them to dominate others so they become feared and rejected. Ultimately these nurses band together and punish others as well as themselves.

Those professional nurses who think highly of

FIGURE 11–6. Management Plan Worksheet

Problem Objectives:

Activities	Target Dates	Person(s) Responsible	Accomplishments

themselves and believe that others do too, take risks in their personal relationships. They give and seek praise, love, support, and participation. All grow stronger and feel more worthy.

Many professionals depend on their jobs as a large source of self-esteem. For this reason nurse managers should aspire to building a milieu to develop and enhance the self-esteem of all nurses. Such a milieu promotes outstanding performance.

Praise is even more important when the environment is beset with shortages and stresses. Managers gain self-esteem from the success of their employees. They must supplement it with outside activities such as sports, hobbies, recreation, volunteer work, and work in service and professional organizations.[36]

Recognition can be made with a special plaque, commendation in a local paper or other medium, group social activities, gifts, and group service activities. Consider the benefits of scheduled versus surprise recognition activities. Nave and Thomas suggest fifty specific techniques to boost employee morale;[37] see Figure 11–7.

Many simple things can be done to improve the working environment. Involving the best workers in the decision-making process rewards the best performers and alerts others. One group had a monthly "warm fluffy day" when they complimented each employee and gave them a cotton ball on a pin. It produced spirit![38]

Though people will participate in team building they still want to retain their individuality. Nurse managers provide leadership that is flexible, fair, mindful of tasks and people, inspires, and models the role of professional nurse.[39]

DEVELOPING AN ORGANIZATIONAL STRUCTURE

An organizational structure for a division of nursing must meet the needs of that division as written in the statements of mission, philosophy, and objectives. Most existing institutions already have an organizational structure. Before the structure is changed, the nurse manager(s) should engage in a systematic analysis as well as some sound thinking about altering its design and structure, starting with objectives and strategy.

Objectives have already been discussed. Strategy covers the key activities of nursing that determine the purpose of the organizational structure.

FIGURE 11–7.   Fifty Specific Techniques to Boost Employee Morale

Listed below are 50 of the techniques identified. In reviewing them, remember that there is no best answer for anyone. That is best which best suits your organization.

1. Supervisors greet employees with a handshake as the employees begin their shifts.
2. Supervisors write personal notes such as "Thank You" or "Happy Birthday" on payroll checks.
3. Members of employee groups meet regularly with management representatives to promote understanding, and carry out activities of mutual interest.
4. Employees and management work side by side once a year on a community help project.
5. Employers are personally congratulated by supervisors when they exceed their goals.
6. Supervisors personally introduce new hires to each employee.
7. An employee's years of service are noted each year on the anniversary date of employment in a plaque or poster in the lobby.
8. When department supervisors enter the employee lounge, they treat all employees who happen to be there to a cup of coffee.
9. Supervisors personally hand employees in their department a silver dollar at Christmas as a "little something extra."
10. Relations with retired employees are maintained by means of an annual breakfast and personal delivery by the supervisors of a box of Christmas candy each year.
11. A cash reward is given each month to the employee with the "best idea" for the firm.
12. Part-time employees are invited to all social events.
13. The chief executive officer periodically has "brown bag" luncheon discussions with employees at which their concerns are addressed.
14. Employees are allowed to accept telephone calls at any time.
15. Letters of commendation are sent to employees for performance above and beyond normal expectations. Copies of the letter are included in the employees' personnel files.
16. The plant manager cooks at the supervisor's picnic. At another firm, supervisors serve the food at a company picnic.
17. Birthday cards are signed by the president of the firm or immediate supervisor and are sent to the employees' homes.
18. Free popcorn is always available for employees and customers.

19. Employee birthdays are celebrated with cake and by singing "Happy Birthday."
20. The safety department issues a monthly "safety for the family" newsletter that is mailed directly to the employees' home.
21. Free meals are provided in the company cafeteria for employees working on special days such as Christmas, Thanksgiving, and the like.
22. At irregular intervals managers provide food for employees to munch in the break area.
23. Softdrinks, coffee, and/or snacks are provided for staff at departmental meetings.
24. Flexible working hours are permitted during slow work times.
25. Morale-building meetings are held at which management informs employees of the firm's successes.
26. Brief meetings are scheduled for all new employees with staff from the business office, security, facilities management, and the like to familiarize new hires with policies and procedures.
27. A worker is recognized by being named "Employee of the Week" or "Employee of the Month." The recognition takes many forms, including presentation of a plaque, lunch with the president or supervisor, gifts, and mention in the company newsletter.
28. An activities committee has been established to plan social events, and new employees are introduced to a member of this committee so they become aware of company activities.
29. Snacks are available during employees' first break each day.
30. Employees missing one day or less due to illness or injury during the year receive a gift.
31. Factory eating areas are decorated on special occasions.
32. Free coffee is provided on special days.
33. Once a quarter, ten to 12 employees selected by random drawing are taken on a guided tour of all plant facilities and have lunch on the house in the plant cafeteria.
34. A Halloween costume contest is held each year, employees wear their costumes the work day, and the winner receives one day off with pay.
35. Receptions are given for every employee who retires.
36. In each month that new accounts exceed an established figure, all employees are taken out for dinner.
37. An annual awards banquet is held for employees on the last working day before a holiday.

FIGURE 11–7.   Fifty Specific Techniques to Boost Employee Morale (*continued*)

38. Annual parties for occasions such as Christmas are given by the company.
39. An appropriate gift is distributed to all employees daily, weekly, or monthly, when a production record is established.
40. A cash drawing is held each month that there is no employee time lost due to accident. Variation: A drawing is held each month for employees who have not missed time due to injury or illness.
41. An annual employee appreciation dinner is given by the company.
42. Lunch and entertainment are provided "on the grounds" for all employees two or three times each year.
43. Some food for snacking is supplied by the company on a daily basis.
44. Positive comments on an employee by a customer result in the employee receiving a silver pin. Three such compliments during the year earn a gold pin.

45. Special food items are given to all employees on occasions such as Thanksgiving or Christmas.
46. Occasional boat rides on a cruiser are made available to all employees.
47. Company-wide potluck luncheons are held.
48. One firm sponsors a daily 15-minute radio program on which one of the employees is recognized/spotlighted.
49. When a new safety record is reached, employees receive a small memento and attend a "cook-out" hosted by management.
50. Lunch is provided for all employees on the last working day before a holiday.

Nursing strategy will indicate the present business of nursing, its future business, and what its business should ideally be. The organizational structure allows, supports, and promotes nursing functions consistent with the organizational mission, philosophy, and objectives.

A newer concept in the theory of organizations is that the organizational structure affects the strategic decision-making process. Historically, changes in organizational structure have followed changes in strategy such as unit volume, geographic dispersion, and vertical and horizontal integration. The organizational form determines the decision-making environment: it delimits responsibilities and communication channels, controls decision-making environment, and facilitates information processing.[40]

Strategic decision making requires wide expertise from numerous levels. In nursing, managers must seek broad input from clinical nurses. This can be done through task forces, committees, project teams, or ad hoc groups. Nurse executives must make conscious decisions to delimit centralization, formalization, and complexity, particularly in large organizations. The object is conscious integration.

Decentralization and participation are discussed in another chapter.

Work Activities and Functions

Work activities and functions that will be analyzed and encompassed in identifying the building blocks of organization include:

1. Operating work at the unit level, including primary nursing care (the basic mission, not the method or modality of nursing); operational nursing management, commonly referred to as head nurse and/or charge nurse activities; and support activities essential to the application of primary nursing care, such as training, clerical work, and others. Management at the unit level includes management of the clinical component of direct nursing care and management of non-nursing or indirect activities.

2. In a fair-sized or big-business type of nursing organization there may be a need for middle managers, commonly referred to as supervisors or clinical coordinators. This would occur in a large univer-

sity health-care complex or a medical center complex. The division of nursing may even be big enough to require a management team for clinical services, organized as departments, such as medical and pediatric nursing. The functions identified will determine the design and the structure and how many people are needed for top management or middle management jobs. An assistant chair will be part of the top management group.

3. In any health-care institution there will be top management functions to be performed. In a small division the nurse manager will be top manager of the department and a member of top management of the institution. Within a large division with multiple missions and objectives there will likely exist enough functions and activities for a top management team in the division of nursing. The chair will still be a member of top management of the institution, functioning at the strategic planning level in both instances.

4. A technostructure of staff of varying size, depending upon the size of the institution, will support the management and clinical components of the nursing organization. These will include experts in infection control, staff development, oncology nursing, quality assurance, and others. In some organizations they are labelled consultants.

5. A need for innovative work would be identified and planned for in designing the organizational structure. It could be assigned to operating level, top management level, or a staff function, the latter being a support activity not in the direct line of authority. It will need top management support but a strategy separate from the management strategy with its own mission, objectives, operational plans, and measurements.

Context

There are contextual variables that relate to an organization's structure, such as size, technology, organizational charter or social function, environment, interdependence with other organizations, structuring of activities, concentration of authority, and line of control of work flow.[41]

Organizational Charter or Social Function.
Nursing organizations exist within institutions that are either government-owned, private not-for-profit, or private for-profit. Government-owned organizations are impersonally founded and highly centralized, with concentrated authority. Impersonality of origin increases the level of control of work flow. Since many health-care organizations are impersonal in origin they are highly centralized with increased line control of the work flow of professional nurses.

In a study of a random sample of forty-six organizations stratified by size and product or purpose it was concluded that:

1. Public accountability did not affect structuring of activities, including the line of control of work flow.
2. Public accountability increased concentration of authority by standardization of personnel policies but relied upon professional line subordinates for work-flow control.
3. Increased accountability decreased or dispersed concentration of ownership with control.
4. Impersonally founded organizations are more dependent upon the founding organization. Publicly accountable organizations are more dependent on external power.
5. High dependence is associated with impersonally founded, publicly accountable, or vertically integrated organizations; contracted specialties; smallness of units; low status; and little representation in policy making.
6. Low dependence is associated with personal foundation, low public accountability, little vertical integration, few contract specialties, and the unit being the parent organization.[42]

Since professional nurses want autonomy of decision making in their clinical practice, these findings need to be substantiated by nursing research. There is empirical evidence to substantiate them in the initiation of nursing administration strategies. Nursing is an occupation with a history of public accountability, a desirable characteristic. Nurse managers, knowledgeable of the impersonality aspects of public accountability, will initiate strategies to increase and allow the desired autonomy and accountability of clinical nurses in order to increase their independence, their status, and their representation on policy-making entities. This is especially true in an environment in which health-care organizations are pursuing vertical integration and mergers that decrease independence.

Size. Larger organizations tend to have more specialization and more formalization than small ones. The larger the size, the more decentralized the organization and the more standardized the procedures for selection and advancement of personnel. Bureaucracy increases with increased size and decreased personal integration.[43]

Increased size of an organization requires that managers differentiate employees into work groups, functions, departments, or work centers with described tasks. They are also differentiated into hierarchical levels. These differentiations are done to exercise management control, coordination, or integration. They are also done to buffer the core technology of an organization and to prepare it to respond to variety in the external environment.[44]

Contingency theory was used to study the technology, size, environment, and structure in 157 nursing subunits located in twenty-four hospitals in the Canadian province of Alberta. The theory postulated that the wide range of differences in organizational structure vary systematically with such factors as technology, size, and environment. It was found that increased subunit beds decreased the R.N. ratio and increased the measure of bureaucratization of professionals. There was no relationship between decentralization of the subunit and size and little relationship between size and role specificity.[45] These findings would support those of Pugh and others who found no relationship between size and concentration of authority, between size and line control of work flow, or between size and autonomy.[46]

Technology. Technology is defined as "the sequence of physical techniques used upon the work flow of the organization, even if the physical techniques involve only pen, ink, and paper." The more rigid and highly integrated the technology, the greater is the structuring of activities and procedures and the more impersonal the control. Complex technology emphasizes administration.[47]

Within nursing subunits uncertainty in the technology *decreased* role specificity and decentralization and *increased* decentralization from the head nurse. A lack of an adequate knowledge base by nurses was related to their perceptions of the uncer-

tainty in the technology. This led to intuitive care for complex social-psychological problems. Increased instability and uncertainty of technology increased the R.N. ratio. Uncertainty in the technology decreased specificity and decentralization from physicians while increasing decentralization from the head nurse. Bureaucracy increased with decreased R.N. ratio and clerical ratio.[48]

Roznowski and Hulin found in a study of four nonunionized hospitals in central Illinois that sophisticated technology increased perceptions of complexity and of increased use and development of skills, thereby creating higher job satisfaction.

This finding was generalized across services with similar technology levels and across organizations. Higher technology leads to higher job satisfaction, a possible reason for nurses aspiring to work in areas of critical care.[49]

Such findings give credibility to nursing management education. Nurse managers can use them to justify differential practice, since complex technology requires more advanced education and by inference staff development that sustains more advanced knowledge and skills. Education can thus be related to performance and pay.

Other Contextual Variables. Age does not relate to structuring of activities or line of control of work flow. Older organizations tended to be more decentralized and to have more autonomy.[50]

Product is related to control of work flow. If the product is nonstandard goods there is impersonal control of work flow. If the product is a standard consumer service there is decreased supervisor line control of work flow.[51] Health-care organizations produce both standard and nonstandard consumer services.

Technology, size, and environment do not operate totally independently in their interaction with structure. More research is needed to discover the combination of contextual variables that interact with specific political processes to produce structure. Nurse managers need to be experienced and competent and to exert powerful leadership that will establish the context within which nurses' values can be implemented. Such a context will include more highly educated R.N.s, less bureaucratization, more clerks, increased documentation using information technology, and increased decentralization.

Forms of Organizational Structure

There are two common forms of organizational structures, hierarchical and free-form. A mixture of both is needed in nursing.

Hierarchical Structures. A hierarchical structure is commonly called a line structure. It is the oldest and simplest form and is associated with the principle of chain of command, bureaucracy and a multi-tiered hierarchy, vertical control and coordination, levels differentiated by function and authority, and downward communications. These structures have all of the advantages and disadvantages of a bureaucracy. Most line structures have added a staff component. In nursing organizations both line and staff personnel will usually be professional nurses.

Line functions are those that have direct responsibility for accomplishing the objectives of a nursing department (or service or unit). For the most part, they include registered nurses, licensed practical nurses, and nursing technicians. Staff functions are those that assist the line in accomplishing the primary objectives of nursing. These include clerical, personnel, budgeting and finance, staff development, research, and specialized clinical consultants. The relationships between line and staff are a matter of authority. Line has authority for direct supervision of employees, while staff provide advice and counsel. There may be line authority within a staff section.

Line sections may act in a staff capacity when they give advice or consultation to another line section. Authority for decision making may be based on staff recommendations but is a line function.

To make staff effective, top management assures that line and staff authority relationships are clearly defined. Personnel of both must work to make their relationships effective; they attempt to minimize friction by increasing mutual trust and respect.

Functional authority occurs when an individual or department is delegated authority over functions in one or more other departments. This has occurred in the development of infection control and quality assurance systems where professional nurses have line authority to hospital management and staff authority to nursing management or line authority to nursing management and staff authority to other divisions. They do this through delegated authority to consult and prescribe procedures and sometimes policies, for the function as it is to be carried out in the other departments. These delegated authority functions are clearly defined and carefully restricted. They are usually limited to procedures and time frames and do not include personnel or content. They should not weaken or destroy the authority and thus the effectiveness of line managers. For example, staff personnel might be assigned to recruit nurses, with line managers retaining final authority over hiring. The nurse administrator should ensure effective use of staff functions by line managers so as to make effective use of the advise of experts and reduce duplication of effort of line managers. Staff give information that will facilitate the solution of problems. Such information is sought by line managers in an effective and cooperative relationship.

Service departments are not necessarily staff in their authority relationships. Usually, they are responsible for a grouping of activities that facilitate the work of other departments through their operating functions. An example is the maintenance department of a hospital. It provides the service of a functioning plant in which patient services are provided. It has the authority for performing its functions. It may provide some staff advice. Within a hospital, as in any business, there may be many such service departments such as word processing centers, learning resource centers, and the like. Activities are grouped together to provide for economical specialization. There may be service units for labor relations, contracts, legal matters, or purchasing. They may have functional authority, but care must be taken to keep them from causing divided loyalties, from delaying performance, and from displaying arrogance. They should provide for uniformity of procedures, policies, and standards; for skilled service and a smooth operation.[52] Figure 11–8 shows a set of standards for evaluation of the effectiveness of line and staff relationships within a nursing division, department, or unit.

Free-Form Structures. Free-form organizational structures are called *matrix* organizations. The matrix organization design enables timely response to external competition and facilitates efficiency and effectiveness internally through cooperation among disciplines.

Characteristics of a matrix organization include:

FIGURE 11–8. Standards for Evaluation of the Effectiveness of Line and Staff Relationships

---

Standards

1. Line authority relationships are clearly delineated and defined by the organizational and/or functional charts and policies.
2. Staff authority relationships are clearly delineated and defined by the organizational and/or functional charts and policies.
3. Functional authority relationships are clearly delineated and defined by the organizational and/or functional charts and policies.
4. Staff personnel are providing consultation, advice, and counsel to line personnel.
5. Service personnel functions are clearly understood by line and staff personnel.
6. Line personnel seek and effectively use staff services.
7. Appropriate staff services are being provided by line nursing personnel and other organizational departments or services.
8. Services are not being duplicated due to line and staff authority relationships.

---

1. Maintenance of old-line authority structures.
2. Specialist resources obtained from functional areas.
3. Promotion of formation of new organizational units.
4. Occurrence of decision making at the organizational level of group consensus, the middle management level.
5. The matrix manager exercising authority over the functional manager.
6. Cooperative planning of program development and allocation of resources to accomplish program objectives.
7. Assignment of functional managers to teams that respond to the chief of the functional discipline and matrix manager.[53]

Advantages of matrix nursing organizational structures include:

1. Improved communication through vertical and horizontal control and coordination of interdisciplinary patient care teams.

2. Increased organizational adaptability and fluidity to respond to environmental changes.
3. Increased efficiency of resource use with fewer organizational levels and decision making closer to primary care operations.
4. Improved human resource management because of increased job satisfaction with achievement and fulfillment, improved communication, improved interpersonal skills, and improved collegial relationships.[54]

Disadvantages of matrix nursing organizational structures include:

1. Potential conflict because of dual or multiple lines of authority, responsibility, and accountability relationships.
2. Role ambiguity.
3. Loss of control over functional discipline due to multidisciplinary team approach.[55]

Adhocracy. "Adhocracy" models of organization are like matrix models. There are simple teams or task forces that exist on an ad hoc basis. They are formed, complete their goals, and are disbanded; new groups are then formed to meet changing and dynamic mission and objectives.[56]

Matrix and adhocracy models employ participatory management. Xerox is an example of a company that has successfully used self-managing work teams. They once exceeded cost reduction targets of $3.7 million by $1 million. The expert is the authority that leads the team. They are consultative organizations that delegate rather than tell. They encourage maverick behavior and reward results. Of 360 manufacturing companies studied, the forty-one that were most successful had fewer employees per sale; encouraged risk taking; had fewer headquarters staff; had decentralized decision making; and had self-contained units or cost centers.[57]

The Organization of Work

Work is organized according to the stages in a process. In some areas the work moves to the skills and tools, a good example being coronary care nursing or operating room nursing. Sometimes a team moves different skills and different tools to the work—for example when an operating room team moves to a delivery room to perform a cesarean section. We certainly find combinations in nursing.

Much of the work in nursing is accomplished by a functionally structured organization. Clarity is an advantage of the functional structure, since the individuals know where they stand and they understand their tasks. Functional structures are usually stable. A disadvantage is that sometimes the task neither relates to the whole structure nor does it contribute to the common purpose. Functional structures are rigid and frequently neither prepare nurses for the future nor train and test them.

Functional organizations become costly when friction builds up and requires coordinators, committees, meetings, troubleshooters, and special dispatchers. Functional organizations make low psychological demands on people; people in such organizations tend to focus on their own efforts only. Small functional organizations are economical and foster good communications. These organizations are good when one kind of work is done. Usually they require that decisions be made at the top. Nurses within them have narrow visions, skills, and loyalties. Employees of such organizations focus on function rather than results and performance. The functional process does not usually apply to top management positions or to performance of innovative work by employees.

The team organization has been tried in nursing for the past 25 years. It has been used mainly at the operating or primary care level rather than at top or middle management levels. "A team is a number of people—usually fairly small—with different backgrounds, skills, and knowledge, drawn from various areas of the organization (their home), who work together on a specific and defined task. There is usually a team leader or team captain."[58]

In health-care institutions, patients see the physician as team leader. However, the team leader uses the resources of the entire organization; in many cases it is the nurse who identifies, recommends, and coordinates these resources.

A team must have a continuing mission, which nursing has. The team should be highly flexible without a rigid chain of command. Like all organizational structures, in business, industry, or health-care institutions, the team organization needs clear and sharply defined objectives. Leadership decides on decision and command authority, and the team is responsible for accomplishing the tasks or mission. Team members know each other's function, but leadership must first establish clarity in the objec-

tives and in everybody's role. Everyone must know the whole work and be adaptable and receptive to innovation. The team leader gives continuing attention to clear communications and clear decision making. A team should be kept small for top management work and for innovative work. Otherwise the team design complements the functional design. A combination may consist of employees who work in teams but produce work organized on the functional principle. This approach seems to work best in nursing, and is probably better than either organizational structure in its pure form.

Knowledge work is best for team design. Use of a functional axis manages people and their knowledge, whereas use of a team axis manages work and task. The team may be the key to making functional design effective. Team organization is a difficult structure requiring great self-discipline.

Another organizational form is known as *federal decentralization*. In this form each unit is autonomous. Units usually have a functional organization but may use teams. Like other organizational forms, this one starts with the results to be achieved. Next, decisions are made regarding the work and key activities to be established. Each unit has an autonomous manager. Tasks of top management are clearly defined and concentrate on direction, strategy, objectives, key decisions for the future, technologies, markets and products, businesses to start and abandon, and the basic values, beliefs, and principles of the company. Capital and people are controlled by these basics. This type of organization needs centralized controls, common measurements, and coordinated planning. Among health-care organizations few would be large enough for this form of organization, although some university hospital complexes and county or state institutions may be. There are principles of organizations that would apply to the development of a functional or team structure for this organized form.

Tall (Vertical) versus Flat (Horizontal) Organizations

Line organizations are considered to be tall or vertical organizations, while matrix and adhocracy models are considered to be flat or horizontal organizations. In a study of the effects of tall versus flat organizational structures on job satisfaction of managers, flat organizations were found to decrease need deficiencies in selected indicators of self-esteem and self-actualization. Tall organizations decrease need deficiencies for selected indicators of security, social needs, and self-esteem. Overall there was "no difference between tall and flat organizations in terms of perceived need deficiencies." Flat organizations are not superior to tall organizations for managers.[59] Research is needed along these lines for practicing nurses.

Guest predicts that future organizations will be unstructured, flat, flexible, and decentralized; that authority will come from competence; and that leaders will change with goals. There will be no formal job descriptions. Employees will be salaried collegial groups of equals who will respond quickly to change.

Vertical integration will diminish with microprocessor technology in communication through artificial intelligence and robotization. People will go from manufacturing to service, transportation, communication, and recreation industries. Employees will telecommute from their homes. Telecommuting programs already exist in 450 companies. The mother and/or father will be able to stay at home and have an improved quality of work life.[60]

Mechanistic versus Organismic Structures

Organismic structures maximize flexibility and adaptability. They emphasize greater use of human potential and greater human worth and importance. Within organismic structures job design stresses personal growth and responsibility. There is decentralization of decision making, control, and goal-setting processes. Communication flows in all directions. Generalization is emphasized in a climate that is informal.[61]

Mechanistic organizations support many of the opposite characteristics: group formality, external pressures, structuring of activities, and centralization of authority with high control. Structural variables do not necessarily relate to work satisfaction. Mechanistic organizations can produce high satisfaction among coworkers in formal groups. The classic dysfunctions of bureaucracy do not necessarily exist at lower levels of organizational structure. Organismic structures probably lead to more flexible and innovative managerial behavior.[62]

ANALYZING ORGANIZATIONAL STRUCTURE IN A DIVISION OF NURSING

There are six main steps in analyzing the organizational structure of a division of nursing. They should be used when major organizational problems occur, such as friction among department heads over authority, staffing problems, and the like. These steps also apply to organizing a new corporation, division, or unit and to reorganizing.

Step 1. Compile a list of the key activities determined by the mission and objectives of patient care. The written philosophy will help by indicating important values to be considered. Once this list is completed it must be analyzed. Group similar activities together. What are the central load-carrying elements? Most will be related to primary care; philosophy will usually dictate that excellence of patient care is a requirement for the accomplishment of objectives.

Whenever the strategy changes, the organizational structure should be reviewed and analyzed. This includes changes in mission, philosophy, objectives, and the operational plan for accomplishing the objectives. The analysis of key activities can be done according to the kinds of contributions made. These will include the following:

1. Results-producing activities related to direct patient care, such as training, recruiting, and employment.
2. Support activities, which may include those related to vision or future, values and standards, audit, advice, and teaching.
3. Hygiene and housekeeping activities.
4. Top management activities, including "conscience" activities such as vision, values, standards, and audit as well as managing people, marketing, and innovation.

Service staffs such as those performing advisory and training support should be limited. They should be required to abandon an old activity before starting a new one. Prevent them from building empires as a career. Informational activities are the responsibility of top management though they stem from support activities such as controller and treasurer. There must be a system for disseminating information. Hygiene and housekeeping need the attention of nurses if they are to be done well and cheaply. This does not mean that nurses will do these tasks; rather nurses should recognize their importance and support and facilitate their being done by the appropriate departments. Contract services are the answer in some instances.

Consider whether the groups of key activities should be rank-ordered in a sequence in which they will occur.

Step 2. Based on the work functions to be performed, decide on the units of the organization. Decision analysis will be important here, since it must be determined which kinds of decisions will be required and who will make them. Decisions involving functions of future commitments may have to be a top management function, depending on the degree of futurity of a decision and the speed with which it can be reversed. It will be necessary to analyze the impact of decisions on other functions, the number of functions involved being an important factor. Qualitative factors such as decisions involving ethical values, principles of conduct, and social and political beliefs will have to be analyzed. The frequency of the decision will influence its placement: Is it recurrent, or is it rare? In principle, all decisions should be placed at the lowest level and as close to the operational scene as possible.

Step 3. Decide which units or components will be joined and which separated. Join activities that make the same kind of contribution. This will require relations analysis and will be related to the sequence of key activities or functions.

Step 4. Decide on the size and shape of the units or components.

Step 5. Decide on appropriate placement and relationships of different units or components. This will result from the relations analysis. There should be the smallest possible number of relationships, with each being made to count.

Step 6. Draw or diagram the design and put it into operation. This will result in an organizational chart or schema.

Steps 3, 4, and 5 involve *departmentation*, the grouping of personnel according to some characteristic. Departmentation is an organizing process.

For departmentation purposes, functional specialties are formed from clusters of units with similar goals. In most health-care institutions, the functions of nursing are grouped into a division or department. Within that division or department are further groupings of nursing personnel by specialization such as medical, surgical, pediatric, or obstetric. Sometimes the grouping is further broken down into areas of subspecialization. This process is termed *functional departmentation*. Clients may also be grouped according to degree of illness such as minimal, intermediate, or intensive care.

There are advantages and disadvantages of functional departmentation. Among the advantages are focus on the basic activities of the enterprise through a logical and time-proven method of organizing, efficient use of specialized personnel, simplified training, and tight control by top administration. A big disadvantage for nursing is that people tend to develop tunnel vision about their specialty and the service or unit within which they work.

Time departmentation is common within health-care organizations. Personnel are grouped by shift. This has important implications for administration as the activities of shifts have to be grouped according to qualifications and numbers of personnel on any shift.

Territorial departmentation involves grouping activities according to geography or physical plant. This is more common in organizations with geographically separated units. Some activities, such as staff development, may be assigned by territory and specialization as well as being grouped by function.

Territorial departmentation should encourage participation in decision-making in provision of health services to a wider population base and be of a nature that will prevent illnesses and injuries. There may be justification for the exploration and formation of consortiums using the principle of territorial departmentation. For example, several small hospitals in an area could contract for consultant services in research, clinical nurse specialist services, or nursing education services.

In addition to functional, time, and territorial departmentation, there is the fourth option, *product departmentation*. This approach has important implications for health care, although its ultimate achievement may not always be immediately practical. Increasingly, the products of nursing care are focused on the health needs of populations—those who need not only the illness care but the care that keeps aging populations healthy; that maintains health and prevents injury and disease in the large group who take voluntary risks such as smoking, reckless driving, poor eating, poor exercising, or using artificial mood changers; that provide health care promoting a clean environment; that modify the health risks associated with human reproduction; and that decrease the need for illness care. In the vertically integrated organization product line departmentation is common in today's health-care institutions.

Departmentation could be done on the basis of consumer needs or demands. There is a distinct possibility that health-care institutions will offer people a choice of services in the future, thereby giving them the opportunity to select those services that will be covered by third-party payers and those that will be paid for out of pocket. Also, the times these services will be given and who will be giving them may well be part of the choice.

There may be no pure form of departmentation that will work in the health-care institution. It may be more important to look at all the variables in order to group people to facilitate successful production of health-care services. In the matrix organization, product and functional forms of departmentation are combined. Projects have managers who move products through production stages in coordination with managers of each production stage. We will see more use of matrix organizations in nursing as health care takes on new dimensions.

At the present, nursing services are usually organized using a mix of departmentations. So long as the system is based on logic, it will provide a viable and efficient organization. Use Figure 11–9 to evaluate departmentation of nursing service activities and personnel.

ORGANIZATION CHARTS

Most nursing organizations have made graphic representations of the organizing process in the form of organization charts. These charts usually show reporting relationships and communication channels. Line charts show supervisor and supervisee relationships from top to bottom of the nursing organi-

FIGURE 11–9. Standards for Evaluation of Departmentation

1. Nursing activities have been grouped to attain goals and sustain the enterprise.
2. Nursing activities have been grouped for intradepartmental and interdepartmental coordination.
3. Personnel roles have been designed to fit the capabilities and motivation of persons available to fill them.
4. Personnel roles have been designed to help employees contribute to departmental or unit objectives.
5. Personnel roles provide optimum and economic job enlargement.
6. Nursing activities have been grouped for full use of resources, people, and material.
7. Nursing activities have been grouped for optimum cost benefits.
8. Nursing activities have been grouped to match special skills to special needs.
9. Nursing activities have been grouped to achieve an optimum management span.
10. Nursing activities and personnel have been grouped for optimum correlation for decision-making and problem-solving.
11. Nursing activities have been grouped to achieve minimal levels of management by providing for delegation of responsibility and authority to the lowest competent operational level.
12. Nursing activities and personnel have been grouped to eliminate duplication of staff services and centralized services of specialists.
13. Nursing activities and personnel have been grouped to facilitate production of products and services that will promote health of individuals and groups.
14. Nursing activities and personnel have been grouped to promote soundness of industrial relations programs and fiscal policies and procedures.
15. Nursing activities have been grouped to fulfill time demands of shifts.
16. Nursing activities have been grouped to achieve priorities and allow for change and flexibility in achievement of objectives.
17. Nursing activities have been grouped to facilitate training of employees.
18. Nursing activities have been grouped to facilitate communication.

zation. These are hierarchical relationships on which communication channels follow the line of authority to and through the chief nurse executive. Figure 11–10 offers an example.

Staff charts show the advisory relationship of specialists or experts who are extensions of the nurse administrators. These types of charts usually depict the title or rank of each line and staff officer position in the authority relationship structure. They denote the delegation of authority and responsibility as well as the direction of accountability for the goals of the nursing division. Figure 11–11 illustrates a staff chart.

Some organization charts depict dual reporting relationships of functional staff, as shown in Figure 11–12. Figure 11–13 depicts a matrix organizational chart.

Organization charts distribute the nursing responsibilities. These responsibilities may be divided according to one or a combination of functions: contiguous geography, similar techniques, similar objectives, or like clientele.

Organization charts are sometimes referred to as schemas. Decentralized schemas are flatter since there are fewer levels of control or management. Managers have more freedom to act and the emphasis is placed on results.

There are advantages to having a current organization chart. Such charts show clear relationships. They show employees who their supervisor is and supervisors who they supervise. They can facilitate coordination and communication. They can prevent intrigue, frustration, and duplication of effort, and promote decision making, efficiency, and adherence to policy. They can tie the structure together and show inconsistencies and complexities. One must remember that organization charts have limitations. They will show formal authority structure only; they will show what was rather than what is if they are outdated and obsolete. Organization charts may confuse authority with status.

Figure 11–14 shows how to evaluate an organization chart of a nursing division or department or unit.

THE INFORMAL ORGANIZATION

Every formal organization has an informal one. The informal organization meets the needs of individuals with similar backgrounds, values, hobbies, inter-

ests, and physical proximity. It meets their needs for gregariousness—for sharing experiences and feelings. Some administrators try to hinder the effects of informal organizations since they facilitate the passing of information. The information may be rumor, but the best way to combat rumor is by free flow of truthful information. Only that information which might violate individual privacy or the survival and health of the enterprise should be kept from subordinates. The informal organization can help to serve the goals of the formal organization if it is not made the servant of administration. It should not be controlled. A major shortcoming in its use is that not all employees are part of the informal organization.[63]

Nurse managers should encourage and nurture informal organizations that:

1. Provide a sense of belonging, security, and recognition.
2. Provide methods for friendly and open discussion of concerns.
3. Maintain feelings of personal integrity, self-respect, and independent choice.
4. Provide an informal and accurate communication link.
5. Provide opportunities for social interaction.
6. Provide a source of practical information for managerial decision making.
7. Are sources of future leaders.

Problems can include creation of conflicting loyalties, restricted productivity, and resistance to change and management's plans.[64]

MINIMUM REQUIREMENTS FOR AN ORGANIZATIONAL STRUCTURE

1. *Clarity*—Nurses need to know where they belong, where they stand in relation to the quality and quantity of their performance, and where to go for assistance.

2. *Economy*—Nurses need as much self-control of their work as they can possibly be given. They need to be self-motivating. There should be the smallest possible number of overhead personnel necessary

FIGURE 11–10. Line

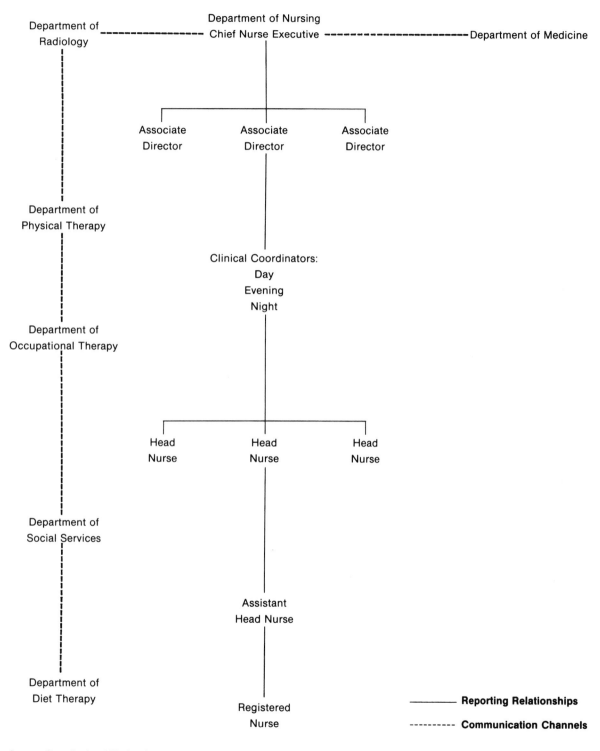

SOURCE: Organizational Models for Nursing Practice, published by the American Hospital Association, 1986.

FIGURE 11–11.   Line and Staff

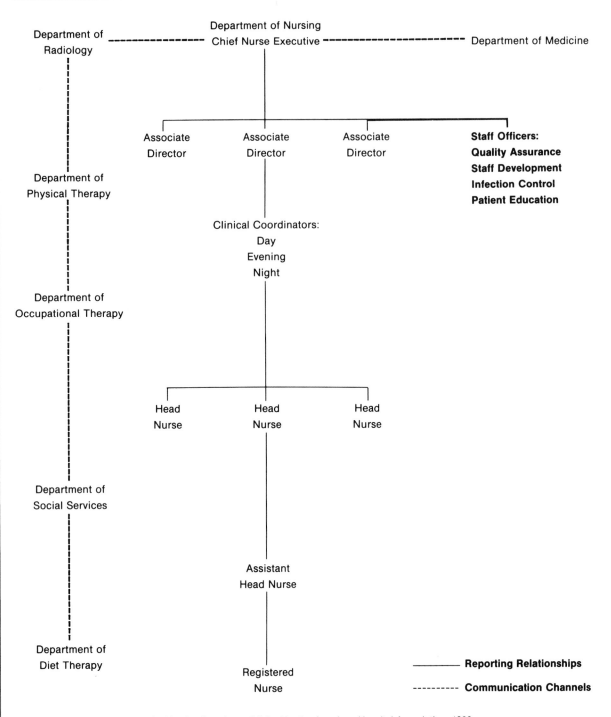

SOURCE: Organizational Models for Nursing Practice, published by the American Hospital Association, 1986.

FIGURE 11–12. Functional

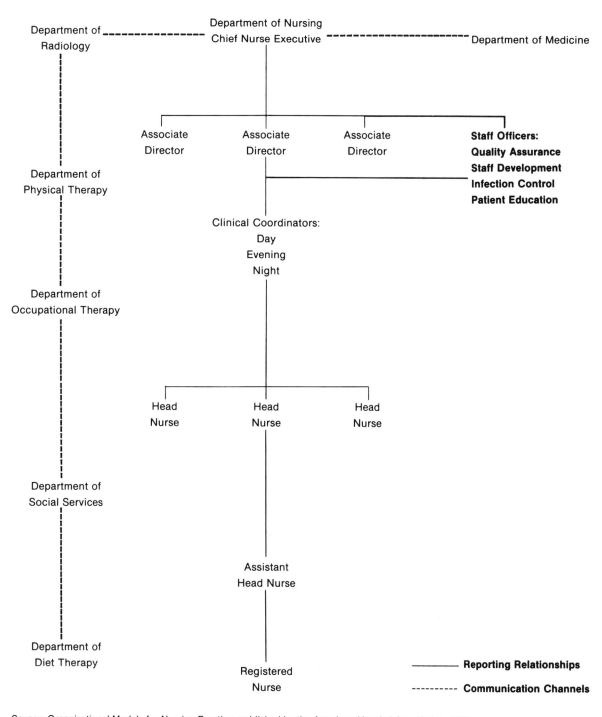

SOURCE: Organizational Models for Nursing Practice, published by the American Hospital Association, 1986.

FIGURE 11–13. Matrix

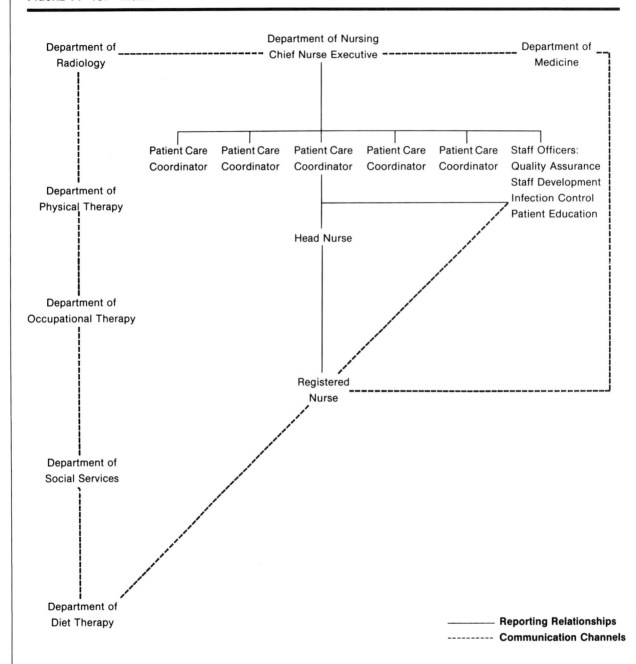

SOURCE: Organizational Models for Nursing Practice, published by the American Hospital Association, 1986.

FIGURE 11–14. Standards for Evaluation of an Organization Chart

1. An organization chart or schema exists for the nursing division or service or unit.
2. The chart is up to date.
3. The chart clearly depicts line and staff authority relationships within the nursing division service or unit.
4. The chart serves as a reference for delegation of authority, for specifying responsibility and accountability, for supervision, and for channels of communication.
5. The chart is familiar to all employees of the nursing division or service or unit.
6. There are organization charts available that depict coordination and communication relationships between the nursing division and other departments or units of the overall organization.

to keep the division and units operating and well maintained.

3. *Direction of vision*—Nurse managers need to direct their vision and that of their employees toward performance, toward the future, and toward strength. Nurse persons need to understand their own tasks and the common tasks, the common ones being those of the organization. They should see that their tasks fit the common tasks of the organization so that the structure helps communication.

4. *Decision making*—Nurses should be organized to make decisions on the right issues and at the right levels. They should be organized to convert their decisions into work and accomplishments. The chair of the department of nursing and the staff should make all nursing decisions and see that the nursing work is done.

5. *Stability and accountability*—Nurses should be organized to feel community belongingness. They can adapt to show objectives requiring changes in their functions and productivity.

6. *Perception and self-renewal*—Nursing services should be organized to produce future leaders. The organizational structure should produce continuous learning for the job each nurse holds and for promotion.

To apply design principles that are appropriate, the nurse manager uses a mixture of all that are productive.

Principle: Organizational needs derive from the statements of mission and objectives and from observation of work performed.

Principle: Organizational design and structure develop to fit organizational needs, so that people perform and contribute to achieving the work of the division of nursing.

Principle: A formal organization should be flexible and based on policy that promotes individual contributions to the achievement of organizational objectives.

Principle: A formal organization is efficient when it promotes achievement of objectives with a minimum of unplanned costs or outcomes. Most results should be planned for, should give satisfaction to supervisors and employees, and should not occasion waste and carelessness. When grouping activities for organizing purposes, the supervisor or administrator should examine the benefits and disadvantages of alternative groupings.

ORGANIZATIONAL EFFECTIVENESS

The product or output of an organization is termed organizational effectiveness (OE). There should be a relationship between organizational effectiveness and organizational performance (OP). Nurse managers define the goals and provide the resources for both OP and OE. They have many dimensions, which can include:

1. Patient satisfaction with care.
2. Family satisfaction with care.
3. Staff satisfaction with work.
4. Staff satisfaction with rewards, intrinsic and extrinsic.
5. Staff satisfaction with professional development: career, personal, and educational.
6. Staff satisfaction with organization.
7. Management satisfaction with staff.
8. Community relationships.
9. Organizational health.

These dimensions of OE are controlled by nurse administrators. Proactivity is more successful in developing them than is reactivity.[65]

The organizational effectiveness of hospitals could be improved if administrators would enter into general or limited partnerships with nurses. Hospitals have moved to vertical integration to capture the lost revenues of retrospective reimbursement. General hospitals have entered into services such as home care, long-term care, psychiatric care, rehabilitation, hospice care, rental and sale of durable medical supplies, and many other profit-making services. While they call for general or limited partnerships with physicians, they ignore nurses as a potential source of partnerships for profit. Instead the not-for-profit status of hospital inpatient beds is reputed to be maintained by policies that tie nursing to charity and idealism rather than to viability and profitability. This tie is validated by such statements as "keeping nursing care in the not-for-profit hospital corporation preserves the oldest tradition of hospitals—their role in serving the needy."[66]

Nurses can overcome this attitude by themselves becoming proactive. As an example nurses could plan a limited partnership that would provide contract nurses through a staffing agency owned by them. They could offer a hospital a contract to provide needed personnel on a first priority basis, surplus personnel being provided for other institutions. The contract could provide for up-to-date continuing education of the agency nurses through cooperative arrangements with the contracting hospital. Profits would be shared and nurses would perceive that the hospital supported nursing entrepreneurship, thus contributing to their morale and professional esteem. Other ventures could be added to improve OP as well as OE and to give nurses a sense of ownership.

Vertical integration, mergers, linkages, and multihospital systems have created more and new corporate nurse roles. The corporate nurse is physically and organizationally removed from daily nursing service operations. As such, the corporate nurse reviews data from a number of hospitals and organizations, comparing outcomes. Having access to much data, many specialties, and serving on corporate committees, the corporate nurse creates a personal power base. She or he can develop systems for member organizations in such areas as management education, nursing disivion policy, search and selection of nurse executives, research, quality assurance, risk management, and others.[67]

SYMPTOMS OF MALORGANIZATION

A symptom of malorganization is recurring problems. They indicate the focus is on the wrong elements of the business when it should emphasize key activities, major business decisions, performance, and results rather than secondary problems. Another symptom of malorganization is too many meetings attended by too many people. Such meetings are poor tools for accomplishing work. An alternative is to give individual assignments and only meet to report and avoid duplication. Committees are instruments of participation and communication and must be made productive. Too many management levels is another symptom of malorganization.

Principle: Build the least possible number of management levels and forge the shortest possible chain of command. This eliminates stresses and levels of friction, slack, and inertia.

If people always have to worry about other people's feelings, there is overstaffing. If the organization is put together to get the job done, layers of coordinators are not needed. Fit the chart to the organization and its needs rather than drawing a chart and building the organization to support it.

SUMMARY

There is no best design for a nursing organization, nor are there universal design principles. Nurse managers need to work for an ideal organizational structure and they need to be pragmatic. They should build, test, concede, compromise, and accept. They should design the simplest organization for getting the job done. They should focus on key activities to produce key results. The organization is productive when the people are performing care that meets client needs and for which employees have a sense of accomplishment.

An organization can be shaped through:

1. Job enlargement that is qualitative—meaningful, interesting, and intellectually rewarding.
2. Making the structure more manageable. Increasing clinical nurses' autonomy reduces the organization's size.

3. Increasing the span of control of the manager.
4. Shortening the hierarchy.
5. Involving the employees in participation.
6. Decentralization.
7. Increasing the employee's stake in his or her own performance.
8. Increasing creativity while maintaining fiscal responsibility.
9. Replacing direction and control with advice.
10. Meeting employees' needs.

The nursing management function of organizing is an evolving one. It evolves as nurse managers learn and apply the knowledge gained from research and experience in business and industry. They further develop the organizing function through nursing research and experience in nursing management.

NOTES

1. C. Argyris, "Personality and Organization Theory Revisited," *Administrative Science Quarterly*, V. 18 1973, 141–167.
2. H. Fayol in *General and Industrial Management* by C. Storrs (London: Sir Isaac Pittman & Sons, 1949), 53–61.
3. L. Urwick, *The Elements of Administration* (New York: Harper & Row, 1944), 37–39.
4. J. L. Gibson, J. M. Ivancevich, and J. H. Donnelly, Jr., *Organizations: Behavior, Structures, Processes*, 5th ed. (Plano, TX: Business Publications, 1985), 488–491.
5. R. H. Hall, "The Concept of Bureaucracy: An Empirical Assessment," *The American Journal of Sociology*, July, 1963, 32–40.
6. Ibid.
7. R. H. Hall, "Professionalization and Bureaucratization," *American Sociological Review*, February 1968, 92–104.
8. J. R. Rizzo, R. J. House, and S. I. Lirtzman, "Role Conflict and Ambiguity in Complex Organizations," *Administrative Science Quarterly*, V. 15, 1970, 150–162.
9. D. Dunphy, "Personal and Organizational Change—Status and Future Direction," *Work and People*, Feb. 1983, 3-6.
10. J. Johnson and K. Luciano, "Managing by Behavior and Results—Linking Supervisory Accountability to Effective Organizational Control," *Journal of Nursing Administration*, Dec. 1983, 19–26.
11. E. C. Dayani, "Professional and Economic Self-Governance in Nursing," *Nursing Economics*, July-Aug. 1983, 20–23.
12. C. Argyris, op. cit.
13. D. S. Ridderheim, "The Anatomy of Change," *Hospital & Health Services Administration*, May/June 1986, 7–21.
14. D. J. del Bueno and P. M. Vincent, "Organizational Culture: How Important Is It?," *Journal of Nursing Administration*, Oct. 1986, 15–20.
15. Ibid.
16. W. G. Dyer and W. G. Dyer, Jr., "Organizational Development: System Change or Culture Change?," *Personnel*, Feb. 1986, 14–22.
17. R. L. Desatnick, "Management Climate Surveys: A Way to Uncover an Organization's Culture," *Personnel*, May 1986, 49–54, 14–22.
18. D. J. del Bueno and P. M. Vincent, op. cit.
19. W. G. Dyer and W. G. Dyer, Jr., op. cit.
20. R. L. Desatnick, op. cit.
21. M. Holt Ashley, "Motivation: Getting the Medical Units Going Again," *Nursing Management*, June 1985, 28–30.
22. M. B. Guthrie, G. Mauer, R. A. Zawacki, and J. D. Conger, "Productivity: How Much Does This Job Mean?" *Nursing Management*, Feb. 1985, 16–20.
23. L. R. Campbell, "What Satisfies . . . and Doesn't?," *Nursing Management*, Aug. 1986, 78.
24. R. L. Jenkins and R. L. Henderson, "Motivating the Staff: What Nurses Expect from Their Supervisors," *Nursing Management*, Feb. 1984, 13–14.
25. T. K. Crout and J. C. Crout, "Care Plan for Retaining the New Nurse," *Nursing Management*, Dec. 1984, 30–33.
26. R. L. Desatnick, op. cit.
27. B. Schneider, "The Preceptor of Organizational Climate: The Customer's View," *Journal of Applied Psychology*, Mar. 1973, 248–256.
28. C. Joiner, V. Johnson, J. B. Chapman, and M. Corkrean, "The Motivating Potential in Nursing Specialties," *Journal of Nursing Administration*, Feb. 1982, 26–30.
29. B. Conway-Rutkowski, "Labor Relations: How Do You Rate?" *Nursing Management*, February 1984, 13–16.
30. R. L. Desatnick, op. cit.
31. G. K. Gordon, "Developing a Motivating Environment," *The Journal of Nursing Administration*, December 1982, 11-16.
32. E. E. Lawler, III, D. T. Hall, and G. R. Oldham, "Organizational Climate: Relationship to Organizational Structure, Process, and Performance," *Organizational Behavior and Human Performance*, Nov. 1974, 139–155.
33. D. L. Niehouse, "Job Satisfaction: How to Motivate Today's Workers," *Supervisory Management*, Feb. 1986, 8–11.
34. M. H. Cohen and M. E. Ross, "Team Building: A Strategy for Unit Cohesiveness," *Journal of Nursing Administration*, Jan. 1982, 29–34.
35. M. Jacobsen-Webb, "Team Building: Key to Executive Success," *Journal of Nursing Administration*, Jan.-Feb. 1985, 16–20.
36. C. Logan, "Praise: The Powerhouse of Self-Esteem," *Nursing Management*, June 1985, 36, 38.
37. J. L. Nave and B. Thomas, "How Companies Boost Morale," *Supervisory Management*, Oct. 1983, 29–33.
38. P. Cornett-Cooke and K. Dias, "Teambuilding: Getting It All Together," *Nursing Management*, May 1984, 16–17.
39. J. W. Frederickson, "The Strategic Decision Process and Organizational Structure," *Academy of Management Review*, Apr. 1986, 280–297.
40. D. S. Pugh, D. J. Hickson, C. R. Hinings, and C. Turner, "The Context of Organization Structures," *Administrative Science Quarterly*, March 1969, 91–114; P. Leatt and R. Schneck, "Technology, Size, Environment, and Structure in Nursing Subunits, *Organizational Studies*, V. 3, No. 3 1982, 221–242.

41. D. S. Pugh, D. J. Hickson, C. R. Hinings, and C. Turner, op. cit.
42. Ibid.
43. M. Roznowski and C. L. Hulin, "Influences of Functional Specialty and Job Technology on Employees' Perceptual and Affective Responses to Their Jobs," *Organizational Behavior and Human Decision Processes*, Oct. 1985, 186–208.
44. P. Leatt and R. Schneck, op. cit.
45. D. S. Pugh, D. J. Hickson, C. R. Hinings, and C. Turner, op. cit.
46. Ibid.
47. P. Leatt and R. Schneck, op. cit.
48. Ibid.
49. M. Roznowski and C. L. Hulin, op. cit.
50. D. S. Pugh, D. J. Hickson, C. R. Hinings, and C. Turner, op. cit.
51. Ibid.
52. R. C. Swansburg, Self-Study Module-27-77: *The Organization Function of Nursing Service Administration* (Hattiesburg, MS: School of Nursing, University of Southern Mississippi, 1977).
53. M. L. McClure, "Managing the Professional Nurse: Part I. The Organizational Theories," *Journal of Nursing Administration*, Feb. 1984, 15–21; M. M. Timm, and M. G. Wavetik, "Matrix Organization: Design and Development for a Hospital Organization," *Hospital & Health Services Administration*, Nov./Dec. 1983, 46–58; American Organization of Nurse Executives, *Organizational Models for Nursing Practice* (Chicago: American Hospital Association, 1984).
54. Ibid.
55. Ibid.
56. B. Fuszard, " 'Adhocracy' in Health-Care Institutions," *Journal of Nursing Administration*, Jan. 1983, 14–19.
57. R. H. Guest, "Management Imperatives for the Year 2000," *California Management Review*, Summer 1986, 62–70.
58. P. F. Drucker, *Management: Tasks, Responsibilities, Practice*, (New York: Harper & Row, 1973), 564.
59. L. W. Porter and E. E. Lawler, III, "The Effects of 'Tall' Versus 'Flat' Organization Structure on Managerial Job Satisfaction," *Personnel Psychology*, Summer 1964, 135–148.
60. R. H. Guest, op. cit.
61. J. L. Gibson, J. M. Ivancevich, and J. H. Donnelly, Jr., op. cit., 491–493.
62. D. C. Pheysey, R. L. Payne, and D. S. Pugh, "Influence of Structure at Organizational and Group Levels," *Administrative Science Quarterly*, V. 16, 1971, 61–73.
63. R. C. Swansburg, op. cit., R. C. Swansburg, *Management of Patient Care Services* (St. Louis: Mosby, 1976).
64. P. E. Han, "The Informal Organization You've Got to Live With," *Supervisory Management*, Oct. 1983, 25–28.
65. K. Cameron, "A Study of Organizational Effectiveness and Its Predictors," *Management Science*, Jan. 1986, 87–112.
66. Ibid.
67. M. Beyers, "Getting On Top of Organizational Change: Part 3. The Corporate Nurse Executive," *Journal of Nursing Administration*, Dec. 1984, 32–37.

REFERENCES

American Nurses' Association, *Standards for Organized Nursing Services and Responsibilities of Nurse Administrators Across All Settings* (Kansas City, MO: American Nurses' Association, 1988).

American Nurses' Association, *Standards of Nursing Practice* (Kansas City, MO: American Nurses' Association, 1973–77).

Brown, D. S., "Shaping the Organization to Fit People," *Management of Personnel Quarterly*, Summer 1966.

Clegg, C. W. and T. D. Wall, "The Lateral Dimension to Employee Participation," *Journal of Management Studies*, Oct. 1984, 429–442.

Dennis, K. E., "Nursing's Power in the Organization: What Research Has Shown," *Nursing Administration Quarterly*, Fall 1983, 47–60.

Donovan, H. M., *Nursing Service Administration: Managing the Enterprise* (St. Louis: C. V. Mosby, 1975).

George, J. R. and L. K. Bishop, "Relationship of Organizational Structure and Teacher Personality Characteristics to Organizational Climate," *Administrative Science Quarterly*, 1971, 467–475.

Heilriegel, D. and J. W. Slocum, "Organizational Climate: Measures Research and Contingencies," *Academy of Management Journal*, June 1972, 255–280.

Hodgetts, R. M., *Management: Theory, Process, and Practice*, Academic Press 4th ed. (Orlando, FL: 1986), 138–231.

_____and R. L. Howe, *Workbook to Accompany Management, Theory, Process, and Practice* (Philadelphia: W. B. Saunders, 1975).

Kanter, R. M. and T. K. Seggerman, "Managing Mergers, Acquisitions and Divestitures," *Newsweek*, October 5 1987, S-14, S-16.

Jablin, F. M., "Formal Structural Characteristics of Organizations and Superior-Subordinate Communication," *Human Communication Research*, Summer 1982, 338–347.

Joyce, W. F. and J. Slocum, "Climate Discrepancy: Refining the Concepts of Psychological and Organizational Climate," *Human Relations* 11, 1982, 951–972.

Krampitz, S. D. and M. Williams, "Organizational Climates: A Measure of Faculty and Nurse Administrator Perception." *Journal of Nursing Education*, May 1983, 200–206.

Locke, E. A., D. M. Schweiger, and G. P. Latham, "Participation in Decision Making: When Should It Be Used?" *Organizational Dynamics*, Winter 1986, 65–79.

Mills, P. K. and B. Z. Posner, "The Relationships Among Self-Supervision, Structure, and Technology in Professional Service Organizations," *Academy of Management Journal*, June 1982, 437–443.

Payne, R. L. and R. Mansfield, "Relationships of Perceptions of Organizational Climate to Organizational Structure, Context, and Hierarchical Position," *Administrative Science Quarterly*, V. 18, 1973, 515–526.

Pritchard, R. D. and B. W. Karasick, "The Effects of Organizational Climate on Managerial Job Performance and Job Satisfaction," *Organizational Behavior and Human Performance* 9, 1973, 126–143.

Schneider, B. and D. T. Hall, "Toward Specifying the Concept of Work Climate: A Study of Roman Catholic Diocesan Priests," *Journal of Applied Psychology*, June 1972, 447–455.

Stevens, B. J., *First-Line Patient Care Management* (Wakefield, MA: Contemporary Publishing, 1976).

Swansburg, R. C., *Nurses and Patients: An Introduction to Nursing Management* (Hattiesburg, MS: Impact III, 1978).

Tushman, M. and D. Nadler, "Organizing for Innovation," *California Management Review*, Spring 1986, 74–92.

Committees

12

COMMITTEES DEFINED

A committee is a group form that evolves out of a formal organization structure. Committees are formed to make collective use of knowledge, skills, and ideas. They blend the good characteristics of several to many individuals, a reason for making careful appointments or selections. The principle of synergy underlies committee activity; putting the thinking power of a selected group together for the most effective outcome. What is the optimum number of people to produce the desired outcome of synergy? The answer is difficult and depends upon the goals to be addressed, the characteristics of committee members, and the environment within which they function. Aim for the best combination of skills and energies.[1]

COMMITTEES AS GROUPS

Because the work of organizations is accomplished by groups, many persons have studied the dynamics of group function. While all groups are not committees, the management of a group of employees in order to accomplish the objectives of an enterprise is similar to the leadership and management of a committee in order to accomplish selective objectives. Already in the 1920s researchers at the Harvard Business School found that worker morale and productivity were positively influenced by small, informal work groups.[2]

In the world of the nurse manager, work is performed by individuals and by groups. Primary nursing has become a much used modality or method of practicing nursing because it gives professional nurses more autonomy than other modalities. It adds accountability through continuous responsibility of nurses for patients from admission through discharge. Case management adds group dynamics to the autonomy, since the case manager is responsible for functioning in a collaborative practice with other professional nurses and physicians. Case management also uses managed care as a medium to keep the patient on the critical path from admission through discharge and can extend through the illness episode to include home care.

Committees are formal groups that can serve useful functions in the organizing process of nursing and organizational administration. In addition to being an organizational entity, committees are planned for and in turn make plans. They are directed by leaders appointed by management or elected by constituents as determined by management. Since professional nurses want autonomy but most are employed by organizations, formal groups, including committees, are a medium for promoting autonomy by giving them a voice in managing the organization. Their effectiveness can be controlled internally and externally. If committees do not serve a useful function they should be evaluated and restructured. When no longer needed they should be selectively abandoned.

There are usually two types of committees, *standing* and *ad hoc* or *special*. Standing committees are advisory in authority, although some may have collective authority to make and implement decisions. They have continuity as organizational entities. Ad hoc committees are formed to fulfill a specific purpose and are disbanded upon achievement of the purpose.

Stevens advocated the use of groups for management and stated that they can greatly increase productivity when used effectively. Nurse managers need to be able to function in groups for the purpose of promoting problem solving and acceptance of responsibility. The group can function within an administrative council and demonstrate being able to manage themselves by preparing agendas, reviewing status of agenda topics, obtaining and using learning aids, and handling meetings. In short, they should be able to structure the business of groups and direct and control the behavior of group members.[3]

Fuszard and Bishop use the term "adhocracy" to refer to the use of ad hoc committees in nursing organizations. They credit Toffler with origination of the term. Applying adhocracy to nursing, a group would be formed to accomplish a specified mission and it would then be dissolved. It could be called a task force, a project team, or an ad hoc committee. Team members would be those nurses with the special qualifications needed to accomplish the task.[4]

In nursing a project team would form around each patient,

each member chosen for special expertise relevant to the patient's unique needs. The team would exist as a group only for a single patient. Its members would solve problems, share expertise, make decisions, implement these decisions, and evaluate their effectiveness, using open systems feedback to monitor and modify the treatment plan. Once the project is completed and the patient discharged, the group of experts would disband to assume roles in other projects needing such expertise.[5]

Adhocracy is associated with primary nursing and case management. It makes all team members equal contributors to decision making. It is group decision making and is associated with the management processes of decentralization and participatory management presented in another chapter. The organizational form is that of the matrix schema in which leadership is fluid. Adhocracy implements an extensive system for communication and coordination for which every member is responsible. The primary purpose of all ad hoc committee meetings is communication.

Fuszard and Bishop conclude:

The operating adhocracy will meet the needs of individual patients and will also benefit professional employees. The nurse will be accountable to the patient, the project team, and the profession and will see the whole effect of professional accountability in assessment, planning, implementation, and evaluation. Nurses will perform nursing functions, rather than secretarial or supervisory functions. Using their professional expertise in interdisciplinary decision making and practicing as equals with other professionals, theirs will be a true professional role. The nursing administrator is in a unique position to help effect this change for the patients, nurses, and the institution.[6]

BENEFITS OF COMMITTEES

What are the benefits of committees? Committees can transmit useful information in two directions—toward administrators or managers and toward employees. They encourage and involve participation of interested or affected employees in the management of the nursing enterprise. Their advice can be helpful, and they can promote understanding of objectives and programs by other employees. They can promote loyalty. Some of the new ideas that keep nursing an open sociotechnical system come from committees. They provide face-to-face meeting of individuals for purposes of gathering information, seeking advice, decision making, negotiation, coordination, and creative thinking to resolve operational problems and improve the quality of services rendered by the organization.

Committees provide a pooling of people with specific skills and knowledge that can be assimilated into plans of action. They can bridge gaps between departments or units. They can use the pooled expertise of specialists and people with special talents and leadership abilities. They give people an opportunity to participate in the social process of group dynamics. They can help reduce resistance to change. Supervision, control, and discipline can be reduced through committee activities. Care quality can be improved, personnel turnover reduced, and harmony promoted through committee work.

All of the positive or beneficial outcomes of committees can be achieved if they are appropriately organized and led. Otherwise they can become liabilities to the organizing process. They can waste time and money; they can defer decisions or provide wrong information for the making of decisions; they can promote too many compromises and stagnation; they can be used to avoid decision making by administrators.

ORGANIZATION OF COMMITTEES

Every committee should have a purpose and short-range objectives and every standing committee should also have long-range objectives. Objectives need to be translated into plans of action with time frames and precise responsibility. Assignments should be given ahead of meeting times so they can be presented during these times. Committee chairs are accountable to a specific administrator who provides guidance to them through consultation. Composition of committees should be addressed to ensure appropriate choice of members for expertise and representativeness. They should be of manageable size for discussion and disagreement. They

should have prepared agendas and effective chairs. Figure 12–1 contains standards for evaluating nursing committees.

Nursing should be represented on most healthcare institution committees and always on those whose activities will affect nursing. They should have representation that will be effective in determining the outcomes of a health team approach to patient care services. In effect, nurses should determine how they will practice nursing. See Appendices 12–1 and 12–2.

GROUP DYNAMICS

Each member of a group plays a role in achieving the work of the group. Since each member has a unique personality and individual abilities, the group leader needs a knowledge of how groups function so as to facilitate their effectiveness. Original studies of group dynamics were done through observations of informal groups. The Hawthorne studies of 1924–1932 were conducted in four phases designed to discover what would make workers increase their output. Employees respond to

FIGURE 12–1. Standards for Evaluation of Nursing Committees

1. The committee has been established by appropriate authority: by laws, executive appointment, or other.
2. There are a stated purpose, objectives, and operational procedures for each committee.
3. There is a mechanism for consultation between chairs and persons to whom they report.
4. There is a published agenda for each committee meeting.
5. Committee members are surveyed beforehand to obtain agenda items including problems, plans, and sharing of news.
6. There is an effective chair for each committee.
7. Recorded minutes of each committee are used to evaluate its effectiveness in meeting stated objectives.
8. Committee membership is manageable and representative of the expertise needed and the people they affect.
9. Nurses are adequately represented on all appropriate institutional committees.

identification with groups and to the interpersonal relationships with members of small groups.

Group members perform task roles, group building and maintenance roles, and individual roles. They do this through interpersonal relationships. In the performance of these roles the group members share the power of the organization and its management.

Group Task Roles

Each member of a group performs a role related to the task of the group or committee. The purpose is to arrive cooperatively at a definition of and solution to a common problem.

Benne and Sheats identify twelve group task roles. Each may be performed by a group member or by the leader, and one person may perform several roles. These roles are:

1. Initiator-contributor—a group member who proposes or suggests new group goals or redefines the problem. This may take the form of new procedures or group restructuring. There may be more than one initiator-contributor functioning at different times within the group's lifetime.
2. Information seeker—a group member who seeks a factual basis for the group's work.
3. Opinion seeker—a group member who seeks opinions that reflect or clarify the values of other members' suggestions.
4. Information giver—a group member who gives an opinion indicating what the group's view of pertinent values should be.
5. Elaborator—a group member who suggests by example or extended meanings the reason for suggestions and how they could work.
6. Opinion giver—a group member who states personal beliefs pertinent to the group discussion.
7. Coordinator—a group member who clarifies and coordinates ideas, suggestions, and activities of the group members or subgroups.
8. Orienter—a group member who summarizes decisions or actions and identifies and questions differences from agreed-upon goals.
9. Evaluator-critic—a group member who questions group accomplishments and compares them to a standard.
10. Energizer—a group member who stimulates and prods the group to act and to raise the level of their actions.
11. Procedural technician—a group member who facilitates the group's action by arranging the environment.
12. Recorder. A group member who records the group's activities and accomplishments.[7]

Group Building and Maintenance Roles

Individual members of the group work to build and maintain group functioning. Again, each may be performed by a group member or by the leader and one person may perform several roles. The seven group-building roles are:

1. Encourager—a group member who accepts and praises the contributions, viewpoints, ideas, and suggestions of all group members with warmth and solidarity.
2. Harmonizer—a group member who mediates, harmonizes, and resolves conflicts.
3. Compromiser—a group member who yields his or her position in a conflict situation.
4. Gate-keeper and expediter—a group member who promotes open communication and facilitates participation to involve all group members.
5. Standard setter or ego ideal—a group member who expresses or applies standards to evaluate group processes.
6. Group observer and commentator—a group member who records the group process and uses it to provide feedback to the group.
7. Follower—a group member who accepts the group's ideas and listens to its discussion and decisions.[8]

Individual Roles

Group members also play roles to serve their individual needs. To keep individual roles from disrupting the group's activities in meeting their objectives, selected group members are frequently trained in group dynamics. This training is particularly important for the group leader. These individual roles are not suppressed but are managed by the leader and each other. These eight roles are:

1. Aggressor—a group member who expresses disapproval of the values or feelings of other members through attacks, jokes, or envy.

2. Blocker—a group member who persists in expressing negative points of view and resurrects dead issues.
3. Recognition-seeker—a group member who works to focus positive attention on himself or herself.
4. Self-confessor—a group member who uses the group setting as a forum for personal expression.
5. Playboy—a group member who remains uninvolved and demonstrates cynicism, nonchalance, or horseplay.
6. Dominator—a group member who attempts to dominate and manipulate the group.
7. Help-seeker—a group member who manipulates members to sympathize with expressions of personal insecurity, confusion, or self-deprecation.
8. Special interest pleader—a group member who cloaks personal prejudices or biases by ostensibly speaking for others.[9]

All groups roles were developed at the First National Training Laboratory in Group Development in 1947. Nurse managers with a working knowledge of group dynamics can use their knowledge to assemble groups. Such knowledge is important to the selection of chairs of committees, task forces, and other groups of clinical nurses. It is equally important to the selection of nurses for organizational committees, so that nursing will gain power and recognition for its contributions to the mission and objectives of the corporate entity.

Group training will give members awareness of the roles they play and opportunity to manage themselves to become more productive. Group training has evolved into a science that contributes to a theory of nursing practice and nursing management. Self-analysis or self-evaluation and development of sensitivity to others to make oneself productive within group settings is a part of these theories. Nurse managers benefit from training in group dynamics and may include it in a continuing staff development program for professional nurses. This can be done with actual role plays of group missions.

Phases of Groups

Groups have a natural history or development. The following are five generally accepted phases of groups:

1. *Forming or orientation phase*—This is a phase in which group members are discovering themselves. They want uniqueness: to belong while maintaining personal identity. They test each other for appropriate and acceptable behavior. It is the time to exchange information, discover ground rules, size each other up, determine fit.

When forming these groups the nurse manager will include experts, affected constituencies, people who will implement the solution, people with different problem-solving styles, and equal numbers of sensing/thinking and intuitive/feeling individuals. The group leader will develop the *explicit* norm of constructive conflict: disagreement, multiple definitions, minority opinions, devil's advocate, professional management, and a "group wins" psychology. *Implicit* norms are avoided as they bring bias to the group process through imposition of individual values and beliefs. The leader helps members fit into the group, providing structure, guidelines, and norms and making them comfortable.

2. *Conflict or storming phase*—During this phase group members jockey for position, control, and influence. There is leadership struggle and increased competition. The leader helps members through this phase, assisting with roles and assignments.

3. *Cohesion or norming phase*—Roles and norms are established with a move toward consensus and objectives. Members reach a common understanding of the true nature of the opportunity. They will diagnose the root cause of the problem, the deviation from expected performance. They will be open to alternative definitions with multiple views. Morale and trust improve and the negative is suppressed. The leader guides and directs as needed.

4. *Working or performing phase*—Members work with deeper involvement, greater disclosure, and unity. They complete the work. The leader may intervene as needed.

5. *Termination phase*—Once goals are fulfilled the group terminates. The leader guides the members to summarize discussions, express feelings, and make closing statements. There is reluctance to break up. A celebration can help.[10]

FIGURE 12–2. Delphi Technique, Round One

	Desirability			Feasibility			Timing probability (year by which probable event will have occurred)		
	High	Average	Low	High	Likely	Unlikely	10%	50%	90%
1. Case management will become dominant in nursing in a majority of hospitals.									
2. A majority of hospitals will have unbundled the hospital bill to cost and charge nursing services.									

SOURCE: Adapted from: R. M. Hodgetts, *Management: Theory, Process and Practice,* 4th ed., Orlando, FL; Academic Press, 1986, 296.

Selected Group Techniques

A number of group techniques have been developed to make groups effective and productive. Among these are the Delphi technique, brainstorming, and the nominal group technique.

The Delphi Technique. Originally developed by the Rand Corporation as a technological forecasting technique, the Delphi technique pools the opinions of experts. This technique can be used in nursing management to pool the opinions of a group of leaders in the field. There are three phases of each round of questioning. For example, the group is polled for input; the inputs are analyzed, clarified, and codified by the investigator and given as feedback to the experts; and the experts are polled for further commentary on the composite of the first round. This process can continue for three to five rounds. See Figure 12–2 for an example of a format for Round one of a nursing management Delphi technique.[11]

Members of a group using the Delphi technique may never meet personally. Most of the activities are done through correspondence.

Brainstorming. As a group technique brainstorming seeks to develop creativity by free initiation of ideas. The object is to elicit as many ideas as possible. Steps in the brainstorming technique are:

1. The leader instructs the group, giving them the topic or problem and telling them to respond positively with any idea or suggestion they have relative to it. No critical responses are allowed or discussed.
2. The leader or chair lists all ideas or responses on a poster or chalkboard as they are given and encourages their generation.
3. Ideas are evaluated only after every group member has contributed all possible ones.

One variation on brainstorming, the Gordon technique, keeps the subject area general to elicit more ideas. Success depends upon the skills of the group leader. A second variation of brainstorming is the Phillips 66 buzz session used for large groups. The large group is broken down into smaller groups of six members. Each conducts a brainstorming session for six minutes and then reports to the large group.[12]

The Nominal Group Technique. In this technique, the problem or task is defined. Members independently write down ideas about it, making their ideas more problem-centered and of higher quality. Each member presents ideas to the group without discussion. The ideas are summarized and listed. Next the members discuss each recorded idea to clarify and evaluate it. They then vote on and give priority to each decision. The results are averaged and the final group decision is taken from the pool. The process takes about 1½ to 2 hours and results in a sense of accomplishment and closure.[13]

Group Leaders

Group leaders may be formal, informal, or specialized. Formal leaders are appointed by management or elected by management directives and carry line authority or power to discipline and control group members. Informal leaders emerge from the group process. Their influence inspires cooperation and mediation and group members reach consensus about their contributions to effective functioning in quest of goals. Specialized leaders are often temporary leaders who have a special skill or ability needed by the group at a particular point in time.

Participatory management requires alignment for individuals to work toward shared goals as well as profitability. A dynamic leader inspires people to put spirit into working for a shared goal. The leader can use symbols, posters, slogans, T-shirts, and memorable events. The leader must believe in people and support McGregor's Theory Y that espouses self-direction, self-control, commitment, responsibility, imagination, ingenuity, creativity, and effort. How the leader behaves toward peer group members will exhibit these beliefs.[14] Leaders can make committees and meetings effective by having an extensive knowledge of group dynamics. They will keep the group on course by convincing each member of the genuine need for input and personal sensitivity to group processes. They will draw in the shy and the quiet. They will politely cut off the garrulous and protect the weak. While controlling the squashing reflex in themselves, they will encourage a clash of ideas by mediating domination by cliques. They will refrain from being judgmental. Being a group leader requires a thinking, skilled performance based on knowledge and ability acquired through management education and training.[15]

MAKING COMMITTEES EFFECTIVE

Purposes of Committees

Organizations, through their meetings, promote communication. In one year the cost of meetings in U.S. companies is several billions of dollars and executives spend as much as 60 percent of their time in them. For this reason nurse managers should evaluate the purposes and functions of committees, particularly of standing committees. Evaluation should be both normative and summative and should determine whether committees are accomplishing their purpose or are wasting the time and talents of the many people who are required to attend their meetings. Are unnecessary meetings being held?

Meetings fulfill deep personal and individual needs. Their effective use by groups improves productivity. Types of committees are determined by organizational objectives and functions. Committees can be effectively used to implement major policy changes, to accomplish a job, and to plan strategically. Problems requiring research and planning are better assigned to individuals. Day-to-day decisions should be handled by line managers.[16]

A major purpose of using committees is to involve personnel in participatory management that gives representation of employees at all levels a share in the decision-making process. According to Dixon this goal can be accomplished by having:

1. Enough groups to ensure representation at all levels.
2. Standing committees, ad hoc committees, town hall meetings, and small meetings, so that all levels feel represented.
3. Visible representation by managers to ensure support.
4. Control of employees.
5. Planned absence of managers at selective meetings to encourage discussion.
6. Stimuli to employee participation; tangible results.
7. Members solicited as volunteers, appointed by managers, or selected by employees.
8. Technical assistance to identify problems, promote hearing, and solve problems.

9. A focus on the power of the group to act on its own recommendations, have its own budget, or access company resources.[17]

American health-care organizations are confronted with a hostile and turbulent environment of expanded demands, inflation, competition, shortages of professional nurses, and intrusion by other groups. Professional nurses are more highly educated with higher expectations for extrinsic reward and intrinsic satisfiers such as autonomy and challenge. They want to participate to impact organizational performance and employee satisfaction positively.

Morhman and Ledford's recommendation for successful employee participation can be used by nurse managers. Success depends upon design and implementation of the participation group process. Participation groups are designed to:

1. Be effective in group problem solving.
2. Be effective within the larger organization as well as within the division or unit of nursing. This can be expanded to include appropriate professional and service organizations.
3. Achieve legitimacy.
4. Acquire resources and approval for their ideas.
5. Motivate others in the organization to accept, implement, and support their group solution.[18]

Advantages of Committees

In addition to participation in decision making, committees allow for group deliberations and coordination. Research comparing two groups of interviews in a public employment agency has shown that the more competitive the group, the less productive it is. On the other hand, the more competitive the individuals in the more competitive group, the more productive they are. A cohesive group reduces anxiety, curbs competitive tendencies, fosters friendly personal relations, and makes the group more productive. Personnel ratings that focus upon production records increase anxiety and decrease cohesiveness and productivity. Supervisors who decrease employee anxiety and increase employee cohesiveness will increase efficiency and productivity. This model could be used in nursing management research on group effect on productivity.[19]

Another advantage of committees is their use as a medium of communication. They should not, however, supplant personal executive action, written communications, individual and conference telephone calls, audio tapes, closed-circuit television, and other techniques.

In addition, meetings provide an opportunity for managers to relate to employees. They bring a collective variety of inputs and a depth of knowledge to make quality decisions. Meetings bring together people who advance more approaches to a problem. They blend concrete experiences, reflective observations, active experiments, and abstract conceptualization. Through group dynamics, committees increase acceptance of solutions and commitment to implementation of their decisions. Also, groups take risks.[20]

Disadvantages of Committees

Committees can waste time. Attendees become cynical, often benefitting more from the recreational than the educational aspects of meetings. Committees do not always use the organization's own experience in a meaningful way. This can be remedied by using organizational personnel and events as part of the program.[21]

Participants complain that committee meetings and conferences do not allow enough individual input, lead to compromise, are expensive, sometimes have weak leaders who are dominated by other members, and act as substitutes for weak executives who cannot make decisions.

If not trained, committee participants may arrive at premature decisions, especially ones that are popular with a majority of members. They may not change decisions when better approaches are found. Without trained leadership they can be dominated by one person and suffer from disruptive conflicts tormented by individuals who must win at all costs.[22]

Improving Committee Effectiveness

Nurse managers can improve the effectiveness of standing and ad hoc committees by establishing minimal ground rules, including:

1. Establish clearly stated objectives. For ad hoc or specialized meetings, discuss the goals before planning the meeting. Base the goals on advanc-

ing the clinical and business goals of nursing (see Appendices 12–1 and 12–2.)

2. Establish a committee structure to support the clearly stated objectives (see Figure 12–3).

3. Plan all meetings and events to meet the goals and objectives.

   3.1 Keep the committee or event to a manageable size. Define membership. *Assemblies* begin at one hundred and increase in size. They see and hear. *Councils* may be forty to fifty persons who listen or comment. *Committees* should include around ten to twelve people who all participate on an equal footing.

   3.2 Draw up a point-by-point agenda and send it to the attendees. Include the purpose of the meeting. Since the sequence of the agenda is important, the following points are helpful:

      3.2.1 Put dull items early and "star" items last.

      3.2.2 Decide whether to place divisive items early or late.

      3.2.3 Plan a time for starting important items.

      3.2.4 Limit committee meetings to two hours or less.

      3.2.5 Schedule meetings to begin one hour before lunch or one hour before the end of work day.

      3.2.6 Avoid extraneous business on the agenda.

      3.2.7 Read the agenda and write in comments before the meeting.

   3.3 Tailor the meeting room to the group and prepare it beforehand.

   3.4 Prepare for the meeting by learning the subject matter and preparing audiovisual materials to support it. Bring input from people who do not attend via videotaped interviews. Make events memorable.

   3.5 Time the agenda items. New or controversial subjects usually take more time. Attention spans diminish after the first hour. Use time efficiently, including mealtimes.

   3.6 Referee and set the pace of the meeting. Summarize and clarify as needed.

   3.7 Promote lively participation by involving attendees in the program with a warm-up "getting acquainted" phase, a conflict phase, and a total collaboration phase.

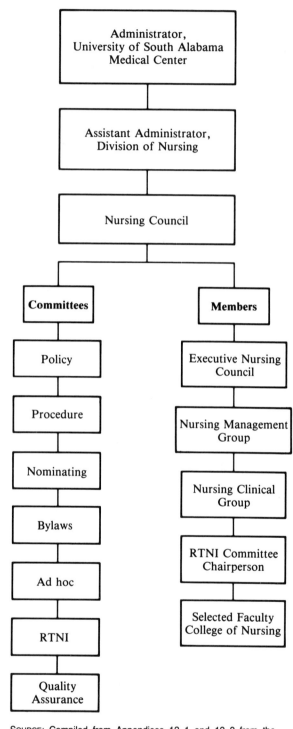

FIGURE 12–3. Committee Structure

SOURCE: Compiled from Appendices 12–1 and 12–2 from the University of South Alabama Medical Center, Mobile, Alabama.

Bring out the personal goals of the individuals.

3.8 Listen to what others say so there will be a sharing of knowledge, experience, judgments, and folklore.

3.9 Bring the meeting to a definite conclusion by obtaining decisions and obtaining commitments.

3.10 Follow up as necessary to eliminate loose ends. Evaluate whether the meeting's purpose was achieved.

3.11 Circulate useful information with the minutes. Keep them brief, listing time, date, place, chair, attendance, agenda items and action, time ended, and the time, date, and place of the next meeting.[23]

A meeting should never be held without a solid reason and an interesting subject on which the attendees will exchange ideas. This subject should meet the needs of the attendees. Leaders of meetings should know how to make them successful. This includes good preparation and a thorough knowledge of the subject area. Useful knowledge is desired by most people. Prepare the meeting place and check to see that directions for setting up facilities are carried out. Everything should be in readiness. In running the meeting, make registration painless and quick and provide identification for the attendees, if needed. Start on time and allow the leader to lead. Meetings should be geared to participants and discussion groups should be kept to small numbers. Discussions should be controlled but lively. Long meetings should have frequent breaks for coffee and stretching. Hold to the schedule. Meetings require critical follow-up review with evaluation by participants as well as those who contributed to planning the meeting. The latter should be thanked in writing. Promised materials should go to the attendees promptly.

GROUPTHINK

Groupthink is inappropriate conformity to group norms. It occurs when group members fail to take risks by disagreeing, by being challenged, or by carefully assessing the points under discussion. The symptoms of groupthink are:

1. Illusions of invulnerability, leading to overconfidence and reckless risk taking.
2. Negative feedback ignored and rationalized to prevent reconsideration.
3. A belief of inherent morality.
4. Stereotyping of the views of people who disagree as wrong or weak and badly informed.
5. Pressure on members to suppress doubts.
6. Self-censorship by silence about misgivings.
7. Unanimous decisions.
8. Protection of members from negative reactions.[24]

Groupthink will not occur when members are aware of its potential. Groups are considered effective when their resources are well used; their time is well used; their decisions are appropriate, reasonable, and error-free; their decisions are implemented and supported by group members; problem-solving ability is enhanced; and group cohesion is built by promoting group norms and structuring cooperative relationships. Teach group members cures for groupthink that include:

1. Acting as a devil's advocate.
2. Considering unlimited alternatives.
3. Thinking critically.
4. Providing increased time.
5. Changing directions.
6. Surveying people affected by the problem under discussion.
7. Seeking other opinions.
8. Constructively challenging group measures.
9. Including people who do not agree with you.[25]

QUALITY CIRCLES

Quality circles are a participatory management technique employing the use of statistical analyses of activities to maintain quality products. The technique was initiated in Japan through the teaching of Dr. Edward Deming, an American, after World War II. The concept is to use statistical analysis to make quality improvements. Workers are taught the statistical concepts and use them through trained, organized, structured groups of four to fifteen employees called *quality circles*. Group members share common interests and problems and meet on a regular basis, usually an hour a week. They represent other employees from whom they gather and bring information to the meetings.[26]

The quality circle process has become widespread in Japan, raising the quality of Japanese manufacturing to worldwide eminence. It involves workers in the decision-making process. Quality circles have spread to major manufacturing companies and to some health-care institutions in the United States.

Quality circles are similar to other elements of participatory management. Employees are trained to identify, analyze, and solve problems. Involved in the process, they make solutions work because they identify with ownership. From being recognized they develop good will towards their employees.

Quality circles are effective when facilitators, leaders, and members are trained in group dynamics and quality circle techniques. Leaders act as peers to generate ideas for operational improvements and problem elimination. In the process all quality circle members reach consensus before decisions are recommended or implemented. Training occurs during regular quality circle meetings and continues during subsequent meetings.[27]

Because quality circles contribute to the knowledge base of human behavior and motivation, the process is important to the development of nursing management theory. This theory will be learned and used by nurse managers concerned with developing job satisfaction of professional nurses to deliver quality nursing care. The objects of quality circles are participation, involvement, recognition, and self-actualization among clinical nurses caring for patients.

Quality circles should meet successful group design guidelines, including:

1. Participation groups must include or have access to the necessary skills and knowledge to address problems systematically. All actors in the process need training. Support people participate only as needed.
2. Formalized procedures enhance the effectiveness of the group. Systematic records should be kept and the formal schedules of meetings adhered to.
3. Participation groups are integrated horizontally and vertically with the rest of the organization to promote communication. Accomplishments are publicized through award dinners and publicity in in-house newspapers. Organized higher-level support groups hear the ideas of lower-level groups. All are limited by usual formal and informal communication mechanisms and routes.
4. Groups are a regular part of the organization and not a special or extra activity. They are composed of members of natural work groups. Results are measured in terms of ongoing organizational objectives and goals.
5. Normal accountability processes operate, using the same skills, habits, and expectations as general organizations.
6. Groups manage themselves and are assisted by leaders and facilitators who are peer group members.
7. Participation occurs in such areas as decisions about job enrichment; hiring; training in problem solving skills, management skills, and business conditions; pay based on skill mastery; gain sharing; and union-management relationships based on mutual interests.[28]

Research indicates that productivity and morale are strongly improved when employees participate in decision making and in planning for change. It is important that participation include goal setting as participation will lead to higher goals and higher levels of acceptance and performance. This research has been supported by meta-analysis. Research also shows that highly nonparticipatory jobs cause psychological and physical harm. *It is an ethical imperative to prevent harm by enabling employees to participate in work decisions.* Mental health is positively influenced by feelings of interest, a sense of accomplishment, personal growth, and self-respect.[29] Nurse managers will use this knowledge in managing clinical professional nurses.

Participation in manager selection by nursing staff increases their support, management knowledge and skills, and ability to write resumes and prepare for interviews. It increases management's knowledge of the nursing staff. It reduces conflict and favoritism and increases the chances of the new manager's power. Such participation by nursing staff can be stressful to managing candidates and it is time-consuming.[30]

SUMMARY

Synergy, putting the thinking power of a selected group together for the most effective outcome, defines a committee's primary function. Committees provide employees a representative voice in the management of organizations.

A standing committee has continuity as an organizational entity, while an ad hoc committee is formed for a purpose and disbanded when that purpose is fulfilled.

"Adhocracy" is a system in which project teams exist for a single purpose and disbands when their purpose is accomplished.

Committees can facilitate communication, promote loyalty, pool special human resources, reduce resistance to change, and give people opportunities to work together. They should have purposes, objectives, and operational procedures.

Chairs of committees need knowledge and skills of group dynamics. This can be provided through staff development programs and to all nurses desiring it.

Groups work in five phases:

1. Forming or orientation phase.
2. Conflict or storming phase.
3. Cohesion or norming phase.
4. Working or performing phase.
5. Termination phase.

Group techniques include the Delphi Technique, brainstorming, and the nominal group technique among others. Group leaders are either appointed (formal leaders) or emerge from the group (informal leaders).

Committees can waste time if they make a premature decision or do not accomplish their objectives. They can be made effective by application of the management functions of planning, organizing, directing (leading), and controlling (evaluating).

Groupthink, in which the entire committee conforms to group norms, should be prevented through training in group processes.

Quality circles have emerged as a participatory management technique using statistical analysis of activities to maintain quality products. Quality circles have the characteristics of groups and use group dynamics but are a regular part of the organization whose members are mature work groups.

Committees can lead to improved productivity.

NOTES

1. R. M. Fulmer and S. G. Franklin, *Supervision: Principles of Professional Management* (2d. ed. New York: Macmillan, 1982), 246–247.
2. E. Mayo, *The Human Problems of Industrial Civilization* (Boston: Harvard Business School, 1946).
3. B. J. Stevens, "Use of Groups for Management," *Journal of Nursing Administration*, Jan. 1975, 14–22.
4. B. Fuszard and J. K. Bishop, " 'Adhocracy' in Health-Care Institutions," in B. Fuszard, *Self-Actualization for Nurses* (Rockville, MD: Aspen, 1984), 90–99.
5. Ibid., 92.
6. Ibid., 99.
7. K. D. Benne and P. Sheats, "Functional Roles of Group Members," *Journal of Social Studies*, Winter 1948.
8. Ibid.
9. Ibid.
10. L. L. Northouse and P. G. Northouse, *Health Communication: A Handbook for Health Professionals* (Englewood Cliffs, NJ: Prentice-Hall, 1985); H. J. Brightman and P. Verhowen, "Running Successful Problem-Solving Groups," *Business*, Apr.-June 1986, 15–23.
11. R. M. Hodgetts, *Management: Theory, Process and Practice*, 4th ed. (Orlando, FL: Academic Press, 1986), 294–300.
12. R. M. Fulmer, and S. G. Franklin, op. cit., 59.
13. Northouse and Northouse, op. cit., 240–241.
14. N. Dixon, "Participative Management: It's Not as Simple as It Seems," *Supervisory Management*, Dec. 1984, 2–8.
15. L. Caramanica, "What? Another Committee?" *Nursing Management*, Sept. 1984, 12–14; A. Jay, "How to Run a Meeting," *Journal of Nursing Administration*, Jan. 1982, 22–28.
16. B. J. Stevens, op. cit.
17. N. Dixon, op. cit.
18. S. A. Morhman and G. E. Ledford, Jr., "The Design and Use of Effective Employee Participation Groups: Implication for Human Resource Management," *Human Resource Management*, Winter 1985, 413–428.
19. P. M. Blau, "Cooperation and Competition in a Bureaucracy," *The American Journal of Sociology*, May 1984, 530–535.
20. R. L. Veninga, "Benefits and Costs of Group Meetings," *The Journal of Nursing Administration*, June 1984, 42–46.
21. R. M. Kanter, "Toward the World's Best Corporate Conference," *Management Review*, May 1986, 7–9.
22. R. L. Veninga, op. cit.
23. A. Jay, op. cit.; B. Y. Auger, "How to Run an Effective Meeting," *Commerce*, Oct. 1967; R. C. Swansburg, *Management of Patient Care Services* (St. Louis: Mosby, 1976) 270–273; R. M. Kanter, op. cit.; B. J. Stevens, op. cit.; B. J. Stevens, *The Nurse as Executive*, 2d ed. (Wakefield, MA: Nursing Resources, 1980); H. S. Rowland and B. L. Rowland, Eds., *Nursing Administration Handbook*, 2d ed. (Rockville, MD: Aspen, 1985) 39–40.

24. E. H. Rosenblum, "Groupthink: The Peril of Group Cohesiveness," *Journal of Nursing Administration*, Apr. 1982, 27–31; H. S. Rowland and B. L. Rowland, op. cit.; M. Leo, "Avoiding the Pitfalls of Management Think," *Business Horizons*, May-June 1984, 44–47.

25. Ibid.

26. The theory of quality circles was actually developed by Frederick Herzberg and E. Edwards Deming of the United States approximately 50 years ago. S. Johnson, "Quality Control Circles: Negotiating an Efficient Work Environment," *Nursing Management*, July 1985, 35A–34B, 34D–34G; A. M. Goldberg and C. C. Pegels, *Quality Circles in Health-Care Facilities* (Rockville, MD: Aspen, 1984).

27. Ibid.

28. S. A. Morhman and G. E. Ledford, Jr., op. cit.

29. M. Sashkin, "Participative Management Remains an Ethical Imperative," *Organizational Dynamics*, Spring 1986, 62–75.

30. N. Ertl, "Choosing Successful Managers: Participative Selection Can Help," *Journal of Nursing Administration*, Apr. 1984, 27–33.

REFERENCES

Baker, K. G., "Application of a Group Theory in Nursing Practice," *Supervisor Nurse*, Mar. 1980, 22–24.

Ganong, W. L. and J. M. Ganong, "Reducing Organizational Conflict Through Working Committees," *Journal of Nursing Administration*, Jan.-Feb. 1972, 12–19.

Golde, R. A., "Are Your Meetings Like This One?," *Harvard Business Review*, Jan.-Feb. 1972, 68–77.

Leebov, W., "Problems, Plans, and Sharing: A Format for Productive Meetings," *Supervisory Management*, June 1984, 35–37.

Llewelyn, S. and G. Fielding, "Forming, Storming, Norming, and Performing," *Nursing Mirror*, July 21, 1982, 14–16.

Llewelyn, S. and G. Fielding, "Under the Influence," *Nursing Mirror*, July 28, 1982, 37–39.

Roberts, V., "The Head Nurse Meeting: Who, What, When, and Where," *Nursing Management*, Aug. 1985, 10, 12.

Rubin, I. M., R. E. Fry, and M. S. Plovnick, *Managing Human Resources in Health-Care Organizations* (Reston, VA: Reston Publishing). 1978.

Swansburg, R. C., *The Organizing Function of Nursing Service Administration* (Hattiesburg, MS: University of Southern Mississippi School of Nursing, 1977).

Webber, J. B. and M. A. Dula, "Effective Planning Committees for Hospitals," *Harvard Business Review*, May-June 1974, 133–142.

APPENDIX 12–1.   Organizational Functions and Entities Nursing Division

1. ASSISTANT ADMINISTRATOR FOR NURSING
   A. Nursing Division
      1. Associate Assistant Administrator for Nursing
         1.1 Directors of Nursing Evenings and Nights
         1.2 Nurse Epidemiologist
         1.3 Clinical Nurse Specialists
         1.4 Staff Development
         1.5 Nursing Service Float Pool
         1.6 Nursing Service Quality Assurance Program
      2. Nursing Departments
         1. Associate Assistant Administrator of Nursing for Special Services
            1.1 Supervisor, Operating Room
               1.11 Head Nurse, Operating Room
            1.2 Supervisor, Emergency Department
               1.21 Head Nurse, Emergency Department
            1.3 Supervisor, CCU/MICU
            1.4 Supervisor, SICU/NTICU
            1.5 Head Nurse, Burn Center
            1.6 Head Nurse, Post Anesthesia Recovery/Emergency Admit Unit/Outpatient Surgery
         2. Director of Nursing for Medical/Surgical Units
            2.1 Head Nurse, 5 North
            2.2 Head Nurse, 5 South
            2.3 Head Nurse, 6th. Floor
            2.4 Head Nurse, 8th. Floor

APPENDIX 12–1. Organizational Functions and Entities Nursing Division (*continued*)

      2.5 Head Nurse, Clinical Research Unit

      2.6 Head Nurse, 9th. Floor

    3. Director of Nursing for Maternal Child Units

      3.1 Supervisor, NICU/PICU

         3.11 Head Nurse, NICU

         3.12 Head Nurse, PICU

      3.2 Head Nurse, Newborn Nursery and Intermediate Nursery

      3.3 Head Nurse, Pediatrics

      3.4 Head Nurse, OB/GYN

      3.5 Head Nurse, Labor & Delivery

    4. Director of Nursing for Community/Mental Health

      4.1 Head Nurse, 7th. Floor

    5. Director of Computerization, Staffing/Special Projects

2. The organizational functions of the division are:

  2.1 Assistant Administrator is responsible to the Hospital Administrator for administering all Nursing Service functions of the University of South Alabama Medical Center.

    2.1.1 Associate Assistant Administrator for Nursing is responsible to the Assistant Administrator for assigned duties and responsibilities of the Assistant Administrator.

      2.1.1.1 Directors of Nursing, Evenings and Nights are responsible for direction of patient care. Perform primary nursing care, technical and consultative services to meet the needs of selected patients who present extremely complex, variable and unstable physiological, psychological, and sociological problems. Participate in inservice of employees, make administrative decisions for hospital in absence of Administrator or Assistant Administrator, and participate in nursing research.

      2.1.1.2 Employee Health Nurse is responsible for management of employee health care to include pre-employment interviews; coordinate annual employee physical exams, assist in evaluating employee injury and illness and visitor injury. Also, functions in liaison with the Nurse Epidemiologist.

      2.1.1.3 Nurse Epidemiologist has the responsibility of supervising the multiple facets of the infection control program in the institution. She is the liaison agent among all departments and the Infection Control Committee.

      2.1.1.4 Clinical Nurse Specialists are professional nurses academically prepared at the master's level with advanced knowledge and competence, capable of exercising highly discriminative judgement in planning, executing and evaluating nursing care based upon assessed needs of patients having one or more common clinical manifestations. They are able to provide expert nursing care and treatment on the basis of scientific knowledge, clinical acumen and professional judgment. They serve as consultants or technical advisors in their clinical specialities to colleagues in nursing, medicine and other health professionals. They conduct and participate in research.

      2.1.1.5 The Director of Nursing for Staff Development is responsible to plan, organize, direct, coordinate and evaluate the staff education program of the nursing service division. He/she provides leadership and management to include program planning, orientation, skill training, and continuing education to nursing service employees with the purpose of improving the care of patients.

        2.1.1.5.1 Clinical Consultants are responsible to the Director for identifying learning needs of division personnel and for planning, coordinating, presenting, directing and evaluating programs to meet these needs.

    2.1.2 Associate Assistant Administrator of Nursing for Special Services and Directors of Nursing are responsible to the Assistant Administrator for administering their units for 24-hour periods. The Associate Assistant Administrator for Special Services will also assume the duties and responsibilities of Assistant Administrator and Administrative Associate Assistant Administrator in their absence.

(*continued*)

APPENDIX 12–1.　Organizational Functions and Entities Nursing Division (*continued*)

Perform primary nursing, care, technical and consultative services to meet the needs of selected patients who present extremely complex, variable and unstable physiological, psychological and sociological problems. Teach in orientation programs, unit staff development programs, and may do clinical teaching in highly complex undergraduate education programs in biological, physical and social sciences. Participate in nursing research.

2.1.2.1 Supervisors and Head Nurses are responsible to the Associate Assistant Administrator for Special Services and the directors for managing all personnel and functions of their respective units on a 24 hour basis.

2.1.3 Secretarial staff are responsible to the Assistant Administrator and provide secretarial support service to the Division of Nursing.

Executive Nursing Council

1. Functions
   1.1 Provide counsel and assistance to the Assistant Administrator in all matters and activities of concern to the division.
   1.2 Assist the Assistant Administrator in identifying and solving problems which influence the effectiveness of the division in achieving its objectives.
   1.3 Strive to build a healthy hospital climate in which employees can work.
   1.4 Set standards and develop policies for the Division of Nursing.
   1.5 Provide a medium for the interchange of ideas and dissemination of information and materials relative to Nursing Service Administration.
   1.6 Identify and define health care issues that effect nursing and establish position statements on these issues.
   1.7 Foster cohesive inter-department relationships.
2. Members
   Assistant Administrator, Associate Assistant Administrators for Nursing, Directors of Nursing, Dean, College of Nursing, Chairman of Nursing Council.
3. Officers
   3.1 Chairman, Vice-Chairman and Secretary
      3.1.1 All officers shall be elected in October of each year and shall serve a one year term.
   3.2 Officers together with the Assistant Administrator shall constitute a Governing Board.
4. Duties of Officers
   4.1 The Chairman shall work closely with the Assistant Administrator and members of the Nursing Council Committee to evaluate systems and methods of nursing management and solve problems which influence the effectiveness of the Division.
   4.2 The Vice-Chairman shall assume duties of the Chairman in his/her absence.
   4.3 Secretary shall record minutes and distribute to members.
5. Meetings
   5.1 Regular meetings shall be held at 7:30 A.M. and 3:30 P.M. alternating on Thursday of each week.
   5.2 Special meetings may be called by the Chairman or Assistant Administrator.
6. Quorum
   A quorum of the Executive Council shall be the majority of the membership.
7. Inter-Department Committees
   7.1 Nursing personnel serve on other hospital committees as appointed by the Administrator or Assistant Administrator.
   7.2 List of Committees
      Medical Records/Utilization Review
      P & T Committee

APPENDIX 12–1. Organizational Functions and Entities Nursing Division (*continued*)

CPR Committee
Nutrition Committee
Safety Committee
Product Evaluation Committee
Disaster Committee
Critical Care Committee
Infection Control Committee
O.R. Committee
Quality Assurance Committee
Blood Transfusion Committee
Radiation Safety Committee
Emergency Department Committee
Tissue Review Committee
Cancer Coordinating Committee
Hospital Policy Committee

Bylaws, Nursing Council

Article I, Name
1.1 The name of this Committee shall be the Nursing Council.

Article II
The Purpose of this Council shall be:
2.1 To ensure excellence in nursing care which will return the patient to his best possible state of health or will enable him to die with dignity.
2.2 To provide a climate which will promote and support the practice of professional nursing.
2.3 To provide a forum for the discussion of management and patient care concerns.

The Function of this Council shall be:
2.4 To ensure excellence in nursing care.
    a. Through the development, implementation and evaluation of tools that measure the quality of nursing care.
    b. Through the development of nursing policies and procedures and the subsequent recommendation to Executive Council.
2.5 To develop nursing service employees to their fullest potential.
    a. Through the provision of a professional climate where the nurse participates in a collaborative relationship with physicians and other health care professionals and is seen as the coordinator of the patient's care.
    b. Through the development and implementation of continuing education programs and a clinical career ladder.
    c. Through the development of policies and procedures and the subsequent recommendation to Executive Council for approval.
2.6 Seek methods to improve communication within the department of nursing and with other departments of the hospital.
2.7 Identify methods of improving management practices to operate within the framework of the budget through proper utilization of personnel and supplies.

Article III, Members
The members of this Council shall be:

3.1 Nursing Management Group, all members of the Executive Council, Nursing Clinical Group, and the Chairman of the RTN I Committee.

(continued)

APPENDIX 12–1. Organizational Functions and Entities Nursing Division (*continued*)

3.2 Associate Dean, Chairman of the Departments of Medical/Surgical Nursing, Community Health, Mental Health and Maternal-Child Nursing in the USA School of Nursing.

Article IV, Officers

The officers shall consist of:

4.1 Chairman, Vice-Chairman and Parliamentarian

    a. All officers shall be elected by secret ballot.

    b. A majority of votes cast will be required to be elected.

    c. In the event a majority of votes is not achieved by the first ballot, a run-off between two candidates having the most votes shall be required.

    d. Ballots shall be counted by Administrative Secretary and the RTN I Committee representative.

    e. Officers shall serve for one year and are eligible for re-election for one consecutive term.

4.2 Officers together with the Assistant Administrator for Nursing shall constitute a Governing Board.

4.3 In the event of a vacancy

    a. The Vice-Chairman replaces the Chairman.

    b. The Parliamentarian shall replace Vice-Chairman.

    c. The new Parliamentarian will be appointed by the governing body.

4.4 Duties of the Officers

    a. The Chairman shall work closely with the other officers of the council. The Chairman and other officers shall meet one week prior to each regular meeting for the purpose of developing and distributing the agenda and establishing time limits for discussion. The Chairman is responsible to the Council for the smooth and effective functioning of its committees. The Chairman is a voting member of the Executive Council and is responsible to the Council for communicating recommendations to Executive Council and is responsible to the Council for communicating recommendations to Executive Council. The Chairman shall function according to the guidelines established in Roberts Rules of Order.

    b. The Vice-Chairman shall assume the duties of the Chairman in his absence and shall serve as Chairman of the nominating committee.

    c. The Parliamentarian shall oversee that the business of Nursing Council is conducted according to Roberts Rules of Order.

4.5 Qualifications for office—Must be members of Nursing Council.

Article V, Meetings

5.1 Regular meetings shall be held quarterly.

5.2 The annual meeting shall be held in November at which time annual reports of officers and chairman shall be read and officers elected.

5.3 Special meetings shall be called by the Chairman. The purpose of the meeting shall be stated in the call and at least 2 days notice will be given.

Article VI, Quorum

A quorum of the Council shall be a majority of the membership. The presence of a quorum shall be documented in the minutes.

Article VII, Committees

7.1 Policy Committee

    a. Purpose—To establish guidelines or policies for personnel of the Nursing Service Department which delineate responsibility and prescribe the action to be taken under a given set of circumstances. To periodically appraise policies followed by nurses if indicated. To develop new policies to meet present and future needs and to recommend necessary revision of policy.

APPENDIX 12–1. Organizational Functions and Entities Nursing Division (*continued*)

  b. Membership
    1. Representatives and alternates shall be elected from each Head Nurse Group (1), Staff Development (1), Clinical Group (1), and Executive Council (1), to serve a two year term beginning December 1 of each year. Each representative may be reappointed for one consecutive term.
    2. The representative or an alternate is expected to attend all meetings.
    3. A member shall be elected from the RTN I Committee. This term shall begin December 1 and this representative is eligible for a one year term only.
  c. Meetings
    1. The Policy Committee shall meet at least twice monthly.
    2. The time, date and place of meetings shall be determined by the chairman.
    3. Minutes of the meeting shall be recorded and kept on file in Nursing Service.
    4. The chairman of this committee shall be elected by its membership.
  d. Duties
    1. To accept written recommendations from an individual or committee regarding the need for a policy.
    2. To identify independently the need for a policy.
    3. To research the literature and other resources to determine common, accepted nursing practice.
    4. To develop policy statements.
    5. To present proposed policies to Nursing Council for vote.
    6. To report to Nursing Council at each regular meeting.
      The report shall include:
      a. A list of all newly received requests for policy.
      b. A list of all policies currently in progress.
      c. A list of policies ready for voting by Nursing Council.
    7. To prepare a written annual report outlining the accomplishments of the committee. The report shall be prepared by the chairman of the committee and submitted to the Chairman of the Nursing Council.

7.2 Procedure Committee
  a. Purpose—To provide instructions for performance of procedures in accordance with current standards of nursing practice. The guidelines are specific and prescribe the precise action to be taken under a set of circumstances.
  b. Membership
    1. Representatives and alternates shall be elected from the Head Nurse Group (1), Staff Development (1), the Executive Council (1), and the Clinical Group (1), to serve a two year term beginning December 1 of each year and may be reappointed for one consecutive term.
    2. A member shall be elected from RTN I Committee. This term shall begin December 1 and this representative is eligible for a one year term only.
    3. The representative and/or alternate is expected to attend all meetings.
    4. The chairman of this committee shall be elected by its membership.
  c. Meetings
    1. The time, date and place of meetings shall be determined by the chairman.
    2. Minutes of the meeting shall be recorded and kept on file in Nursing Service.
    3. The committee will meet at least quarterly or as called by the chairman.
  d. Duties
    1. To accept written recommendations from an individual or committee regarding the need for a procedure.
    2. To identify independently the need for a procedure.
    3. To research the literature and other resources to determine common, accepted nursing practice.
    4. To develop procedure statements.
    5. To present proposed procedures to Nursing Council for vote.

(continued)

APPENDIX 12–1. Organizational Functions and Entities Nursing Division (*continued*)

6. To prepare an annual written report outlining the accomplishments of the committee. This report shall be prepared by the Committee Chairman and submitted to the Chairman of Nursing Council.

7.3 Nominating Committee will meet during the last quarter prior to the annual meeting as called by the chairman. The slate of nominees shall be presented to Council for consideration one month prior to the annual meeting.

7.4 Bylaws
   a. Purpose—To review the by-laws of the Nursing Council and make recommendations to the Council for by-laws revision.
   b. Membership
      1. A Chairman shall be elected from Nursing Council following the annual meeting.
      2. Members shall be volunteers from Nursing Council.
   c. Meetings
      1. The Chairman shall determine the frequency, time, date and place of meetings.
      2. Minutes of the meeting shall be recorded and kept on file in Nursing Service.

7.5 Ad Hoc Committees
   a. Purpose: To provide a vehicle by which specific tasks or programs can be assumed by a committee.
   b. Membership
      1. Membership shall follow the same format as for standing committees, unless the council decides that a smaller, more specific group, will be more appropriate.
      2. Members can be appointed by Nursing Council or the committee may elect its chairman during its first meeting.
   c. Meetings
      1. During the first meeting, the committee shall:
         a. Define their purpose
         b. Outline the necessary steps to achieve the purpose.
         c. Establish a tentative time-table.
         d. Determine the frequency, time, dates and place of future meetings.
      2. Minutes of the meetings shall be recorded and kept on file in Nursing Service.
   d. Duties
      1. The committee Chairman shall report to Nursing Council during regular meetings.
      2. When the committee has completed its task, a final recommendation is made to Nursing Council for approval. Upon acceptance of this final recommendation, the Ad Hoc Committee is dissolved.

7.6 RTN I
   a. Purpose—To provide a forum for the discussion of topics relating to the practice of professional nursing at USAMC.
   b. Duties
      1. To identify problems related to professional nursing and recommend solutions to Nursing Council.
      2. To disseminate information to their coworkers.
      3. To review at monthly meetings all approved new and/or revised policies and procedures.
      4. To accept and assume responsibility for projects delegated by Nursing Council.
      5. To report to Nursing Council at each regular meeting. The report shall include:
         a. Problems identified concerning professional nursing.
         b. Recommendations for the solution of the identified problems.
         c. Progress on delegated projects.
         d. Summary of monthly committee activities.
      6. To prepare an annual written report outlining the accomplishments of the committee. This report shall be prepared by the Committee Chairman and submitted to the Chairman of Nursing Council.

APPENDIX 12–1. Organizational Functions and Entities Nursing Division (*continued*)

7.7 Quality Assurance
    a. Purpose
        1. To routinely gather information to objectively and systematically measure and evaluate the quality and appropriateness of nursing care. This information encompasses the process of delivery of patient care and the appropriateness and outcome of that patient care.
        2. To develop objective criteria to monitor the quality and appropriateness of patient care provided by the Nursing Department/Service and to evaluate and resolve identified concerns and problems.
    b. Membership
        1. Associate Assistant Administrator for Nursing shall assume position of Chairman.
        2. Nursing Directors shall be appointed as the committee members and will be responsible to the committee for their individual departments.
    c. Meetings
        1. Committee will meet at least monthly, or as called by the Chairman.
        2. An annual written report outlining the accomplishments of the committee shall be prepared by the chairman and submitted to the Chairman of Nursing Council.

Article VIII, Parliamentary Authority
The business of the Council shall be conducted according to the Roberts Rules of Order.

Article IX, Amendment
The By-Laws may be amended during the year. Any member of Council may present an amendment for vote. The amendment must be presented one month prior to vote and must be supported by 25% of current Nursing Council members. A two-thirds vote of total membership of Council is required for an amendment to carry.

Bylaws Nursing Management Council

Article I, Name
1.1 The name of this committee shall be Nursing Management Council.

Article II, Purpose
2.1 To provide a forum for the discussion of management and partient-care concern.
2.2 To promote positive attitudes and morale in management.
2.3 To promote and support the practice of nursing in a professional manner.

Article III, Members
3.1 The members of this council shall be Head Nurses, Supervisors, Assistant Administrator for Nursing and Hospital Administrator.

Article IV, Officers
4.1 The officers shall be Chairman, Vice Chairman and Secretary.
    a. All officers shall be elected by secret ballot.
    b. A majority of votes cast will be required to be elected.
    c. In the event a majority of votes is not achieved by the first ballot, a run-off between two candidates having the most votes shall be required.
    d. Ballots shall originally be counted by an ad hoc committee and thereafter by the Vice-Chairman.
    e. Officers shall serve for one year and are eligible for re-election for one consecutive term.

(continued)

APPENDIX 12–1.　Organizational Functions and Entities Nursing Division (*continued*)

4.2 Officers together with Assistant Administrator for Nursing shall constitute a Governing Board.

4.3 In the event of vacancy:

　　a. The Vice-Chairman replaces the Chairman.

　　b. Other vacancies among officers shall be filled by a qualified member elected by plurality vote to serve until the next annual meeting.

4.4 Duties of Officers:

　　a. The Chairman shall preside at all meetings as a voting member.

　　b. The Vice-Chairman shall assume the duties of the Chairman in his/her absence, and shall serve as Chairman of the nominating committee.

　　c. The Secretary is responsible for recording the minutes. Copies will be distributed to all members.

Article V, Meetings

5.1 Regular meetings shall be held on the first Monday of each month.

5.2 The annual meeting shall be held in November at which time officers shall be elected.

5.3 Special meetings may be called by the Chairman, who shall state the purpose of the meeting in a memo with at least two days notice prior to the meeting.

Article VI, Quorum

A quorum shall consist of a majority of members.

Article VII, Standing Committees

The only standing committee shall be the Nominating Committee.

Article VIII, Parliamentary Authority

The business of the committee shall be conducted according to Roberts Rules of Order.

Article IX, Amendments

The by-laws may be amended at any regular meeting by a majority vote.

The proposed amendment must be presented to the Committee in writing one month prior to voting.

Bylaws, Clinical Group of Nursing Council

Article I, Name

The name of this group shall be the Clinical Group of Nursing Council.

Article II

The purpose of this group shall be:

2.1 To ensure excellence in nursing care which will return the client to his optimum state of health or will enable him to die with dignity.

2.2 To provide a climate which will promote and support the practice of professional nursing.

2.3 To provide a forum for the discussion of staff and patient concerns.

The functions of this group shall be:

2.4 To ensure excellence in nursing care

　　a. through the development, implementation, and evaluation of tools that measure the quality of nursing care.

APPENDIX 12–1. Organizational Functions and Entities Nursing Division (*continued*)

---

    b. through participation on nursing policy and procedure committees, and their subsequent recommendations to Nursing Council.

2.5 To develop nursing service employees to their fullest potential

    a. through the provision of a professional climate where the nurse participates in a collaborative relationship with physicians and other health care professionals and is seen as the coordinator of the patient's care.

    b. through the development and implementation of continuing education programs and the clinical career ladder.

    c. through the development of policies and procedures and the subsequent recommendation to Nursing Council for their consideration.

2.6 Seek methods to improve communication within the department of nursing and with other departments of the hospital.

2.7 Identify methods of improving nursing practices to operate within the framework of the budget through proper utilization of personnel and supplies.

Article III, Members

The members of this group shall be the members of Staff Development, the Clinical Consultants of the Department of Nursing, the Chairman of the RTN I Committee, and a representative of the Department Heads of the University of South Alabama College of Nursing.

Article IV, Officers

The officers of this group shall consist of:

4.1 A Chairman, Vice-chairman, and a Secretary.

    a. all officers shall be elected by a secret ballot.

    b. a majority of votes cast will be required to be elected.

    c. in the event that a majority of votes is not achieved on the first ballot, a run-off will be held between the two candidates having the most votes.

    d. ballots shall be counted by a group appointed by the membership at the time of the election.

    e. officers will serve for a term of one year and are eligible for election for one consecutive term.

4.2 In the event of a vacancy:

    a. the Vice-chairman replaces the Chairman.

    b. the Secretary replaces the Vice-chairman.

    c. the new Secretary will be chosen by a majority vote of the membership.

4.3 Duties of the Officers:

    a. the Chairman shall work closely with the other officers of the group. The Chairman is responsible to the group for the smooth and effective functioning of its committees. The Chairman is a voting member of Executive Council and is to be responsible to the group for communicating recommendations to Executive Council. The Chairman shall function according to guidelines established in Roberts Rules of Order.

    b. The Vice-chairman shall assume the duties of the Chairman in her absence. The Vice-Chairman also services as the chairman of the Nominating Committee as well as serving the group as parliamentarian. The Vice-chairman shall see the group functions according to Roberts Rules of Order.

    c. The Secretary shall be responsible for taking the minutes at the meetings, distributing copies of the minutes to the members of the group, distributing notices of the meetings to the members of the group, and maintaining a Master File of the group's business and activities.

4.4 Qualification for Office—must be a member of the Clinical Group of Nursing Council.

(continued)

APPENDIX 12–1. Organizational Functions and Entities Nursing Division (*continued*)

Article V, Meetings

5.1 Regular meetings shall be held at 12:00 noon on the third Tuesday of each month.

5.2 The annual meeting shall be held in November at which time annual reports of the officers shall be read and new officers shall be elected.

5.3 Special Meetings shall be called by the Chairman. The purpose of the meeting shall be stated in the call and at least 2 days notice shall be given.

Article VI, Quorum

A quorum of the group shall be a majority of the membership. The presence of a quorum shall be documented in the minutes.

Article VII, Committees

7.1 Ad hoc Committee

    a. Purpose: to provide a vehicle for which specific tasks or programs can be assumed by a committee.

    b. Membership: membership shall be determined by the group on a voluntary or appointed basis whichever should be most appropriate.

    c. Meetings:

        1. during the first meeting, the committee shall define its purpose.

        2. the committee shall outline steps necessary to achieve its purpose.

        3. the committee shall establish a tentative timetable.

        4. the committee shall determine the frequency, time, dates, and places of future meetings.

        5. the committee shall report to the group during regular meetings and shall submit a written report to the Secretary to be maintained in the Master File.

    d. When the committee has completed its task, a final recommendation shall be made to the group for its approval. Upon acceptance of this recommendation, the Ad Hoc Committee shall be dissolved.

Article VIII, Parliamentary Authority

The business of this group shall be conducted according to the Roberts Rules of Order.

Article IX, Bylaws

The Bylaws may be amended during the year. Any member of the group may present an amendment for a vote. The amendment must be presented one month prior to vote and must be supported by 25% of the current Clinical Group membership. A majority vote of total membership is required for the amendment to carry.

SOURCE: Courtesy of University of South Alabama Medical Center, Mobile Alabama.

APPENDIX 12–2. Bylaws of the RTN I

Article I

Name

The name of this committee shall be RTN I Committee.

Article II

Functions

The function of this committee shall be to provide a forum for assessment of problems and recommendations for potential solutions as pertains to:

2.1 Promoting quality patient care.

2.2 Promoting the problem solving process by:

    A. Identifying problems

    B. Recommending possible solutions to identified problems.

    C. Helping nursing cope with unresolved problems.

2.3 Promoting positive attitudes and morale among nurses.

2.4 Promoting cost-effectiveness.

2.5 Promoting an environment that is conductive to the optimum practice of nursing.

Article III

Membership

The Members of this committee shall be:

3.1 An RTN I, with each active member having one vote.

    A. An active member will be elected by the members of each individual unit and the Float Pool to serve for a minimum term of one year. At the end of one term each unit may keep same representative or choose to hold re-election.

    B. An alternate member may attend all meetings, but will have voting privileges only in the absence of the active member from that unit.

    C. Resigning members shall notify the chairman of intentions in writing two weeks in advance of the next scheduled meeting. At this time the alternate member from that unit will become an active member with voting privileges and a new alternate will be elected by the representative unit.

3.2 Any RTN I may attend meetings as an observer.

3.3 An advisor(s) chosen by the committee may attend meetings by his/her request or by request of the committee and has no voting privileges.

Article IV

Officers

Officers shall consist of a Chairman, Vice-Chairman, Secretary, and Parliamentarian.

4.1 Election of Officers

    A. All officers shall be elected at the annual meeting by secret ballot, plurality vote, with votes being counted by the secretary.

    B. Officers shall serve for a term of one (1) year, and may be eligible for re-election for one consecutive term.

4.2 Vacancies among officers shall be filled by a qualified member elected by plurality vote to serve until the next annual meeting.

4.3 Officers who transfer units shall complete their term of one year office but will have no voting privileges during this time.

4.4 Duties of Officers

    A. The chairman shall preside at all meetings, work closely with advisors toward achieving objectives, and appoint committees.

(continued)

APPENDIX 12–2. Bylaws of the RTN I (*continued*)

    1. The chairman of RTN I Committee shall be a voting member of Nursing Council.
    2. An annual written report outlining the accomplishments of the Committee shall be prepared by the Chairman and Submitted to the chairman of Nursing Council.
B. Vice-Chairman shall assume the duties of the Chairman in his/her absence, and shall serve as Chairman of the Nominating Committee.
C. The Secretary is responsible for recording the minutes and maintaining a record of all committee business. Copies will be distributed to all units in the house.
D. The Parliamentarian shall oversee that the work of the RTN I Committee is conducted according to Robert's Rules of Order, and serve as secretary in the absence of the Secretary.

4.4 Qualifications
    Any active member shall qualify for nomination, except as restricted in Article IV, Section 4.1.

Article V

Meetings
5.1 Regular meetings shall be held on the second Wednesday of every month.
5.2 The Annual Meeting shall be held in November at which time officers shall be elected.
5.3 Special meetings may be called by the Chairman, who will state the purpose of the meeting in a memo, with at least 2 days prior notice to the meeting.

Article VI

Quorum
A quorum shall consist of a majority of members.

Article VII

Standing Committees
The only standing committee shall be the Nominating Committee.

Article VIII

Parliamentary Authority
The business of the Committee shall be conducted according to Robert's Rules of Order.

Article IX

Amendments
The bylaws may be amended at any regular meeting by a majority vote. The proposed amendment must be presented to the Committee in writing one month prior to voting.

Article X

Standing Rule
Standing rules may be amended or deleted by a majority vote at any regular meeting.
10.1 The committee shall meet at 1:00 P.M. on the 2nd Wednesday of every month.

SOURCE: Courtesy of the University of South Alabama Medical Center, Mobile, Alabama.

Decentralization and Participatory Management 13

DECENTRALIZATION

Description

Decentralization refers to the degree to which authority is dispersed downward within an organization to its divisions, branches, services, and units. Decentralization of authority includes dispersal of the management components of planning, organizing, directing, and controlling or evaluating. It involves the delegation of decision-making power, authority, responsibility, and accountability. Decentralization of these functions represents a management philosophy and reflects the management style of the chief executive officer (CEO) and the chief nurse executive. Decentralization within an organization varies in degree but is never total. Top management must bear ultimate responsibility for the success of an organization, achievement of goals and objectives, outcomes, and profit or loss.[1]

The United States Compared with Japan and Europe

In Japan, when workers are asked who is in charge, they respond, "I am!" Japanese management is a fad of the present era. It must be remembered that Japan has an entirely different culture. The Japanese have learned to manage complex organizations. They do it through Theory Z, developed by Dr. William Ouchi after studying Japanese systems and similar management approaches in the United States. Basic management principles of Theory Z are:

- Long-term employment.
- Relatively slow process of evaluation and promotion.
- Broad career paths.
- Consensus decision making.
- Implicit controls with explicit measurements.
- High levels of trust and egalitarianism.
- Holistic concern for people.[2]

The Japanese studied U.S. management and modified it to fit their culture.

Decentralization is a U.S. business strategy that was instituted in the 1960s to aid in the penetration of European markets. It is considered necessary for the successful management of large firms. The Japanese are still constrained from decentralizing into the United States. Both Europe and Japan have more family-held firms. Japanese firms retain collective, centralized, and strongly hierarchical organizational structures. Managerial reward systems in the United States usually emphasize individual rather than group performance.[3]

The United States has more formal business education schools than Europe and Japan. European firms tend to provide management education and training in-house. While U.S. colleges and universities graduate over 60,000 MBAs annually, Japan graduates very few, Great Britain 1,500, and West Germany even fewer.

The United States produces professional managers who switch firms. Japan has strong patterns of corporate loyalty and long-term employment. The United States has professional associations for managers; management is more tolerant of mergers, organizational development, and new ideas such as "strategic planning matrices," "intrapreneurs," and corporate cultures. U.S. firms hire more outside consultants and adopt external management ideas such as worker representation on corporate boards of directors, flextime work schedules, and worker participation in job design. Organized labor is weaker in the United States.[4]

Joiner implemented Theory Z at Chrysler and the Mead Corporation. The following is a summary of some of his activities for implementing Theory Z:

1. *Build a cohesive top management team.* They must trust each other.

2. *Create a strategic vision and communicate it effectively.* The vision of the future will include a strategy to gain a competitive edge. The vision will be exciting and inspiring.

3. *Build strong personnel support systems within the organization.* Such systems should reinforce the company's belief in its people and permit employees to build broad careers. This will give them security by committing them to life-long careers and the workforce will be stable and trained. Primary personnel systems will provide for regular organizational effectiveness surveys to monitor the health of the system. They will reward employees by fair and competitive compensation programs, including bonus or profit-sharing plans. Employees will be involved in a broad formal job selection and placement process. There will be effective regular performance reviews that reflect development of employees. Specific educational opportunities will be reimbursed. Every personnel transaction will be viewed as a significant opportunity to encourage, motivate, and establish trust.

4. *Create a participatory organizational structure to facilitate problem solving and consensus building.* All employees must be motivated to become committed to goals. An outside facilitator may be used. The participatory organization structure can be created by eliminating meddling managers and staff by reducing reporting levels, widening span of controls, and cutting their numbers. People will be given jobs and trusted to do them. Participatory organizational structures are rigid, with agreed-upon forms, operational plans, and timetables of action. The managers manage by "wandering around." Proper forums for participation include committees, policy boards, and task teams.

5. *Provide leadership.* Change requires good common-sense leaders who have strong beliefs in people and are committed to excellence. They will practice group leadership skills including decision by consensus. When the leadership team is prepared they tell the employees where the organization is headed. The leadership will put effort into making the system work, keeping it alive, human, personal, informal, and measured.[5]

Reasons for Decentralization

Health-care organizations are among the most complex organizations in the world. Their complexity increases with size; thus decisions are better managed at the specific site from which they originate. Communication does not have to travel up and down an organizational hierarchy. Sound decisions can be made and action taken more promptly when decision making is decentralized.

The variety and depth of nursing management problems have increased. Patient care must keep moving: delay in a diagnostic procedure or treatment can delay progress toward recovery and discharge, thereby increasing expense. Staffing is a complicated process that must account for many variables: physician absences due to education, vacation, or illness; seasonal fluctuations due to such factors as school vacations for children; the random nature of tertiary care for heart attacks, strokes, trauma, cancer, and other conditions; third-party payer requirements; government rules and regulations related to patients and employees; coordination of multiple activities; increased technology with increased specialization, leading to environmental and human stress; the complexity of managing human beings, including those with dual careers as nurses and homemakers; complaints; quality assurance; staff development; and much more.

The object of decentralizing nursing is to manage decisions in their specific area of origin, thereby facilitating communication and effectiveness. Decentralization also supports role clarification to prevent overlapping and duplication of individual work.[6]

Studies have shown that decentralized decision making increases productivity, improves morale, increases favorable attitudes, and decreases absenteeism. One could conclude that decentralized decision making is good for health-care institutions because it is good for nursing personnel. Research on the decentralization of decision making confirms the hypothesis that it enhances job enrichment and job enlargement.[7]

Decentralization embodies the concept of participatory management, including shared governance.

PARTICIPATORY MANAGEMENT

When top management implements a philosophy of decentralized decision making, the stage is set for involving more people—perhaps even all staff—in making decisions at the level at which the action occurs. Both decentralized management and participatory management delegate authority from top managers downward to the people who report to them. In doing so objectives or duties are assigned, authority is granted, and an obligation or responsibility is created by acceptance. The employee is accountable for results.[8]

In nursing, as in other organizations, delegation fosters participation. A first line manager with delegated authority will contact another department to solve a problem in providing a service. The first line manager does not need to go to a department head, who contacts the department head of that service, creating a communication bottleneck. The people closest to the problem solve it. This is efficient and cost-effective management.

The following sections detail some of the characteristics of participatory management.

Trust

Participatory management is based on a philosophy of trust. This employee is trusted to complete the task, with periodic progress reports and a final review with management. The time and rate of participation should be managed to control stress. The entire task or decision should be delegated as much as possible. More and more professional nurses want to control their nursing practice; the manager can facilitate this by teaching them to make complete operational plans, including structuring priorities and setting deadlines. Such plans provide a documented standard for joint review. Managers who empower and facilitate employee performance communicate trust. This process will demonstrate the employee's capabilities and reveal shortcomings.

Motorola has had a participatory management program in effect since 1968, with almost all of their 57,000 U.S. employees involved in it at some stage. The three basic ideas of their program embody trust:

- Every worker knows his or her job better than anybody else.
- People can and will accept the responsibility for managing their own work if that responsibility is given to them in the proper way.
- Intelligence, perspective, and creativity exist among people at all levels of the organization.[9]

Commitment

Personal involvement in managing a nursing service requires commitment from the chief nurse and other nurse managers. Managers should be highly visible to the staff, supporting and nurturing them in the process. In turn, the staff should also be committed, a characteristic they will develop from association with the committed managers. They gain this commitment from seeing their bosses out at the production level, where patients are being treated, from cooperating with their colleagues and managers in a spirit of teamwork, and from feelings of accomplishment. Nursing commitment comes from knowing that the purpose of the organization is patient care and the managers are working with them to produce that care. Staff share in making decisions and in consensus with the bosses. This experience in participation turns them on and tunes them in and they do not want to be lazy and mediocre or to featherbed. Commitment inspires staff to be industrious, outstanding, and productive. Under participatory management, commitment is elicited, not imposed.

Professional nurses are motivated to develop their human skills resulting in increased individual self-esteem. They have a sense of accomplishment and feel that their accomplishment has been supported by management. They feel they are expanding their worth through their work.

Professional nurses demand professional courtesies. When these are not extended they resort to deviant behavior. They tend to align themselves with colleagues and professional associations for recognition and evaluation. They frequently recommend each other for awards.[10]

Goals and Objectives

Conflict resolution is a major requirement or goal of participatory management. Conflict is inevitable when human beings work together. It is nonproductive during process and in outcomes. In nursing as in other occupations, it produces stress and results in turnover and absenteeism. Employees can be sensitized to deal with potential and real conflict and to take action to reduce its destructive consequences of fear, anger, distrust, jealousy, and resentment. This can be accomplished through establishment of a climate of openness with established procedures for problem solving, persuasion, bargaining, and politicizing. The goal is reduced adversarial relations. It is accomplished through joint planning and problem solving and facilitation of employee consultation.[11] Refer to the chapter on conflict management.

A key goal for a nursing organization is to keep itself healthy. A healthy work environment is encouraged by participatory management. Participation will make maximum use of employees' abilities,

without relinquishing the ultimate authority and responsibility of management. Professional nurses want input into decisions but do not want to do the jobs of managers. They want the support of managers, to be able to talk with them, to be informed. Without this support they develop anger and hostility that results in absenteeism and lower productivity.

Goal-setting activities can occur with reasonably frequent performance review and feedback. Nursing personnel bring their goals and objectives to the conferences. The process is reciprocal, with the manager and employee together developing goals and objectives that are challenging, clear, consistent, and specific. They will both be motivated. Healthy stress will be increased and undesirable stress reduced.

Career development programs for professional nurses help to mediate conflict and inspire loyalty to an organization. Provided with job information, nurses set goals that relate to promotion and to tenure with job security. Differences in work attitudes and personal aspirations are recognized. There is less professional role conflict. New employees who are young and fresh out of college should be given information on the nature of the organization, current and future availability of jobs, career opportunities and career ladders, and management goals and responsibilities. Managers learn the professional nurse employees' aspirations and expectations and should help them set a course and monitor it.[12]

The motivation of professional nurses should be stimulated by incentives. These incentives include rewards of money and recognition for effective involvement. Participation can result in promotion or changes in work assignments. Knowing this keeps nurses working to achieve their goals and objectives.

Autonomy

Autonomy is the state of being independent, of having responsibility, authority, and accountability for one's work as well as one's personal time. Professional employees indicate they want autonomy for practicing their profession, for making decisions about their work. They do not want their decisions made for them by hospital administrators, physicians, or others. They want to be treated as equal partners and colleagues in the health-care delivery system. This desire for autonomy has increased as nurses have become increasingly sophisticated in knowledge and skills and have used them with effective results.

Professional nurses want autonomy over the conditions under which they work, including pace and content. These decisions are often in conflict with management's coordination roles, a conflict that can be mediated by involving professional nurses in delegated activities of coordination.[13]

Professional nurses are willing to assume and accept responsibility, to be held accountable for a charge. They want the authority, the rightful and legitimate power to fulfill the charge. This authority comes from their expert knowledge and skill, their license, their position, and their peers.[14]

The autonomy of professional nurses is evident in an organization in which management trusts them by giving them freedom to make decisions and take actions within the scope of their knowledge. They are free to exercise their authority. This freedom is legitimized in the bylaws of their departments, in job descriptions, in performance appraisals, and in management support of their decisions as binding. Their independent behavior includes acknowledging mistakes and taking action to correct them and prevent them from happening again.

The professional nurse is accountable for the consequences of his or her actions. Accountability is the "fulfillment of the formal obligation to disclose to referent others the purposes, principles, procedures, relationships, results, income, and expenditures for which one has authority."[15] The relationship between responsibility, authority, autonomy, and accountability is depicted in Figure 13–1.

To have autonomy, nursing employees should be allowed to determine their own means of accomplishing their goals. They should be involved in setting their own goals. This principle applies to all nursing employees. When professional nurses work with other nursing employees they should facilitate participation and input from these groups. This approach promotes these persons' interest, trust, and commitment.[16]

Other Characteristics

Participation in management should be inclusive rather than exclusive, but it should be voluntary. The climate of the organization, as set by the philos-

FIGURE 13–1. Interlocking Major Concepts

Concept	Key Aspects
Responsibility	The charge
Authority	The rightful power to act on the charge
Autonomy	Freedom to decide and to act
Accountability	Disclosure regarding the charge

SOURCE: Reprinted from "Clarifying Autonomy and Accountability in Nursing Service: Part 2" by F. M. Lewis and M. V. Batey, with permission of *The Journal of Nursing Administration,* October 1982.

ophy of its managers, will motivate (or fail to motivate) professional nurses to participate at a level consistent with their goals and desires. Participation is increased by facilitators who are enthusiastic and expert.

The participatory management environment promotes change and growth, fostering originality and creativity. The professional nurse recognizes that conditions can be changed, that the changes are real, that managers listen and support, that suggestions are evaluated and are used or are discussed when rejected. In the Motorola participatory management program employees submit "I recommend" suggestions that require posted answers within 72 hours. The answers can be discussed with management, a process that promotes employees' trust of management.[17]

All of these characteristics exact a large investment from professional clinical nurses and their nurse managers. They are required to put great effort into learning new skills and relationships. They must face increased ambiguity and uncertainty about the process, until it is established and working. They must also cope with the psychological pain and discomfort related to changing beliefs and attitudes.

Participation may be temporary when it is specific to a task. It takes time. Since it involves risk many people will not voluntarily choose it, therefore it has to be managed for success. Participatory management will not work automatically and will not work in every situation.

STRUCTURE OF DECENTRALIZED AND PARTICIPATORY ORGANIZATIONS

Flat organizational structures are characteristic of decentralized management. Traditional hierarchical structures with increasingly authoritative levels of management frighten employees, threaten their security, and make them uncomfortable. Economic events of the past decade favor horizontal organizational structures with no rank, no boss, and no seniority. Flat organizational structures are flourishing, increasing management/employee association and commitment, and deemphasizing numbers of managers and manuals ("M&Ms"), titles, and executive suites.[18]

In nursing there are reports of the elimination of head nurse positions, with committees of professional nurses elected by unit staff to manage unit activities. Their efforts are facilitated by the new breed of leaders who are democratic, participative, and laissez-faire or free-rein, involving their followers in the decision process, in setting objectives, in establishing strategies, and in determining job assignments. These leaders put emphasis on people, employees, and followers and their participation in the management process. They are employee-centered and relationship-centered.

Decentralized organizational structures are compatible with primary nursing. Decisions are made, goals are set, there is peer review and evaluation, schedules are made, and conflicts are resolved by primary nurses. Levels of practice are built into staffing.[19]

Each nursing unit in a hospital is usually as big as other departments, such as the medical laboratory or pharmacy, and should be considered a department on the same level. This organizational structure increases accountability and teamwork. The planning of care, staffing, budget, equipment, education, and environment more accurately reflect the needs of the individual unit. Staffing for each unit becomes the responsibility of each department head; floating is eliminated because each unit has its own part-time (float) staff. However, there can still be a central staffing coordinator.

Decentralized organizations call for increased involvement by the staff development department, which can also be decentralized. Each department (unit/specialty) is autonomous, with goals specific to that department. Cooperation and sharing of ideas are increased and goals and output are evaluated. Continuity of care is improved with a single department head and elimination of float personnel from other units. The department head is responsible for hiring, training, performance, evaluation, and termination of personnel.

Top Management

What is the role of top management under a decentralized system with participatory management? Their role is directed toward results. They share in the planning and implementation of the program. Since effective controls are needed to monitor performance of lower-level units, they use computers to assist in making their decisions and in developing controlling techniques for decentralization.

In one research study, eighteen of twenty hospitals had some decentralization, including 77 percent down to the unit level. The overriding purpose was to increase worker satisfaction. Decentralization resulted in increased morale, job satisfaction, and motivation among managers and workers. Personnel development, flexibility, and effective decision making all increased; conflict decreased along with operational costs, negativism of attitudes, and underutilization of managers. The work force stabilized and became more effective and efficient.

The study indicated that most managers do not understand the concept of delegation, are not effective communicators, do not concentrate on goals, and do not delegate according to the abilities and interests of their employees.[20]

With the dynamics of decentralization, each unit works with their own budget, job descriptions are clear, concise, flexible, and current, in-service training is effective, performance standards are clear, employee recognition occurs, and accountability is enforced at all times.

Vertical versus Horizontal Integration

Vertical integration combines decentralization with integration. While businesses and industries decentralize their operations into product lines and subsidiaries, they maintain their partnership and identity within the corporate structure. Prior to the advent of the prospective payment system (PPS) and competition among hospitals, the industry was largely characterized by horizontal integration of departments within divisions, examples being nursing; operations related to patient care services such as pharmacy, physical therapy, occupational therapy, and others; operations related to plant management including housekeeping and others; and finance.

As competition among hospitals increased they began the quest to diversify into new markets. New corporate structures were formed that included umbrella corporate management with subsidiary companies. Among the objectives of vertical integration are:

1. Conversion of internal cost centers into revenue producers. An example is medical supply and durable medical equipment. Heretofore, hospitals would refer discharged patients to hospital or medical equipment companies for purchase of dressings, wheelchairs, and the like. Profits can no longer be made from charges as a lump sum is paid per diagnostic-related group under Medicare. Some hospitals have formed their own companies to sell and rent medical supplies and equipment to ambulatory patients and to other subsidiaries within the corporate structure. Profits go to the hospital subsidiary instead of to the medical supply company.

2. Development of new and expanding markets for hospitals. These include home health care, formerly a referral service to a public health agency or private home health care agency. Referrals have increased dramatically with early discharge of patients. Hospital corporations have also formed health insurance companies as preferred provider organizations (PPOs) or health maintenance organizations (HMOs).

The hospital is struggling for survival and has chosen vertical integration as a means of capturing lost revenues. Whether all efforts at vertical integration will be successful depends upon the market share of products and services captured.

From another viewpoint, that of functions rather than structure, organizations have focused on the vertical dimensions of decentralized decision making. This vertical dimension aims for representation by levels of employees, thereby restricting decentralization to a single function or issue considered to be of primary importance to the organiza-

tion. Recently health care has focused on issues of marketing and quality control, in which decisions are made up or down the hierarchy.

Integration of the decentralization decision-making process horizontally or laterally attends to traditionally separate functional hierarchies. The object here is to improve communication across functions with mutual influence of inputs from different interest groups whose individual values, objectives, and loyalties have been compartmentalized into obstructions to lateral integration. Horizontal integration is important to the success of participation. The organizational structure and functions require adaptation to models that will support participatory processes.[21]

THE PROCESS OF PARTICIPATORY MANAGEMENT

In the process of participatory management, professional nurses are involved in decisions that affect them and in setting their own work standards. This process involves training, changed roles for supervisors, changed roles for unions, and communication. It also involves preparation of managers for changed organizational structures. Participation involves understanding and support of many levels of people in the organization.

As organizations grow they are frequently geographically dispersed. In hospitals this can occur as new services or products are added. Home health care is an example. When the mission is established it is frequently housed in another building and sometimes in another part of the community. Geographic dispersion tends to result from vertical integration and to increase decentralization.

Health-care organizations grow as they establish new missions for wellness, sports medicine, outpatient surgery, freestanding emergency centers and surgical centers, birthing centers, and auxiliary services and clinics of many kinds. The diversity of specialization as well as the geographic distribution encourage decentralization and delegation of decision-making authority, responsibility, and accountability. Decentralization tends to increase if organizational growth is internal rather than external. As these products and services grow it is more difficult to manage them effectively from a central office. It is important to have well-qualified product managers and unit managers, particularly when there is a great diversity of products and services.

Hospitals are highly differentiated entities, as are many functions within them. Political differences emerge as each department or function recruits its own experts. Separate functions produce uncertainty, with output for one phase being input for another. Examples of this dynamic are pharmacy and nursing, or the operating room versus other nursing departments. Matrix management and project management are systems aimed at the improvement of lateral coordination and cooperation.

Within a hierarchy participation based on interaction and influence will succeed to the extent it can operate independently of other parts of the organization. Product management will be done across organizational functions, so managers must attend to the quality of lateral arrangements. This includes integration of line and staff functions such as production and marketing or production and education.

Uncertainty is associated with information processing. One function must know how its inputs affect another's outputs and vice versa. The greater the uncertainty the greater the need for information. Uncertainty leads to a heavy information processing load, leading to differentiation with its subsequent problems and the need for lateral integration.

On the one hand, specialists and experts dominate participatory structures because of their ability to make highly complex technical decisions. On the other hand, circumstances promoting the need for participation encourage the opposite trend, as problems of lateral integration constrain and inhibit participation.

Structurally, the optimum conditions for participation include uncertainty plus facilitation of integration of differentiated interest groups. The participators are approached systematically, the organization being restructured laterally.[22]

Training

Managers at all levels of nursing should subscribe to the philosophy of participatory management if it is to be successful. All managers and employees must unfreeze the present system of attitudes and values. This unfreezing process will require a comprehen-

sive, well-planned training program. Training will promote a sense of job security as it will prepare everyone for changed roles. Staff at every level learn the reasons for participatory management, the advantages, the disadvantages, and the roles they will play.

Managers may be threatened by the concept of participatory management if they perceive their authority as being diminished. Their training program will require that their competencies be assessed. This will include developing their abilities for frankness with employees, being willing to admit past failures, and encouraging contributions from their workers and being influenced by them. Managers need to learn to deal with justifying the existence of their jobs.[23]

More than 1,000 businesses in the United States are involved in some form of participatory management. Many nursing organizations subscribe to the notion to some degree. Centralized management and authority is becoming history in the development of the science of human behavior.[24]

Because they have been subjected to centralized, authoritarian management for so long, nursing personnel will need to be schooled in the process of participatory management. This will include training for their input into collaborative decision making.

With participatory management there is a complementary relationship between managers and practitioners, rather than a hierarchical one. Training is done to prepare staff and prevent insecurity. Availability of managers qualified to function in participatory management increases decentralization. Training of supervisors will focus on changes in their needs as well as their functions. They will learn to gain self-fulfillment from delegating and team building.[25]

Management training of supervisors will include group dynamics, problem solving, planning, and decision making. Such training can occur through conferences, workshops, and seminars. It should be rewarding and continuous to be successful. It will relieve their perceived threats from challenges of employees, from exposure of their weaknesses, from perceived loss of prestige and power, and from "digging in" to keep control.[26]

Changed Roles of Supervisors

Decentralization with participatory management changes roles which have to be defined and coordi-

FIGURE 13–2. Long Beach Community Hospital Education Organizational Chart

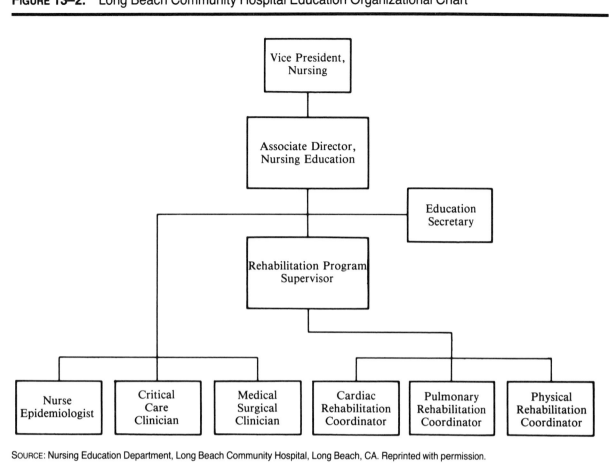

SOURCE: Nursing Education Department, Long Beach Community Hospital, Long Beach, CA. Reprinted with permission.

nated to prevent conflict. Head nurses, charge nurses, and primary nurses have increased management responsibility. For some this will mean decreased hands-on clinical responsibility. Supervisors of head nurses have decreased responsibility for unit management. They become mentors, role models, and facilitators. With a flattened organizational structure some may lose jobs, while others have the overall scope of their responsibility increased.[27]

In an experiment in decentralized patient education, all clinical nurses caring for patients became the teachers. The assistant head nurse became the facilitator—the person responsible for planning and developing objectives for patient education programs and promoting staff interest and participation in all phases. The education department became the resource available to coordinate teaching programs in support of the primary nurse. The advantages of decentralized versus centralized patient education are summarized in Figure 13–2.[28]

As supervisors learn to delegate authority, they modify the climate that promotes deviant behavior by giving professional nurses what they want, the authority to manage themselves. Since this gain gives them initiative in performing their jobs and freedom to question managers, the latter should expect loyalty in return. The profession of nursing does not employ nurses; organizations do. Participatory management is a process in which there must be dialogue with constraints. The nurses will control their profession; management uses its input to set objectives and priorities and to review output. Nurse employees cannot control the enterprise, and management cannot compromise the professional or ethical standards of professional nurses.[29]

In participatory management the supervisor facilitates rather than directs the work force. Traditional supervisory functions are delegated downward. There must be clear delineation of managers' basic responsibilities, as opposed to their behavioral or management style. Managers can gain satisfaction from their ability to make clinical nurses successful and satisfied. The interpersonal skills and conceptual abilities demanded of supervisors will increase. They should be challenged and should have a future. They promote implementation of committee decisions, listen, and offer assistance.[30]

Since there will be fewer supervisors, career development programs for college-educated nurses must provide promotional opportunities as clinical practitioners, managers, teachers, or researchers.

Supervisors are important to the success of decentralization of decision making and employee involvement in management of nursing and the health-care system. They should be taught to manage under employee involvement programs. They need to learn that they will have more time to plan and organize work, to be creative. Their jobs can be expanded upwards but they should keep contact with employees, encouraging participation by everyone.

Changed Roles of Unions

Decentralized decision making and participatory management are not processes that give comfort to unions. Unions may view them as threats to their survival and to membership and as a prelude to efforts to decertify. Plans should include union membership participation that emphasizes the common interests of unions and management. Both entities want mutual trust, quality of work life, and employee involvement. Both want job security for their employees and members; successful participatory management programs give security a high priority.

Some employers will promote decertification of unions while working to bond employees to them through involvement. Others will cooperate with their unions, promoting their active support. In the latter instance, traditional prerogatives of management are sometimes subjected to union influence. The risk-benefit ratio of mutual union-management involvement will have to be weighed by both sides.

The union's role will have to be defined. The goal is good labor-management relations. If they are to play a role, union shop stewards will be trained with supervisors. There will need to be a memorandum of understanding for keeping grievance and contractual issues outside of the employee involvement program.[31]

Communication

Good communication within the nursing organization is essential to an effective employee participation program. Good communication is effective communication, evident in employees who are informed about the business of nursing. They know what management is saying and what management's intentions are. Management knows what employees are saying and how it squares with perceptions management is working to develop. Broken communication contributes to stress and leads to direct economic losses through low productivity, grievances, absenteeism, turnover, and work slowdowns or strikes.

Flat organizational structures promote effective communication. Managers plan the vehicles, content, and intent of effective communication and they monitor the process. Supervisors are important to effective communication and work to ensure its openness as another aspect of their changed roles. Management attitudes should promote truth, frankness, and openness.

Participation enhances commitment and interdepartmental and intradepartmental communication. In medium-sized and large organizations, a communication center will operate 24 hours a day. Message delivery will be facilitated. Computers will be used to communicate instantly, nurse to nurse, nurse to manager, manager to nurse, and nurse to others. Messages will be hand-delivered when necessary.

With direct communication the middle person is eliminated and time is saved. The problem of missing medical laboratory or radiology reports is taken up between the primary nurse or the head nurse and the manager of the other department immediately responsible for the activity, by computer, telephone or direct contact.[32]

Increased representation of clinical nurses on hospital and departmental committees improves communication. The goal is to facilitate the sharing of information, not embody it into the authority of a management position. Management by objectives (MBO), group brainstorming, and quality circles are vehicles of effective communication used in participatory management.

ADVANTAGES OF PARTICIPATORY MANAGEMENT

The following is a list of advantages of participatory management as cited by writers in business, industry, and health care, including nursing:

1. High trust and mutual support.
2. Eliminated full-time-equivalent positions; fewer levels of management; fewer specialized departments.
3. Increased accountability of managers and employees.
4. Reduced ambiguity in work requirements for practitioners and employees, with improved communication.
5. Enhanced role for clinical nurses; self-supervision; active involvement of employees in identifying and solving problems; encouragement of employee contributions; career development.
6. Increased independence of the nursing division.
7. Legal clarity.
8. Increased efficiency of nurse/patient ratio.
9. Teamwork: people become cooperative and independent with increased motivation and initiative.
10. Improved organizational communication, with nurses being briefed on all phases of the nursing business including revenues, costs, and strategic plans, thereby increasing employee understanding of the organization.
11. Decreased absenteeism.
12. Increased effectiveness and productivity. Quality of work done improves; higher level of mastery.
13. Uplifted morale and motivation at work. Increased excitement from fluctuating participation. Participation makes work and values visible.
14. Fresh ideas for management decision making and problem solving.
15. Identification of potential leaders.
16. Fostering within professionals of a strong sense of identification with employer's goals and objectives.
17. Decreased turnover and increased stability of workforce.
18. Increased commitment as attitudes become positive.
19. Less overtime.
20. Lower cost.
21. Better utilization of professional nurses as participants have their skills and talents enhanced and discovered.
22. Increased job satisfaction.
23. Recognition of contributions, because participation increases individual and organizational capacities to learn, adapt, and develop toward higher levels of excellence.[33]

Involvement of employees in the decision-making process creates favorable attitudes and behavior. Employees want to be productive and to learn. Decision-making skills raise their competency levels, preparing them for future opportunities. One way of measuring attitude changes is to survey attitudes before and after implementing an employee involvement program. This can be done on an experimental unit basis before being applied to the entire nursing organization. Research findings support the positive results or advantages of employee involvement in management processes.[34]

Participatory management reduces the potential frustration and loss of significance of the individual nurse. Employees have evidence that their suggestions count.

In the Motorola participatory management program, factory-level employees of Plan I belong to groups of fifty to 250 people who set targets and valid standards that measure current cost, in-process quality, product deliveries, inventory levels, and housekeeping and safety. Representatives belong to working committees that review ideas, recommendations, waste and quality. The committees solve problems and send recommendations to a representative steering committee for review. Committee involvement of workers improves communication. Improved product quality or customer satisfaction is evident in increased sales and profits and results in financial bonuses to employees. In this process, each employee can see the effect of his or her contribution on the group and feels a sense of accomplishment. In one instance, as a result of the participatory management process at Motorola a 4 percent loss of gold went to zero in two months. Volume of production at one plant went up 33 percent with fewer employees. They had team spirit and a sense of cooperation between management and employees, and they worked with less supervision.[35]

Research studies have reported greater motivation and satisfaction when subordinates participate in performance appraisal. Research indicates mutual goal setting improves performances and increases productivity. It satisfies employees' need for fulfillment and self-actualization, and thus contributes to the well-being of the organization. Participatory management develops mature, healthy, self-directed personalities among employees.[36]

DISADVANTAGES OF PARTICIPATORY MANAGEMENT

Some of the disadvantages of participatory management include:

1. There will be occasional failures.
2. Initiation of programs takes time and money.
3. Policies and procedures have to be changed.
4. It is sometimes difficult to determine which responsibilities are whose, even though other ambiguities are reduced.
5. The budget office and other offices or departments have to deal with several units in nursing service rather than a single department.
6. Lacking knowledge of the process, employers do not want it imposed upon them. They give such excuses as that employees have too little attachment to the organization, employees are not interested in work and have a weak commitment to the work ethic, employees and managers don't get along, employees have a poor assessment of their supervisors, and employees have low regard for organization-wide openness.
7. It is difficult to change management style to true participation.
8. Employees who view management as being autocratic perceive participatory performance appraisal as being insincere, patronizing, and manipulative. The person who initiates it has gone "soft."

9. Self-evaluation is threatening as the employee feels exposed to the view of others.[37]

All of these disadvantages will be overcome by a committed chief nurse executive (CNE) who prepares and implements a plan with supervisors who are prepared psychologically, politically, and technically. The CNE selects and develops key people who are the human beings developing human beings, works at a long-range future, and is accessible.

ACTIVITIES INVOLVING NURSES IN PARTICIPATORY MANAGEMENT

Some of the activities that can be used to involve nurses in participatory management include job enrichment, personalization, gainsharing, participation, primary nursing, and response to identified factors causing job dissatisfaction.

Job Enrichment

Job enrichment satisfies the motivational force for higher-order need fulfillment. This includes variety within and among jobs and a strategy that challenges with performance output stressed over job processes. Job enrichment creates jobs with greater responsibility and more flexibility and promotes personal development.

Enrichment requires preparation and careful implementation. It makes maximum use of employee skills and expands them with focus on the whole job. It includes decision-making authority. Growth from job enrichment prevents apathy, burnout, and alienation. Individuals can choose to assume more responsibility for particular assignments. Lateral transfers are supported with job postings and project assignments. Output is evaluated, not the process used to produce it. Professionals respond to orders from other professionals, an indication that professional nurses will respond best to enrichment from competent professional nurse managers with management styles that promote participation and involvement. Enrichment works best with hard workers who like to work best with friendly people.[38]

Personalization

Personalization is a strategy that focuses on people and knowledge, not numbers and politics. Its users stress empathy and involve professionals in critical decisions that affect them. Career development opportunities are facilitated by advertising jobs, allowing transfers, giving feedback to job applicants, allowing and providing liberal training and development, and promoting based on objective measures.[39]

Primary Nursing

Primary nursing as a modality of nursing care delivery makes nursing worthwhile work, enhances the self-esteem of performing a complete function, produces results of personal endeavor, and realizes collegial and collaborative relationships.[40] In a hospital setting where primary nursing is practiced, decentralization of patient care delivery systems provides the maximum efficiency of nursing care. Primary nurses are accountable. Primary nursing with a stable, mature, self-directed, skilled, and committed staff trained in leadership skills is the ideal environment for self-governance.[41]

Other nursing modalities that are compatible with participatory management are modular nursing, team nursing, case management, and collaborative practice models.

Entrepreneurship

There is a great opportunity for professional nurses to be involved in entrepreneurship, with decentralization and vertical integration strategies being implemented in health-care organizations. Nurses can form small companies with the support of government agencies and private businesses. They require venture capital which can be obtained from government and the private health-care industry. As an example, in the face of greater professional nurse shortages, hospitals could find it advantageous to contract with the corporate nurse agencies or personnel spin-offs through vertical integration that produces nurse staffing subsidiaries, durable medical goods subsidiaries, clinical nursing care subsidiaries, and others.

College students indicate they are more interested in money, power, and status than in the humanities. They do not want to be dehumanized and robotized. Practicing nurses may be telling potential students to major in other fields for these same reasons. Students want to be able to use entrepreneurial skills. They want freedom on the job. Large companies cannot recruit and retain them unless they change their cultures and climates. The implications for health care are obvious.

Small companies are creating jobs, innovations in the marketplace, product diversity for customers, and competition for old-line firms. Self-employed enterprises increased from three million employees in 1976 to 3.9 million in 1982, 28 percent of the self-employed being women in 1982. Fifty-one percent of all new jobs created between 1976 and 1980 were by small businesses.[42]

Levinson recommends the following strategies to promote entrepreneurship:

1. Decentralize.
2. Give actual responsibility and authority to key executives.
3. Let executives express their managerial skills and give them a chance to make their own business mistakes on the road to excellence.
4. Monitor these executives and encourage them to make business decisions on their own, so that they can measure the results of these decisions not only in dollars and cents, but in terms of the effects on the people involved.
5. Establish a basic corporate policy that people are the biggest asset of the company, and make it clear that the development of these people will contribute greatly to the company's strength.[43]

Entrepreneurship in nursing will be good for professional nurses and the health-care industry, as it will create independent thinkers motivated to be productive, creative, and more competitive in the marketplace. They will become like other business people who have a strong desire to control their own careers.

Gainsharing

Gainsharing is a group incentive program in which employees share in the financial benefits of improved performance. It has many of the same advantages and disadvantages as other methods of participatory management, top management being sensitive to employee's goals and employees identifying with the organization through greater involvement.

Initiation of gainsharing takes a long-term plan that includes application of these three phases of the change process:

1. Unfreezing: organizational diagnosis, management questionnaire on gainsharing, bonus calculation, and employee attitude survey.
2. Moving: establish employee ownership with a task force of employees, meetings, training of employees and managers. Involve everyone at once.
3. Refreezing: institutionalize plan, continued training, improved motivation and communication, goals, periodic reviews, periodic elections to task force or committee, and annual reviews.[44]

The results are measurable: savings, improved labor-management relations, fewer grievances, less absenteeism, and reduced turnover. Gainsharing adds money to intrinsic rewards. Stock ownership and profit sharing are economic rewards similar to gainsharing. Gainsharing, stock ownership and profit sharing may not be legally possible in not-for-profit organizations. However increased financial benefits can be made available through legal means such as merit pay, certification pay, and clinical promotions. Also, vertically integrated corporations have profit-making ventures under their corporate umbrellas.

Pay Equity

Pay equity between management and employees is an issue of participatory management. Employees resent announcements of huge salary increases, fringe benefits, and perquisites for top management. Incentive programs for employees are a part of participatory management programs. While employees receive intrinsic satisfaction from public recognition and praise, they also obtain extrinsic rewards from financial bonuses, stock options, and profit sharing.[45]

Professional nurses, like other professional workers, frequently respond negatively to the strategy of linking financial benefits to promotion into management. They want financial rewards for accomplishing personal and organizational objectives that increase productivity and reduce turnover and absenteeism. This can be nonmanagerial advancement with salary, status, recognition, autonomy, and responsibility. It is accomplished through dual ladders, clinical promotions that match management promotions. It preserves their professional career opportunities with financial rewards based on graduated pay scales that can be objectively measured through levels of achievement culminating in mastery.

SUMMARY

Decentralization disperses authority and power downward to the operational units of an organization. Japanese organizations practice decentralization by eliciting consensus of decision making in their management. Decentralization in nursing organizations facilitates communication and effectiveness of decisions and clarifies roles.

Increased productivity, improved morale, increased favorable attitudes of people, and decreased absenteeism are the products of decentralized decision making. Decentralization supports participatory management, the characteristics of which are trust, commitment, involvement of employees in setting goals and objectives, autonomy, inclusion of employees in decision making, change and growth, originality, and creativity.

Decentralized and participatory organizations are usually flat or horizontal: employee-centered and relationship-centered. They are also vertically integrated to enhance revenue production by developing new markets for health-care organizations.

Training is essential to the success of participatory management, as managers are threatened by loss of authority. They have to be prepared for their new roles. Practicing nurses need to be able to perform as collaborators in the management of the nursing organization and the health-care institution. With their new roles comes increased accountability for practicing nurses. Managers become facilitators.

Decentralization and participatory management are consistent with union participation. A memorandum of agreement is needed to keep grievance and contractual issues outside the employee involvement program. Some employers will opt to promote union decertification while bonding employees to the organization through participatory management.

Increased participation of nurses on organizational boards and committees will improve communication. Communication among units and departments becomes direct and hence faster and more accurate.

While there are numerous benefits or advantages of participatory management, there are also some disadvantages. Among these disadvantages are occasional failures, occasional difficulty in fixing responsibilities, and difficulty in changing employee perceptions of previously authoritarian management.

Nurses can be involved in participatory management through such activities as job enrichment, personalization, primary nursing, case management, entrepreneurship, gainsharing, and pay equity.

NOTES

1. L. C. Megginson, D. C. Moseley, and P. H. Pietri, Jr., *Management: Concepts and Applications*, 2d ed. (New York: Harper & Row, 1986), 266; H. Shoemaker and A. El-Ahraf, "Decentralization of Nursing Service Management and Its Impact on Job Satisfaction," *Nursing Administration Quarterly*, Winter 1983, 69–76.
2. C. W. Joiner, Jr., "SMR Forum: Making the 'Z' Concept Work," *Sloan Management Review*, Spring 1985, 57–63.
3. R. Edfelt, "A Look at American Management Styles," *Business*, Jan.-Mar. 1986, 51–54.
4. Ibid.
5. C. W. Joiner, Jr., op. cit.
6. B. J. A. Simons, "Decentralizing Nursing Service—Six Months Later," *Supervisor Nurse*, Oct. 1980, 59–64; R. B. Fine, "Decentralization and Staffing," *Nursing Administration Quarterly*, Summer 1977, 59–67.
7. H. Shoemaker and A. El-Ahraf, op. cit.
8. L. C. Megginson, D. C. Moseley, and P. H. Pietri, op. cit. 266–267.
9. W. J. Weisz, "Employee Involvement: How It Works at Motorola," *Personnel*, Feb. 1985, 29–33; G. W. Poteet, "Delegation Strategies: A Must for the Nurse Executive," *The Journal of Nursing Administration*, Sept. 1984, 18–27.
10. J. A. Raelin, C. Sholl, and D. Leonard, "Why Professionals Turn Sour and What to Do," *Personnel*, Oct. 1985, 28–41.
11. R. B. Fine, op. cit.; R. E. Walton, "From Control to Commitment in the Workplace," *Harvard Business Review*, Mar.-Apr. 1985, 77–84.
12. J. A. Raelin, C. Sholl, and D. Leonard, op. cit.
13. Ibid.
14. M. V. Batey and F. M. Lewis, "Clarifying Autonomy and Accountability in Nursing Services: Part I," *The Journal of Nursing Administration*, Sept. 1982, 13–17.
15. F. M. Lewis and M. V. Batey, "Clarifying Autonomy and Accountability in Nursing Services: Part 2," *The Journal of Nursing Administration*, Oct. 1982, 10.
16. J. E. Bragg and I. R. Andrews, "Participative Decision Making: An Experimental Study in a Hospital," in B. Fuszard, *Self-Actualization for Nurses* (Rockville, MD: Aspen, 1984), 102–110.
17. W. J. Weisz, op. cit.
18. G. Klaus, "Corporate Pyramids Will Tumble When Horizontal Organizations Become the New Global Standard," *Personnel Administrator*, Dec. 1983.
19. E. A. Elpern, P. M. White, and A. F. Donahue, "Staff Governance: The Experience of the Nursing Unit," *The Journal of Nursing Administration*, June 1984, 9–15.
20. H. Shoemaker and A. El-Ahraf, op. cit.
21. C. W. Clegg and T. D. Wall, "The Lateral Dimension to Employee Participation," *Journal of Management Studies*, Oct. 1984, 429–442.
22. Ibid.
23. W. J. Weisz, op. cit.
24. R. E. Walton, op. cit.
25. B. J. Simons, op. cit.
26. M. H. Schuster and C. S. Miller, "Employee Involvement: Making Supervisors Believers," *Personnel*, Feb. 1985, 24–28.
27. B. J. A. Simons, op. cit.
28. S. Malkin and P. Lauteri, "A Community Hospital's Approach—Decentralized Patient Education," *Nursing Administration Quarterly*, Winter 1980, 101–106.
29. J. A. Raelin, C. Sholl, and D. Leonard, op. cit.
30. R. E. Walton, op. cit.
31. Ibid.; M. H. Schuster and C. S. Miller, op. cit.
32. C. L. Cox, "Decentralization: Uniting Authority and Responsibility," *Supervisor Nurse*, Mar. 1980, 28, 32.
33. H. Shoemaker and A. El-Ahraf, op. cit.; M. P. Lovrich, "The Dangers of Participative Management: A Test of Unexamined Assumptions Concerning Employee Involvement," *Review of Public Personnel Administration*, Summer 1985, 9–25; W. J. Bopp and W. P. Rosenthal, "Participatory Management," *American Journal of Nursing*, Apr. 1979, 671–672; J. A. Fanning and R. B. Lovett, "Decentralization Reduces Nursing Administration Budget," *Journal of Nursing Administration*, May 1985, 19–24; G. W. Poteet, op. cit.; C. L. Cox, op. cit.; R. E. Walton, op. cit.; S. R. Hinkley, Jr., "A Closer Look at Participation," *Organizational Dynamics*, Winter 1985, 57–67.
34. J. E. Bragg and I. R. Andrews, op. cit.
35. W. J. Weisz, op. cit.
36. M. P. Lovrich, op. cit.; M. H. Schuster and C. H. Miller, op. cit.
37. H. Shoemaker and A. El-Ahraf, op. cit.; M. P. Lovrich, op. cit.; W. J. Weisz, op. cit.; C. L. Cox, op. cit.
38. J. A. Raelin, C. Sholl, and D. Leonard, op. cit.; H. Shoemaker and A. El-Ahraf, op. cit.; R. E. Walton, op. cit.
39. J. A. Raelin, C. Sholl, and D. Leonard, op. cit.
40. J. E. Bragg and I. R. Andrews, op. cit.
41. M. R. Probst and J. M. Noga, "A Decentralized Nursing Care Delivery System," *Supervisor Nurse*, Jan. 1980, 57–60; E. A. Alpern, P. M. White and A. F. Donahue, op. cit.

42. R. E. Levinson, "Why Decentralize?," *Management Review,* Oct. 1985, 50–53.

43. Ibid.

44. L. L. Hatcher and T. L. Ross, "Organizational Development Through Productivity Gainsharing," *Personnel,* Oct. 1985, 42, 44–50; R. E. Walton, op. cit.

45. R. E. Walton, op. cit.

The Directing Process

14

INTRODUCTION AND BACKGROUND

In describing the functions of management, Fayol stated that the manager must know how to handle people and must be able to defend his or her point of view with confidence and enthusiasm. The manager must learn continuously and must educate people at all levels for success in their assigned tasks.[1]

Fayol stated that command occurs when the manager gets "the optimum return from all employees of his (sic) unit in the interest of the whole concern."[2] To do this the manager must know the personnel, eliminate the incompetent, be well versed in binding agreements with employees, set a good example, conduct periodic audits, confer with chief assistants to focus on unity of direction, not become mired in detail, and have as a goal unity, energy, initiative, and loyalty among employees.[3] Fayol defined coordination as creating harmony among all activities to facilitate the working and success of the unit.[4] In modern management, command and coordination are labelled "directing."

According to Urwick, it is the purpose of command and the function of directing to see that individual interests do not interfere with the general interest.[5] Command (directing) protects the general interest and should ensure that each unit has a competent and energetic head. Command functions to promote esprit de corps and to carefully select a staff that can be of most service.[6] It was Urwick's premise that bringing in new blood rather than promoting from within may excite resentment. He indicated the need for a grievance procedure, for common rules to be observed by all, and for regulation that allows for self-discipline. Managers should explain regulations and cut red tape. They should "decarbonize," clean out rules and regulations as needed.[7]

Rowland and Rowland stated that directing is "closely interrelated with leadership."[8] They suggested that a manager's choice of leadership style will be the major factor in exercising the directing function. Among the activities of directing are delegation, communication, training, and motivation.[9]

Kron used the term "implementing" as a synonym for "directing." The activities noted under this function include supervision, making assignments and giving directions, observation, evaluation, and leadership and interpersonal relationships with co-workers, maintaining morale, and supervision.[10]

Douglass provided the following definition:

> Directing is the issuance of assignments, orders, and instructions that permit the worker to understand what is expected of him or her, and the guidance and overseeing of the worker so that he or she can contribute effectively and efficiently to the attainment of organizational objectives.[11]

Douglass considered interpersonal relationships and communication to be directing functions, leadership and management taking effect through communication. According to Douglass, there are twelve technical activities or objectives related to the directing function at lower or first-level management. These activities are part of the directing function of the nurse manager and include:

1. Formulating objectives for care that are realistic for the health agency, patient, client and nursing personnel.
2. Giving first priority to the needs of the patients/clients assigned to the nursing staff.
3. Providing for coordination and efficiency among departments that provide support services.
4. Identifying responsibility for all activities under the purview of nursing staff.
5. Providing for safe, continuous care.
6. Considering the need for variety in task assignment and for development of personnel.
7. Providing for the leader's availability to staff members for assistance, teaching, counsel, and evaluation.
8. Trusting members to follow through with their assignments.
9. Interpreting protocol for responding to incidental requests.
10. Explaining procedure to be followed in emergencies.
11. Giving clear, concise formal and informal directions.
12. Using a management control process that assesses the quality of care given and evaluates individual and group performance given by nursing personnel.[12]

Fulmer and Franklin defined a manager or supervisor as "someone who is responsible for directing the performance of one or more workers so that organizational goals are accomplished."[13] Rubin, Fry, and Plovnick wrote of directing in terms of theories of leadership effectiveness, group dynamics, values and value conflicts, effective interpersonal transactions, working with teams, and managing teams in organizations.[14] Barrett referred to development of personnel and supervision of work; Alexander to communication, assignments, and staffing.[15]

According to Donovan, standards are a basis for directing and controlling. They provide direction for performance. Other sources for direction are procedure manuals and policy manuals. A nurse manager orients a new worker to the use of these manuals and thereby facilitates the following of standards in the performance of nursing work. Other sources of standards are job descriptions arrived at through job analysis. They subsequently form the basis for personnel evaluation. Donovan indicated that nursing care plans, nursing care conferences, and patient care conferences are the vehicles for directing nursing care. Directing is also influenced by the physical plant, how the facilities are organized, and by patient distribution according to degree of illness.[16]

DIRECTING AND NURSING MANAGEMENT

Directing is a physical act of nursing management, the interpersonal process by which nursing personnel accomplish the objectives of nursing. To understand fully what it entails, the nurse manager examines the conceptual functions of nursing management, i.e., planning and organizing.[17] From the statement of mission or purpose, the statement of beliefs or philosophy, and the written objectives, the nurse manager develops management plans, the process by which methods and techniques are selected and used to accomplish the work of the nursing unit. Directing is the process of applying the management plans to accomplish nursing objectives. It is the process by which nursing personnel are inspired or motivated to accomplish work. Three of the major elements of directing are embodied in supervision of nursing personnel; motivation, leadership, and communication.[18] These elements are discussed in succeeding chapters.

Nurse managers will learn something of the nature of human beings. Subordinates are hired as total human beings and have to be managed as total human beings who respond to many institutions within society: church, school, government, family, service organizations, professional societies, and all of the other social groupings. There are similarities and differences between supervisors and subordinates. Both are complex human beings with known and conscious needs for food, safety, sex, and human associations. People react to the stresses and strains of a fast-paced society and may need some time for solitude if they are to function effectively and survive. Most individuals place their own concerns before those of others. They enjoy work from which the benefits exceed the costs, and they take a job that meets their established priorities for income, and, maybe, social life.

People can be led and will accept leadership for various reasons, among them admiration, power, income, and safety. The zest with which they pursue achieving the objectives of the nursing division, department, service, or unit will correspond to the leader's ability to create an internal environment that inspires them to work at the levels of their capabilities. It is inherent in the acceptance of an administrative position that the person develop and use leadership abilities. These include:

1. Identification of personal training needs of individuals and establishment of programs to meet them.
2. Establishment of a system of performance appraisal to identify personal competencies and assignment and promotion based on competency.
3. Development of trust and subsequent delegation of responsibility and authority for decision making.

A good leader will contribute to creating a work environment that has the following properties:

1. Jobs that offer a living wage as well as adequate work.
2. Group identity and group purpose—the opportunity to work with others.
3. Pleasant surroundings and coworkers.
4. Interesting work.
5. Recognition that employees' work is valued and well done.
6. Opportunity for accomplishment and challenge.
7. Harmony between organizational and individual goals: equality of opportunity to be safe and secure, to achieve differently, to have choices about shifts, to have job enlargement, and to be recognized as an individual.

Like other human beings, a nurse leader who is also a nurse manager is in many ways different from subordinates. He or she is the one who persuades the group to work to achieve organizational objectives. The nurse leader knows more about organizational policies, goals, new programs, and plans for change. He or she is believed to have good judgment based on a breadth of experience. He or she controls the careers of subordinates. The nurse leader is expected to behave in a socially acceptable manner, to exhibit personal qualities acceptable to subordinates, and to demonstrate skill in leadership, communication, and motivation techniques.

Effective directing increases subordinates' contributions to achievement of nursing management goals. Effective directing creates harmony between nursing management goals and nursing workers' goals. Effective directing operationalizes the principle of unity of command; a subordinate is answerable to one boss as completely as possible.[19]

DELEGATING

Delegating is a major element of the directing function of nursing management. It is an effective management competency by which nurse managers get the work done through their employees. One of the criticisms of new nurse managers is that they emerge from clinical nurse roles and fail to develop identification with their management roles. They have been rewarded for their nursing, not for their skill in leading nurses. Delegation is a part of management requiring professional management training and development to accept the hierarchical responsibilities of delegation. Nurse managers need to be able to accept delegation of some of their own duties, tasks, and responsibilities as a solution to overwork leading to stress, anger, and aggression.

As nurse managers learn to accept the principle of delegation they become more productive and come to enjoy relationships with the staff. They learn to delegate by purposefully thinking about the delegation process, by doing careful planning for it, by gaining knowledge of clinical nurses' capabilities, by planning and implementing effective interpersonal communications, and by being willing to take risks. As they learn to delegate they become freed of daily pressures and time-consuming chores and have time to manage.

The following is a list of ways for nurse managers to delegate successfully:

1. Train and develop subordinates. It is an investment. Give them reasons for the task, authority, details, opportunity for growth and written instructions if needed.
2. Plan ahead. It prevents problems.
3. Control and coordinate the work of subordinates. Do not peer over their shoulders. Develop ways of measuring the accomplishment of objectives with communication, standards, measurements, and feedback to prevent errors. Nursing employees want to know the nurse manager's expectations of them. They understand expectations where there are clear, consistent messages and behavior that prevents confusion. They understand expectations from clearly defined jobs, work relationships, and expected results.
4. Visit subordinates periodically. Spot potential problems of morale, disagreement, and grievance.
5. Coordinate to prevent duplication of effort.
6. Solve problems and think about new ideas. Emphasize employees solving their own problems.
7. Accept delegation as desirable.
8. Specify goals and objectives.
9. Know subordinates' capabilities and match the task of duty to the employee. Be sure the employee considers it important.
10. Agree on performance standards. Relate managerial references to employee performance.
11. Take an interest.
12. Assess results. Expect what is clearly and directly asked for as the deadline set for completing and reporting arrives. The nurse manager should accept the fact that employees will perform delegated tasks in their own style.
13. Give appropriate rewards.
14. Do not take back delegated tasks.[20]

Build professional nurses' self-esteem by delegating as much of the authority for nursing practice as possible. Professional nurses want authority over their practice and can be educated to perform management tasks related to it. Nurse managers will determine what authority to delegate through communication with clinical nurses. Authority should be commensurate with assigned responsibility. As professional nurses gain individual self-esteem, organizational self-esteem follows. Employees respond to participation in decision making and gain satisfaction with their jobs and the organization.

Organizational self-esteem will be built by:

1. Managerial interest in employees' well-being, status, and contributions and concern and support for their personal problems, personal development, and comfort.
2. Job variety from delegation that provides job enlargement, autonomy, significant work, and use of skills and abilities the employees value. Delegating that enlarges an employee's job develops his or her sense of responsibility, general understanding, and job satisfaction.
3. A climate or work environment that bolsters cohesiveness and trust.
4. Management faith in and recognition of the rewards of self-direction.[21]

Reasons for Delegating

Five reasons for delegating include:

1. Assigning routine tasks.
2. Assigning tasks for which the nurse manager does not have time.
3. Problem solving.
4. Changes in the nurse manager's own job emphasis.
5. Capability building.[22]

The nurse manager should be careful not to misuse the clinical nurse by delegating tasks that can be done by non-nurses or nonlicensed personnel. This error can be avoided by consulting with clinical nurses to determine what authority they want.

Techniques for Delegating

Nurse managers at all levels can prepare lists of duties that can be delegated, from nurse executive to department head, from department head to unit head, and from unit head to clinical nurse. Delegation includes authority to approve, recommend, or implement. The list of duties should be ranked by time required to perform them and their importance to the institution. One duty should be delegated at a time.

When Not to Delegate

Do not delegate the power to discipline, responsibility for maintaining morale, overall control, a "hot potato," jobs that are too technical, or duties involving a confidence.[23] These are complicated areas of nursing management requiring specialized knowledge and skills. Nurse managers who handle them should be well educated in the sciences of management and behavioral technology. Delegating these duties and responsibilities will cause clinical nurses to assume that managers are incompetent to handle these areas of nursing leadership and management.

Barriers to Delegating

Barriers to delegating are listed in Figure 14–1.

MANAGEMENT BY OBJECTIVES

Management by objectives (MBO) as a directing element was first advocated by Peter Drucker and made famous by George Ordiorne, who defined it as:

> a process whereby the superior and subordinate managers of an organization jointly identify its common goals, define each individual's major areas of responsibility in terms of the results expected of him (sic), and use these measures as guides for operating the unit and assessing the contribution of each of its members.[24]

Ordiorne further defines MBO as a system for making organizational structure work, to bring

FIGURE 14–1. Barriers to Delegating

Barriers in the Delegator

1. Preference for operating oneself.
2. Demand that everyone "know all the details."
3. "I can do it better myself" fallacy.
4. Lack of experience in the job or in delegating.
5. Insecurity.
6. Fear of being disliked.
7. Refusal to allow mistakes.
8. Lack of confidence in subordinates.
9. Perfectionism, leading to excessive control.
10. Lack of organizational skill in balancing work loads.
11. Failure to delegate authority commensurate with responsibility.
12. Uncertainty over tasks and inability to explain.
13. Disinclination to develop subordinates.
14. Failure to establish effective controls and to follow up.

Barriers in the Delegatee

1. Lack of experience.
2. Lack of competence.
3. Avoidance of responsibility.
4. Overdependence on the boss.
5. Disorganization.
6. Overload of work.
7. Immersion in trivia.

Barriers in the Situation

1. One-person-show policy.
2. No toleration of mistakes.
3. Criticality of decisions.
4. Urgency, leaving no time to explain (crisis management).
5. Confusion in responsibilities and authority.
6. Understaffing.

SOURCE: Reprinted by permission of publisher from, *The Time Trap*, by R. Alex MacKenzie © 1972 AMACOM, a division of American Management Association, New York. All rights reserved.

about vitality and personal involvement in the hierarchy by means of statements of what is expected from everyone involved and measurement of what is actually achieved. It stresses ability and achievement rather than personality.[25]

MBO allows the individual nurse to contribute to the common goal of the enterprise while nurse managers focus on the business goals. It promotes high standards, focusing on the job and not on the manager or the worker. Applying Drucker's MBO theory accomplishes this as nurse managers are the persons who know what to expect of employees. Just like their managers, nursing staff should know for what they will be held accountable.[26]

MBO spells out the results expected of the clinical nursing unit and of the unit in relation to other units. It emphasizes teamwork and team results. It will include short-range and long-range objectives, as well as tangible and intangible objectives. Intangible objectives include development of the individual, performance and attitude of workers, and public responsibilities. Objectives should include those that indicate the contributions to higher levels of the enterprise.

MBO allows people to control their own performance, to measure themselves, and to exercise self-control. Through MBO clinical nurses make demands of themselves. Nurse managers will assume that clinical nurses want to be responsible, want to contribute, want to achieve, and have the strength and desire to do so. According to Drucker:

> What the business enterprise needs is a principle of management that will give full scope to individual strength and responsibility as well as common direction to vision and effort, establish team work, and harmonize the goals of the individual with the commonweal. Management by objectives and self-control make the commonweal the aim of every manager. It substitutes for control from outside the stricter, more exacting, and more effective control from inside. It motivates the manager to action, not because somebody tells him (sic) to do something or talks him into doing it, but because the objective task demands it. He acts not because somebody wants him to but because he himself decides that he has to—he acts, in other words, as a free man.
>
> I do not use the word "philosophy" lightly; indeed I prefer not to use it at all; it's much too big a word. But management by objectives and self-control may properly be called a philosophy of management. It rests on a concept of the management group and the obstacles it faces. It rests on every manager, whatever his level and function, and to any organization whether large or small. It

ensures performance by converting objective needs into personal goals. And this is genuine freedom.[27]

Procedure and Process

Training. Begin the training for the MBO process with the nurse managers of the enterprise. They will learn the characteristics of the process, the objectives of initiating an MBO program, the procedures to be used, and methods for evaluating its effectiveness. During this training program nurse managers can simulate the procedures to be used.

Once nurse managers are trained, all nursing employees are given similar training. Employees will be made aware of the necessity for writing and working towards their personal objectives as they seek to achieve those of the organization. They will be taught the value of synergism of personal and organizational objectives. They will bring their written lists of objectives to the first meeting with their superiors (see Figure 14–2).

First Meeting. The first MBO meeting should be held in quiet surroundings, with sufficient time for discussion. The nurse manager should set the employee at ease. Most survival and safety needs of nurses are reasonably satisfied. Their social, ego, and self-fulfillment needs are predominant at this time. As they present each personal objective the nurse manager relates it to an objective of the enterprise. Thus they create the conditions for them to fulfill these needs. This includes the removal of obstacles, encouragement of growth, and provision of guidance.

Nurses, like other workers, do not have their higher-level needs met by their employers. They meet these higher-level needs themselves by using their capabilities, having responsibility, being active, having meaningful work, being self-controlled and self-directed, and being treated as mature adults. They want to participate by setting their own targets and evaluating themselves in obtaining them.[28] Nurse managers can facilitate these processes by establishing a climate and environment that supports achievement of the higher-level needs of clinical nurses.

Nurses are professionals and will not be controlled. Nurse managers and clinical nurse employees can explain their jobs to each other during the MBO process. The nurse manager may learn that the clinical nurse wants management to promote dignity and personal responsibility, peer status and acceptance, and recognition for achievement and creativity. The clinical nurses may learn that the nurse manager represents an organization that will create the conditions for them to achieve their own goals by directing their efforts toward the goals of the organization.[29]

During this first meeting nurse managers and clinical nurses set goals that are specific, promote teamwork, are measurable in terms of being quantified or described qualitatively, and are attainable. Goals should involve enough risk to challenge but not defeat. They should include objectives that are routine, problem solving, creative or innovative, and for personal development.[30]

At the end of the first meeting both nurse manager and clinical nurse should be satisfied with the written objectives. Each will have a copy. They will part with an understanding of how future meetings will progress and mutual expectations, including a time for the next meeting.

Actions. Between meetings employees perform work that meets their agreed-upon objectives. They should periodically review these objectives and summarize their accomplishments.

Second Meeting. Conditions for the second MBO meeting will be as for the first meeting. It will be a time for evaluation of results, review, appraisal, and setting further goals.

The employee should be encouraged to spell out gratifying and exhilarating experiences, to do self-examination, and to relate his or her thoughts about work. The nurse manager should listen and make the employee feel safe while helping him or her to have a person-organization fit.

The superior examines his or her own reactions without criticizing the subordinate. They build trust and confidence as well as an ethical relationship. In doing so they establish an organizational climate for personal and organizational achievement.[31]

MBO should include appraisal of managers by subordinates. The latter will appraise how well the manager helps employees do their jobs, supports them, assists with problems, and demonstrates proficiency and visibility.[32]

Both nurse manager and employee should exit this meeting with a sense of accomplishment. This does not mean they will not be made aware of

deficiencies or shortcomings. It will be recognized in the form of needed additions or changes, increased progress and even deletions. All will be tied to patient care and organizational development. It is the feedback process that tells employees what is expected and when they make errors.

This process will be repeated at intervals, with dates and times agreed upon at each meeting. At the end of an appraisal period a performance results contract will be signed off and sent to the personnel department for the employee's record. This performance appraisal can be used to identify promotion potential and determine merit pay increases.

Problems with MBO

MBO must be viewed as genuine and fair by all employees. It must allow for errors and for adjustments due to work constraints and individual capabilities. Specific problems of MBO include:

1. *Top management nonsupport.* To be effective MBO must be supported and carried out at all levels. It must be monitored closely.

2. *Inconsistency among managers.* This can be fixed or avoided by awareness of both parties. Periodic summative evaluation conferences can help uncover these inconsistencies.

3. *Goals either too easy or unattainable.* Employees sometimes fear that they will be subjected to goals of increasing difficulty. Frank discussion will help resolve this problem. Employees have a need to meet increasing personal needs as they climb the career ladder. These can be recognized and satisfied through MBO.

4. *Conflict of goals and policies.* When this occurs, policies should give way to goals unless they would violate a safety or legal standard.

5. *Accountability beyond control of subordinates.* When this occurs the nurse manager helps modify the goal and makes allowance for the difference. This can be done by decreasing accountability or increasing authority. Factors beyond the employee's control should not be evaluated.

6. *Lack of commitment of subordinates.* Determine the cause if possible and produce interactions that will

FIGURE 14–2. Summary of MBO Cycle

Phase	Key Activities	Participants
Planning	Identify and define key organizational goals.	Manager
	Identify and define key departmental goals that stem from overall goals.	
	Identify and define performance measures (operational goals) for employees.	
	Formulate and propose goals for specific job.	Subordinate
	Formulate and propose measures for specific jobs.	
	Participate in management conferences.	Manager and
	Achieve joint agreement on individual objectives and individual performance.	subordinates
	Set up timetable for periodic meetings for performance review.	
Performance review	Continue to participate in management conferences.	Manager and
	Adjust and refine objectives based on feedback, new constraints, and new inputs.	subordinates
	Eliminate inappropriate goals.	
	Readjust timetable as needed.	
	Maintain ongoing comparison of proposed timetable and actual performance through use of control monitoring devices, such as visible control charts.	
Feedback to new planning stage	Review overall organizational and departmental goals for the next planning period, such as the next fiscal year.	Manager

Reprinted from *Management Principles for Health Professionals* by J. G. Liebler, R. E. Levine, and H. L. Dervitz, p. 253, with permission of Aspen Publishers, Inc., © 1984.

increase commitment. Discuss the problem frankly and encourage the subordinate to be specific in a plan to cope with it. Do not threaten.

Organizational Development

MBO is needed for organizational development (OD) and vice versa. It allows the organization to be managed against goals and for results. OD occurs as management skills and organizational processes are applied to shape and develop the conditions for human effectiveness. These are:

1. Interpersonal competence. The individual has high expectations, respect for the individual, honest relationships, freedom to act, and a team orientation.
2. Meaningful goals. The goals are understandable, desirable, attainable, and synergistic. The individual influences the goals.
3. Helpful systems. Users understand them and control them because they are goal-oriented and

provide feedback. Users adapt to them and adopt them.
4. Achievement/self-actualization. As the organization grows the individual grows. People are committed to goals, are highly motivated, and have high trust and minimal dissatisfaction.[33]

The philosophy of management should permit these conditions for human effectiveness to occur. In addition it should emphasize meaningful work in which the doers are involved in all aspects of the job. Managers should delegate decisions, ensuring that they are made, that limits are known, that support is provided, and that accountability is met through evaluation of results. MBO is a total management process that includes planning, organizing, directing, and controlling.

Figure 14–2 illustrates the MBO process and Figure 14–3 is a list of standards for evaluating the directing function of nursing management.

A theory of nursing management explores the cause-effect relationship between clinical nurses

FIGURE 14–3. Standards for Evaluation of the Directing Function

1. Managers have established a medium by which nursing workers feel free to ask for advice, counsel, and consultation.
2. Needed written directions are available in the form of policies, procedures, standards of care, job analysis, job descriptions, job standards, and nursing care plans. They are clearly stated and current.
3. A training program is in effect that meets nursing employees' needs as they perceive them. They participate.
4. Supervisors are competent in needed knowledge and skills of administration and clinical specialization.
5. Nurse managers periodically work evening, night, weekend, and holiday shifts to keep abreast of clinical and administrative behaviors peculiar to these shifts.
6. The nurse administrator has operationalized ANA *Standards for Organized Nursing Services* and *Responsibilities of Nurse Administrators Across All Settings.*
7. The nurse managers have operationalized the ANA *Standards of Nursing Practice.*
8. Nurse managers are knowledgeable about and apply the appropriate Standards of the Joint Commission on Accreditation of Healthcare Organizations, National League for Nursing, and Medicare and Medicaid.
9. The nurse administrator uses techniques of operations analysis. (This service is available at no charge to member hospitals of the American Hospital Association and its state affiliates.)
10. Nurse managers use a system of management by objectives.
11. The nurse administrator works with the consent and knowledge of patients and solicits input from consumers regarding nursing services desired.
12. Nursing unit personnel are organized into and working as direct care personnel and clerical personnel.
13. Nurse managers use the physical plant to the best advantage for patients and personnel.

and their performances. It has as object the removal of controls that create distrust, fear, and resentment and the promotion of conditions (climate) that provide opportunities for clinical nurses to achieve their goals.

SUMMARY

Effective directing will result in greater harmony in the actions of supervisors and subordinates and in the achievement of the objectives of personnel as well as of the enterprise. Directing will be most effective when a subordinate has a single superior who gives direct personal contact. Direction that encourages leadership, motivation, and communication techniques and which emphasizes the human aspects of managing individuals is most desirable. It can be fostered by nursing administrators who desire to improve their directing activities.

NOTES

1. H. Fayol, trans., *General and Industrial Management,* by C. Storrs (London: Sir Isaac Pitman & Sons, 1949), 82–96.
2. Ibid., 97.
3. Ibid., 97–98.
4. Ibid., 103.
5. L. Urwick, *The Elements of Administration* (New York: Harper & Row, 1944), 77.
6. Ibid., 81–82.
7. Ibid., 90–96.
8. H. S. Rowland and B. L. Rowland, Eds., *Nursing Administration Handbook,* 2d ed. (Rockville, MD: Aspen, 1980), 7.
9. Ibid., 8.
10. T. Kron and A. Gray, *The Management of Patient Care: Putting Leadership Skills to Work,* 6th ed. (Philadelphia: W. B. Saunders, 1987), 155–176.
11. L. M. Douglass, *The Effective Nurse: Leader and Manager* (3rd ed. Saint Louis: C. V. Mosby, 1988), 115.
12. Ibid., 117–118.
13. R. M. Fulmer and S. G. Franklin, *Supervision: Principles of Professional Management* (2d. ed. New York: Macmillan, 1982), 6.
14. I. M. Robin, R. E. Fry, and M. S. Plovnick, Eds., *Managing Human Resources in Health Care Organizations* (Reston, VA: Reston Publishing, 1978), 128–29, 154–61, 182–89, 198, 236–43.
15. J. Barrett, *The Head Nurse: Her Changing Role* (New York: Appleton Century Crofts, 1968), 310–32; E. L. Alexander, *Nursing Administration in the Hospital Health Care System,* 2d ed. (Saint Louis: C. V. Mosby, 1978), 198–246.
16. H. M. Donovan, *Nursing Service Administration: Managing the Enterprise* (Saint Louis: C. V. Mosby, 1975), 128–54.
17. C. Arndt and L. M. D. Huckabay, *Nursing Administration: Theory for Practice with a Systems Approach,* 2d ed. (Saint Louis: C. V. Mosby, 1980), 92–106.
18. H. Koontz, C. O'Donnell and H. Weihrich, *Essentials of Management* (4th ed. New York: McGraw-Hill, 1986), 392.
19. R. C. Swansburg, *The Directing Function of Nursing Service Administration* (Hattiesburg, MS: University of Southern Mississippi School of Nursing, 1977), 3–5.

20. B. B. Beegle, "Don't Do It—Delegate It!," *Supervisory Management*, Apr. 1970; J. K. Matejka and R. J. Dunsing, "Great Expectations," *Management World*, Jan. 1987, 16–17.

21. J. K. Matejka and R. J. Dunsing, op. cit.

22. H. S. Rowland and B. L. Rowland, op. cit., 54–57.

23. Ibid.

24. R. M. Hodgetts, *Management: Theory, Process and Practice* (4th ed. Orlando, Fl.: Academic Press, 1986), 575.

25. Ibid.

26. P. F. Drucker, *Management: Tasks, Responsibilities, Practices* (New York: Harper & Row, 1973, 1974), 430–442.

27. Ibid., 441–442.

28. D. McGregor, *Leadership and Motivation* (Cambridge, MA: MIT Press, 1966).

29. Ibid.

30. M. L. Bell, "Management by Objectives," *Journal of Nursing Administration*, May 1980, 19–26.

31. H. Levinson, "Management by Whose Objectives?," *Harvard Business Review*, July-Aug. 1970, 125–134.

32. Ibid.

33. A. C. Beck, Jr., and E. D. Hillman, "OD to MBO or MBO to OD: Does It Make a Difference?," in A. T. Hollingsworth and R. M. Hodgetts, *Readings in Basic Management* (Philadelphia: W. B. Saunders, 1975), 190–196.

REFERENCES

Gibson, J. L., J. W. Ivancevich, and J. H. Donnelly, Jr., *Organizations: Behavior, Structure, Processes*, 6th ed. (Homewood, Il.: Richard A. Irwin, Inc., 1988.)

Holley, W. H. and K. M. Jennings, *Personnel Management: Functions and Issues* (New York: Dryden Press, 1983), 237–240.

Leadership

15

SHARON FARLEY, Ph.D., R.N.,
Associate Professor,
School of Nursing
Auburn University at Montgomery
Montgomery, Alabama

Florence Nightingale, after leaving the Crimea, exercised extraordinary leadership in health care for decades with no organization under her command.[1]

One of the purest examples of the leader as agenda-setter was Florence Nightingale. Her public image was and is that of the lady of mercy, but under her gentle, soft-spoken manner, she was a rugged spirit, a fighter, a tough-minded system changer. In mid-nineteenth century England a woman had no place in public life, least of all in the fiercely masculine world of the military establishment. But she took on the establishment and revolutionized health care in the British military services. Yet she never made public appearances or speeches, and except for her two years in the Crimea, held no public position. She was a formidable authority on the evils to be remedied, she knew exactly what to do about them, and she used public opinion to goad top officials to adopt her agenda.[2]

Florence Nightingale was both leader and manager.

LEADERSHIP DEFINED

Researchers have studied leadership for decades, but experts still do not agree on exactly what it is. Many persons use the term leadership as if it were a magic quality, almost as if one must be born with it or as if one simply has a talent for it. However, like talent for music and art, leadership requires much knowledge and disciplined practice. Many definitions of leadership have been written, among them that of Stogdill, who defines it as "the process of influencing the activities of an organized group in its efforts toward goal setting and goal achievement."[3] There is a difference in responsibilities among group members, and each influences the groups' activities. A leader is one others follow willingly and voluntarily.[4]

Stogdill's definition of leadership can be applied to nursing. In nursing practice, goals of patient care are set. Each patient has a nursing care plan that lists the problems that interfere with achieving physical, emotional, and social needs. For each problem a goal is set and an approach or nursing prescription is written. An interdisciplinary team may identify problems, set goals, and write prescriptions. They are influenced by the most highly skilled nurse available, the registered nurse who coordinates the care. Each interdisciplinary team member assumes different responsibilities in performing the total team functions. This process holds true when the modality of team nursing is practiced or when there is a mixed staff of R.N.s, L.P.N.s, and nursing assistants.

The same principles may be applied to the entire division of nursing. Usually the head of the division is titled assistant administrator, vice-president, chair, or director of nursing services. This person is responsible for influencing all nursing employees in achieving the stated purpose and objectives of the division of nursing. The nurse administrator is influenced by a stated philosophy or statement of beliefs about the kinds of services to be rendered by the personnel of the division of nursing. The total staff includes personnel in different job categories, including head nurses, charge nurses of shifts and clinical nursing personnel, each with differing nursing responsibilities.

Gardner defines leadership as "the process of persuasion and example by which an individual (or leadership team) induces a group to take action that is in accord with the leader's purposes or the shared purposes of all."[5] Numerous other definitions of leadership exist. Embodied in these definitions are the terms leader, follower or constituent, group, process, and goals. One would conclude that leadership is a process in which a person inspires a group of constituents to work together using appropriate means to achieve common mission and common goals. They are influenced to do this willingly and cooperatively, with zeal and confidence and to their greatest potential.[6]

Merton described leadership as a social transaction in which one person influences others. He stated that people in authority do not necessarily exert leadership. Rather, effective people in authoritative positions combine authority and leadership to assist an organization to achieve its goals. Merton described effective leadership as satisfying four primary conditions: (1) a person receiving a communication understands it; (2) this person has the resources to do what is being asked of him or her in the communication; (3) she or he believes the behavior being asked is consistent with her or his personal interests and values; and (4) he or she believes it is consistent with the purposes and values of the organization.[7]

According to McGregor, "There are at least four major variables now known to be involved in leadership: (1) the characteristics of the leader; (2) the attitudes, needs, and other personal characteristics of the followers; (3) the characteristics of the organization, such as its purpose, its structure, the nature of the task to be performed; and (4) the social, economic, and political milieu."[8] McGregor said that leadership is a highly complex relationship that changes with the times, such changes being brought about by management, unions, or outside forces. In nursing, changes in leadership are wrought by nursing management, nursing educators, nursing organizations, unions, and the expectations of the clientele—patients and their families.

Talbott said, "Leadership is the vital ingredient that transforms a crowd into a functioning, useful organization."[9] The theme seems always to be the same: "Leadership is the process of sustaining an initiated action. It is certainly not a matter of pointing in a direction and just letting things happen. Leadership is the conception of a goal and a method of achieving it; the mobilization of the means necessary for attainment; and the adjustment of values and environmental factors in the light of the desired end."[10]

In all of these definitions, leadership is viewed as a dynamic, interactive process that involves three dimensions—the leader, the followers, and the situation. Each of the dimensions influences the others. For instance, the accomplishment of goals depends not only on the personal attributes of the leader but also on follower needs and the type of situation.[11]

LEADERSHIP THEORIES

Trait Theories

Much of the early work on leadership focused on the leader. This research was directed toward iden-

FIGURE 15–1.   Traits Associated with Leadership Effectiveness

Intelligence	Personality	Abilities
Judgment	Adaptability	Ability to enlist cooperation
Decisiveness	Alertness	Popularity and prestige
Knowledge	Creativity	Sociability (interpersonal skills)
Fluency of speech	Cooperativeness	Social participation
	Personal integrity	Tact, diplomacy
	Self-confidence	
	Emotional balance and control	
	Independence (nonconformity)	

Adapted from B. M. Bass, *Stogdill's Handbook of Leadership* (New York: Free Press, 1982), 75–76, in J. Gibson, J. Ivancevich, and J. Donnelly, *Organizations: Behavior Structure, Processes* 6th ed., Homewood, IL.: Richard D. Irwin, 1988, 375.

tifying intellectual, emotional, physical, and other personal traits of effective leaders. The underlying assumption was that leaders are born, not made.

After many years of research, no particular set of traits have been found that predict leadership potential. There are some possible reasons for this failure to find specific traits. According to McGregor, "research findings to date suggest that it is more fruitful to consider leadership as a relationship between the leader and the situation than as a universal pattern of characteristics possessed by certain people."[12] This statement implies that leadership is a human relations function and that different situations may require quite different characteristics from a leader. Is it not to a large degree universally accepted in nursing that authoritarian power is effective in times of crisis but that it otherwise promotes instability?

In spite of the shortcomings of the trait theory, some traits have been identified which are common to all good leaders. A summary of some of the most widely researched traits is shown in Figure 15–1.

Intelligence.   Traits related to intelligence include knowledge, decisiveness, and fluency of speech. Perceived knowledge and competence in a specific job is one of the most important factors in a leader's effectiveness. A competent leader has expert power when it is used to inspire subordinates to excel in performance. Leaders who are competent and expert have greater latitude in their relationship with subordinates.

Research has been designed to examine the effects that a leader's expertise has on subordinates' role perceptions of leaders. This approach is related to the path goal theory of leadership: people are attracted to discerning leaders. The sample was 101 employees of a large nonprofit organization attending a planning conference. The "results suggest that leaders with expertise decrease ambiguity when they provide structure for their subordinates, while leaders who lack expertise increase ambiguity when they provide structure for their subordinates."[13]

From this study it could be inferred that nursing leaders who want to be effective should maintain their knowledge and expertise in clinical nursing. This condition has important implications for nursing management education and practice, since even policies and procedures must be perceived as expert in source. While this study has limited use, similar studies could be done by researchers in nursing management.[14]

A requirement of leadership is a gift for language. To influence people, leaders must communicate with them and must do so truthfully. Otherwise their credibility is questioned. Brower said, "A leader, then, must tell and act the truth about himself (sic)."[15]

Traditional systems of communication are through suggestion systems, a house organ or newspaper, and staff meetings. Some behavioral scientists believe that T-group methods may improve communication by helping people establish real and meaningful relationships. Sensitivity training has become more commonplace in nursing as nursing leaders have recognized the need for improved communications.

Leaders are decisive. They take command rather than waiting to be given direction, while remaining mindful that command is contantly in need of ratification by the constituents.

Leaders know the goals of the organization and its employees and how to achieve them. They make the mission important, exciting, and possible. They evaluate all of the resources available to their use in achieving goals. They must then allocate these resources based on priorities. This is important for both organizational growth and employee career development.

Personality.   Personality traits such as adaptability, self-confidence, creativity, and personal integrity are associated with effective leadership. A leader is effective and knows how to motivate workers to achieve the goals of the organization.

"Leaders facilitate the adaptive capacity of social systems. They initiate change that is responsive to both the internal and external environments of the system."[16] As the nursing environment changes, the nursing leader helps personnel adapt to the changing environment. As an example, the nurse manager of today must help nursing personnel adapt to role changes that not only focus upon being a manager of a clinical practice discipline, but upon goals of productivity and profitability in a prospective payment environment. In this changing environment the nurse manager must help staff to develop their new roles while performing the primary functions of nursing as clinicians or practitioners.

A person who motivates others must have emotional balance and control and personal integrity. Jennings describes a leader as having a mission in life, the mission being to overcome mass feelings of alienation and self-inadequacy. He says the mission begins with a struggle with self. The leader develops a personal set of values, courage, and self-control. The leader disciplines herself or himself to wholeness, to acquire inner strength and become a superior type of person.[17] Leaders will not blame others for their failures; they accept responsibility. When they have to, they "eat crow," a bird with a rank taste that can become a mite palatable when results show that people respond to honesty and humility. They have courage and persistence and are believed.

Abilities

A leader has sufficient popularity and prestige and interpersonal skills to symbolize, extend, and deepen collective unity among members of the system. In most nursing situations, the leader is appointed by the hospital or nursing administrator. Without losing authority and control, an appointed leader has to demonstrate understanding and achieve the workers' understanding of and motivation for achieving the goals of the organization. Too often the supervisor has been appointed because of technical and administrative talents rather than leadership abilities or acceptance by the group. This fact points up the relative emphasis given to leadership abilities and attitudes.

All of these traits and characteristics can be used by leaders either to inspire or to deflate morale and esprit de corps. Nurse managers need to develop those nurses who inspire high morale and esprit de corps.

Although it may be that leaders are made, not born, there are some persons who are natural leaders. They emerge from a group in which they have made known their talents for representing and articulating group values and goals. These natural leaders have plans for meeting the personal needs of the group, and thus the group willingly accepts their direction. *The group gives the person in the leadership role influence.* According to Holloman, "Leadership results when the appointed head causes the members of his (sic) group to accept his directives without any apparent exertion of authority or force on his part."[18]

Gardner's Leadership Studies

John W. Gardner is writing a definitive study of leadership. Two major areas of his writings that relate to the traits of leadership are *The Tasks of Leadership* and *Leader-Constituent Interaction.* A brief summary of his ideas on these topics follows.[19] Gardner identifies nine tasks to be performed by leaders:

1. *Envisioning goals.* These include a vision of the best a group can be, solving problems, and unifying constituencies. Goals may involve extensive research. They may be shared and they come from many sources. Long-term goals lend greater stability.

2. *Affirming values.* Communities have "shared assumptions, beliefs, customs, ideas that give meaning, ideas that motivate." These include "norms" or "values." Values embody religious beliefs and secular philosophy. Society celebrates its values in art, song, ritual, historic documents, and textbooks. People will strive to meet standards that affirm their values and motivate them. Values must be continually rebuilt or regenerated, with leaders assisting to rediscover and adapt traditions to the present. Leaders reaffirm values verbally, through policy decisions, and through their conduct.

3. *Motivating.* Leaders stimulate people to serve society and solve its problems. They balance positive attitudes and acts with reality. They look toward the future with confidence, hope, and energy. Loss of confidence breeds rigidity, fatalism, and passivity. Poverty affects morale, learning, and performance negatively. Leaders correct the circumstances of negative attitudes and defeat. Involving employees in decisions gives them a sense of power and ownership. Leaders bring resolve to failure, frustration, and doubt and use intuition and empathy to solve problems.

4. *Managing.* Leadership and management overlap. Leaders set goals, plan, fix priorities, choose means, and formulate policy. They also build organizations and institutions that outlast them. Leaders keep the system functioning by setting agendas and making decisions. Leaders mold public opinion and exercise political judgments.

5. *Achieving workable unity.* Leaders function in a pluralistic society in which conflict is necessary if there are grievances to be settled. Conflict is also necessary in commercial competition, settling civil suits, and bringing justice to the oppressed. Conflict must be resolved to achieve cohesion and mutual tolerance, internally and externally. Society is fragmented and must not be polarized. Conflict resolution requires political skills: brokering, coalition formation, mediating conflicting views, de-escalation of rhetoric and posturing, saving face, and seeking common ground. People must trust each other most of the time to prevent or resolve conflict. Leaders raise the level of trust.

6. *Explaining.* Leaders must communicate effectively. They teach.

7. *Serving as a symbol.* Leaders speak for others. They represent unity, collective identity, and continuity.

8. *Representing the group.* All human systems are interdependent. Leaders view events affecting them broadly.

9. *Renewing.* Leaders blend continuity with change. They are innovators who awaken the potential of others. They visit the front lines and keep in touch. Leaders sustain diversity and dissent, and they change the social order.[20]

Leader-Constituent Interaction

Charismatic leaders. Gardner defines charisma as the quality that sets one person apart from others: supernatural, superhuman, endowed with exceptional qualities or powers. Charismatic leadership can be evil. Charismatic leaders emerge in troubled times and in relation to the state of mind of constituents. They eventually run out of miracles and "white horses" even though they are magnetic, persuasive, and spellbinding.

Masses of people will often follow the charismatic leader. Such masses have historically been labelled unstable. The worry of mob rule and instability still exists. Social disorder is embodied in our constitution as human beings.

Influence of constituents on leader. Constituents and leaders have an equal influence on each other. Constituents confer the leadership role. Good constituents select good leaders and make them better. In politics constituents may follow any leader unless they are bureaucratic constituents (such as government employees) who feel constrained to mute their support. Loyal constituents support leaders who help meet needs and solve problems.

Influence of leader on constituents. Leaders choose to be leaders. They must adapt their leadership style to the situation and to their constituents. In doing so they weigh these considerations: the degree of structure they want in relationships with constituents; the degree or hierarchy of authority; formality; disciplines; constraints; controls; and the amount of focus on task versus people.

Leaders influence their superiors and their subordinates and have the courage to defy their constituents. Sam Houston was a leader of this type. He opposed the secession of Texas from the United States, going contrary to his constituents. A leader may show different faces to pluralistic groups of constituents, including special interest groups.

Transforming leaders. Transforming leaders respond to the basic needs, wants, hopes, and expectations of people. They may transcend the political system or even attempt to construct it in order to operate within it. Transforming leadership is innovative and evolutionary.

The best leadership may be that which focuses on self-development and self-actualization. Leaders should develop the strengths of constituents and make them independent.[21]

Behavioral Theories

Among the behavioral research and theories are those of Douglas McGregor's Theory X and Theory Y, Rensis Likert's Michigan Studies, Blake and Mouton's managerial grid, and Kurt Lewin's studies. Each of these is described in more detail below.

McGregor's Theory X and Theory Y. McGregor's Theory X and Theory Y are discussed elsewhere in this book. McGregor related his theories to the motivation theories of Maslow.

McGregor stated that each person is a whole individual living and interacting within a world of other individuals. What happens to this person happens as a result of the behavior of other people. The attitudes and emotions of others affect this person. The subordinate is dependent upon the superior and desires to be treated fairly. A successful relationship is desired by both and depends upon the action taken by the superior.

Security is a condition of leadership. Subordinates need security and will fight to protect themselves against real or imagined threats to their needs in the work situation. Superiors must act to give subordinates this security through avenues such as fair pay and fringe benefits. Unions act to solidify job security.

A superior provides a further condition for effective leadership by creating an atmosphere of approval for subordinates. This atmosphere is created through the leader's manner and attitude. Given the genuine approval of their superior, sub-ordinates will be secure. Otherwise they will feel threatened, fearful, and insecure.

Knowledge is another condition of effective leadership espoused by McGregor. A person has security when she or he knows what is expected of her or him, including:

1. Knowledge of overall company policy and management philosophy.
2. Knowledge of procedures, rules, and regulations.
3. Knowledge of the requirements of the subordinate's own job—duties, responsibilities, and place in the organization.
4. Knowledge of the personal peculiarities of the subordinate's immediate superior.
5. Knowledge by the subordinate of the superior's opinion of her or his performance.
6. Advance knowledge of changes that may affect the subordinate.[22]

Consistent discipline is another condition for effective leadership. People are met with approval when they do their jobs according to the rules. They should know what to expect in terms of disapproval when they break these rules. Superiors should be consistent in setting standards and expecting subordinates to meet them. Even discipline must occur in an atmosphere of approval.

Security encourages independence, another condition for effective leadership. Insecurity causes a reactive fight for freedom. Security that stimulates independence is desired. Subordinates need to be actively independent by becoming involved in contributing ideas and suggestions concerning activities that affect them. When workers are secure and are encouraged to participate in solving the problems of work, they provide new approaches to solutions of problems. They work to achieve the goals of the organization and feel they are a part of the organization.

With security and independence, subordinates develop a desire to accept responsibility. The level of responsibility can be increased at a pace commensurate with preservation of their security. It will give them pleasure and pride. Superiors need security before they can delegate responsibility to subordinates.

All subordinates need provision for appeal, for an adequate grievance procedure by which they take their differences with their superiors to a

FIGURE 15–2. Likert's Leadership Systems

Authoritative		Democratic	
System I: Exploitive-Authoritative	System II: Benevolent-Authoritative	System III: Consultative-Democratic	System IV: Participative-Democratic
Top management makes all decisions	Top management makes most decisions	Some delegated decisions made at lower levels	Decision making dispersed throughout organization
Motivation by coercion	Motivation by economic and ego motives	Motivation by economic, ego, and other motives such as desire for new experiences	Motivation by economic rewards established by group participation
Communication downward	Communication mostly downward	Communication down and up	Communication down, up, and with peers
Review and control functions concentrated in top management	Review and control functions primarily at top	Review and control functions primarily at the top but ideas are solicited from lower levels	Review and control functions shared by superiors and subordinates

SOURCE: Adapted from R. Likert, *The Human Organization* (New York: McGraw-Hill, 1967), 4–10. Reprinted with permission of McGraw Hill Book Co. © 1967.

higher level in the organization. Superiors who do the jobs expected of them, who treat subordinates in ways to meet their needs and give them security, achieve self-realization and self-development.[23]

Likert's Michigan Studies. Likert and his associates at the Institute for Social Research at the University of Michigan did extensive leadership research. They identified four basic styles or systems of leadership: exploitive-authoritative, benevolent-authoritative, consultative-democratic, and participative-democratic. These systems are summarized in Figure 15–2.

A measuring instrument for evaluating an organization's leadership style was developed by Likert's group. It contains fifty-one items and encompasses variables of the concepts of "leadership, motivation, communication, interaction-influence, decision-making, goal setting, control, and performance goals."[24]

It is generally conceded that leadership behav-

ior improves in effectiveness as it approaches System IV.

Blake and Mouton's Managerial Grid® The managerial Grid® is a two-dimensional leadership model. Dimensions of this model are tasks or production and employee or people orientations of managers.

Grid® synopsis. Two key dimensions of managerial thinking are depicted on the Grid®: *Concern for Production* on the horizontal axis, and *Concern for People* on the vertical axis. They are shown as nine-point scales, where 1 represents low concern, 5 represents an average amount of concern, and 9 is high concern.

These two concerns are interdependent; that is, while concern for one or the other may be high or low, they are integrated in the manager's thinking. Thus, both concerns are present to some degree in any management style. Study of the Grid® enables one to sort out various possibilities and the attitudes,

FIGURE 15–3A. The Managerial Grid®

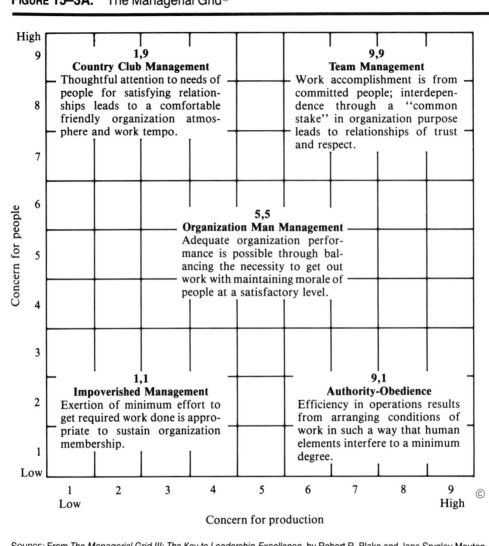

SOURCE: From *The Managerial Grid III: The Key to Leadership Excellence,* by Robert R. Blake and Jane Srygley Mouton. Houston: Gulf Publishing Company. Copyright © 1985, page 12. Reproduced by permission.

values, beliefs, and assumptions that underlie each approach. When one is able to objectively see personal behavior in contrast to the soundest approach, it provides motivation to change in order to more closely approximate the soundest management. When group members come to share 9,9 values, beliefs, attitudes, and assumptions, they develop personal commitment to achieving group goals as well as their individual goals. In doing so, they develop standards of mutual trust and respect that cause them to elevate cooperation and communication.

Blake and Mouton contend that the 9,9 style is the one most likely to achieve highest quality results over an extended period of time. The 9,9 style, unlike the others, is based on the assumption that there is no inherent conflict between the needs of the organization for performance and the needs of people for job satisfaction.

Finally, as an orienting framework, the Grid®

FIGURE 15–3B. The Nurse Administrator Grid®

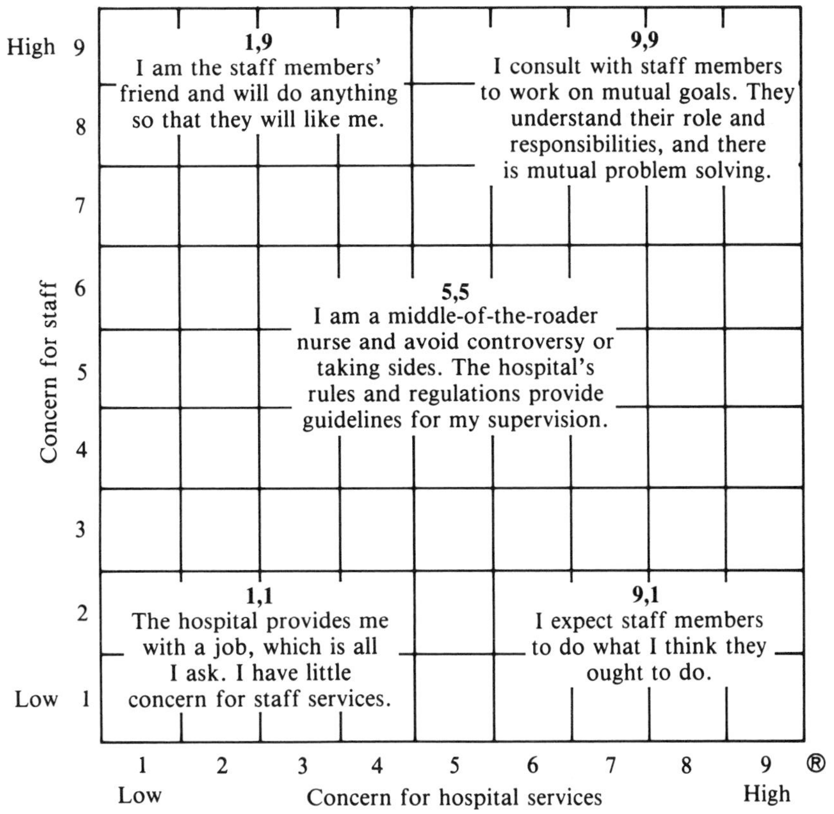

SOURCE: From *Grid Approaches for Managerial Leadership in Nursing,* by Robert R. Blake, Jane Srygley Mouton, and Mildred Tapper. St. Louis: C.V. Mosby Company, Copyright © 1981, page 2. Reproduced by permission.

serves as a roadmap toward more effective ways of working with and through others. When group members have this common frame of reference for what constitutes an effective or an ineffective approach to issues of mutual concern, they are able to take corrective action based on common understanding and agreement about the soundest approach and objectivity when actions taken are less than fully sound.[25]

Figure 15–3a illustrates general management application of the Grid®, while Figure 15–3b illustrates its application to the job of the nurse administrator.

Kurt Lewin's Studies. Lewin's leadership studies were done in the 1930s. He examined three leadership styles related to forces within the leader, within the group members, and within the situation. These three leadership styles are summarized in Figure 15–4.

Other behavioral studies include the Ohio State studies using a quadrant structure that relates leadership effectiveness to initiating structure, with emphasis on the task or production, and consideration, with emphasis on the employee. These studies identified four primary leadership styles, as illustrated in Figure 15–5.

These researchers used the Leader Behavior Description Questionnaire. Items related to "initiating structure" and "consideration" describe how

FIGURE 15–4. Kurt Lewin's Studies of Leadership Styles

Autocratic. Leaders make decisions alone. They tend to be more concerned with task accomplishment than with concern for people. Autocratic leadership tends to promote hostility and aggression or apathy and to decrease initiative.

Democratic. Leaders involve their followers in the decision-making process. They are people-oriented and focus on human relations and teamwork. Democratic leadership leads to increased productivity and job satisfaction.

Laissez-faire. Leaders are loose and permissive and abstain from leading their staff. They foster freedom for everyone and want everyone to feel good. Laissez-faire leadership results in low productivity and employee frustration.

SOURCE: Adapted from L. C. Megginson, D. C. Moseley, and P. H. Pietri, Jr., *Management: Concepts and Applications* (New York: Harper & Row, 1986), 397.

Most questionnaire-based leadership research has been conducted in laboratory settings. The results are biased by the fact that some conditions do not exist in typical field settings. Research participants do not know or have contact with the target leader; thus the behavioral-level accuracy of their responses is limited. Phillips and Lord make the following suggestions to improve research techniques of existing behavioral description questionnaires:

1. Assess whether the level of accuracy required for the purpose is classification or behavioral.
2. Assess whether the level of accuracy produced by the chosen measurement technique is classification or behavioral.
3. Evaluate the research setting for potential biases "such as rote knowledge of performance, leniency in describing superiors, or other relevant rater characteristics."
4. If biases exist, judge whether they are likely to be confounded with substantive variables of interest to the user.
5. Collect global measures of leadership and leniency during the measurement process.

Leadership questionnaires are useful if used and interpreted appropriately.[28]

leaders carry out their activities. Both factors are considered simultaneously rather than on a continuum. As to which combination works best, the situation determines the style.[26]

Problems With Leadership Questionnaires. According to Phillips and Lord, the accuracy of leadership questionnaires is debatable. Yet they are often the only feasible way to measure leadership in real-world settings. Some researchers consider reliable questionnaires accurate. However these authors contend that any systematic sources of variance, such as leniency error, halo, or implicit theories, can produce high internal consistency. Factor structures produced solely on the basis of implicit leadership theories do not tell users of these questionnaires anything about accuracy.

The Leader Behavior Description Questionnaire was flawed by having subjects form an overall leadership impression before completing it. Questionnaires can be improved by requiring "observers to distinguish between the presence and absence of specific, conceptually equivalent behaviors in video-taped stimulus materials."[27]

FIGURE 15–5. Ohio State Leadership Quadrant

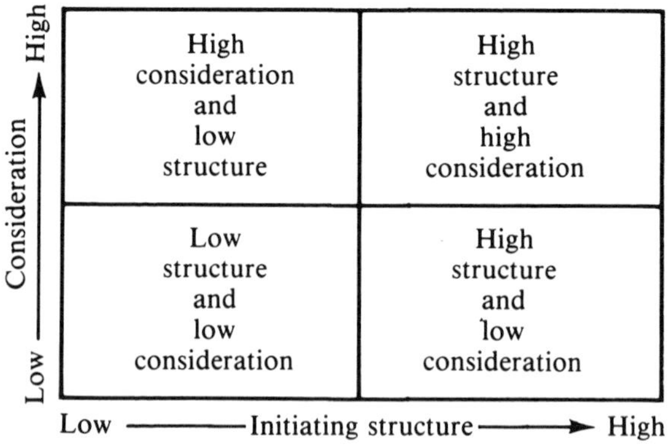

	Low ——————— Initiating structure ————→ High
High **Consideration** Low	High consideration and low structure	High structure and high consideration
	Low structure and low consideration	High structure and low consideration

SOURCE: From *Management: Concepts and Applications*, page 410, by Myguire, Mosley, and Pietri. Copyright © 1986 by Harper & Row, Inc. Used with permission of the publisher.

FIGURE 15–6. Life-Cycle Theory of Leadership

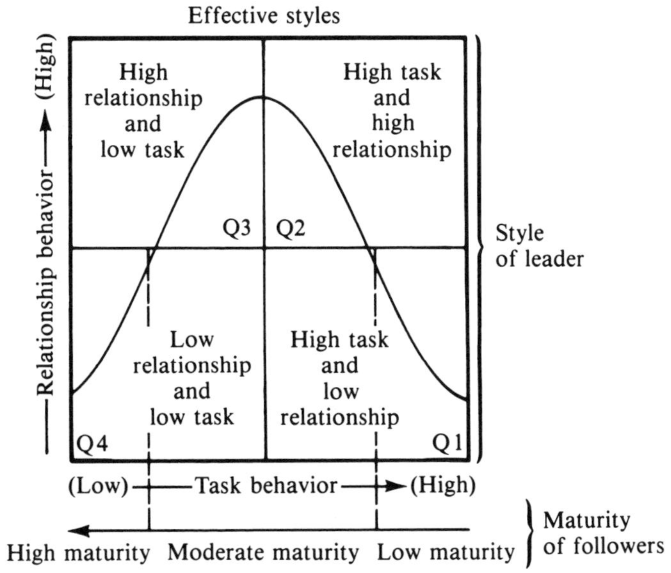

SOURCE: P. Hersey and K.H. Blanchard, *Management of Organizational Behavior* (3rd. ed. Englewood Cliffs, NJ: Prentice-Hall, 1977). Used with permission of Leadership Studies.

LEADERSHIP STYLE

Other studies of leadership focus on style. These include contingency-situational leadership models that focus upon a combination of factors such as the people, the task, the situation, the organization, and a number of environmental factors. Such approaches combine the theories of Fred F. Fiedler, William J. Reddin, Paul Hersey and Kenneth H. Blanchard, William Ouchi, and John W. Gardner, whose contributions are discussed in the following sections.

Fiedler's Contingency Model of Leadership Effectiveness

There must be a group before there can be a leader. Fiedler indicates three classifications that measure the kind of power and influence the group gives its leader. The first and most important of these is the relationship between the leader and the group members. Personality is a factor but its influence depends on the group's perception of the leader. Second is the task structure, the degree to which details of the group's assignment are programmed. If the assignment is highly structured, the leader will have less power. If it requires planning and thinking, he or she will be in a position to exert greater power. Third is the positional power of the leader; it should be noted that greater power does not yield better group performance. The best leader has been found to be one who has a task-oriented leadership style. This style works best when the leader has either great influence and power or no power over group members. When the leader has moderate influence over group members, a relationship-oriented style works best.

The organization shares responsibility for the leader's success or failure. Leaders can be trained to learn in which situations they do well and in which they fail. The job can be fitted to the leader. The appointee can be given a higher rank or can be assigned subordinates who are nearly equal in rank and status. Most appointees can be given sole authority or can be required to consult with the group. The appointee can be given detailed instructions or independence. A highly successful and effective leader will avoid situations in which failure is likely. That leader will seek out situations that fit his or her

FIGURE 15–7. Reddin's Three-Dimensional Management Styles

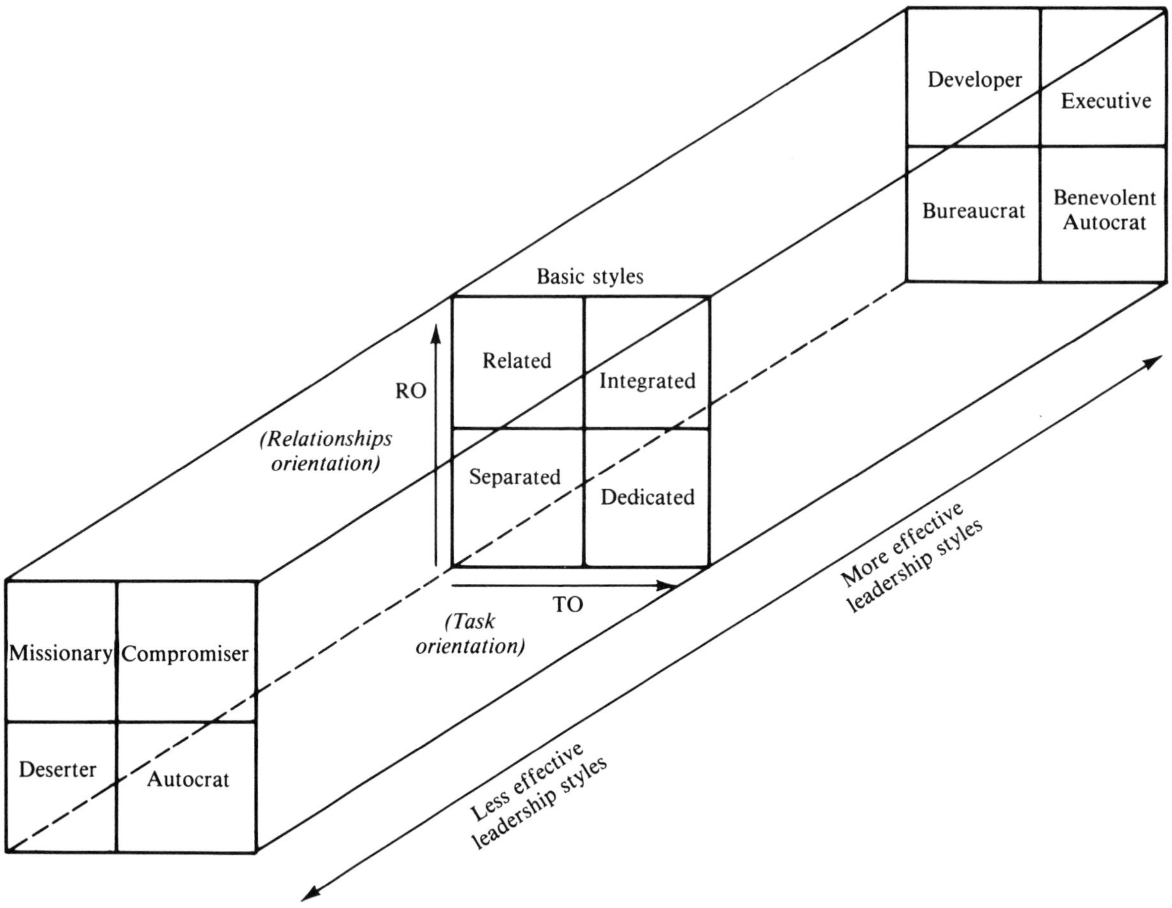

SOURCE: W.J. Reddin, *Managerial Effectiveness* (New York: McGraw-Hill, 1970), 230. Reprinted with permission.

leadership style. Knowledge of strengths and weaknesses will help in choosing this style.[29]

Fiedler's theory is one of situations. Leadership style will be effective or ineffective depending upon the situation.

The Life-Cycle Theory of Hersey and Blanchard

Blanchard and Hersey follow a situational approach to leadership. This theory predicts the most appropriate leadership style from the level of maturity or immaturity of the constituents.

With immaturity the leadership style will focus on the task, constituents being relatively passive and dependent. The leadership style will focus on rela-

tionship behaviors as the constituents become more mature, active and independent.[30] This theory is illustrated in Figure 15–6.

Reddin's Three-Dimensional Theory of Management

Reddin combined Blake and Mouton's managerial grid with Fiedler's contingency leadership style theory. The outcome was a three-dimensional theory of management, the dimensions being adapted from:

1. Managerial Grid® theory.
2. Contingency leadership style theory.
3. Effectiveness theory.

The possible combinations result in four basic leadership styles (see Figure 15–7).

1. *Separated,* in which both task orientation and relationship orientation are minimal.
2. *Dedicated,* in which task orientation is high and relationship orientation low. Dedicated leaders are dedicated only to the job.
3. *Related,* in which relationship orientation is high and task orientation is low. Related leaders relate primarily to their subordinates.
4. *Integrated,* in which both task and relationship orientation are high. Integrated leaders focus on managerial behavior combining task orientation and relationship orientation.

These management styles are graphically represented by the first two dimensions of Figure 15–7. The third dimension of effectiveness represents the degree of the leader's achievement of position objectives and is situational:

- "Executive" leaders are integrated and more effective than "compromiser" leaders who are less effective integrated leaders.
- "Developer" leaders are related and more effective than "missionary" leaders who are less effective related leaders.
- "Bureaucrat" leaders are separated and more effective than "deserter" leaders who are less effective separated leaders.
- "Benevolent autocrat" leaders are dedicated and more effective than "autocrat" leaders who are less effective dedicated leaders.

The range of effectiveness is a continuum. As in other theories of leadership, the effective behavior of the leader is relative to the situation. Effective leaders apply leadership styles after assessing situations.[31]

Theory Z Organizations

Theory Z organizations focus upon consensual decision making. The leadership style is a democratic one that includes decentralization, participatory management, employee involvement, and quality of life. Leaders are managers who concentrate on developing and using their interpersonal skills. These theories have been attributed to William Ouchi.[32]

LEADERSHIP AND POWER

Gardner defines power as "the capacity to ensure the outcomes one wishes and to prevent those one does not wish."[33] Power is dispersed in a pluralistic society. The desirable social dimension of power brings about intended consequences and behavior that benefits people. The intended consequences and behavior can sometimes become malevolent even in a democratic society.

Power Bases

French and Raven suggested five interpersonal bases of power: legitimate, reward, coercive, expert, and referent.[34]

Legitimate Power. Legitimate power is a person's ability to influence because of her or his position. A person with a higher organizational position has power over people below. Legitimate power is dependent on subordinates. A supervisor who tries to coerce employees to contribute to a favorite political candidate may find that only some people comply.

Reward Power. A leader with legitimate power can use rewards to gain the cooperation of subordinates. Followers may respond to directions or requests if a leader can provide valued rewards such as raises, bonuses, or a choice job assignment. For example, a head nurse who can reward employees with requested time off or merit pay increases can exert reward power.

Coercive Power. Coercive power is the power to punish. Followers may comply because of fear. Managers may punish employees by blocking promotions or pay raises or by harassment. Even though coercive power may be used to correct nonproductive behavior in organizations, it often brings about the opposite effect. Those being punished may attempt to escape or avoid (through absenteeism or turnover) or show hostility toward management (through sabotage).

Referent Power. Charisma is the basis of referent power. A charismatic leader can influence people because of his or her personality or behavior style. Even though charisma is often used in reference to politicians, actors, or sports figures, some managers are regarded as charismatic by their employees.

Expert Power. A person with special expertise that is highly valued has expert power. Expert power is not tied to rank. A ward secretary can have high expert power if he or she knows details of how the nursing unit functions. A staff nurse, because of years of employment, may have more information or job-specific expertise than a new head nurse and so may have more power.

The five types of interpersonal power are interdependent because they can be used in various combinations and each can effect the other.[35] For example, a nursing supervisor may lose referent power if she or he punishes staff by cancelling merit pay increases.

People use power to accomplish goals and to strengthen their positions in the organization. The use of power is legitimate when used in a fair and ethical way to achieve organizational, group, and individual objectives. Good managers desire power to influence the behavior of employees for the good of the organization, not for personal gain.

Differences between Leadership and Management

Managers come from the headship (power from position) category. They hold appointive or directive posts in formal organizations. They can be appointed for both technical and leadership competencies, usually needing both to be accepted. Managers are delegated authority, including the power to reward or punish. A manager is expected to perform such functions as planning, organizing, directing, and controlling.

Informal leaders, by contrast, are not always managers performing those functions required by the organization. Leaders often are not part of the organization. Florence Nightingale, after leaving the Crimea, was not connected with an organization but was still a leader.

Zaleznik indicates that the manager is a problem solver who succeeds because of "persistence, tough-mindedness, hard work, intelligence, analytical ability, and, perhaps most important, tolerance and good will."[36]

Managers focus on results, analysis of failure, and tasks. These management characteristics are desirable for nurse managers. Effective managers also need to be good leaders. Managers who are leaders choose and limit goals. They focus on creating spirit and in doing so they develop committed followers. Manager-leaders do this by seeking advice and solutions to problems. They ask for information and provide positive feedback. Leaders understand the power of groups. They empower their constituents making their subordinates strong—the chosen ones, a team infused with purpose. Mistakes are tolerated by manager-leaders who challenge constituents to stretch their potentialities.

Managers emphasize control, decision making, and decision analysis. As manager-leaders they are concerned with modeling appropriate behavior as symbols of values and norms. Effective manager-leaders are technically capable and provide assurance in crises.

Managers focus inward but add the leadership dimension of connecting their group to the outside world, focusing intense attention on important issues. They escalate issues and complaints up the organization to be handled quickly and appropriately rather than trying to control issues and complaints.[37] While managers are sometimes described in less glowing terms than leaders, successful managers are usually successful leaders. Leadership is a desirable and prominent feature of the directing function of nursing management.

Similarities between Leadership and Management

Gardner asserts that first-class managers are usually first-class leaders. Leaders and leader/managers distinguish themselves beyond the general run of managers in six respects:

1. They think longer-term—beyond the day's crises, beyond the quarterly report, beyond the horizon.
2. They look beyond the unit they are heading and grasp its relationship to larger realities—the larger organization of which they are a part, conditions external to the organization, global trends.
3. They reach and influence constituents beyond their jurisdiction, beyond boundaries. Thomas Jefferson influenced people all over Europe. Gandhi influenced people all over the world. In an organization, leaders overflow bureaucratic boundaries—often a distinct advantage in a world too complex and tumultuous to be handled "through channels." Their capacity to rise above jurisdictions may enable them to bind together the fragmented constituencies that must work together to solve a problem.

4. They put heavy emphasis on the intangibles of vision, values, and motivation and understand intuitively the nonrational and unconscious elements in the leader-constituent interaction.

4. They have the political skill to cope with the conflicting requirements of multiple constituencies.

6. They think in terms of renewal. The routine manager tends to accept the structure and processes as they exist. The leader or leader/manager seeks the revisions of process and structure required by ever-changing reality.[38]

Good leaders, like good managers, provide visionary inspiration, motivation, and direction. Good managers, like good leaders, attract and inspire. People want to be led rather than managed. They want to pursue goals and values they consider worthwhile. Therefore, they want leaders who respect the dignity, autonomy, and self-esteem of constituents.[39] Effective nurse executives combine leadership and management.

Mitchell describes five major requirements for every executive, implying that being an executive requires the attributes of a leader:

1. Adjustment to a complex social environment of several or many units.
2. Ability to influence and guide subordinates.
3. Emotional and intellectual maturity as a preparation for leadership.
4. Ability to think through and make decisions and to translate decisions into effective action.
5. Capacity to see beyond the immediate or surface indications and, with experience, to acquire perspective.[40]

Effective nurse leader-managers will work to achieve these same qualities.

That a relationship between leadership and management exists seems scarcely arguable. Leadership is a subsystem within the management system. It is included as an element of management science in management textbooks and other publications. In some texts the term "leading" has replaced the term "directing" as a major function of management. In such a context communication and motivation would be elements of leadership, a concept that could be debated according to management theorists' philosophical bent.

Management includes written plans, clear organizational charts, well-documented annual objectives, frequent reports, detailed and precise job descriptions, regular evaluations of performance against objectives, and the administrative ordering of theory.[41] Nurse managers who are leaders can use these tools of management.

HEADSHIP VERSUS LEADERSHIP

A job title does not make a person a leader, nor does it cause a person to exercise leadership behavior over subordinates. This is as true of nurses as it is of personnel in industry or the military services. It is a mistake to refer to the dean of a college, a professor of nursing, a nurse administrator, a supervisor, a head nurse, or any nurse as a leader by virtue of position. That person is in a headship position rather than a leadership one, since "leadership is more a function of the group or situation than a quality which adheres to a person appointed to a formal position of headship."[42] A person's behavior will indicate whether that person also functionally occupies a leadership position.

Gardner writes that people in position of high status are not all leaders. Some are chief bureaucrats or custodians. Their high status does have "symbolic values and traditions that enhance the possibility of leadership" since people have higher expectations of people in headship positions.[43] Authority embodied in a title or position of headship is legitimized power, it is not leadership.[44] Leadership is an attempt to influence groups or individuals without the coercive form of power.

Appointed heads are not selected by persons they will direct. Appointed heads frequently work toward organizational goals while ignoring the personal goals of employees. Their authority comes from above and not from their influence within the group.

In cases in which heads are elected by the group, they keep their positions only as long as they satisfy the members' needs for affiliating with the organization. They are responsible to the group only, while the appointed head is usually responsible to both the appointive authority and the group. Nurses who are elected to chair committees or preside over professional organizations will not be re-elected unless they satisfy the members' needs.

Appointed heads may lack the freedom to choose relationships with subordinates because their supervisors do not allow it. They will have authority and power without being accepted by the group. If appointed nurse managers are allowed to and can exercise their leadership abilities, they can be accorded leadership status by the group. The nurse managers will understand and motivate employees so as to be trusted by them.[45]

Preparation of Leaders as Managers

Young nurse managers need to be entered into a leadership-management development program. Such a program would teach them to recognize the worth and feelings of employees while having employees evaluate their personal goals in relation to those of the organization. This is one reason for agreement on a set of job standards and for the cooperative process of management by objectives. Principles that are applicable here include:

1. People need to know the standards expected of them. These standards should be flexible with details negotiated. If a person does not meet a standard, that person should be helped to plan a program to meet it.
2. People should know where they stand; they should be helped to improve when necessary.
3. People should be praised when they deserve it. A person should not be praised publicly unless it is important that others know the manager has a high opinion of the person.
4. Managers should show caring for people.
5. People should be made independent by helping them achieve their fullest potential.
6. Managers should be tactful, polite, and diplomatic.
7. Managers can learn from employees.
8. Managers should show confidence in themselves and in personnel.
9. People should be allowed freedom of expression.[46]

Organizational managers including nurse executives will teach managers the nature of leadership. They will train nurse managers in leadership skills. They will put managers in the proper environment to learn leadership. This will include "starting up an operation, turning around a troubled division, moving from staff to line, working under a wise mentor, serving on a high-level task force, and getting promoted to a more senior level of the organization."[47]

Nurse executives and managers should be trained to coach their subordinates on leadership skills. Subordinates can be trained to help managers in leadership. Leaders can listen and articulate, can persuade and be persuaded, can use collective wisdom to make decisions, and can teach subordinates to relate or communicate upward.

Persons who are only managers control. Managers who are leaders create commitment. They create a work unit that stands out, with culture and values that distinguish it from others. Forward-looking businesses are developing leadership at the lower levels. Most governments are not.[48]

Males versus Females

Levenstein has stated that nursing supervisors differ in leadership from women who reach managerial posts in industry. He supported this premise by stating that head nurses described themselves lower on consideration or orientation to relationships than did women managers in industry. Since industry is more production oriented, women employees would be expected to be more structure oriented than nurses. General duty nurses described themselves as more considerate than businesswomen. Consideration was "defined as the supervisor's ability to display warmth, mutual respect, concern for the needs of the subordinates, and a desire to encourage participation in decision making."[49]

A study comparing subordinates' perceptions of leadership behavior of male supervisors versus female supervisors showed no significant difference in subordinates' satisfactions. The Ohio State Leader Behavior Description questionnaire was used. The twelve leadership qualities analyzed were representation, demand reconciliation, tolerance of uncertainty, persuasiveness, initiating structure, tolerance of freedom, role assumption, consideration, production emphasis, predictive accuracy, integration, and superior orientation.

There were differences between men and women on individual qualities. The conclusion was that leadership differences between the sexes are culturally imposed. Since the myth frequently surfaces that subordinates work better for male supervisors, this single-hospital research should be replicated to further dispel the myth.[50]

LEADERSHIP AND NURSING

Nursing is usually conspicuous by its absence from lists of national leaders. National consumers do not perceive nurse leaders as having power. Cutler's perspective on nursing educators and nursing service personnel is that they have been the product of directive and authoritarian leadership.[51]

Historically, nurses have avoided opportunities to obtain power and political muscle. The profession now understands that power and political savvy will assist in achieving its goals, which are to improve health care and to increase nurses' autonomy. Milio believes that nurses have the capacity for power to influence public policy and recommends the following steps to prepare:

1. Organize.
2. Do the homework: learn to understand the political process, interest groups, specific people and events.
3. Frame arguments to suit the target audience by appealing to cost containment, political support, fairness and justice, and other data relevant to particular concerns.
4. Support and strengthen the position of converted policy makers.
5. Concentrate energies.
6. Stimulate public debate.
7. Make the position of nurses visible in the mass media.
8. Choose as the main strategy the most effective one.
9. Act in a timely fashion.
10. Maintain activity.
11. Keep the organizational format decentralized.
12. Obtain and develop the best research data to support each position.
13. Learn from experience.
14. Never give up without trying.

Nurses in leadership positions are most influential.[52]

Leadership Research Applicable to Nursing

To answer the question of which leadership behaviors will predict effectiveness of supervisors (or will produce the best subordinate outcomes), Jones developed a list of twenty-two control strategies. These were methods that could be adapted by supervisors to change the effectiveness of the work group for which they are responsible. Each control strategy had four dimensions: obtrusive versus inobtrusive control, situational versus personal control, professional versus paternalistic control, and process versus output control.

This study indicates that a behavior control strategy evaluates the subordinate's behavior. Outcome control strategy involves rewards such as promotion, based on current performance. There are numerous dimensions of leadership. The leader chooses the control strategy, behavioral or outcome. During this process the leader employs a cost-benefit analysis strategy that weighs intrinsic plus extrinsic outcomes and employee satisfaction versus performance or profits. In choosing the strategy to fit the situation, leaders match a form of leader behavior to the subordinate and the tasks, considering situational characteristics to maximize benefits and minimize costs.

This research, while theoretical, could be beneficial to nurse managers. They could identify their own leadership behaviors including those for decision making. Then they could adjust their behavior to achieve desired outcomes.[53]

Campbell developed and used a questionnaire to determine whether management styles affected burnout. When leadership skills are mastered by nurse managers, stress and burnout are reduced. Nurse managers need to master the skills of leadership.[54]

Buffering

Nursing leaders (managers) can act as buffers or advocates for nurses. In doing so they will protect subordinates from the internal and external pressures of work. Nurse managers can keep employees from being confronted and reduce barriers to clinical nurses completing their clinical work.

Buffering protects practicing clinical nurses from external health system factors, from the health-care organization, from other supervisors and employees, from top administrators, from the medical staff and from themselves when their behavior jeopardizes their careers. It is another facet of the theory of leadership related to management. It requires leadership training.

The nurse practitioner, the extended-role nurse, staff nurses, and ancillary personnel can be protected by buffering action by nurse managers. Professional nurses do not want jobs to be delegated to them if they are already under severe pressure and stress. Delegation of decision making is power; delegation of work is drudgery. Professional nurses should be involved in a way designed to motivate, not dissatisfy.

Smith and Mitry suggest three methods of buffering:

1. Work coordination—support services, standardized records.
2. Insulation by intervening with pressure groups, unity of command.
3. Evaluating the impingement.

The benefits will be improved performance, better morale, increased loyalty, a healthier organization, and respect for leaders.[55]

While management writers say there is a difference between leadership and managers, their textbooks and writings on the subject all include leadership content. It can be stated unequivocally that professional nurses want to be led, not directed or controlled. Also, nurse managers can learn the concepts, principles, and laws that will assist them in becoming effective leader-managers.

Different situations require different leadership styles. The leader manager assesses each situation and exercises the appropriate leadership style. Some employees want to be involved; others do not. There must be a fit between leader and constituents. The leader demonstrates this by changing style and training others until a transition is made. A flexible leadership style is necessary and vital.

SUMMARY

The theory of nursing leadership is a part of the theory of nursing management.

Leadership is a process of influencing a group to set and achieve goals. There are several major theories of leadership. One of the earliest theories of leadership is the trait theory. This theory infers that leaders have many intellectual, personality, and ability traits. Trait theory has been succeeded by other leadership theories indicating that managers, including nurse managers, can learn the knowledge and skills requisite to leadership competencies.

Behavioral theories of leadership include McGregor's Theory X and Theory Y, Likert's Michigan studies, Blake and Mouton's managerial grid, and Lewin's studies.

Other studies of leadership focus on contingency-situational leadership styles and factors such as people, tasks, situations, organizations, and environmental factors. Theorists include Fiedler, Reddin, Hersey, Blanchard, Ouchi, and Gardner.

John W. Gardner is working on a definitive study of leadership that includes the nature of leadership, identification of leadership tasks, leader-constituent interaction, and the relationship between leadership and power.

Nurse managers should learn to practice leadership behaviors that stimulate motivation within their constituents, practicing professional nurses and other nursing personnel. These behaviors will include promotion of autonomy, decision making, and participatory management by professional nurses. It should be noted that these behaviors are facilitated by effective nurse manager–leaders.

NOTES

1. J. W. Gardner, *The Nature of Leadership: Introductory Considerations* (Washington, DC: Independent Sector, 1986), 8.
2. J. W. Gardner, *The Tasks of Leadership* (Washington, DC: Independent Sector, 1986), 15; E. Huxley, *Florence Nightingale* (New York: G. P. Putnam's Sons, 1975).
3. C. R. Holloman, "Leadership or Headship: There Is a Difference," *Notes & Quotes* No. 365, 1969, 4; C. R. Holloman, " 'Headship' Versus Leadership," *Business and Economic Review*, Jan.-Mar. 1986, 35–37.
4. L. B. Lundborg, "What Is Leadership?," *The Journal of Nursing Administration*, May 1982, 32–33.
5. J. W. Gardner, *The Nature of Leadership*, op. cit., 6.
6. C. R. Holloman, " 'Headship' Versus Leadership," op. cit.; A. Levenstein, "So You Want to Be a Leader?," *Nursing Management*, Mar. 1985, 74–75; G. R. Jones, "Forms of Control and Leader Behavior," *Journal of Management*, Fall 1983, 159–172; D. McGregor, *Leadership and Motivation* (Cambridge, MA: MIT Press, 1966), 70–80.
7. R. K. Merton, "The Social Nature of Leadership," *American Journal of Nursing*, December 1969, 2614–2618.
8. D. McGregor, op. cit., 73.
9. C. M. Talbott, "Leadership at the Man-to-Man Level," *Supplement to the Air Force Policy Letter for Commanders*, No. 8, Aug. 1971, 13.
10. D. G. Mitton, "Leadership—One More Time," *Industrial Management Review*, Fall 1969, 77–83.
11. J. Kilpatrick, "Conservative View," *Sun-Herald* (Biloxi, MS), Feb. 2, 1974, 4.
12. D. McGregor, op. cit., 75.
13. P. M. Podsakoff, W. D. Todor, and R. S. Schuler, "Leader Expertise as a Moderator of the Effects of Instrumental and Supportive Leader Behaviors," *Journal of Management*, Fall 1983, 173–185.
14. Ibid.

15. B. Brower, "Where Have All the Leaders Gone?" *Life,* October 8, 1971, 70B.
16. R. K. Merton, op. cit., 2626.
17. E. E. Jennings, "The Anatomy of Leadership," *Notes & Quotes* No. 274, Mar. 1962, 1, 4.
18. C. R. Holloman, "Leadership or Headship: There Is a Difference," op. cit., 4.
19. J. W. Gardner, *The Tasks of Leadership,* op. cit.; *The Heart of the Matter: Leader-Constituent Interaction;* and *Leadership and Power* (Washington, DC: Independent Sector, 1986).
20. J. W. Gardner, *The Tasks of Leadership,* op. cit., 7.
21. J. W. Gardner, *The Heart of the Matter: Leader-Constituent Interaction,* op. cit.
22. D. McGregor, op. cit., 55–57.
23. Ibid., 49–65.
24. R. Likert, *The Human Organization* (New York: McGraw-Hill, 1967), 4–10.
25. The Grid® synopsis was furnished courtesy of Scientific Methods, Inc., Box 195, Austin, Texas 78767.
26. L. Megginson, D. Mosley, and P. Pietri, Jr., *Management: Concepts and Applications* (New York: Harper & Row, 1986) 397.
27. J. S. Phillips and R. G. Lord, "Notes on the Practical and Theoretical Consequences of Implicit Leadership Theories for the Future of Leadership Measurement," *Journal of Management,* Spring 1986, 33.
28. Ibid.
29. F. E. Fiedler, "Style or Circumstance: The Leadership Enigma," *Notes & Quotes* No. 358, Mar. 1969, 3; L. Megginson, D. Mosley, and P. Pietri, Jr., op. cit., 419–422.
30. P. Hersey and K. H. Blanchard, *Management of Organizational Behavior,* 3d ed. (Englewood Cliffs, NJ: Prentice-Hall, 1977).
31. W. J. Reddin, *Managerial Effectiveness* (New York: McGraw-Hill, 1970), 230; R. M. Hodgetts, *Management: Theory, Process and Practice* (4th ed. Orlando, Fl.: Academic Press, 1986), 319–320.
32. W. G. Ouchi, *Theory Z* (Reading, MA: Addison-Wesley, 1981).
33. J. W. Gardner, *Leadership and Power,* op. cit., 3.
34. J. French and B. Raven, "The Basis of Social Power" in *Studies in Power,* D. Cartwright, Ed. (Ann Arbor: Institute for Social Research, University of Michigan, 1959).
35. J. Gibson, J. Ivancevich, and J. Donnelly, Jr., *Organizations: Behavior, Structure, Processes,* 6th ed. (Homewood, Il.: Richard D. Irwin, Inc. 1988), 335–337.
36. A. Zaleznik, "Managers and Leaders: Are they Different?," *Harvard Business Review,* May-June 1977, 68.
37. J. H. Zenger, "Leadership: Management's Better Half," *Training,* Dec. 1985, 44–53.
38. J. W. Gardner, *The Nature of Leadership,* op. cit., 12.
39. J. H. Zenger, op. cit.
40. W. N. Mitchell, "What Makes a Business Leader?," *Notes & Quotes* No. 350, July 1968, 2.
41. J. H. Zenger, op. cit.
42. C. R. Holloman, "Leadership or Headship: There Is a Difference," op. cit.
43. J. W. Gardner, *The Nature of Leadership,* op. cit. 6.
44. Ibid.
45. C. R. Holloman, " 'Headship' Versus Leadership," op. cit.
46. M. R. Feinberg, *Effective Psychology for Management* (Englewood Cliffs, NJ: Prentice-Hall, 1965), 133–141.
47. J. H. Zenger, op. cit.
48. Ibid.; J. W. Gardner, *The Nature of Leadership,* op. cit.
49. A. Levenstein, "Where Nurses Differ," *Nursing Management,* Mar. 1984, 64–65.
50. A. Levenstein, "So You Want to Be a Leader," *Nursing Management,* Mar. 1985, 74–75.
51. M. J. Cutler, "Nursing Leadership and Management: An Historical Perspective," *Nursing Administration Quarterly,* Fall 1976, 7–19.
52. N. Milio, "The Realities of Policymaking: Can Nurses Have an Impact?" *The Journal of Nursing Administration,* Mar. 1984, 18–23.
53. G. R. Jones, "Forms of Control and Leader Behavior," *Journal of Management,* Fall 1983, 159–172.
54. R. P. Campbell, "Does Management Style Affect Burnout?," *Nursing Management,* Mar. 1986, 38A-38B, 38D, 38F, 38H.
55. H. L. Smith and N. W. Mitry, "Nursing Leadership: A Buffering Perspective," *Nursing Administration Quarterly,* Spring 1984, 45–52.

REFERENCES

Catton, J. J., "Applying Leadership to People Problems," *Supplement to the Air Force Policy Letter for Commanders,* No. 9-1971, Sept. 1971, 30.

Dunning, H. F., "Nobody Can Give You Leadership," *Notes & Quotes,* Sept. 1963, 3.

Davis, C. K., D. Oakley, and J. A. Sochalsk, "Leadership for Expanding Nursing Influence on Health Policy," *Journal of Nursing Administration,* Jan. 1982, 15–21.

Glucksberg, S., "Some Ways to Turn on New Ideas," *Think* (IBM), Mar.-Apr. 1968.

Goldberg, D., "What Makes a Leader?," *Mississippi Press,* Nov. 23, 1978, 6D.

Jennings, E. E., "The Anatomy of Leadership," *Notes & Quotes,* No. 274, Mar. 1962, 1, 4.

Kaprowski, E. J., "Toward Innovative Leadership," *Notes & Quotes* No. 351, Aug. 1968, 2.

Koontz, H., "Challenges for Intellectual Leadership or Management," *Notes & Quotes* No. 315, Aug. 1965, 1, 4.

Levenstein, A., "Leadership Under the Microscope," *Nursing Management,* Nov. 1984, 68–69.

Lundborg, "What Is Leadership?," *Journal of Nursing Administration,* May 1982, 32–33.

Pike, O., "Rutan, Yeager Showed What Leadership Is About," *Mobile Press Register,* Jan. 1987, 4A.

Smith, H. L., F. D. Reinow, and R. A. Reid, "Japanese Management: Implications for Nursing Administration," *Journal of Nursing Administration,* Sept. 1984, 33–39.

Yanker, M., "Flexible Leadership Styles: One Supervisor's Story," *Supervisory Management,* Jan. 1986, 2–6.

Motivation

16

THEORIES OF MOTIVATION

Introduction

Motivation is a concept used to describe both extrinsic conditions that stimulate certain behavior and intrinsic responses that demonstrate that behavior in human beings. The intrinsic response is sustained by sources of energy, termed "motives." They are often described as needs, wants, or drives. All living people have them. Motivation is measured by observable and recorded behaviors. Deficiencies in needs stimulate people to seek and achieve goals to satisfy their needs.

Why do some registered nurses pursue an area of nursing specialization to the extent of continuously acquiring new knowledge and skills that enable them to make rapid and accurate nursing diagnosis and prescription? Why does a pediatric nurse pursue development of a role in which professional practice is extended into such areas as teaching parents to enjoy their children, providing follow-up health observations of high-risk newborns, and health teaching of their parents after they have been discharged to their homes? Why does that nurse go a step further and teach others to extend themselves and then write articles to provide the information for all?

Why does a mental health nurse pursue a role as a co-therapist of a group even in off-duty time and in addition to rotating shifts as a staff nurse? Why does another work to sell the concept and then conduct a psychodrama therapy program and ask for the privilege of answering mental health consultations for medical and surgical patients? Why does a professional nurse work many hours as a committee member for a district nurses' association?

Why does a professional nurse contribute numerous hours of volunteer work to community organizations? Why does that nurse continuously pursue off-duty education courses for academic credit to update clinical practice?

Why does one professional nurse pursue any of these activities without watching the clock or setting limits to accepting responsibility for patient care?

Why do some nurses perform in a positive manner and others negatively?

Why do some people always act with truthfulness and integrity to support principles they believe in, whereas others remain silent and passive?

Why are some nurses goal-oriented and others not? Why are some nurses actively dedicated to improving their quality of life, whereas others merely exert minimal effort to maintain it?

What makes some nurses come on duty on time, work hard and without error, maintain a pleasant demeanor, and meet all standards of performance, appearance, and behavior, whereas others do just the opposite? Some persons do not do well in an organization. This does not mean these persons are no good; the organization may be lacking the means of making them productive, useful, satisfied employees.

The answer to all these questions is motivation. Some nurses are motivated to excel and be creative, whereas others put forth just enough effort to do their job.

Theories of motivation have been classified into content theories and process theories.[1]

Content Theories of Motivation

Content theories of motivation focus on factors or needs within a person that energize, direct, sustain, and stop behavior. The most widely recognized work in motivation theory is that of Maslow. While not universally accepted because of its lack of scientific evidence or research base, it is universally known and many managers attempt to use it as they turn to a human behavior approach to management.

Much has been said in support of Maslow's theories of motivation relative to human needs and goals. Like every science, nursing is a human creation stemming from human motives, having human goals, and being created, renewed, and maintained by human beings called nurses.

Nurses are motivated as are other scientists by physiological needs including that for food; by needs for safety, protection, and care; by social needs for gregariousness, affection, and love; by ego needs for respect, standing, and status leading to self-respect or self-esteem; and by a need for self-fulfillment or self-actualization of the idiosyncratic and species-wide potentialities of the individual human being. Many but not all are also motivated by cognitive needs for sheer knowledge and understanding, voraciously questioning others, reading textbooks, journals, and patients' charts and continuously pursuing courses in their specialty and in the liberal arts, particularly the humanities. Others are motivated by aesthetic needs for beauty, symmetry, simplicity, completion, and order and by their need to express themselves. How many of these needs are related to a nurse's need for continuing to learn and to apply new knowledge and skills? What can the nurse administrator do to spark the motive of curiosity in a nurse that sets in motion a desire to understand, explain, and systematize? These and many other human needs may serve as the primary motivations for pursuing a career in nursing and updating and expanding knowledge and skills. The need may be a feeling of identification and belongingness with people in general, a feeling of love for human beings, a desire to help people, the need to earn a living, a means of self-expression, or a combination of all these needs working at the same time. Certainly the diversity in needs is individualistic.[2]

A second content theory of motivation was developed by Alderfer who reduced Maslow's hierarchy of needs from five to three levels, existence (E), relatedness (R), and growth (G)—thus the term ERG theory. Comparing Alderfer's scheme with Maslow's, existence needs would equate to physiological and safety needs; relatedness needs would equate to belongingness, social, and love needs; and growth needs would equate to self-esteem and self-actualization.

Whereas Maslow's theory proposed that the next level emerged when the predominant (satisfaction-progression) ones were fulfilled, Alderfer's theory proposed the addition of a frustration-regression process. When higher-level needs are frustrated, people will regress to satisfaction of lower-level needs.[3]

There is limited research available to support or sustain the ERG theory. As with other theories of motivation, nurse managers should become familiar with it and use its implications as appropriately as possible.

Herzberg did research on a third content theory, which he labelled a two-factor theory of motivation. One factor is labeled extrinsic conditions, hygiene factors, or dissatisfiers. These include salary, job security, working conditions, status, company procedures, quality of technical supervision, and quality of interpersonal relations among peers, with supervisors, and with subordinates. They must be maintained in quantity and quality to prevent dissatisfaction. They become dissatisfiers when not equitably administered, causing low performance and negative attitudes. The other set of factors are labeled intrinsic conditions, motivators, or satisfiers. They include achievement, recognition, responsibility, advancement, the work itself, and the possibility of growth. They create opportunities for high satisfaction, high motivation, and high performance. The individual must be free to attain them. Herzberg's research was criticized for its limited sample of accountants and engineers and for being simplistic.[4]

McClelland proposed and researched a fourth content theory of motivation closely associated with learning concepts. There are three primary groups of learned needs acquired from the culture: the need for achievement, the need for affiliation, and the need for power.

McClelland used the Thematic Apperception Test (TAT) to measure the need for achievement. He contended that needs can be learned through organizational and nonorganizational meetings. Persons high in the need for achievement want to set their own performance goals, which they prefer to be moderate and achievable. They want immediate feedback and they like responsibility for solving problems.[5]

Many nursing personnel enjoy working together and are motivated by their affiliations. In some situations, such as nursing homes, they do not receive the recognition they need from clients, so they look for it from colleagues. Many nursing personnel want to talk to and socialize with each other on the job. They enjoy and prefer group-centered work activities, teamwork, interdependence, dependability, and predictability. The nurse manager works with them to maintain this affiliation need at a mutually acceptable level.[6]

Process Theories of Motivation

Four process theories of motivation are reinforcement theory, expectancy theory, equity theory, and goal setting. Most behavior within organizations is learned behavior: perceptions, attitudes, goals, emotional reactions, and skills. Practice that occurs during the learning process results in a relatively enduring change in behavior.

Skinner advanced a process theory of motivation called operant conditioning. Learning occurs as a consequence of behavior. This is also called behavior modification. Behaviors are the operants and are controlled by altering the consequences with reinforcers or punishments, as illustrated in Figure 16-1.

Positive or desired behaviors should be rewarded or reinforced. Reinforcement motivates, increasing the strength of a response or inducing its repetition. Continuous reinforcement speeds up early performance. Intermittent reinforcement at fixed or variable ratios sustains performance. Research indicates higher rates of response with ratio rather than interval schedules. Reinforcers tend to weaken over time and new ones have to be developed.

Undesirable organizational behavior should not be rewarded. Negative reinforcement occurs when desired behavior occurs to avoid negative consequences of punishment. Although frequently used, punishment creates negative attitudes and can increase costs. Behaviorists believe that people will repeat behavior when consequences are positive.

Behavior modification research uses a scientific approach. Application of behavior modification is occurring in large companies. Benefits or results claimed include improved attendance, productivity, and efficiency and cost savings. Reinforcers center on praise, recognition, and feedback. The problem-solving method is used to apply behavior modification:

- Identify and define (observe and measure) the specific behavior.
- Measure or count the occurrences.
- Analyze the antecedents, behaviors, and consequences (ABCs) of the behavior.
- Perform positive reinforcement, negative reinforcement, punishment, or extinguish the behavior. Positive reinforcement is best as people repeat behavior that is rewarded and avoid that which is punished. Identify by asking employees or through an attitude survey.
- Evaluate changes. Provide feedback for reinforcement or correction. Give positive reinforce-

FIGURE 16–1. Reinforcement Theory

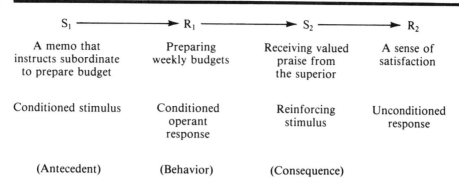

SOURCE: Adapted with permission from J. Gibson, J. Ivanovich, and J. Donnelly, *Organizations: Behavior Structure Processes*, 6th ed. Homewood, IL: Richard D. Irwin, Inc. 1988.

ment while discussing areas that need improvement. Give feedback at all steps of performance, not just at outcomes. Follow-up reinforcement motivates people to put plans into effect because of the attention generated: somebody cares and is paying attention. Structured follow-up can include review sessions between clinical nurse and nurse manager, interdisciplinary or intradisciplinary team review of outcomes, review of instrumented data, or direct consultation.

Critics of the behavior modification theory consider rewards to be bribes.[7]

A second process theory of motivation is the expectancy theory of Vroom. This theory postulates that most behaviors are voluntarily controlled by a person and are therefore motivated. There is an effort-performance expectancy or belief by a person that a chance exists for a certain effort to lead to a particular level of performance. The performance-outcome expectancy or belief of this person will have certain outcomes. Given choices, the individual selects the choice with the best expected outcome. Research on expectancy theory is increasing although not systematic or refined. It is a complicated process in which unconscious motivation is avoided.[8]

Equity theory is a third process theory. People believe they are being treated with equity when the ratio of their efforts to rewards equals those of others. Equity can be achieved or restored by changing outputs, attitudes, the reference person, inputs or outputs of the reference person, or the situation. Research on equity theory has focused on pay.[9]

A fourth process theory of motivation is the goal-setting theory of Locke. This theory is based on goals as determinants of behavior. The more specific the goals, the better the results produced. Research indicates goals are a powerful force. They must be achievable. The difficulty level of goals should be increased only to the ceiling to which the person will commit. Goal clarity and accurate feedback increase security.[10]

Maslow

Maslow's theory of motivation is a positive one and is based on a holistic-dynamic theory.

At the base of a needs system are physiological needs. These are based on homeostasis, which is a condition of constancy of body fluids, functions, and states; the constancy is maintained automatically by uniform interaction of counteracting processes. It should be noted that human beings do not just eat; they eat selectively to maintain homeostasis. The same is probably true of other physiological needs. Not all physiological needs are homeostatic, and they are relatively independent of each other while at the same time interdependent; for example, smoking may satisfy the hunger need in some persons. Some are in opposition, such as the tendency to be lazy at the same time one has a desire to be industrious.

Physiological needs are the most prepotent or strongest of human needs when unsatisfied. A starving person will steal food and perform other acts that threaten safety. Dominance of a physiological need changes the individual's philosophy for the future.

Human needs are organized in a hierarchy of prepotency: higher ones emerge as lower ones are satisfied. When the physiological needs are satisfied, the human being is no longer motivated by them. However, when deprived of a long-satisfied need, that person tolerates it better than one who has been long or previously deprived.

Safety needs are the second group in the hierarchy. Among these are security, protection, dependency, and stability; freedom from anxiety, chaos, and fear; need for order, limits, structure, and law; strength in the protector, and others. Their satisfaction influences a person's philosophy of life and of values. What threatens the safety of nursing? Are nurses threatened by increased consumer interest in their shortcomings, which may lead to consumer control of practice? What motivates people? Is it a fear of the high cost of extended illnesses and poor results of care? The average person likes law, order, predictability, and organization, and this may be one reason people resist change. Insurance programs, job tenure, and savings accounts are expressions of safety needs. People prefer familiar to unknown things. Today's managers are often threatened by the new generation of personnel who question regulations and use the law to achieve their goals.

Once the physiological and safety needs have been satisfied, the needs for love, affection, and belongingness emerge. Most individuals in nursing today have had their physiological and safety needs satisfied, although there are notable exceptions, the nonpromoted workers being among them. Now they want to be part of a group or family with love, acceptance, friendliness, and a feeling of belonging. Are these needs thwarted by frequent moves? How are the needs of the individual as well as those of the organization satisfied? A society that wants to survive and be healthy will work to satisfy these needs. Otherwise people will be maladjusted and will exhibit severe emotional and behavioral pathology.

Two categories emerge under the fourth set of needs—the esteem needs. All people share these needs. First they desire strength, achievement, adequacy, mastery and competence, confidence before the world, independence, and freedom. Second, they desire reputation or prestige, status, fame and glory, dominance, recognition, attention, importance, dignity, or appreciation. A person whose self-esteem is satisfied has feelings of self-confidence, worth, strength, capability, adequacy, usefulness, and being needed in society. For it to be stable and healthy, self-esteem must be based on known or deserved respect. The reason for it must be known and recognized within the recipient.

Finally, at the pinnacle of the hierarchy of needs is the emotional gold—the need for self-actualization, the effort of people to be what they can be. Nurses want to become everything that they are capable of becoming, to achieve their potential, to be effective as nurse persons, to be creative, and to meet personal standards of performance.

Certain conditions are prerequisites for basic need satisfaction. When basic needs are thwarted, the individual is threatened. These conditions include:

1. Freedom to speak—communication.
2. Freedom to do what one wishes to do without harming others—choice of jobs, friends, and entertainment.
3. Freedom to express oneself—creativity.
4. Freedom to investigate and seek for information.
5. Freedom to defend oneself; justice, fairness, honesty, and orderliness in the group.

Human beings want to gain new knowledge, to solve problems, to bring order, and to explore, and they will voluntarily face dangers to do so.

The hierarchy of needs is not a simple classification. Individuals put their needs into different orders, some placing self-esteem before love. Others place creativity before all else. Certain people have low levels of aspiration. Permanent loss of love needs results in a psychopathic personality.

A long-satisfied need may become undervalued; having never been deprived, a person does not regard such a need as being important. If two needs emerge, a person will probably want the more basic one satisfied first. People who have loved and been well loved, and who have had many deep friendships, can hold out against hatred, rejection, or persecution.

Most normal people in our society have partial satisfaction and partial dissatisfaction of all of their basic needs at the same time. They have a higher partial satisfaction of physiological needs and correspondingly lower partial satisfaction of self-actualization needs. Emergence of new needs is gradual. Needs are more often unconscious than conscious.

Basic needs are common throughout different cultures. Most behavior is multidetermined—all of the basic needs are involved. A single act of an individual could be analyzed to show how it addresses physiological needs, safety needs, love needs, esteem needs, and self-actualization needs. Not all behavior is internally motivated; some is stimulated externally. Some is highly motivated, some weakly, and some not at all. Some is expressive and some rote. A gratified or satisfied need is not a motivator of behavior. Healthy persons are primarily motivated by the need to develop and actualize their fullest potentialities and capacities.

Usefulness to Nurse Managers

Although there are many theories and much has been written about motivation, there is no easy way to motivate employees. Human motivation is diverse, subtle, and complex. To use the available information on motivation effectively, the nurse manager will read it and select and use those elements that appear to be practical and workable.

Some theories of motivation are contradictory. They provide useful knowledge when used selectively and carefully. Theories of motivation are really constructs and not theories, as motivation cannot be directly observed and measured.[11]

Knowledge of motivation theories is essential to improving job performance of employees. Individual employees have different needs and goals. Nurse managers will learn and use motivation theories selectively.

DISSATISFACTIONS

There are many dissatisfactions in nursing and many have been enumerated in nursing studies. A summary of the major studies is given in Appendix 5–3.

The following paragraphs relate to dissatisfaction among nurses. Dissatisfaction can be alleviated by learned approaches to change by nurse managers within nursing organizations.

Productivity

Nurses respond negatively and become dissatisfied when managers use force, control, threats, and repeated applications of institutional power. Productivity decreases or stagnates. The new breed of nurses question authority and give loyalty to those who earn it. An attitude of mutual respect between clinical nurses and managers is essential to productivity.

To promote mutual respect there must be free interaction and communication in which expectations are clarified, feedback on performance is given, and promises that cannot be delivered are avoided. There must be role modeling of expected and desired performance. In more than seven out of ten working relationships, the employee does not know what is expected of her or him. Expectations must be clear. In a Productivity Attitude Test developed and administered to production workers by Pryor and Mondy over a 2-year period, 75 percent of respondents said that their supervisors did not keep promises they made. Broken promises anger employees and decrease productivity.[12]

Nurse managers are powerful models for staff. They are emulated, whether their example is good or bad. The obvious inference is that nurse managers should do self-assessment and modify their behavior to assume roles beneficial to both staff and organization.

Like other workers, all nurses work to survive, to meet their needs and aspirations. The complexity of the technological environment for patient care can lead to specialization and the depersonalization of jobs and work. This alienates nursing employees and the quality of their work declines.

The Nurse as Knowledge Worker

Drucker indicates that knowledge workers are productive only with self-motivation, self-direction, and achievement. We have wasted over 200 years learning this. There is no one dominant dimension to working. People are motivated to work based on Maslow's hierarchy of needs. Even though satisfied, a human need remains important. Economic rewards that are not properly taken care of create dissatisfaction with work. They become deterrents.[13]

Nurses are knowledge workers. Their basic economic needs are related to other human needs or human values. Performing work of equal difficulty, they want economic rewards of equal value to those of other knowledge workers. Pay is part of the social or psychological dimension of nurses. They also want increased rank, power, and status, commensurate with other knowledge workers.

Education makes fear a demotivator. Educated people are mobile. Nurses can move laterally to jobs in other organizations. The role of discipline is to take care of marginal friction. If used to drive nurses, discipline causes resentment and resistance; it demotivates. Direction and control are useless in meeting ego needs.

The nurse as knowledge worker is self-directed and takes responsibility. Rewarding and reaffirming self-direction and responsibility produce learning; fear produces resistance. Psychological manipulation is only a replacement for the carrot-and-stick approach to management. It does not work.

Thwarted needs or deficiencies lead to sick or negative behavior. Focus on already satisfied needs is ineffective; however, employees will demand more of what they already have unless attention is given to self-esteem and self-actualization. In such a situation money becomes the only means available of satisfying needs. Nurses want it to purchase material goods and services. Inflation increases the demand as it takes more money to satisfy other desires. However, this increased demand for money and material rewards destroys their usefulness as incentives and managerial tools.

Nurses are adults and as such have outgrown dependence. They want to be independent. They want to be treated as adults and partners with dignity and respect. It is the practicing clinical nurses who achieve health-care productivity gains, not capital spending and automation.

Nursing personnel retreat from association and identification with organizations in which they cannot meet their perceived care requirements. While more believe themselves competent and able to do good work, they are dissatisfied because they cannot live up to the standard of care they want to provide. They care and because they care they are dissatisfied.

SATISFACTIONS

The Science of Human Behavior

How do we apply the knowledge of the social sciences so that our human organizations will be truly effective? We have the knowledge, just as we have the knowledge of physical sciences to develop alternative sources of energy such as solar, tidal, atomic, and geothermal energy. Application of vast knowledge in both physical and social sciences is expensive and time-consuming.

Theory X and Theory Y

Although Douglas McGregor died in 1964, his theories of leadership and motivation live on. Unfortunately his Theory X has not been replaced by his Theory Y. Theory X, as he noted it to be in the world of business, was summarized into these points:

1. Management is responsible for organizing the elements of productive enterprise—money, materials, equipment, people—in the interest of economic ends.
2. With respect to people, this is a process of directing their efforts, motivating them, controlling their actions, modifying their behavior to fit the needs of the organization.
3. Without this active intervention by management, people would be passive—even resistant—to organizational needs. They must therefore be persuaded, rewarded, punished, controlled—their activities must be directed. This is management's task—in managing subordinate managers or workers. We often sum it up by saying that management consists of getting things done through other people.

Behind this conventional theory there are several additional beliefs—less explicit, but widespread:

4. The average man (sic) is by nature indolent—he works as little as possible.
5. He lacks ambition, dislikes responsibility, prefers to be led.
6. He is inherently self-centered, indifferent to organizational needs.
7. He is by nature resistant to change.
8. He is gullible, not very bright, the ready dupe of the charlatan and the demagogue.[14]

How many nurse managers demotivate practicing nurses by falling into the trap of voicing the very statements embodied in Theory X? How may nurse managers motivate practicing nurses by following the contrasting precepts of Theory Y:

1. Management is responsible for organizing the elements of productive enterprise—money, materials, equipment, people—in the interest of economic ends.
2. People are not by nature passive or resistant to organizational needs. They have become so as a result of experience in organizations.
3. The motivation, the potential for development, the capacity for assuming responsibility, the readiness to direct behavior toward organizational goals are all present in people. Management does not put them there. It is the responsibility of management to make it possible for people to recognize and develop these human characteristics for themselves.
4. The essential task of management is to arrange organizational conditions and methods of operation so that people can achieve their own goals *best* by directing *their own* efforts toward organizational objectives.[15]

Nurse Managers and Motivation

The first manager to tackle the problem of productivity was Robert Owen (1771–1858) in his textile mill in Lanark, Scotland in the 1820s. Owen is pictured as a manager who was a real person relating to the work, the worker, the enterprise, and the manager.[16]

Nurse managers should apply techniques, skill, and knowledge, including knowledge of motivational theory, to help people obtain what they want out of nursing work. At the same time these techniques must be directed to achieve the objectives of the institution and the division of nursing.

To be persuaded to apply their skills to the achievement of nursing and organizational goals requires brilliance and a sensitivity to people on the part of the nurse manager. It requires energy and negotiating skill. It requires gaining people's attention so that their aspirations and emotions are melded with the leader's and with that of the profession and the organization for which they work. It requires integrity so that people will be controlled only to the point needed.

To successfully lead today's nurses toward accomplishing the goals of nursing, nurse leaders must do motivational research or at least be aware of the findings of motivational research and apply them to personnel management. This is a prime subject for continuing education for nurse leaders.

Through intuition, observation, and knowledge, the nurse's objectives are mixed with those of leaders (and thus of nursing management and the nursing profession). They will be restated so that when ratified by the group they are seen as desirable objectives to attain. This process requires intellectual skills that open nurses' hearts and minds, analysis of their perceptions, and synthesis of their perceptions with those of leadership. To achieve results will require mental agility, emotional intensity, and communicative and negotiative skills.

According to O. William Battalia's theories of leadership,

> to accomplish a true union of aspirations, a true blending of goals, a true melding of motivation, [the leader] must initiate compensatory moves— to balance off the weak and the strong, the meek and the brash, the glib and the tight-mouthed, the too ambitious and the indolent, the bright and the dull. These moves to create harmony will include cutting down and building up—cutting off and adding on.[17]

The big secret is *listen.*

Several authors make a good case for saying that one person cannot motivate another and that motivation lies within the individual. Everyone has it. If one can study, accept, and apply theories of motivational psychology, such an approach is compatible with the knowledge that human beings have needs that motivate them.

The choice of action lies with the individual. Incentives must be meaningful to the individual and motivation must be stimulating on an individual basis. The organization has a set of standards it wants met relative to providing care that is satisfactory to patients. Nurses want remuneration for providing that care. They provide it best as part of an organized group. An interaction between employee and employer is essential to a contract. To be successful there must be rapport and involvement. It depends on the employer's authority to give or withhold rewards and the employee's level of aspiration. Does the nurse want to advance if risks increase? To find out the nurses' needs and aspirations, ask them. Note their individual responses to a variety of work assignments and incentives. A person will seldom respond to being a number. Personnel policies must provide support to supervisors. Communication that identifies needs is not an invasion of privacy but rather a realistic approach that leads to mutual trust and frankness between people.[18]

Motivation is an emotional process, being psychological rather than logical. Learn how a nurse wants to feel and help this nurse use the tools that will permit achievement of those feelings. Such feelings may relate to associations with people on the job that make the nurse feel accepted, performance of those acts for which she or he is highly skilled, and recognition for a satisfactory performance, among other things.

As previously stated, motivation is basically an unconscious process. When asked why she or he did a certain thing, a nurse may not be able to give the answer. Even though people's basic motives are hidden and intangible, their actions or behavior makes sense to them.

Each person is unique, the key to behavior lying within the self. A supervisor must use judgment to figure out why each person reacts in a given way to any situation.

Within each unique individual motivating needs differ from time to time. The key lies in figuring out which need is currently predominant.

People shape a nurse's needs and actions, making the nurse a social being and motivation a social success. People help satisfy these needs.

Motivational patterns are learned early and followed for years. There is no conscious selection, judgment, or decision involved in 95 percent of what people do.

Perhaps with hard work, nurse managers may be able to influence the motivational processes that cause practicing nurses to do things that will benefit the organization. In evaluating nurses the supervisor will observe how well each one defines and solves problems on the job. They will be tested on their capacities to generalize—to tie facts together and predict the outcome; to see degrees of difference—what make one solution better than another; and ability to abstract—to weed out the inessential. They will be tested on their abilities to depart from orderliness and demonstrate creative and imaginative solutions to problems. They will be tested for their feelings, emotions, and attitudes to determine the stability of their individual personalities. All nurses will be tested for their social skills. They will be tested for their insight as well as their insight into others. Can they look objectively and thoughtfully at the actions of both?

They will be tested for their ability to use good work habits and to discriminate among tasks.

They will be tested on their individual philosophy of life and the code of standards they set and follow for themselves. Can you as a nurse manager influence all the aspects of individual nurses so as to meet their inner drives or needs? Perhaps a better question would be, can you provide those things from the outside world that will satisfy the inner drives or needs of the individual? Actions will earn respect, self-satisfaction, and love. Money usually cannot buy loyalty, creativity, or morale. Positive motivation and consistent fairness are the marks of good leadership. Satisfied employees will be happy and as productive as their capacities allow. The secret of success, then, is to enable them to achieve an exciting and satisfying life by doing the things that you need to have done. Successful people usually are well motivated.[19]

Human beings, including nurses, motivate themselves. The nurse manager will provide practicing nurses the opportunity for satisfaction of their needs, or deprive them of it.

> The motivational theory under discussion asserts that man (sic)—if he is freed to some extent, by his presence in an affluent society, from the necessity to use most of his energy to obtain the necessities of life and a degree of security from the major vicissitudes—will by nature begin to pursue goals associated with his higher-level needs. These include needs for a degree of control over his own fate, for self-respect, for using and increasing his talents, for responsibility, for achievement both in the sense of status and recognition and in the sense of personal development and effective problem solving. Thus freed, he will also seek in many ways to satisfy more fully his physical needs for recreation, relaxation, and play. Management has been well aware of the latter tendency; it has not often recognized the former, or at least it has not taken into account its implication for managerial strategy.[20]

Hard versus Soft Approach to Nursing Management. What are the effects of a hard approach to personnel management such as coercion and disguised threats, close supervision, and tight controls over behavior? Experience has shown that such an approach causes counterforces, including the restriction of output, militant unionism, and subtle but effective sabotage of the objectives of management.

Nurses turn to labor organizations when they fail to achieve results with their supervisors. They do this when authoritarian managers manage from the top down with job descriptions, performance standards and evaluations, rules, pay incentives, promotions, management objectives, and dismissal threats. They are not consulted on any of these management tools and activities.

The soft approach to personnel management, such as permissiveness, satisfying people's demands, and achievement of harmony, has been proven to cause indifferent performance, with expectations of receiving more and giving less. As a consequence, many managers try to take a middle-of-the-road approach.

Observation and evidence of the social sciences indicate that employees' behavior shapes itself to management perceptions. This behavior does not result from inherent human nature but from the nature of organizations, management philosophy, policy, and practice.

The nursing leader looks for simple, practical, immediate ideas to solve personnel problems. There are no magic wands, but that does not mean there are no solutions.

Solutions

Career Planning. Career planning is a continuous process of self-assessment and goal setting. It is a cooperative venture between the organization and the employee, the career counselor (who could also be a mentor or sponsor) and the individual nurse. Career planning is an organized system with short-term and long-term career goals fitted to those of the organization.

To build a career development program requires major effort. The following outline stresses the major activities:

1. Assess the future goals and labor power needs of the nursing organization relative to recruitment, promotion, hiring, placement, retention, and turnover.
2. Develop job structures with career paths and qualifications including career opportunities within the nursing organization.

3. Recruit qualified applicants, including those already employed within the nursing organization.
4. Assess each applicant for personal expectations: Why are they making this career choice? What are their needs, motivators, and job satisfiers? What stresses make them frustrated and dissatisfied? What stresses excite them? What are their career goals? How does their present performance relate to their career goals? What are their competencies and interests? What potential performance will be needed to achieve their career goals?
5. Develop an individual career development plan for the individual nurse.
6. Provide developmental opportunities for the individual nurse to achieve career goals.

There can be a career development program advisory committee. Staff development personnel can be career counselors. The real goal is self-development of a career plan for every nurse fostered by the nursing organization. For this reason the individual nurse is best involved in the entire career development program from its inception. Most nurses will benefit from participation in a career development program, even if it only improves the quality of their working lives.[21]

Communication. To produce quality nursing products and services requires highly motivated practicing nurses. Nurse managers can motivate nurses by sharing information about the organization. Consultative managers consult with nurses on problems, solutions, and decisions and share information about results.

Communication involves giving feedback as information and as reinforcement. It avoids surprising nurses by keeping them informed of changes. Communication media are used to recognize nurses, thereby improving their self-esteem and to clarify expected behavior and job performance. They can be part of an effective open door policy and complaint system, and they can be used to inform nurses about a workable career ladder and educational opportunities to upgrade their knowledge and skills. Communication media implement uniform grievance procedures.

Effective communication by nurse managers, along with other motivators, boosts morale and keeps practicing nurses from turning to labor organizations for need satisfaction that includes security.[22] Communication is discussed more fully in a separate chapter.

Teamwork. Nurse managers can motivate practicing nurses by encouraging teamwork. Teams can be built from work groups for discussion and resolution of work-related issues. Teams should have identifiable output, inclusive membership, leaders with carefully circumscribed authority, agreement on purpose, rules of procedure, and measurable goals, resources, and feedback.

Allender suggests the following ways to enhance productivity through teamwork:

1. Form teams by common activity and include all people associated with each activity from top management to lowest level.
2. Manager chooses a results-oriented leader who is a motivator, compassionate, respected, and organized. This leader keeps the team on schedule as its chair and summarizes and distributes the minutes. The leader ensures that decisions are reached by consensus.
3. The team develops a written statement of team purpose with which members totally agree. This agreement is reached through discussion.
4. Meeting times are set to accommodate all members, usually about an hour every one to two weeks.
5. The team develops measurement criteria for team performance, uses them, and records the results on charts.
6. The team gathers data on past and present performance and sets goals. It displays the performance data of graphs at each meeting.
7. The team identifies indirect issues of the work environment and attends to them. Completion addresses concerns of team members as items are never left hanging.

Through using teams, Hewlett-Packard has cut labor costs, reduced defects, solved vendor problems, eliminated jobs, decreased inspections, cut scrap production, and reached targets ahead of schedule. Teamwork achieves personal recognition, raising self-esteem, motivation, and commitment. It is stimulated by trust, support, completion, acknowledgment, communication, and agreement.[23]

Cornett-Cooke and Dias describe the use of teamwork to raise the spirits of nurses during a time of economic recession, cutbacks, and curtailment of capital expenditures. They identified that teamwork could be used to clarify the purpose or mission of a department or unit, to define a vision of the process and product of team effort, to identify blocks and barriers to their vision, to look at ways the work group members support each other, to make requests and agreements about how each can better work together with others on the team, and to plan the team's work goals and activities and commit each member to accomplishing them. The result would be an effective team with personally satisfied members.

This strategy was used to build a team. They made a schedule of their sessions to include one on team building. They planned for input from representatives of all shifts. Their kickoff included posters, including one of each nurse team member's graduation picture and school on a U.S. map.

They had a productive session in which they agreed on ground rules including what the manager would do and what the manager would ask the staff to do. They explored such vision areas as patient care, staffing, interpersonal communication, and professional relationships. They analyzed problems and set about solving them with action plans. Each month they recognized each other with "warm fluffy days," giving each team member a compliment and a cotton ball on a pin. They even had an intrashift team session to share experiences when they became curious about each other. They developed spirit through teamwork.[24]

Teamwork recognizes people as worthy. It provides support and commitment of goals leading to productivity. It motivates practicing nurses. Nurse managers can develop it.

Self-Esteem. Self-esteem is having a stable, firmly based, usually high evaluation of oneself, having self-respect, and being self-confident from being able to act independently, from achieving one's personal and professional goals, and from competence in personal and professional skills and knowledge. Being held in esteem by others by reason of one's personal accomplishments and reputation gives a person status and recognition. It makes one feel appreciated and respected and increases one's self-esteem. It satisfies the desire for having strength among family, friends, colleagues, supervisors, patients, visitors, and others.[25] See Figure 16–2 for examples of self-esteem based in strength.

Self-esteem is also satisfaction of the desire for achievement of personal, professional and organizational goals, as illustrated in Figure 16–3.

Self-esteem comes from satisfaction of the desire for adequacy, feeling worthwhile as a person in society and as a worker, as illustrated in Figure 16–4.

Self-esteem involves satisfying the desire for mastery and competence in the knowledge and skills needed to perform a role in clinical practice, management, education or research, as a member of a family, and as a citizen, as shown in Figure 16–5.

Self-esteem comes from acquiring a feeling of confidence in the face of the world, as in Figure 16–6.

Self-esteem involves satisfying the desire for independence and freedom. To satisfy the need for self-esteem, a person must be free to speak, free to act without hurting others, free to express herself or himself, free to investigate and seek information, and free to defend herself or himself. Each person must be treated with justice, fairness, honesty, and orderliness in the group; see Figure 16–7.

There are other terms that can be used to describe self-esteem. These include valuing oneself or estimating one's worth. Our goal is to value ourselves highly, to consider ourselves favorably, to appreciate and think well of ourselves. We also want

FIGURE 16–2. Examples of Self-Esteem through Strength

1. Head nurses have strength when they know that other employees want to hire them because of their demonstrated influence with nurses, physicians, and others. They have self-esteem when this gives them satisfaction.
2. Nurse administrators have strength when chosen by top management to expand their spheres of responsibility to direct other departments and when recognized by other administrators for skills and knowledge—being consulted by legislators, or leaders in nursing and health care. They have self-esteem when this gives them satisfaction.

FIGURE 16–3. Examples of Self-Esteem through Achievement of Goals

1. A professional nurse satisfies the desire for self-esteem by running for and winning a government office or an office in some service or professional organization.
2. A professional nurse satisfies the desire for self-esteem by achieving credentials such as certification, an advanced degree, or the skill of using a computer.
3. A professional nurse manager satisfies the desire for self-esteem by lowering the absenteeism and turnover rates of personnel in the nursing division.

FIGURE 16–4. Examples of Self-Esteem through Adequacy

1. A professional nurse feels that she is a good wife and mother because she can work a schedule compatible with her husband's, be involved in the activities of her family, and save money for a future college education for her children.
2. A staff nurse in the recovery room feels that she has time to assess, plan, and give good care and attend to good documentation of care. She even has opportunity to obtain reading references she needs to keep her knowledge and skills updated.

FIGURE 16–5. Examples of Self-Esteem through Mastery

1. A nurse manager involves clinical nurses in preparing strategic objectives for a unit. The plan is approved by the organization's administrators.
2. A clinical nurse is selected to implement a theory of nursing about which she is considered an authority.

others to have a high regard for us, to honor and admire us.

In terms of Maslow's hierarchy of needs, self-esteem is a higher-level need in the ego category. It emerges after physiological, safety, and belongingness and love needs are fairly well gratified. Al-

FIGURE 16–6.   Examples of Self-Esteem through Confidence

1. A professional nurse goes to work confident that she can perform as well as any other nurse, and better than some; that she can learn anything she needs to learn to do a job well; that other people recognize her abilities and give her credit for them, that she will earn full merit pay; and that she will do this while meeting standards of her employers, the ANA, the JCAHO, and other internal and external agencies.
2. A professional nurse decides that she has the capacity to win support for her candidacy and wages a successful campaign.

FIGURE 16–7.   Examples of Self-Esteem through Independence

1. A supervisor decides she would like to know something about joint practice as a modality of nursing. She obtains information and writes a position paper on it. Her administrator tells her to go ahead with making a plan to practice it. She sets a specific schedule to orient and gain approval of the clinical nurses and then the physicians who use the unit.
2. Clinical nurses are given complete freedom to manage the care of their patients including coordination with personnel of x-ray, medical laboratory, nutrition, and food service; with physicians; and with others.

though self-actualization needs are higher in the hierarchy, this hierarchy of needs does not follow the same order in everyone. Self-esteem needs are rarely fully satisfied.

People want a good reputation and to have prestige (respect or esteem) from others. They want to be recognized, to have attention, to be important, and to be appreciated.

People meet their esteem needs in different ways. They are influenced by culture, including the culture of the organization in which they work. The ends or results of achieving self-esteem and the esteem of others are more important than the roads taken to achieve those ends. All human beings want esteem, unless they are pathological. Persons lacking self-esteem feel inferior, weak, helpless, and discouraged. They become indolent, passive, resistant to change, lacking in responsibility, and unwilling to follow a dialogue. They focus on salary and fringe benefits, making unreasonable demands for economic benefits. They can become neurotic or emotionally sick when they have a deficiency in self-esteem.[26]

Meeting the self-esteem needs of employees is of great significance to management, in nursing as everywhere. Most nurses work in bureaucratic organizations such as hospitals, home health-care agencies, nursing homes, clinics, and the like. In these bureaucratic organizations work is organized to meet many concerns, including those of the organization and the physicians and the routines and personnel of other departments. The lower levels of

the hierarchy have few opportunities to meet their ego needs. Nurses must schedule care of their patients around everyone else. They are the servants of the organization.

Direction and control are useless methods of motivating professional nurses where social, ego, and self-fulfillment needs are predominant. Intellectual creativity is a characteristic of professional nurses. They do not get ego satisfaction from wages, pensions, vacations, or other benefits of work. The job itself must be satisfying and fun if professional nurses are to satisfy their self-esteem needs. They get their ego needs met by having a voice in decision making. Professional nurses will commit to organizational objectives when allowed to determine the steps to take to achieve them. They want to collaborate with other professionals, both internally and externally to the environment in which they work.

Full utilization of their talent and training is another desire of professional nurses. They want attention paid to the nature of nursing as a critical practice discipline, to the organization of nursing functions and job challenges. They do *not* want close and detailed supervision. One reason for the success of primary nursing has been the control professional nurses have over the nursing process of patients who are their primary nursing responsibility. This success will not continue unless management gives attention to a career development plan. Such a plan is the logical evolution into joint practice in which physicians and nurses collaborate to give total care to patients. Professional nurses want opportunities to develop within their professional careers *as clinical nurses.* Career ladder progression must relate to clinical practice.

Professional nurses want status, internally and externally. This includes publication with clerical support services from employers. It includes participation in the affairs of professional societies to which employers pay annual dues and expenses of attending meetings for at least representative groups.[27]

What can management do? Management can set the conditions under which professional nurses become committed to organizational goals and exercise self-control and self-direction. This leads to creativity.

Strategic planning by top management can involve professional clinical nurse participation. Is not the end result accomplished through professional nursing? The strategic plan can then be submitted to the department level for input by clinical nurses and other professionals. They will contribute to it by critiquing it, strengthening it, and making it a plan to which they can commit. This management process will be a difficult task, the accomplishment of which gives professional nurses new knowledge and skills, opportunity for creativity, and recognition and prestige in other peoples' eyes, meeting their ego needs for self-esteem. In the area of performance evaluation, nurse managers can again set the stage for meeting the self-esteem needs of professional nurses who want to be evaluated, promoted, rotated, and transferred in terms of their clinical or other personal career motivations. Self-evaluation in which individuals plan and appraise their contributions to organizational objectives promotes self-esteem. Conventional performance appraisal attacks self-esteem.[28]

It is obvious that management can create the conditions for professional nurses being able to meet their esteem needs. They can make nurses feel good about themselves by providing adequate staffing to give good nursing care, by correct placement and orientation to achieve mastery, independence, and freedom, by respecting them for a job well done, and by promoting deserved respect from coworkers and employees.[29]

Managers can give professional nurses freedom to do something besides quit. They can give them a KITA (kick in the ____) that will be psychologically positive and will increase their self-esteem. When they do this professional nurses will gain basic confidence in their managers.[30]

What do manager get from their jobs—freedom? Social satisfaction? Opportunities for achievement? Knowledge? Ability to create? Who gets the reward and for what? Who must provide the opportunities for increased dignity, achievement, prestige, and social satisfaction?

Self-esteem involves the personhood of all professional nurses, be they managers, clinical nurses, researchers, or teachers. Each should enrich the esteem of the other person, should be the peer pal, mentor, sponsor, and guardian of the person within the profession. Esteem results in leading and influencing. One can listen to other people, treat them as individuals, show earnest exhilaration in responding to their creativity, offer ideas for improvement, and share the excitement of their success with victories and wins. Success gives a good self-image. It builds self-esteem. It avoids the pain of failure.[31]

Self-Actualization

Self-actualization was defined by Maslow as an ego need at the top of the needs hierarchy. It does not exist by itself and in some persons may be no stronger than the love and belonging need or the self-esteem need.

Self-actualized people are better able to distinguish the real world, seeing reality more clearly. Comfortable with the unknown, self-actualized people are attracted to it. All are creative in whatever they do and perceive.

Accepting and adjusting to their own shortcomings, self-actualized people are less defensive and less artificial. They feel guilty if they are not doing something about improvable shortcomings, prejudice, jealousy, envy, and the other shortcomings of humanity. They have autonomous codes of ethics, yet are the most ethical of people. They conform when no great issues are involved.

In the area of values, self-actualized people accept their own nature, human nature, the realities of social life, and the constraints of physical reality. Self-actualized people are problem-centered, not ego-centered. Their values are broad, universal, and time-wide. Being deeply democratic as opposed to authoritarian by nature, they respect people and have a strong sense of right and wrong, of good and evil. Self-actualized people are not interested in hostile humor. Their humor is of a philosophical bent, stated only to produce a laugh.

Self-actualized people like solitude and privacy. They are detached and objective under conditions of turmoil. They are self-movers with more free will. While they generally want to help the human race and can sometimes feel like strangers in a strange land, their relationships with people are more profound and their circle of friends small. They love children and humanity but can be briefly hostile to others when it is deserved or for the others' good. In social terms, self-actualized people are godly but not religious.

While they are not conventional, they conform to social graces with toleration. They can be radical.

Maslow indicates that living at the higher need level is good for growth and health, both physically and psychologically. Self-actualized people live longer, have less disease, sleep and eat better, and enjoy their sexual lives without unnecessary inhibitions. For them life continues to be fresh, thrilling, exciting, and ecstatic. They count their blessings.

Self-actualized people have mystic or peak experiences. These are natural experiences. Happiness can cause tears. It comes from appreciation of the transcendence of poetry, music, philosophy, religion, interpersonal relationships, beauty, or politics. They can have the peak experience from doing or sensing.

Self-actualized people merge or unify dichotomies such as selfishness, considering every act to be both selfish and unselfish. They perceive work as play, duty as pleasure, and so on. The purpose of higher needs is a "healthward" trend—when people experience them they place a higher value on them.

Self-actualized people are "metamotivated." Their motivations are for character growth, character expression, maturation, and development. They place more dependence upon self-development and inner growth than the prestige and status of others' honors.

Self-actualizing people are not perfect. They can be (or can be perceived to be) joyless; mundane; silly, wasteful, or thoughtless in their habits; boring, stubborn, or irritating; superficially vain or proud; partial to their own productions, family, friends, or children; temperamental; ruthless; strong and independent of others' opinions; shocking in language and behavior; concentrated to the point of absent-mindedness or humorlessness; mistaken; or

needing improvement. They can feel guilt, anxiety, sadness, self-castigation, internal strife, and conflict.

Self-actualized people develop detachment from the culture. They become autonomous and accepting.

The satisfaction of higher needs requires more preconditions, such as more people, larger scenes, longer runs, more means and partial goals, and more subordinate or preliminary steps. To achieve the higher needs requires better environmental conditions.

Pursuit and gratification of higher needs have desirable civic and social consequences: loyalty, friendliness, civic consciousness. People who are living at this level make better parents, spouses, teachers, public servants, and so on. They also create greater, stronger, and truer individualism. They are synergistic.

A conclusion could be that the self-actualized person achieves a highly satisfactory quality of life and that this quality of life extends from the gratified self-actualized person into society. Gratification or satisfaction of the higher-level needs can be positively influenced by the social environment of work, family, community, government, and the like.

Applying these insights to nursing, the nurse manager would selectively apply knowledge and skills to the social and behavioral sciences to creating an environment or climate in which practicing nurses could become self-actualized. In so doing nurse managers themselves become self-actualized and the products and services of nursing increase in quantity and quality.

While critics of Maslow's work say it is based on too narrow a population, it is widely accepted and used. He analyzed the profiles of sixty subjects including Lincoln, Jefferson, Einstein, and Frederick Douglass. Maslow suggested that our population may be limited to being from 5 to 30 percent self-determined, another forecast criticized by other scientists.[32]

SUMMARY

To summarize:

1. A person is motivated.
2. A person has goals.
3. Management has goals.

4. A condition or environment needs to be established whereby a person can achieve personal goals by achieving management's goals (or vice versa).

5. The person will be rewarded by work achievements that are successful. Management will have provided the setting for success through managerial practices, perhaps by removing restraints or giving other intrinsic rewards. High-level ego needs are met on the job.

6. There will be a cooperative interaction between manager and employee, since the latter will be participating in decisions that affect her or him.

7. Motivation occurs.

8. Personal and motivational goals are met as the nurse is motivated to be ambitious and responsible, to show initiative, to be proud of fellow nurses and the employing institution, to welcome change, and to demonstrate individual abilities.

This law will apply to successful leadership in nursing; find out where nurses want to go and what they want to accomplish, and bring these wants into line with those of the organization. Then nurses will accomplish organizational goals as their own.

NOTES

1. R. M. Hodgetts and D. F. Kuratko, *Management* (2d. ed. New York: Harcourt Brace Jovanovich, 1988), 285, 294.

2. A. H. Maslow, *Motivation and Personality*, 2d ed. (New York: Harper & Row, 1970).

3. J. L. Gibson, J. M. Ivancevich, and J. M. Donnelly, *Organizations: Behavior, Structure, Processes* (6th ed., Homewood, IL.: Richard D. Irwin, Inc., 1988), 116.

4. R. M. Hodgetts and D. F. Kuratko, op. cit., 287–289. D. McGregor, *Leadership and Motivation* (Cambridge, MA: MIT Press, 1966).

5. J. M. Ivancevich, J. H. Donnelly, Jr., and J. L. Gibson, (4th ed. Homewood, IL.: BPI/Irwin, 1989), 373–376.

6. E. C. Murphy, "What Motivates People to Work?," *Nursing Management*, Feb. 1984, 58, 61–62; G. K. Gordon, "Developing a Motivating Environment," *Journal of Nursing Administration*, Dec. 1982, 11–16.

7. J. M. Ivancevich, J. H. Donnelly, Jr., and J. L. Gibson, op. cit.

8. J. M. Ivancevich, J. H. Donnelly, Jr., and J. L. Gibson, op. cit. 381–384.

9. Ibid.

10. Ibid.

11. G. K. Gordon, op. cit.

12. K. L. Roach, op. cit.; M. G. Pryor and W. Mondy, "Mutual Respect Key to Productivity," *Supervisory Management*, July, 1978, 10–17.

13. P. F. Drucker, *Management: Tasks, Responsibilities, Practices* (New York: Harper & Row, 1973–74), 176, 195–6.

14. D. McGregor, op. cit., 5–6.

15. Ibid., 15.

16. P. F. Drucker, op. cit., 23.

17. O. W. Battalia, "Style Changes in the Way Men Lead Men," *Psi Phi Quarterly*, Fall 1971, 4–7.

18. J. Lancaster, "Creating a Climate for Excellence," *Journal of Nursing Administration*, Jan. 1985, 16–19; L. Ackerman, "Let's Put Motivation Where It Belongs—Within the Individual," *Personnel Journal*, July 1970.

19. M. Miller, "Understanding Human Behavior and Employee Motivation," *Notes & Quotes*, 1968; D. McGregor, op. cit., 211–212.

20. Ibid.

21. M. K. Kleinknecht and E. A. Hefferin, "Assisting Nurses Toward Professional Growth: A Career Development Model," *The Journal of Nursing Administration*, July-Aug. 1982, 30–36; J. C. Crout, "Care Plan for Retaining the New Nurse," *Nursing Management*, Dec. 1984, 30–33; R. C. Swansburg and P. W. Swansburg, *Strategic Career Planning and Development for Nurses* (Rockville, MD: Aspen, 1984).

22. B. Conway-Rutkowski, "Labor Relations: How Do You Rate?" *Nursing Management*, Feb. 1984, 13–16; W. L. Ginnodo, "Consultative Management: A Fresh Look at Employee Motivation," *National Productivity Review*, Winter 1985–86, 78–80.

23. M. C. Allender, "Productivity Enhancement: A New Teamwork Approach," *National Productivity Review*, Spring 1984, 181–189.

24. P. Cornett-Cooke and K. Dias, "Teambuilding: Getting It All Together," *Nursing Management*, May 1984, 16–17.

25. A. H. Maslow, op. cit.

26. B. Fuszard, Ed., *Self-Actualization for Nurses: Issues, Trends, and Strategies for Job Enrichment* (Rockville, MD: Aspen, 1984), 140.

27. D. McGregor, op. cit.

28. B. Fuszard, op. cit., 140.

29. Ibid., 40.

30. Ibid., 58.

31. Ibid., 207.

32. A. H. Maslow, op. cit.

384–385; K. L. Roach, "Production Builds on Mutual Respect," *Nursing Management*, Feb. 1984, 54–56; R. B. Youker, "Ten Benefits of Participant Action Planning," *Training*, June 1985, 52, 54–56.

Communications 17

Between two beings there is always the barrier of words. Man has so many ears and speaks so many languages. Should it nevertheless be possible to understand one another? Is real communication possible if word and language betray us every time? Shall, in the end, only the language of guns and tanks prevail and not human reason and understanding?

—Joost A. M. Meerloo[1]

COMPONENTS OF COMMUNICATION

In answering the question of who is involved in communication, one could simply answer, everyone! However, there are several aspects to be considered. The first of these is that the person who wants to be heard is involved in communication. For example, the Bantam fried chicken facility wants to sell chicken and wants people to know that it has chicken to sell. Its manager will therefore advertise in an effort to communicate this desire to sell an appetizing product. She will do this through such media as newspapers, billboards, radio, and television. All kinds of tempting pictures will be portrayed in these advertisements. If she is successful and people buy lots of Bantam fried chicken as a result of these advertisements, then they have received the message, and she has communicated to them.

A second type of communication occurs when a person seeks out desired information. Suppose a working wife is just plain tired of cooking and wants Bantam fried chicken to serve her family for Sunday dinner. She knows where the nearest location is, since she has heard it advertised on TV or seen it on a billboard. She may have driven by the facility and seen the sign and markings that identify the product. She may have been reminded of it in the Sunday paper as she sipped her cup of coffee that morning. And even if she can't remember the address, she can always refer to the Yellow Pages for an address and phone number or call directory assistance. When she wants the information, she has many sources from which to obtain it. All these sources are media of communication.

Elements of Communication

At least two people are involved in communication, a sender or provider and a receiver. A sender usually has something he wants to communicate, although he could conceivably have to provide information of a nature distasteful to him. A receiver usually has need of some information, good or bad. Regardless of the medium, information is transmitted from sender to receiver and a communication occurs.

Regardless of whether money is involved, there is always a buyer or seller involved in a communication. The buying or selling is based on a need. Sometimes the receiver's need to hear is not as acute as the sender wants it to be. An example of this is the communication between a parent and a child or vice versa. The parent can tell the child to be in by midnight on Saturday, but she has said the same thing before, and when the child did not return by midnight, nothing happened. Now the child does not even hear the parent, since he has no reason for listening. When he returns after midnight and is told he will not be allowed out after 8:00 P.M. for 4 weeks, he has a reason to listen. Communication now takes place, since he finds there is sufficient reason for listening.

Communication is a human process involving interpersonal relationships—and therein lies the problem. Some managers view their knowledge of events as power; they see sharing knowledge through communication as sharing power and they do not want to. Other managers do not realize the importance of communication in an information age because they are not up to date on the advantages of decentralization and participatory management. They frequently fall into crisis management, treating the symptoms of poor communication and never identifying the root causes. A third group of managers recognize that communication is like the central nervous system. It directs and controls the management process.

Over 80 percent of a higher-level manager's time is spent on communication: 16 percent reading; 9 percent writing; 30 percent speaking; and 45 percent listening. Is there any question that communication skills are absolutely essential to career advancement in nursing?[2]

There are three basic principles for successful communication:

1. Successful communication involves a sender, a receiver, and a medium.
2. Successful communication occurs when the message sent is received.
3. Successful nurse managers achieve successful communication.

Climate for Communication

Organizational climate and culture are discussed in the chapter entitled "Organizing Nursing Services." The communication climate should be in harmony with the corporate culture and should be used to encourage positive values among nursing employees. These include values of quality, independence, objectivity, and client service. Communication is used to support the mission (purpose or business) and vision of the nursing organization. It is used to tell the consumers or clients that nursing is of high quality. The media used will include performance, nursing records, and marketing. It will be objective when it is accurately portrayed with descriptions of factual outcomes judged on the basis of objective outcome criteria.

Nursing literature abounds with evidence of nurses' desire for autonomy. Nurse managers will use this knowledge to communicate their support of autonomy. They will also provide a climate in which the nursing business remains as free of political constraints as possible. When political considerations are imperative, the imperative will be communicated to employees. Employees make decisions based on the institution's values and beliefs.

While organizational culture is more difficult to change than organizational climate, both can be modified with managerial effort and skill. The first step for nurse managers is to sample employees' attitudes or ideas of how they receive information and effect communication. Managers and employees know the formal structure, including roles and modes of operation used to inform and communicate. What is the informal structure? It involves people who are heroes or role models who can be involved in communication if they are positive and enthusiastic. Otherwise they may have to be replaced, particularly if they are destructive.

Cultural Agendas. Cultural agendas publicize the mission or business of the organization. They tell what the organization stands for. They will tell what the nursing division, department, or individual unit places value on.

Cultural agendas are used to communicate promotions, new hires, marriages, deaths, and other personal news about personnel. Heroes are highlighted with features that illustrate support of desired values and beliefs: the nurse who presents a paper, authors a book, achieves prominence in the profession or in the community; the nurse who is a champion bowler, an elected officer in an organization, an appointed official in the health-care system; the nurse who is a volunteer in community activities. The cultural agendas are used to publicize nursing units and special achievements such as ongoing research in burn care or rehabilitation.

Various media are used to publicize cultural agendas including newsletters, memorandums, awards ceremonies, and external communications via publications, radio, television, and organizational meetings. Such communications will be most effective when they depict the people who are directly involved in the publicized events.

Cultural agendas can be effectively used to change the organizational climate and culture.[3] The nurse manager has to establish the climate for effective communication. Wlody recommends:

Step I: Review your own communication technique.
Step II: Concentrate the staff's attention on communication as a needed skill which everyone can develop.
Step III: Lead the staff into more positive interaction within the unit.
Step IV: Make daily rounds with the whole team.
Step V: Form a group to reduce stress.[4]

Nature of Communication Climate. Important communication occurs between supervisor and employees at the work level where climate is set. A supportive climate encourages employees to ask questions and give solutions to problems. Figure 17–1 summarizes characteristics of supportive and defensive communication climates. Nurse manag-

ers would strive for a supportive climate. There is a strong relationship between good communication skills and good leadership.

Joblin reported "a study of the effects of formal structural attributes of organization upon certain characteristics of superior-subordinate communication."[5] Although research in this area has been limited and the results inconclusive, there is some evidence that organizational size (number of employees) influences communication among subordinates but not between superiors and subordinates.

Joblin determined that "subordinates in the lower levels of their organizational hierarchies perceive significantly less openness in superior-subordinate communication than subordinates at higher levels of their hierarchies."[6] Joblin studied the communication climate of fifteen different organizations located in several cities in the midwestern United States, including two health-care organizations. The climate was more open at the top, where higher-level supervisors involved subordinates more in decision making. Openness decreased as organizations increased in size, particularly over 1,000 employees. Communication increased in quantity with increased organizational size but employees perceived it to be increasingly closed: more communication, less openness. Although a narrow span of control increases communication between supervisor and subordinate, increased span of control was not perceived to decrease openness, indicating quality of interaction may be more important than quantity.[7]

Analytic Approach. A supportive climate will produce clear communication to support productive nursing workers and effective teamwork. It will provide for identification of communication problems. These will be substantiated by designing instruments to collect data during specified periods of time. Real communication patterns and problems will be diagnosed from analysis of the data. They can be related to communication climate and solved by using problem-solving techniques. (See chapter on "Decision Making and Problem Solving").

When disagreements about the intent of a communication occur, negotiation is indicated to prevent conflict, resignation, or avoidance between supervisor and employee. When there is lack of confidence between supervisor and employee or among employees, nurse managers can solve the communication problem through a climate of open-

FIGURE 17–1. Supportive versus Defensive Communication Climate

Supportive Climate	Defensive Climate
1. The individual is free to talk to managers at any level of the organization without fear of retribution of any kind. Opportunities for this are planned and made known to the entire staff.	1. The individual works within traditional management principles of chain of command, line of authority, and span of control.
2. Equality: management by objectives (MBO) supports equality by encouraging two-way communication in which both supervisor and employee evaluate progress and make future plans.	2. Superiority: pyramids, hierarchies, and chains of command support superiority.
3. Descriptive evaluation with management analysis and employee input. The employee gets information at specific intervals and when indicated.	3. Traditional evaluation with one-way communication done on an annual basis.
4. Spontaneity.	4. Strategy is kept at managerial planning level.
5. Problem orientation emphasizes joint view, bringing employee into the process.	5. Control emphasizes supervisor's view.
6. Provisionalism encourages adaptation and experimentation.	6. Certainty is dogmatic; it squelches.
7. Empathy indicates concern and respect. Use to counteract neutrality by using nontraditional management techniques.	7. Neutrality indicates nonconcern. It is fostered by orientation to numbers as in outcomes, profits, and even standardization of orientation procedures.

SOURCE: Adapted from C. E. Beck and E. A. Beck, "The Manager's Open Door and the Communication Climate," *Business Horizons*, Jan.–Feb. 1986, 15–19.

ness that restores confidence through agreement and promotes individual autonomy as well as esprit de corps.[8]

Open-Door Policy. Communication climate influences the success of an open-door policy. An open-door policy of a nurse manager implies that an employee can walk into that person's office at any time. Usually, the one who does will find the manager has a schedule and it is more convenient for both for the employee to make an appointment.

The communication climate associated with some organizations has made employees wary of the open-door policy. Line managers are threatened when they see their employees in the boss's office. They find out the reason for the visit by any means possible. Some punish the employee by telling them to use the chain of command. Some adjust performance evaluations, ostracize, adjust pay increases, or work to fire the employee. This climate quickly

teaches the employee not to use the open-door policy.

A nurse manager who believes in the open-door policy will clearly state the rules. They will include whether the employee needs anyone's permission to make an appointment with the manager. A democratic manager who believes in setting a climate for open communication will encourage visits. Such a manager knows how to deal with confidential communication to protect employees and their supervisors.

COMMUNICATION AS PERCEPTION

In nursing as in other disciplines, communication is perception. Sound is created by the sensory perceptions people have associated with it. The noise aspect of communication is voice. There is communication only if the receiver hears, and the person hears or perceives only that which she is capable of hearing. It is important that the communication be uttered in the receiver's language, and the sender must have knowledge of the receiver's experience or perceptual capacity.

Conceptualization conditions perception: a person must be able to conceive to perceive. In writing a communication, the writer must work out his or her own concepts first and ask whether the recipient can receive it. The range of perception is physiological, since perception is a product of the senses. However, the limitations to perception are cultural and emotional. Fanatics cannot receive a communication beyond their range of emotions.

Different people seldom see the same thing in a communication, since they have different perceptual dimensions. Drucker has said that to communicate, the sender must know what the recipient, the true communicator, can see and hear and why. Perhaps if we focus on the recipient as the true communicator, we will improve communications. The unexpected is not usually received at all or is ignored or misunderstood. The human mind perceives what it expects to perceive. To communicate, the sender must also know what the recipient expects to see and hear. Otherwise the recipient has to be shocked to receive the intended message.[9]

People have selective retention by emotional association and receive or reject based on good or bad experiences or associations. Communications make demands on people. It is often propaganda and so creates cynics. It demands that the recipient become somebody, do something, or believe something. It is powerful if it fits aspirations, values, and goals. It is most powerful if it converts, since conversion demands surrender.

Leveling with Employees

Leveling is being honest with employees. It makes all information known to them, both the good and the bad. It gives them a chance to improve. Managers can control the content of negative information, not by concealing it but by sharing ideas, feelings, and information with affected employees. Nurse managers address issues as they arise. They focus on employee needs, offering help as indicated. Communication is a major factor in performance evaluation (see the chapter on "personnel evaluation").[10]

Conflict Management

Conflict is often a result of poor communication. Supervisors might react to employee outbursts by:

1. Overriding their better judgments.
2. Becoming defensive.
3. Reprimanding the individual.
4. Cutting off further expression of feelings.
5. Monopolizing the conversation.

The result is increased frustration for both employee and manager, the latter being ineffective.

Baker and Morgan suggest the following techniques for dealing with employee outbursts:

1. Tune into the real message the employee is trying to communicate. Interpret it correctly and direct a response at the feeling level of the employee.

2. Determine the nature of the feelings being expressed. Be sensitive to them. They are subjective and express the employee's values, needs, and emotions. Feelings are neither right nor wrong but to the individual, they represent absolute truth. Usually, they are disguised as factual statements. Determine if they disguise anger, frustration, hurt, or disappointment.

3. Let the feelings subside by encouraging ventilation. Listen and give emotional support. Then summarize what you have heard and interpreted from the outburst.

4. Clarify issues with questions that can be answered "yes" or "no."

5. When impasses occur try "linking" the ideas or feelings the employee has expressed.

6. Allow face saving.

7. Be sure your perceptions are accurate by summarizing them and checking them with the employee.

8. Verbalize your feelings as a supervisor by using positive "I" statements.[11]

Refer to the chapter on "Conflict Management."

COMMUNICATION DIRECTION

For effective communication the place to start is with the perceptions of the recipients. Listeners do not receive the communication if they do not understand the message. Know what they can perceive, what they expect to perceive, and what they want to do. Then formulate the message. Many nurse managers focus on what they want to say and then cannot understand why it is not understood by the recipients.

The information load should be kept down. This will help to increase communication. Management by objectives focuses on perceptions of both recipients and senders. Recipients have access to the experience of the manager. The communicative process focuses on aspirations, values, motivations: the needs of the subordinates. Performance evaluation or appraisal should focus on the recipient's concerns, perceptions, and expectations. Communication then becomes a tool of the recipient and a mode of organization, since it is used by the employee.

Feedback

Feedback completes or continues communication, making it two-way. Today's workers are better managed under a climate that promotes Theory Y and participation or involvement. Most are more affluent, better educated, have increased leisure, and retire earlier, all indications of their changed values.

Feedback is one of the most important factors influencing behavior. People want to know what they have accomplished and where they stand. Feedback works best when specific goals are set to specify the improvements sought, with measurable targets, specific deadlines, and specific methods of attaining goals.

Effective communication includes giving and receiving suggestions, opinions, and information. If this two-way interaction does not occur, there is little or no communication. Communication requires mutual respect and confidence.

One-way communication prevents input or feedback and interaction. It causes nurses to depersonalize their relationships with patients and families. It serves as a barrier between nurses and physicians. It causes distorted communications that result in distorted and inaccurate feedback; scapegoating of peers, patients, and families; and emotional blowups, skepticism of all messages, frustration, stress, delay of therapeutic intervention, and negative socioeconomic consequences.[12]

Research on Feedback

Feedback increases productivity. One study showed an 83 percent increase in productivity as measured by staff treatment programs and client hours using the technique of private group feedback. The experiment covered 15 to 23 weeks in sixteen departments of a state hospital. Using the technique of public group feedback, productivity increased 163 percent in 38 weeks.

When suggestions were answered promptly in a mental health organization of eighty employees, they increased 222.7 percent over a 32-week period. In other studies, feedback plus training have been found to be even more effective. A review of twenty-seven empirical studies indicated that objective feedback worked in virtually every case.[13]

A study was done to test the effect of feedback on "process" versus "outcomes" of reality orientation in a psychiatric hospital serving elderly patients. Subjects were psychiatric nurses. They were divided into three groups, two being given appropriate feedback while the third group did not receive any. The "process feedback" group showed "substantial increases" in process behavior over the control group that did not receive feedback. They had increased patient contacts but it was not determined that their patients had increased reality orientation.[14]

Innovation and experimentation may be reduced by feedback that causes people to concentrate on process, methods, and procedures. Nurse managers should focus on outcomes or accomplishments that indicates clinical nurses have been creative. New ideas should be encouraged as well as application of results of nursing research and clinical nurses should be supported to develop proposals and conduct new nursing research studied. Levenstein recommends:

1. Be clear in your own mind about the criteria you are using to assess staff performance.
2. Clarify ends, and the means are more likely to fall into place.

3. Emphasize flexibility in getting results rather than ritualistic observance of rules and procedures.[15]

INFORMATION

Although they are interdependent, communication and information are different. Communication is perception; information is logic. Information is formal and has no meaning. It is impersonal and not altered by emotions, values, expectations, and perceptions.

Computers allow us to handle information devoid of communication content, an example being personal information. Information is specific and economical. It is based on need by a person and for a purpose. Information in large amounts beyond that which meets a person's needs is an overload. Communication may not be dependent on information; it may be shared experience. Information should be passed to the person who needs to know it, and that person must be able to receive it and act on it. Perception and communication are primary to information, and as the latter increases the communicator or receiver must be able to perceive its meaning.[16] In the interest of time management nurse managers need skills that sort information according to its import, skills that require clear communication and acute perception.

LISTENING

Communications take place between employer and employee, and herein lies the crux of the situation. An employer must hear what employees are saying as well as what they are *not* saying. That employer must do so to have satisfied, productive employees. To hear them requires concentration since most people speak at 125 to 150 words per minute. It is just like church on Sunday. While the preacher talks, the congregation hears only by concentrating. Otherwise they are planning next week's work. Many managers do not listen effectively to what people are saying to them. They shut off the person who wants to say something about a problem but knows that it either will not be heard or will have no effect.

Because a person can listen four times as fast as words are spoken is one reason personnel have a problem listening to the change-of-shift report. As a consequence they forget to give a person a message about an appointment or to do something for a patient. It is usually more efficient to read change-of-shift reports or to listen to tape-recorded reports.

According to Haakenson, a working person is engaged in some form of verbal communication 70 percent of her waking day, or approximately 11 hours and 20 minutes out of 16 hours. Of that time, 45 percent is spent listening to what is 50 percent forgotten within 24 hours. Another 25 percent is forgotten in the next 2 weeks.[17] If this is true of nursing personnel, you will forget 75 percent of what you hear today within the next two weeks. Others claim we remember only 50 percent of what we hear immediately after a 10-minute speech. Twenty-five percent is considered a good retention level.[18]

Causes of Poor Listening Habits

Remember that it is a bad habit to call a subject uninteresting or boring. Listen for useful information from what is considered a dull subject. Sift and screen, separate wheat from chaff, and look for something useful. Be an interested person and make the subject interesting. Good listeners attempt to hear what is said.

It is a bad habit to criticize the delivery. Concentrate on finding out what the speaker has to say that is interesting or useful. Keep from being overstimulated by the subject. Otherwise you mentally prepare an argument or rebuttal and miss what the speaker says. Hear the speaker out before making judgments. Listen for the main idea rather than the facts and identify principles, concepts, and generalizations. Facts merely support the generalizations. Accept the face value of the message rather than evaluate it.

Avoiding the speaker's eye contact is a bad habit as it decreases trust. Remember that 60 percent of a message is nonverbal.

Defensive listening occurs when the speaker's message threatens the listener with blame or punishment for something. It is a bad habit as it prevents accurate listening and perceptions. Defensive listening is stimulated when a person's speech implies a listener's behavior is being evaluated. Defensive response is reduced when the speaker describes behavior objectively.

Speech that indicates the sender is trying to control the receiver evokes defense. People don't want their values and viewpoints controlled and will shut such messages out. They want to have freedom to choose. When the sender solicits the collaboration of the receiver in solving mutual problems, the receiver responds positively.

Receivers defend themselves against perceived strategies to change their behaviors or control them, which they regard as deceitful. They respond to spontaneity and honesty that they perceive as free of deceit.

Speech perceived as unconcerned about a group's welfare evokes defense. Speech perceived as empathetic evokes acceptance. People want to hear speech that indicates they are valued. Gestures communicate neutrality or empathy.

Speech, verbal or nonverbal, that indicates superiority evokes defense, while speech indicating equality is accepted and supported. Certainty indicates dogmatism and evokes defense. Defensiveness is reduced by professionalism in speech. It indicates the sender wants help, information, data, or input from the listener.[19]

Other reasons supervisors give for not listening include:

1. Thinking employees do not expect them to listen.
2. Thinking employees have nothing of value to say.
3. Thinking listening is not part of their jobs.
4. Thinking employees should listen to them.
5. Thinking employees will change their minds and they will have to reevaluate them.[20]

Techniques to Improve Listening

There are many ways of improving listening ability. Summarize what is being said for better understanding and retention. Give empathetic attention to the speaker and try to understand the substance of what is being said. Seek to be objective and to apply creativity. Go beyond the speaker's dialect, stance, gestures, and attire to understand the meaning of the speaker's words. Try to counter your own emotionality or prejudice even though you may have opposite convictions.

It is important to discriminate in those to whom you listen. Listen to people who keep you informed and lighten your workload or save time. Listen to those who argue constructively and force them to sharpen your judgment. Know the kind of people who want to listen to you and the situation in which they will try to make you hear. Learn to recognize when you are prone to listen and when not. Some people give good information and one should listen to them. They are trusted trouble-shooters, line managers in charge of the bread-and-butter functions of primary patient care, staff specialists delegated special tasks such as the staff development specialist, and those who need the decisions only you can make. Graciously avoid exaggerators, opportunists, office politicians, gossips, and chronic complainers.[21]

Things said by the speaker, appearance, facial expression, posture, accent, skin color, or mannerisms can all turn off the listener. So, if a person wants to hear, that person must put aside all preconceived ideas or prejudices and give the speaker full attention so that the speaker will be motivated to do a better job of attempting to communicate. While the person is talking, the listener analyzes what is being said for ideas and facts. The receiver must also listen for feelings, which appear in what a person says in relation to background and performance, tone of voice, gestures, and facial expressions.

Mnemonics. A mnemonic is a devise used to assist the memory. The following are two examples of mnemonics:

1. AIDA: Capture *a*ttention, sustain *i*nterest, incite *d*esire, and get *a*ction.
2. PREP: *P*oint, *r*eason, *e*xample, *p*oint.[22]

These formulas are useful for preparing impromptu comments. The AIDA formula causes the speaker to focus on the listener—needs, interests, and problems. The PREP formula is ideal for spur-of-the-moment speaking. The first point is intended to cause the speaker to clearly express a point of view on the subject. In giving the reason, the speaker explains why this is her point of view. These reasons should be illustrated with specific examples that are as quantitative as possible. The speaker should use statistics, personal experiences, authoritative quotes, examples, analogies, anecdotes, and concrete illustrations to clarify and substantiate the point. For the final point, the speaker brings the speech to a close with a restatement of the initial point of view. These formulas are intended to gain the attention of the listeners so that the responses to the communication will be positive.

Other Practical Suggestions. The literature abounds with examples of practical suggestions for encouraging people to listen. Listening shows respect and value for employees. It encourages their cooperation and their acceptance of change. It helps to relieve stress and prevent burnout. A manager who talks and listens to an employee helps that person to figure out how to do the job.

Listening elicits suggestions that lead to profitability. It prevents operating deficiencies and cuts costs. Listening saves disciplinary actions and jobs when it reveals the real cause of an error. It promotes loyalty.[23] Poor listening can cost millions of dollars.

Practical suggestions for encouraging people to listen if you are the speaker include:

1. Be prepared; answer the questions "who and what?"
2. Identify and evaluate the purpose of your remarks.
3. Organize and outline the report or speech to convey the facts.
4. Make efficient notes and use them. Outline.
5. Remember that you are part of the package.
6. Make your voice work for you with proper breathing and pitch.
7. Communicate with your eyes.

Results

The results of effective listening are that (1) two people hear each other, (2) beneficial information is furnished on which to base right decisions, (3) a better relationship between people is established, and (4) it is easier to find solutions to problems.[24]

MEDIA OF COMMUNICATION

Meetings

Meetings of all kinds are a medium for communication, often for purposes of dissemination of information as well as true communication. Refer to the chapter on committees.

Supervisors

Supervisors or managers at all levels are also a media for communication; refer to the chapter on supervision.

Questions

Questions are an important part of communications. They are asked to obtain information; the goal is mutual understanding. The tone of voice must encourage confidence and trust from the person questioned. Facial expression is important, as is the physical conduct of the questioner. Always go beyond the answer to a primary question: do not flatly agree or disagree with the answer. Types of questions to use include:

1. Open questions that give the other person the opportunity to freely express thoughts and feelings, rather than close-out questions that force a receiver to become the sender of information. Questions that can be answered "yes" or "no" do not give information or explanation. In the courtroom, attorneys use them to trap people or clarify a point.

2. Leading questions that give direction to the reply, rather than loaded ones that restrict by putting the respondent into a hot spot.

3. Cool questions that appeal to reason, rather than heated ones reflecting the emotional state of asker and answerer.

4. Planned questions that are reflective and asked in logical sequence, rather than impulsive ones that just happened to occur to the asker.

5. Complimentary or "treat" questions that tell the respondent he can make an important contribution to the asker's views, rather than trick ones that place the respondent on the spot.

6. Window questions that elicit the respondent's true thoughts and feelings, rather than mirror ones that reflect the point of view of the questioner.

Successful questioning consists of creating and maintaining a climate for communication, asking the right questions asked in the right way and listening to the responses.

Questions can be used to improve listening. Their use serves to clarify unclear statements. The questioner should take care not to overawe or threaten the speaker. Questions could be worded and spoken in a nonthreatening way: "I am sorry I did not hear your comment clearly. Would you mind repeating it, please?" Or: "I do not quite understand what you mean by 'capital resource.' Would you explain further, please?"

A listener should never be embarrassed to ask questions that improve her understanding of a person's communication. Serious questions that inform or clarify information will prevent lack of comprehension. They will clarify incorrect perceptions and help senders and receivers. If the medium of communication is an oral presentation, questions can be written down for use at appropriate times such as question periods, breaks, after meetings, and even later interviews. This allows the listener to construct thoughtful questions.

When questions are used to clarify a point made by the sender, they can be closed yes-or-no questions. An example might be, "Do you support the position on nursing autonomy you have just described?"[25]

Oral Communication

Oral communication is the most common form used by executives, who spend 50 percent to 70 percent of their time listening and talking and as much as 80 percent communicating. Since oral communication takes so much of a nurse manager's time, one should use the most effective words. Verbal messages are said to be 7 percent verbal (word choice), 38 percent vocal (oral presentation), and 55 percent facial expression.[26]

An advantage of face-to-face communication is that each person can respond directly to another or to others. The larger the group, the less effective is face-to-face communication. An effective message requires a knowledge of words and their various meanings as well as the contexts within which they can be used. In short, effective communication may depend on use of the dictionary for effective vocabulary. Many people cannot adequately read or write the English language. They can improve their ability by reading books and articles on techniques of effective speaking and writing, by using dictionaries and grammer books, and by taking courses that teach the skills of speaking and writing. The com-

municator of messages should learn to transmit them so they will be understood by the recipients, who are the true communicators. The sender should know their backgrounds, interests, and motives so that the message will give the desired meaning and motivate the recipients. Courtesy, tact, and finesse are more effective than giving orders. The listener must listen for understanding of the meaning of the message being conveyed by the speaker. The listener must keep his mind from straying and must grasp the main ideas, organize them, and translate them into an order for future action.

When giving a speech, remember that the members of the audience are usually informed and sophisticated and have access to information. They want the speaker to talk things over with them. You as speaker must be sincere and must respect the listeners. Develop an outline and hold to four or five main ideas. Put others under them as subordinate ideas. Open with an introduction and close with a brief summary. Type the speech for easy reading and practice reading it. Maintain eye contact and keep your voice and manner informal and conversational. After learning your speech, practice it without notes. Plan, organize, develop, and practice. A speaker should know the audience and their knowledge on the subject, their intellectual level, their attitudes and beliefs. Former Vice-President Hubert Humphrey said, "The necessary components to build a speech are full understanding of the facts of the subject, thorough understanding of the particular audience, and a deep and thorough belief in what you are saying."[27]

Figure 17–2 summarizes other techniques to use in preparing and giving an oral presentation.

Written Communication

Writing is one of the most common media of communication, not only in nursing but in society in general. It comes in massive proportions: publications and memos to be read and passed on even if they go into the wastebasket; letters that need to be answered. How should one go about handling all this material? First, make a mental decision: It must be dealt with, so organize yourself and attend to it. A system must be established for assigning priorities to the mass of written communications. Go through them by scanning, and then answer or delegate that which can be handled immediately. Lay aside whatever can be taken care of at a future date, but do not

FIGURE 17–2. Techniques for Effective Public Speaking

1. Prepare carefully. What is the goal of your presentation? Is it to inform? Persuade? Entertain? It can be a combination of these and to be effective should probably combine at least two, such as entertainment with information or persuasion.
2. Prepare the presentation carefully. Make an outline and develop the content to fit the outline. Start well in advance so that you can read and adjust the material for a smooth flow of ideas.
   2.1 What is the purpose of the presentation? Did you select the topic or was it given to you? In both instances clarify the purpose with the organizers of the event or whoever has engaged you to do the presentation.
   2.2 Prepare an introduction that will gain the attention of the audience. Spark their interest. Humor often helps but be careful of using cynicism or making derogatory remarks. References to religion, sex, and other controversial subjects should be carefully selected, if used at all. They are better avoided if you wish to persuade or inform, unless they are a part of your topic. Remember, words convey feelings, attitudes, opinions, and facts. Use them to turn the audience on, not off.
   2.3 Make the main points in the body of the presentation. Support them with appropriate and specific examples.
   2.4 Prepare or select visual aids to support the key points of the presentation effectively. They are an extension of your presentation designed to appeal to the senses and increase reception.
   2.5 Know who the audience will be and tailor the message to it. Provide useful material.
   2.6 Plan for audience participation with questions or appropriate exercises to involve listeners.
   2.7 Tie the message together with interval summaries and an effective conclusion. How do you want to leave the audience?
   2.8 If you plan to speak extemporaneously, make notes on cards or put outlines on a visual aid such as a poster, a chalkboard, an overhead transparency, or a slide projection screen.
3. Prepare the environment beforehand. Surroundings are important and should be as attractive as possible. Bear this in mind when you have input into selection.
   3.1 If you want to speak from a podium, make sure it is in place. If you want to sit, have a table and chair in place.
   3.2 Check lighting and sound equipment.
   3.3 Check audiovisual equipment.
   3.4 Remove unneeded barriers such as screens, furniture, and other movable objects. If pillars are in the way, rearrange your position or the audience seating if this is possible. Arrange your proximity to the group to facilitate a feeling of closeness.
   3.5 Prepare your person for the presentation. Wear clothes that present you best. Conventional clothes are best as the audience focus on your words rather than your appearance. Be well-groomed.
   3.6 Good preparation will help you to be relaxed. Get a good night's sleep the night before the presentation. Plan your schedule so as not to be excited beforehand. Eat and drink moderately. Sit and do deep breathing exercises immediately before.
4. Be on time and use time effectively.
5. Speak to be heard.
   5.1 Use your voice, varying pitch, volume, rate and tone for planned effect.
   5.2 Practice pronouncing words with which you have trouble.
   5.3 Pause to enhance your delivery. Short silences emphasize points and allow the audience to think about them.
   5.4 Make your presentation sound natural even if you read it.
6. Use body language effectively.
   6.1 Develop the audience's awareness of your nonverbal behavior slowly. Be aware of it yourself.
   6.2 Maintain eye contact.
   6.3 Plan your movement: walking, standing. Your posture should convey energy, interest, approval, confidence, warmth, and openness.
   6.4 Keep the space between you and the audience open.
   6.5 Use positive gestures. They are positive in themselves.
   6.6 Use head movements for effect.
   6.7 Use facial expression for effect.
   6.8 Know where your hands and feet are at all times.

SOURCE: Adapted from J. Lancaster, "Public Speaking Can Be Improved," *The Journal of Nursing Administration,* Mar. 1985, 31–35; D. Caruth, "Words: A Supervisor's Guide to Communications," *Management Solutions,* June 1986, 34–35; W. D. St. John, "You Are What You Communicate," *Personnel Journal,* Oct. 1985, 40–43.

FIGURE 17–2. Techniques for Effective Public Speaking (*continued*)

6.9 Be genuine! An audience can quickly identify a fake.
7. Adapt to audience feedback, being sensitive to listeners' interests and moods.
   7.1 Listen for unrest, shifting in seats, whispering, muttering.
   7.2 Watch for nonverbal responses. Pay attention to body language, facial expressions, gestures, body movements. Leaning backward or away is perceived as a negative response.

7.3 Be prepared to answer questions if there are breaks in the presentation. You may want to plan for them. Repeat them before answering whether they are oral or written. You are giving additional information.
7.4 Treat your audience with respect in every way and they will view you as genuine.

---

put things where you will forget them. You can put them in a folder in priority sequence until you can attend to them.

You are writing to the receiver: a reader, viewer, listener, observer, or member of an audience. They are not interested in you as the author, only the message you are sending. Write everything to the reader or listener, the receiver. Use good marketing techniques and sell your product.[28]

Figure 17–3 lists nine rules to follow when writing.

Words are an important part of written communication. Put the reader's interest first. Begin with a provocative question or striking statement to jar them. Go right to the point: the purpose of the letter and the request for action. A personal letter is always better than a form letter. People like personal letters. Use a personal, friendly tone, with first names and personal pronouns. You are expressing interest in the reader. Contractions such as "aren't" should, however, be used with discretion.

Use active voice verbs for strength. About 10 percent of total words should be verbs. Use strong nouns. Use the subject and main verb early in the sentence. Avoid overuse of adjectives and adverbs and be specific when using adjectives. State the specific amount such as "100" instead of "much," "any" or "a lot."

Be as brief as possible. Use short rather than long words. Use sentences that contain one idea and are no longer than sixteen to twenty words. Vary the sentence length. Write naturally, using friendly, conversational language.

Reread and revise written communication. Look at the nouns and verbs; the simplicity or wordiness of your sentences. Have you stated what you intended? Do you mean what you say? Eliminate unneeded words. You may want to add a personal, handwritten note to the bottom.[29]

Evaluate your written communication using the Gunning Mueller Fog Index presented in Figure 17–4.

Written Reports

Written reports should indicate how the objectives of the division of nursing are being met. If a 24-hour nursing report is made from the patient units to the director of nursing, the information provided should show progress in relation to the achievement of ward and department objectives. The information should be provided in a manner that is simple, functional or practical, and qualitative rather than complex and quantitative. In providing information, the reporter should consider its relative value and purpose, eliminate any overlap or duplication, and put the report in perspective. The report should indicate the workload and state pertinent facts describing patients' status, why they are hospitalized, and the nursing diagnosis and prescription.

Other factors to consider in writing useful reports are:

1. Size and cost should not exceed their need or strength.
2. A strong report will not be contaminated with individual bias. For that reason a computer printout has value over a hand-prepared report.

FIGURE 17–3.   Nine Rules to Follow When Writing

1. Empathize—be sensitive to the needs and desires of those who will read what you are writing. Arouse and maintain the reader's interest by appealing to the mind and emotions. For example, compose a message that will transmit respect for the nurse while offering a credible and unique inspiration to take nursing histories or prepare nursing care plans. When you give orders, tell the person why you are having her do something. You-centered rather than I-centered communications are interesting to the reader or listener. Give people honest and deserved praise, the kind of flattery that makes them feel they are worth flattering. If you are addressing a particular person, a unique human personality, put that person's name in the salutation as well as in the body of the letter or memo. Make an effort to please the receiver by using tact, respect, good manners, and courtesy.

2. Attempt to avoid the COIK fallacy ("clear only if known" to the reader or listener already). Think of the misunderstandings that could occur in a written message using abstract terms. Your aim should be to create mental pictures using language that is suitable to the experience and knowledge level of the receiver.

3. Do not repeat anecdotes frequently or the reader will be insulted. Avoid overcommunication, overdetailing, and redundancy. Necessary repetition can be achieved by using pleasant and meaningful examples, illustrations, paraphrasing, and summaries. Repetition is essential to the mastery of a skill.

4. Express yourself in clear, simple language. Lincoln's Gettysburg Address contains 265 words, three fourths of them of one syllable. Abstract, technical-sounding jargon, cliches, and trite platitudes may cover up insecurity in a writer afraid of committing himself in writing. Avoid archaic commercial expressions, specialized in-house jargon, and fading journalese by writing clearly and concisely.

5. Make yourself accessible to the reader by positively and courteously requesting a response. You can ask a direct question and expect a reply by a certain date. You can also encourage response by giving a special return address, a private box or phone number, writing instructions, a postcard, or a return envelope. Make it easy, desirable, and pleasant for the reader to reply.

6. Use the format of the newspaper story: accuracy, brevity, clarity, digestibility, and empathy. Arouse the reader with a headline opener. Follow it with a summary that tells significant highlights in the opening paragraph. Then tell the details. Here is an example of a memo form that has worked for others.

Date _____   Time _____
To: _____   Subject: _____
From: _____
Objective: _____
1. _____
   _____
2. _____
   _____
3. _____

7. Break up a solid page of print with a variety of forms: underline, space, italicize, capitalize, enumerate, indent, box, summarize, and illustrate. Make your reading attractive and digestible.

8. Back up what you write by what you do; build a reputation for integrity.

9. Organize your material.
   9.1 Outline key points.
   9.2 Compile data into groups according to commonality.
   9.3 Arrange materials in a logical sequential order:
       9.3.1 Chronological.
       9.3.2 Cause-effect relationship.
       9.3.3 Increasing complexity.
   9.4 Tie the groups together using transitional devices:
       9.4.1 Time-order words (first, later, finally).
       9.4.2 Guide words (as a result, therefore, on the other hand).
   9.5 Link the communication with the previous message by referring to:
       9.5.1 Date.
       9.5.2 Subject.
       9.5.3 Sender of correspondence.
   9.6 Furnish appropriate excerpts from past correspondence.

FIGURE 17–4. The Fog Index

The Gunning Mueller Fog Index presents a way to measure the reading ease of a piece of writing. It produces a number that approximates the grade level at which a person must read to comprehend the material. Here is how to use it.

Take a 100-word sample of your writing and:

1. Find the average number of words per sentence. (If the final sentence in the sample runs beyond the hundredth word, use more than 100 words for this step.)
2. In the first 100 words, count the number of words that contain three or more syllables. Do not count proper nouns, combinations of short words like "bookkeeper" or "manpower," or verbs made into three syllables by adding "-ed" or "-es."
3. Add the average number of words per sentence and the number of words containing three or more syllables. Multiply the sum by 0.4.

The result tells you the grade level of the writing sample. Remember, the average person reads at about a ninth grade level, and anything above a seventeenth grade level is difficult for college graduates.

Caution: Do not let the formula restrict your writing. Use it only to spot-check your writing periodically. Slavish devotion to the formula could result in choppy writing.

SOURCE: Reprinted with permission of *Communications Briefings*, "How to Write to Be Understood," *Business*, Jan.-Mar. 1985, 39–40.

---

3. A strong report will be useful to many people, providing them with vital information to run the operation.
4. A strong report will have authentic and reliable sources of information—people with knowledge and the skills that are required to judge what information needs to be transmitted. Some information can be given by clerks, some by technicians, and some must of necessity be given by the charge nurse.
5. If the report is going to be a group of people with limited time, such as a board of directors, add an executive summary to the beginning. Highlight what it is you want the readers to act on. This may speed up their response to you.

Sometimes there is a tendency to eliminate reports. Although the busy nurse manager may hope they would all go, doing so without consensus sometimes drives them underground. Since they tend to proliferate, every report or form should have an elimination date, at which time it will be eliminated unless it is rejustified.

Special request reports fill a void in communications. They fill a hole in the information channel, sometimes for someone with little to do except keep apprised of all that goes on regardless of whether it serves any useful purpose. It cannot be overemphasized that nursing management's objectives should be well defined and in writing. Objectives should be coordinated at all levels—unit or ward, department, division, and institution.

Reports are a form of communication or vision. As they rise toward top administration, they should adequately depict what is below without all of the minute details. Each factor should be reported in summary form so that the basic picture emerges clearly.

Reports should be built on a planned base, which is a responsibility of management.

Time is an element common to all reports. The "perpetual report" shows up-to-date events for a full year. As the latest month or quarter is added, the oldest is dropped. This time base deals with the realities of the present and provides consistency, completeness, and effectiveness in reporting.

If top management cannot extract the information it wants from the reports, then either the information is unncessary or the procedures need to be improved.

People who design reports and reporting procedures must do the following:

1. Gain access to all documents listing the short- and long-range objectives of the unit, department, division, and institution. Objectives should be in agreement and clearly stated in writing. Progress is reported.
2. Establish priorities for reports.
3. Categorize them, indicating which objectives are supported by each.
4. Determine what top management needs and wants to know, then screen reports.
5. Test reports for logical patterns that avoid complexity and unwieldy clumsiness.
6. Classify them according to frequency.
7. Determine the levels through which they will pass.
8. Determine the point of origin.

9. Coordinate reports with the organizational structure.
10. Check for accuracy and consistency.
11. Account for the total cost of reporting.
12. Obtain the concurrence of all levels of management.

Reports form the nucleus of all management communications, and successful communications are dependent on an intelligently conceived reports structure.

Interviews

Interviewing is a basic tool of communication. A prospective employee is interviewed. If good counseling and guidance techniques are practiced, interviews are used to apprise the employee of performance. An interview is essential to practicing management by objectives. In disciplining an employee, it is necessary to interview the individual. When an employee leaves, an exit interview is desirable to learn why the person is leaving and gain suggestions for strengthening the personnel management program. Questions for these interviews should be worded to obtain the most beneficial information.

1. Use plain and direct language rather than technical, professional, or slang terms.
2. Keep questions short.
3. Use familiar illustrations.
4. Don't assume the interviewee knows something. Check the extent of her knowledge beforehand.
5. Avoid improper emphasis so as not to indicate the answer you hope to elicit.
6. Be sure the interviewee gives words the same meaning as you do.
7. Be precise in picking words. Use accurate synonyms.
8. Use words with one pronunciation.

Refer to the chapter on personnel management for more discussion of interviewing.

Organizational Publications

Barnard stated that the first function of an executive was to develop and maintain a system of communication.[30] The bigger the organization, the more difficult it is for the director of nursing to communicate to the employees who give direct care to patients. This problem is further complicated by the requirement for 24-hour-a-day, 7-day-a-week services. One medium for communication between nurse executives and employees is an organizational publication. This does not have to be confined to nursing but can be supported and used by nursing. Certainly the nurse executive will have input into the development and evaluation of an organizational publication.

According to Tingey a successful organizational publication will fulfil six requirements:

1. It will meet clearly stated objectives related to the process of communications. These objectives will state what the executives of the institution or organization, including nursing, want to accomplish through the publication.

2. The publication will need a competent editor who can do professional editing and who will ensure the objectives are met.

3. The editor will need access to the ideas of top management. This means that the nurse executive will provide the editor with the information needed to inform nursing personnel of changes in policy and procedures.

4. Like management of any area, the objectives of the publication will be developed into a master management plan. This plan will indicate articles and story themes that will be used to accomplish each objective.

5. Information about future events will provide personnel with articles that give an anticipatory viewpoint. In nursing this could include the organization's role in supporting continuing education, expected problems involved in collective bargaining, changes in organizational structure, and changes that will affect practice—new equipment, new supply products, and new support activities.

6. The editor must know the audience—their educational level, interests, problems, and attitudes. The publication must be interesting to family members and contacts. An unread publication is useless.[31]

Specific objectives of the publication will be related to the internal technological environment, the internal social environment, the external environment, company social responsibilities, and organizational dynamics.

OBTAINING INFORMATION

Receivers have a responsibility for obtaining information. Every professional employee feels some conflict between personal needs and the demands of the organization. Communication, the giving of information, helps the employee to control or tolerate this conflict. Assume that management controls information that will be given to employees. A conservative manager will give employees as little information as possible, since that manager considers that it will be distorted or misunderstood.

A director of nursing stated that although the registered nurse in the recovery room was totally competent, she would not give her the title of charge nurse and bring her to charge nurse meetings because she would misinterpret the statements made there. The enlightened manager will be direct and honest, believing that employees need all the information they can have to do their jobs. Bad news usually leaks, and trying to keep it covered up only creates distrust and anxiety.

Poor communication is caused by caution and preoccupation with running the department. Some middle managers tend to treat information as private property. Geography and size effect communication. People tend to protect their egos and their prejudices, and employees have to seek out information.

Communication of information is a joint responsibility of employer and employee. So if you need to know something, go find out—ask. Gather intelligence. Find out how your organization is developing and what its future prospects are. Will its requirements continue to be compatible with your personal goals?

THE FUTURE

Since the success pattern of the industrial age is a liability to the information age, corporations will have to reshape their policies and structures to recruit employees in the information age of the 1990s. We are not on the threshold but have entered the information age and will be in it for the next 50 years.

During this time the following changes have started and will continue to occur:

1. Agriculture will be reduced in people and productivity.
2. Only 10 percent of the population will be employed in manufacturing.
3. Sixty-five to 70 percent of the workforce will be employed in the service industries.
4. The information/electronic industry is creating 4 to 4.5 million jobs a year.
5. Education will be a dominant industry, since services are education-intensive.
6. Total training budgets will be $10 trillion per year.
7. There will be 350 million people in the United States.
8. Income will be $40,000 per capita at a 2 percent per year compound model of growth in the gross national product.
9. A new accounting system will evolve to depreciate people. Education will become the capital to replace losses.
10. There will be more organizations with fewer employees per organization.[32]

People as Capital

Specialization, division of labor, and economies of scale do not work in a service organization. People are the capital resource and the return on people is the measurable outcome, not capital in building and machines. The cost basis of service organizations will continue to be in people.

What will organizations be like?

■ Those that foster personal growth will attract the best and brightest people. Work enlargement yields greater productivity from such people. They want health and fitness and education programs from their employers. They want work integrated into their lives. They want to work in environments that are democratic and allow them to network and to work in small teams. They want work to be fun.

- Good employees want ownership. They want to own stock in the company. They also want psychic ownership in the company. They believe they are entrepreneurs. Within the corporation, "intrapreneurship" is already creating new products and new markets, revitalizing companies from the inside out.

- The service economy produces to meet unique human needs. Ideas come from employees with a rich mix of cultures. Customer demands and needs spur intuition and creativity leading to new products and services. Medical problems including nursing are not neatly packaged. They are organic and interdependent, requiring workers who will integrate the specialists to meet the needs of the people.

- Capital has to be compounded through education and software. Training and education will reduce general and administrative costs to maintain and increase competition. Information should be bought as direct cost since a productive employee must be up to date and have information to be competent and productive.

Organizations

To grow and profit, organizations will have to eliminate their hierarchical orientation and become team-oriented. They will have to emulate the positive and productive qualities of small business. The infrastructure of the organization will give way to networking and people orientation.

Many businesses are striving for monopoly through mergers, acquisitions, and coalitions to control their environments. While success evolves from market feedback, market forces demand change from people and are brutally destructive when they fail. The market will become the arbiter of power, obliterating layers of bureaucracy unless seized by political means.

Managers

Managers should be retrained to be coaches and facilitators. Some organizations are already doing this. W. L. Gore & Associates have thirty-eight plants, 5,000 employees, and no plant managers. Plant size is limited to 150 employees. As employees develop a following they become the chosen leaders. Employees have sponsors when they are employed. If a job is not learned within 90 days, the employee is no longer paid. Advocate sponsors are consulted by a compensation sponsor to determine salary based on accomplishment.

Thirty-five percent of American corporations pay managers more than they deliver as value added, the increased production and profit they add as a result of their performance. The manager's new role is that of coach, teacher, and mentor.[33]

Technology

Technology will be linked to the service orientation of surviving, adaptive, customer-oriented organizations. It will shift the cost curve, with labor continuing to have high income because of increases in productivity.

Quality will be paramount, requiring that the organizational design and the technology be brought together as enablers for human resources. Computers can supplement, not replace, human capital.

Technology will become overhead. Information technology will be used to solve problems where there is little intelligence and very little collective knowledge. When available information should be bought, not generated directly, to decrease both overhead costs and hierarchy. Otherwise managers have to establish entire teams of experts to develop and implement a system that may already be available. It will be cheaper to pay the experts by the minute, as many will be available electronically. Thus contract or consultative labor will replace hired labor, especially in the technological sphere.

Artificial intelligence will be a key enabler that will create generalists. It replaces experts and encapsulates and capitalizes knowledge. Knowledge is added to machines to become an extension of the user. There will be a symbiotic relationship between the manager and the expert machine.

Survival in the information age will depend upon a combination of technology and strategic insights. Service organizations will have to find people who heed services and deliver them. During the past 6,000 years information has belonged to the power structure. They did not trade it, market it, or give it away. The service industries of the information age will market services that are heavily information-based.

Technology is always in arrears as both people and systems quickly become obsolete in developing data bases. Managers should go after strategic, not technical, gains. They should not computerize what does not work nor maintain obsolete technology in hiring people. The people have to be developed and updated, adjusted to the system. They will career hop within and without the organization. Turnover is expensive as it throws away assets. Human resource assets generate more value added when they are managed, enriched, and involved in the enterprise.[34]

SUMMARY

Communications occur between government and governed, between governments, between buyers and sellers, between manufacturers and consumers, between pupils and teachers, between parents and children, and between neighbors, but most important communication occurs between people *only if they want it to.* The products of lack of communication are too costly to accept: misinformation, misunderstanding, waste, fear, suspicion, insecurity, and low morale.

People have difficulty accepting the fact that communication is not the answer to all problems of human relations and personnel management. There is a gap between senders and receivers that must be recognized before it can be bridged—a gap in background, experience, and motivations.

Good communication is frequently an illusion. It is not achieved with open doors, geniality, or jokes. It is helped by listening to what people are really saying and perceiving what they are projecting through their words, their facial expressions, their tones of voice, and their actions. They may be worrying about what is on the boss's mind. To induce greater numbers of people to accept direction and not undermine it, they must participate. They will listen for genuineness in the word of the boss as demonstrated by actions.

NOTES

1. J. Anderson, "What's Blocking Upward Communication?," *Personnel Administration,* Jan.-Feb. 1968, 5ff.
2. P. Morgan and H. K. Baker, "Building a Professional Image: Improving Listening Behavior," *Supervisor Management,* Nov. 1985, 34–36; J. A. Griver, "Communication Skills for Getting Ahead," *AORN Journal,* Aug. 1979, 242–249.
3. W. J. Corbett, "The Communication Tools Inherent in Corporate Culture," *Personnel Journal,* Apr. 1986, 71–72, 74.
4. G. S. Wlody, "Communicating in the ICU: Do You Read Me Loud and Clear?," *Nursing Management,* Sept. 1984, 24–27.
5. F. M. Joblin, "Formal Structural Characteristics of Organizations and Superior-Subordinate Communication," *Human Communication Research,* Summer 1982, 338–347.
6. Ibid.
7. Ibid.
8. P. S. O'Sullivan, "Detecting Communication Problems," *Nursing Management,* Nov. 1985, 27–30. Research report.
9. P. F. Drucker, *Management: Tasks, Responsibilities, Practices* (New York: Harper & Row, 1973), 483.
10. W. D. St. John, "Leveling with Employees," *Personnel Journal,* Aug. 1984, 52–57.
11. H. K. Baker and P. Morgan, "Building a Professional Image: Using 'Feeling-Level' Communication," *Supervisory Management,* Jan. 1986, 20–25.
12. G. S. Wlody, op. cit.
13. A. Levenstein, "Feedback Improves Performance," *Nursing Management.* February, 1984, pp. 64, 66.
14. A. Levenstein, "Back to Feedback," *Nursing Management,* Oct. 1984, 60–61.
15. Ibid.
16. P. F. Drucker, op. cit., 487–489.
17. R. Haakenson, "How to Be a Better Listener," *Notes & Quotes* No. 297, Feb. 1964, 3.
18. P. Morgan and H. K. Baker, op. cit.
19. J. R. Gibb, "Defensive Communication," *The Journal of Nursing Administration,* Apr. 1982, 14–17.
20. D. E. Shields, "Listening: A Small Investment, A Big Payoff," *Supervisory Management,* July 1984, 18–22.
21. N. Stewart, "Listen to the Right People," *Nation's Business,* Jan. 1963, 60–63.
22. J. Guncheon, "To Make People Listen," *Nation's Business,* Oct. 1967, 96–102.
23. D. E. Shields, op. cit.
24. N. B. Sigband, "Listen to What You Can't Hear?," *Nation's Business,* June 1969, 70–72.
25. E. D. Nathan, "The Art of Asking Questions," *Personnel,* July-Aug. 1966, 63–71; Pulick, M. A. "How Well Do You Hear?"; *Supervisory Management* November, 1983, 27-31, and P. Morgan and H. K. Baker, op. cit.
26. W. D. St. John, "You Are What You Communicate," *Personnel Journal,* Oct. 1985, 40–43; D. Caruth, "Words: A Supervisor's Guide to Communication," *Management Solutions,* June 1986, 34–35.
27. H. P. Zelko, "How to Be a Better Speaker," *Notes & Quotes* No. 311, Apr. 1965, 3.
28. R. Wilkinson, "Communication: Listening from the Market," *Nursing Management,* Apr. 1986, 42J, 42L.
29. R. Dulik, "Making Personal Letters Personal," *Supervisory Management,* May 1984, 37–40.
30. C. I. Barnard, *The Functions of the Executive* (Cambridge, MA: Harvard University Press, 1938), 226.
31. S. Tingey, "Six Requirements for a Successful Company Publication," *Personnel Journal,* November 1967, 638–642.
32. P. A. Strassman and S. Zuboff, "Conversation with Paul A. Strassman," *Organizational Dynamics,* Fall 1985, 19–34; A. J. Rutigliano, "Naisbitt & Aburdene on 'Re-Inventing' the Workplace," *Management Review,* Oct. 1985, 33–35.

33. Ibid.
34. Ibid.

REFERENCES

Auger, B. Y., "How to Run an Effective Meeting," *Commerce,* Oct. 1967.

Gelfand, L. I., "Communicate Through Your Supervisors," *Harvard Business Review,* Nov.-Dec. 1970, 101–104.

"Is Anybody Listening?," *Fortune,* Sept. 1950, 77ff.

Lynch, E. M., "So You're Going to Run a Meeting," *Personnel Journal,* January 1966, 22ff.

Finsher, S., "Rework, Revise, Rewrite," *Business,* July-Sept. 1985, 54–55.

Nursing Management Information Systems

18

RICHARD J. SWANSBURG, B.S.N., M.S., R.N.
Health Systems Coordinator
University of South Alabama Medical Center
Mobile, Alabama

INTRODUCTION

Communication is important in a health-care institution because many departments are involved in patient care. Hospitals spend $7 to $10 billion a year on communication.[1] Since hospitals are only one part of the health-care industry, the total price for communication in the industry could be in the vicinity of $25 billion.

Nursing services and nurse administrators have entered the information age, an age that is here to stay. Already the computer is absolutely essential to the management of:

1. An increasingly complex financial environment.
2. Reporting requirements of numerous agencies.
3. Communication needs of a diverse health-care team.
4. Knowledge related to all areas of patient care.[2]

Computers are affecting practice, administration, education, and research, and their impact will continue to spread. The information age is the biggest social and technological change in recent history, and it will continue to shape how people live and work for decades. This chapter is intended as a brief overview of computers, focusing on aspects which relate to nursing management. (See Appendix 18-1 for a Glossary of Commonly Used Computer Terms.)

HISTORICAL PERSPECTIVE

The electronic computer was introduced about 50 years ago. The first computers of the 1940s and 1950s were bulky machines which used vacuum tubes for calculation and control. In the late 1950s the transistor replaced the vacuum tube, making computers smaller, more reliable, and more efficient.

A big break came in the early 1960s with the introduction of integrated circuits. The first integrated circuits combined hundreds of transistors on a single silicon chip as small as a fingertip. Then in the 1970s large-scale integrated circuits containing thousands or tens of thousands of transistors were introduced. These large-scale integrated circuits started the microcomputer revolution.

Hospitals were slow to catch on to the computer revolution. In a 1962 survey only 39 hospitals reported using computer services. By 1974 this figure had grown to almost 6,000 hospitals that were using some type of computer services.[3] Today almost every hospital uses computer resources, at least for financial management.

Nursing has been even slower to experience the benefits of computerization. Early attempts at nursing computerization in the late 1960s and 1970s included:

1. Automation of nurses' notes to describe the patient status and care.[4]
2. Storage of census and nursing staff figures to analyze for future staffing trends.[5]

In the middle 1970s, the idea of hospital information systems (HISs) caught on and nursing began to experience the benefits of management information systems. Finally the 1980s brought extremely powerful microcomputers and specialized software for nursing known as nursing management information systems (NMISs).

THE STATE OF THE ART IN NMIS

"State of the art" is a phrase commonly used by salespeople and consultants. It means that something is as advanced as is technologically possible. More often than not, what is state of the art today is old technology tomorrow.

Hardware

Computers are the hardware of NMISs. They are devices that accept numbers or alphabetical characters, otherwise known as data, process these data in some way, and then record the processed data. Data that have been processed or manipulated are called information. Information can be viewed on a screen and/or printed; see Figure 18–1. Information is stored temporarily in the computer's memory. For permanent storage, it is recorded on magnetic tapes or disks. The computer is like a factory with a work area, storage area, tool crib, and administration.[6]

The stored information is the data base, which is used as a source for decision making by nurse managers. The data are processed by the computer at the request of users. Computers organize and communicate data quickly. Since nurse managers will facilitate the use of NMISs they need knowledge and skills in computer use. With computers involved in more than 75 percent of all jobs, nurse managers need to take the initiative in making computer applications to nursing.[7]

Hardware is extremely diverse. Large mainframe computers are being used as system controllers. They run the hospital information systems and may be connected to, or interfaced with, smaller minicomputers and microcomputers. Minicomputers are utilized to run the smaller departmental subsystems such as central supply, laboratory, and pharmacy. For example, if a hospital has over 300 beds, a mainframe computer may not be able to handle its total information needs. Only the information useful to all areas of the hospital will be located on the mainframe, such as admissions, medical records, business office records, and order management applications. These applications are basic to all HISs. Areas such as central supply, pharmacy, nursing, and the laboratory have complex additional needs not shared by all other areas of the hospital. Therefore applications in these areas may run on their own dedicated computer, with information that needs to be shared passing from one computer to another via an interface.

In smaller hospitals the entire system may be run by a mainframe or, in some situations, by a minicomputer. For example, in hospitals with 100 to 300 beds a mainframe computer is capable of handling all the information needs of all areas. In a hospital of 100 beds or less a minicomputer may be all that is needed. The two factors determining the size of computer needed are:

1. The amount of information that needs to be managed and stored.
2. The number of users that will be working with the computer.

The more people that use the system and the more information that needs to be managed, then the larger the computer needs to be.

FIGURE 18-1. U.S.A. Medical Center Patient Classification Summary

Run Date 06/05/89

NS	Total Type 1	2	3	4	Total C/NC		Total Census	Avg. Acuity	Hrs Per Pat Day	Wkld Indx	Hrs Per Wkld Indx	Required Staffing	Req. Staff 7-3	Req. Staff 3-11
BURN	00	00	02	03	05	01	06	4.0	13.0	20.0	3.2	8.5	2.9	2.8
CCU	00	00	04	02	06	01	07	3.3	10.3	20.0	3.1	8.2	2.8	2.7
CRU	00	00	02	01	03	01	04	3.3	10.3	10.0	3.1	4.1	1.4	1.4
ICN1	00	00	07	05	12	01	13	3.5	11.1	42.5	3.1	17.5	6.0	5.8
ICN2	00	00	09	00	09	00	09	2.5	7.0	22.5	2.8	8.4	2.9	2.8
L&D	00	00	00	00	00	04	04	.0	.0	.0	.0	.0	.0	.0
MICU	00	00	00	05	05	00	05	5.0	17.0	25.0	3.4	11.3	3.8	3.7
MINU	00	00	00	00	00	02	02	.0	.0	.0	.0	.0	.0	.0
NBN	00	00	00	00	00	23	23	.0	.0	.0	.0	.0	.0	.0
NTIC	00	00	00	03	03	00	03	5.0	17.0	15.0	3.4	6.8	2.3	2.2
PICU	00	00	00	00	00	00	00	.0	.0	.0	.0	.0	.0	.0
PN	00	00	13	00	13	00	13	2.5	7.0	32.5	2.8	12.1	4.8	3.6
SICU	00	00	00	04	04	00	04	5.0	17.0	20.0	3.4	9.0	3.1	3.0
SINU	00	00	03	00	03	00	03	2.5	7.0	7.5	2.8	2.8	1.0	.9
3	02	00	00	00	02	21	23	.5	1.0	1.0	2.0	.2	.1	.1
4	00	00	00	00	00	19	19	.0	.0	.0	.0	.0	.0	.0
5N	00	03	10	00	13	02	15	2.1	6.0	28.0	2.8	10.4	4.7	3.1
5S	05	03	12	00	20	02	22	1.7	4.9	35.5	2.7	12.7	5.7	3.8
6	00	00	00	00	00	26	26	.0	.0	.0	.0	.0	.0	.0
7	00	08	24	00	32	01	33	2.1	6.0	68.0	2.8	25.3	12.7	8.9
8N	00	00	00	00	00	12	12	.0	.0	.0	.0	.0	.0	.0
8S	00	00	00	00	00	10	10	.0	.0	.0	.0	.0	.0	.0
9N	00	02	13	00	15	02	17	2.3	6.4	34.5	2.8	12.8	5.1	4.5
9S	01	06	07	00	14	02	16	1.7	4.8	24.0	2.8	8.9	3.6	3.1

(continued)

FIGURE 18–1. U.S.A. Medical Center Patient Classification Summary (*continued*)

Nursing Station MICU

** PROBE CONTINUE FOR STAFFING **

Number of Patients Classified as Type 1 = 00
Number of Patients Classified as Type 2 = 00
Number of Patients Classified as Type 3 = 00
Number of Patients Classified as Type 4 = 05

Total Number of Patients Classified   = 05
Total Number of Patients Not Classified = 00

Total Number of Patients   = 05

CONTINUE   RE-INQUIRE   MASTER

SNC1CSUM
NURSING STATION STAFFING SUMMARY   06/05/89   1340

Nursing Station MICU

Average Acuity   = 5.0   Required Staffing (7-3) = 3.8
Hours per Patient Day   = 17.0   Required Staffing (3-11) = 3.7
Workload Index   = 25.0   Required Staffing (11-7) = 3.7
Hours per Workload Index = 3.4   Required Staffing (24 hrs) = 11.3

Actual Staffing:	RN	LPN	NA	NU FTE	WC	TOT FTE
11-7	00.0	00.0	00.0	00.0	00.0	00.0
7-3	00.0	00.0	00.0	00.0	00.0	00.0
3-11	00.0	00.0	00.0	00.0	00.0	00.0
24 Hours	00.0	00.0	00.0	00.0	00.0	00.0

PAGE BWD   RE-INQUIRE CENSUS   MASTER

SNI1CSTF

Source: University of South Alabama Medical Center, Mobile, Alabama. Reprinted with permission.

Microcomputers are capable of running departmental subsystems by themselves. Currently there are systems on the market for pharmacy, nursing, radiology, medical records, and central supply that run on microcomputers. These microcomputer subsystems are intended to meet special departmental needs and to provide a degree of independence from the mainframe HIS. Often some information must be shared between these systems. Today much attention is being focused on this information sharing and the micro-to-mainframe link. In actuality, microcomputers are still predominantly being used to do word processing, spread sheets, and file/data base management. Even so, microcomputers are fast becoming the machines of choice for running nursing management information systems.

Personal computers or microcomputers are the computers of the 1980s and beyond. These computers are extremely powerful and are becoming more so every year. Today some microcomputers are capable of doing the same work as minicomputers and smaller mainframe computers. The only thing holding them back is the lack of adequate operating system software.

Microcomputers can run software applications for personal productivity, and they can interface to the NMIS and to the HIS. For approximately two to three times the price of a single mainframe terminal, a nurse manager can have a microcomputer with a hundred times the capability and functionality.

Laser Scanners and Bar Code Readers

The biggest advance in functional hardware has come with the refinement of laser scanners or bar code readers. This technology allows for quick, reliable identification and tracking of central supply items, medical records, and x-ray films, to name just a few possibilities. These units are small enough to be held in the hand, portable enough to be carried anywhere, and thoroughly reliable.

In central supply bar codes are already on almost every chargeable item. Bar codes can also be enumerated to indicate a patient name and account number. Nursing personnel can use the bar code reader to identify the patient and the central supply item and determine whether the item is to be charged or credited. This is done by passing the reader over the bar codes. The information is stored in the bar code reader and transferred to the computer at a later time for patient billing and inventory control. Complete inventory can also be done easily and in a matter of hours, whereas before it may have taken days.

In medical records and x-ray, the bar code reader simplifies the identification of a medical record or an x-ray film. This facilitates the issuing and returning of these items. In this era of nursing shortages nurse managers will attempt to develop systems to assign these activities to clerical personnel.

SOFTWARE

There are many areas where microcomputers are better suited than mainframes to assist nursing functions. Such applications include scheduling, report writing, unit budget planning, unit policy and procedure documentation, research, unit-specific personnel records, continuing and in-service education records, programmed instruction, and clinical support.[8]

Although more are appearing, there are still relatively few specialized nursing application programs for microcomputers. Most nursing applications are incorporated into NMISs.

Nursing administrators should not let the lack of a specialized program prevent them from reaping the benefits of a microcomputer, especially if they have easy access to one. There are many general-purpose programs available which can be used to meet nursing needs,[9] such as spreadsheet programs, word processing programs, file/data base management programs, and graphics programs.

Spreadsheets

A spreadsheet is a tool used to record and manipulate numbers. Originally spreadsheets were paper ledgers used for business accounting such as the recording of debits and credits. With the coming of the microcomputer revolution, electronic spreadsheets were developed.

An electronic spreadsheet is a software package that turns a microcomputer into a highly sophisticated calculator. Huge quantities of numbers can be recorded, manipulated, and stored quite simply and easily. Nurse managers could use spreadsheets to maintain statistics, create graphics, plan budgets,

FIGURE 18-2. Report of Emergency Department Statistics

	Oct 88	Nov	Dec	Jan 89	Feb	Mar	Apr	May	Jun	Jul	Aug	Sep
Triage Out	482	428	524	515	510	412	356	353	358	346	301	342
Treated & Released	1862	1761	1637	1599	1553	1853	1766	2043	1962	2064	1868	1983
Admitted	503	510	548	499	523	584	514	540	482	566	549	546
DOA	8	10	3	10	7	8	2	0	4	4	2	2
ED DEATH	8	8	10	6	7	2	7	12	9	8	7	6
OB	360	362	338	342	269	300	303	329	351	358	425	381
Total	3223	3079	3060	2971	2869	3159	2948	3277	3166	3346	3152	3260

Year to Date:	Oct 88	Nov	Dec	Jan 89	Feb	Mar	Apr	May	Jun	Jul	Aug	Sep
Year to Date:	3223	6302	9362	12333	15202	18361	21309	24586	27752	31098	34250	37510
TO%	14.96	13.90	17.12	17.33	17.79	13.04	12.08	10.77	11.31	10.34	9.55	10.49
TR%	57.77	57.19	53.50	53.82	54.13	58.66	59.91	62.34	61.97	61.69	59.26	60.83
A%	15.51	16.56	17.91	16.90	18.23	18.49	17.44	16.48	15.22	16.92	17.42	16.75
DOA%	0.25	0.32	0.10	0.34	0.24	0.25	0.07	0.00	0.13	0.12	0.06	0.06
DEATH%	0.25	0.26	0.33	0.20	0.24	0.06	0.24	0.37	0.28	0.24	0.22	0.18
OB%	11.17	11.76	11.05	11.51	9.38	9.50	10.28	10.04	11.09	10.70	13.48	11.69

	Oct 88	Nov	Dec	Jan 89	Feb	Mar	Apr	May	Jun	Jul	Aug	Sep
Triage Out	300	346	365	435	409	328	312	276	223	237	279	255
Treated & Released	2098	1840	1887	2016	1972	1957	2205	2318	2218	2392	2397	2125
Admitted	551	547	612	706	607	589	577	562	592	576	558	613
DOA	4	4	5	8	0	1	2	1	3	3	3	4
ED DEATH	13	13	13	13	12	8	10	16	12	15	15	8
OB	370	353	423	388	364	318	340	382	376	396	393	419
Total	3336	3103	3305	3566	3364	3201	3446	3555	3424	3619	3645	3424

Year to Date:	Oct 88	Nov	Dec	Jan 89	Feb	Mar	Apr	May	Jun	Jul	Aug	Sep
	3336	6439	9744	13310	16674	19875	23321	26876	30300	33919	37564	40988
TO%	8.99	11.15	11.04	12.20	12.16	10.25	9.05	7.76	6.51	6.55	7.65	7.45
TR%	62.89	59.30	57.10	56.53	58.62	61.14	63.99	65.20	64.78	66.10	65.76	62.06
A%	16.52	17.63	18.52	19.80	18.04	18.40	16.74	15.81	17.29	15.92	15.31	17.90
DOA%	0.12	0.13	0.15	0.22	0.00	0.03	0.06	0.03	0.09	0.08	0.08	0.12
DEATH%	0.39	0.42	0.39	0.36	0.36	0.25	0.29	0.45	0.35	0.41	0.41	0.23
OB%	11.09	11.38	12.80	10.88	10.82	9.93	9.87	10.75	10.98	10.94	10.78	12.24

	Oct 88	Nov	Dec	Jan 89	Feb	Mar	Apr	May	Jun	Jul	Aug	Sep
Triage Out	161	152	128	223	220	211	160	242	229	0	0	0
Treated & Released	2390	2182	2252	2238	2287	2444	2378	2497	2512	0	0	0
Admitted	662	570	551	559	567	626	580	577	600	0	0	0
DOA	1	5	2	4	6	2	7	5	2	0	0	0
ED DEATH	11	9	17	14	15	16	10	14	16	0	0	0
OB	331	374	331	377	316	313	248	293	326	0	0	0
Total	3556	3292	3291	3415	3411	3612	3383	3628	3685	0	0	0

Year to Date:	Oct 88	Nov	Dec	Jan 89	Feb	Mar	Apr	May	Jun	Jul	Aug	Sep
	3556	6848	10129	13544	16955	20567	23950	27578	31263	0	0	0
TO%	4.53	4.62	3.90	6.53	6.45	5.84	4.73	6.67	6.21	0	0	0
TR%	67.21	66.28	68.64	65.53	67.05	67.66	70.29	68.83	68.17	0	0	0
A%	18.62	17.31	16.79	16.37	16.62	17.33	17.14	15.90	16.28	0	0	0
DOA%	0.03	0.15	0.06	0.12	0.18	0.06	0.21	0.14	0.05	0	0	0
DEATH%	0.31	0.27	0.52	0.42	0.44	0.44	0.30	0.39	0.43	0	0	0
OB%	3.31	11.36	10.09	11.04	9.26	8.67	7.33	3.08	3.35	0	0	0

Source: University of South Alabama Medical Center, Mobile, Alabama. Reprinted with permission.

FIGURE 18–3. Computer-Generated Graphic Display

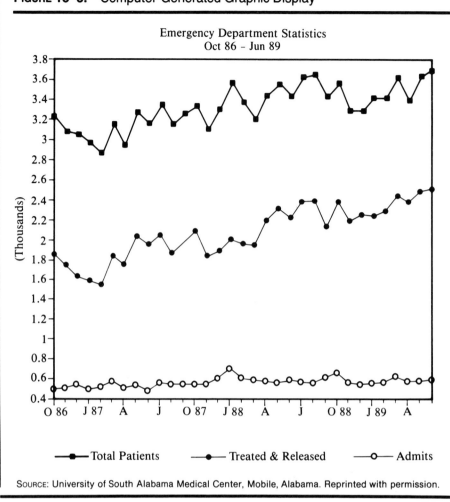

Emergency Department Statistics
Oct 86 – Jun 89

——■—— Total Patients ——●—— Treated & Released ——○—— Admits

SOURCE: University of South Alabama Medical Center, Mobile, Alabama. Reprinted with permission.

and evaluate quality assurance. See Figures 18–2 through 18–5 for examples.

A spreadsheet is made up of columns and rows of memory cells. These cells can be variable in size to allow for small or very large numbers. Besides numbers, cells can store text and formulas. Text is used in a spreadsheet to allow for titles, column and row headers, comments, and instructions. Formulas are used to perform the actual mathematical manipulation of memory cells and their numbers, such as addition, subtraction, multiplication, and division.

Formulas are what really make a spreadsheet a powerful number-crunching tool. For example, a formula can be inserted in the last cell of a column to add all the numbers in that column and display the total (see Figure 18–6). The formula could just as easily have added the cells, divided that number by the number of cells in the column, and given an average. Formulas can also be inserted to subtract one cell from another or multiply one cell by another.

Spreadsheets also have functions for copying, moving, inserting, and deleting cells. One of the most important spreadsheet functions is graphing, which allows numbers to be displayed in the form of a line graph, a bar graph, or a pie graph (see Figure 18–7).

Although electronic spreadsheets are a relatively new tool for nurse managers, they are the best tool to use in situations that require the management of a lot of numbers. For this reason they are particularly pertinent to financial management,

FIGURE 18–4. University of South Alabama Medical Center Report of Patient Account Audit

Patient Name _____   Date of Audit _____

Account # _____   Audit Firm _____

Sgical Record # _____   Auditor _____

Admission Date _____/_____/_____

Discharge Date _____/_____/_____

Department	Amount Billed	Undocumented		Unbilled		Adjusted	
		Amount	Percent	Amount	Percent	Amount	Percent
Anesthesia							
Blood Bank							
Burn Center							
Cath Lab							
Central Supply							
Circulation Tech.							
Dialysis							
EEG							
EKG							
Emergency Department							
Enterostomal Therapy							
Fiber Optic Lab							
GI Lab							
Guest Charges							
L & D Charges							
Laboratory							
Operating Room							
Orthopedics							
Pharmacy							
Physical Therapy							
Pulmonary Function							
Radiology							

(continued)

FIGURE 18–4.   University of South Alabama Medical Center Report of Patient Account Audit (*continued*)

Department	Amount Billed	Undocumented		Unbilled		Adjusted	
		Amount	Percent	Amount	Percent	Amount	Percent
Radiology—US/NM/MAM							
Recovery Room							
Respiratory Therapy							
Room Charges							
Transport							
Vascular Lab							
Total							
Comments							

SOURCE: University of South Alabama Medical Center, Mobile, Alabama. Reprinted with permission.

where they speed up the processes of budgeting, forecasting, developing tables and schedules, and so on.

Middleton recommends teaching employees to use spreadsheets before word processing and data base management programs, although word processing is often used more. He suggests the following tips for learning spreadsheet software use:

1. Use the package immediately.
2. Apply it to something practical such as mortgage payments or personal budgets.
3. Take a course if it is self-training.
4. Find the learning method best liked: manual, audiocassette, interactive video.
5. Decide whether to take the course or do self-study.
6. Set a schedule and keep it.
7. Share the results with a friend or colleague.
8. Keep up to date and include reviews.
9. Avoid plateaus.
10. Enjoy it![10]

Word Processing

Word processing is the manipulation of words and special characters to produce a printed document. Examples are memorandums, letters, policies/procedures, forms, labels, instruction sheets, manuals, signs, books, and others. See Figures 18–8 through 18–11 for examples.

A word processor is a specialized software package that allows a computer and a printer to do word processing. In a sense, a word processor makes a computer and a printer act like a super deluxe typewriter. Some advantages of a word processor are:

1. A document can be visualized on a computer display screen exactly as it will look when printed.
2. A document can be modified or changed very quickly and easily without having to redo it.
3. A document can be printed numerous times with the same material in different formats.

FIGURE 18–5. University of South Alabama Medical Center Audit Summary
Report, June 1989

Total Number of Records Audited — 17
       AUDIT FIRM AUDITS — 8
         PATIENT AUDITS — 9
NUMBER OF INCORRECT BILLS — 17

Department	Amount Billed	Undocumented		Unbilled		Adjusted	
		Amount	Percent	Amount	Percent	Amount	Percent
Anesthesia	$4,957.00	$299.75	6.05%	$72.25	1.46%	($227.50)	−4.59%
Blood Bank	$4,733.50	$0.00	0.00%	$0.00	0.00%	$0.00	0.00%
Burn Center	$0.00	$0.00	0.00%	$0.00	0.00%	$0.00	0.00%
Cath Lab	$0.00	$0.00	0.00%	$0.00	0.00%	$0.00	0.00%
Central Supply	$25,737.25	$652.50	2.54%	$500.25	1.94%	($152.25)	−0.59%
Circulation Tech.	$1,021.62	$0.00	0.00%	$0.00	0.00%	$0.00	0.00%
Dialysis	$0.00	$0.00	0.00%	$0.00	0.00%	$0.00	0.00%
EEG	$833.75	$0.00	0.00%	$0.00	0.00%	$0.00	0.00%
EKG	$286.00	$0.00	0.00%	$31.25	10.93%	$31.25	10.93%
Emergency Department	$1,705.25	$390.50	22.90%	$0.00	0.00%	($390.50)	−22.90%
Enterostomal Therapy	$0.00	$0.00	0.00%	$0.00	0.00%	$0.00	0.00%
Fiber Optic Lab	$0.00	$0.00	0.00%	$0.00	0.00%	$0.00	0.00%
GI Lab	$0.00	$0.00	0.00%	$0.00	0.00%	$0.00	0.00%
Guest Charges	$15.00	$0.00	0.00%	$0.00	0.00%	$0.00	0.00%
L & D Charges	$1,497.18	$0.00	0.00%	$0.00	0.00%	$0.00	0.00%
Laboratory	$19,200.50	$46.75	0.24%	$169.25	0.88%	$122.50	0.64%
Operating Room	$10,580.63	$148.50	1.40%	$0.00	0.00%	($148.50)	−1.40%
Orthopedics	$0.00	$0.00	0.00%	$0.00	0.00%	$0.00	0.00%
Pharmacy	$27,058.73	$4,782.78	17.68%	$7,322.60	27.06%	$2,539.82	9.39%
Physical Therapy	$2,451.95	$261.25	10.65%	$117.50	4.79%	($143.75)	−5.86%
Pulmonary Function	$13,955.75	$0.00	0.00%	$110.50	0.79%	$110.50	0.79%
Radiology	$12,920.50	$295.00	2.28%	$57.25	0.44%	($237.75)	−1.84%
Radiology—US/NM/MAM	$373.75	$0.00	0.00%	$0.00	0.00%	$0.00	0.00%
Recovery Room	$1,302.50	$415.00	31.86%	$0.00	0.00%	($415.00)	−31.86%
Respiratory Therapy	$39,046.25	$1,764.00	4.52%	$2,152.75	5.51%	$388.75	1.00%
Room Charges	$55,470.75	$140.00	0.25%	$115.75	0.21%	($24.25)	−0.04%
Transport	$218.95	$0.00	0.00%	$0.00	0.00%	$0.00	0.00%
Vascular Lab	$0.00	$0.00	0.00%	$0.00	0.00%	$0.00	0.00%
	$41.75	$0.00	0.00%	$0.00	0.00%	$0.00	0.00%
Total	$223,408.56	$9,196.03	4.12%	$10,649.35	4.77%	$1,453.32	0.65%
Total-Ancillary Only	$167,937.81	$9,056.03	5.39%	$10,533.60	6.27%	$1,477.57	0.88%

SOURCE: University of South Alabama Medical Center, Mobile, Alabama. Reprinted with permission.

FIGURE 18–6.　Output from Spreadsheets

Ed Admits
Jan 89 to Jun 89

Jan	559
Feb	567
Mar	626
Apr	580
May	577
Jun	600
Total	3509

Ed Admits
Jan 89 to Jun 89

Jan	559
Feb	567
Mar	626
Apr	580
May	577
Jun	600
Total	3509
Average	585

SOURCE: University of South Alabama Medical Center, Mobile, Alabama. Reprinted with permission.

4. Special graphics can be used to enhance or high-light the content of a document.
5. Multiple documents (up to 350 types pages) can be stored as compressed electronic files with a removable and transportable magnetic disk as small as 3 1/2 inches square by 2 millimeters deep. See Figure 18–12 as an example of an electronic file listing.

Some word processors have facilities for multi-ple document profiles. The document's profile es-tablishes:

1. Line spacing, such as single, double, or triple.
2. Character pitch, such as pica, elite, or com-pressed (number of characters per inch).
3. Font or type style such as script, italics, or standard.

FIGURE 18–7.　Graphs

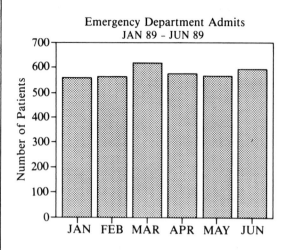

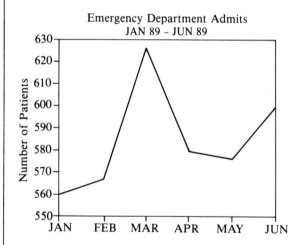

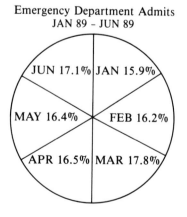

SOURCE: University of South Alabama Medical Center, Mobile, Alabama. Reprinted with permission.

FIGURE 18–8. Word Processor–Generated Memo

May 7, 1986

TO: Assistant Administrator, Finance

FROM: Health Systems Coordinator
           Data Processing

SUBJECT: H.I.S. Orientation and Training for New Employees

I would like to recommend that all new hospital employees, who are issued an ID to use the H.I.S., be required to attend an orientation class in use of the computer and the H.I.S. An ID would not be issued until the employee had attended this class and had been instructed in areas of H.I.S. security, user signon, information confidentiality, terminal operation, and H.I.S. overview. Also, I would like for you to consider additional training which is departmental specific. Objectives for this training would be developed jointly between the department heads and myself. Records of all employee training should also be maintained.

RJS:djm

SOURCE: University of South Alabama Medical Center, Mobile, Alabama. Reprinted with permission.

---

4. Number of lines per inch, such as 6 or 8 lines per inch.
5. Margins and tabs.
6. Page headers or footers.
7. Footnote or outline formats.
8. Printer types, such as letter-quality or graphics.
9. Paper size and type.
10. Different keyboard types.

Different profiles can be set up and used when different documents are to be produced.

Most word processors have utilities for checking spelling within a document. These utilities usually contain a standard dictionary to which the text in a document can be compared. Often words can be added to the dictionary. When the dictionary is called, words that are misspelled can be highlighted for correction. If the word is not recognized, then a list of words that are similar can be generated and the user can choose the correct word.

Utilities for performing block functions are also standard in most word processors. It is easy to insert, move, copy, or delete words, sentences, paragraphs, or pages of text within a document. Simple insertion or deletion of characters can be accomplished with a few keystrokes. A particular word or sentence can be searched for and found anywhere within a document by a simple request.

A document can be paginated after it is completely typed. This function can justify the text within set margins; hyphenate words which are too long for a line; establish a set number of lines per page; and establish page numbers for the document's pages.

Shell documents can be created where the main content of a document never changes, but some areas are reserved for text that will change each time the document is printed. The best examples of this are in memorandums and letters, where the same memo or letter goes to many different people. The document and the list of variable information can actually be created separately and then merged at printing time.

In a division such as nursing where there are many different typing tasks, changing to a word processor could greatly improve document-handling efficiency.

File/Data Base Management

Electronic files and data bases are the computer counterparts to the standard file cabinet and its contents. They are used to store data and are manipulated for information much like paper files. Nurse managers could use a computer and a data base software package, in place of a manual filing system, to handle many of their information and record-keeping needs. Examples might include personnel records, education records, and equipment inventory.

A microcomputer data base program allows for data bases to be created by defining their record layouts and data fields. When a data field is defined, its maximum length is set and the type of data that can be stored in it established. Data types can be character (allowing letters, numbers, and special symbols), numeric (allowing only numbers), logical (allowing only yes or no; true or false), or date

FIGURE 18–9. Word Processor–Generated Form

University of South Alabama Medical Center
Personal Computer Inventory Form

Date: _____

Department: _____ Contact: _____ Phone: _____

Location: _____ Use: _____

PC Model: _____ SN: _____ Date Purchased: _____

System Board Memory: _____ Expanded Memory: _____ Total Memory: _____

System Board Slots: _____ Slots Used: _____ Slots Available: _____

Display Type: _____ SN: _____ Date Purchased: _____

Keyboard Type: _____

Floppy Disk Drives:

Type	*Disk Size*	*Memory Capacity*	*Drive Height*
_____	_____	_____	_____
_____	_____	_____	_____
_____	_____	_____	_____

Hard Disk Drives:

Type	*Memory Capacity*	*Drive Height*
_____	_____	_____
_____	_____	_____

Tape Backup: _____ Expansion Unit: _____

Expansion Unit Board Slots: _____ Slots Used: _____ Slots Available: _____

Attached Printers:

Type	*Model*	*Graphics*	*Letter Quality*
_____	_____	_____	_____
_____	_____	_____	_____

FIGURE 18–9.   Word Processor–Generated Form (*continued*)

Add On Circuit Boards:

Type	Use	SN	Date Purchased	Main/ Expansion Unit	Slot
1. _____	_____	_____	_____	_____	____
2. _____	_____	_____	_____	_____	____
3. _____	_____	_____	_____	_____	____
4. _____	_____	_____	_____	_____	____
5. _____	_____	_____	_____	_____	____
6. _____	_____	_____	_____	_____	____
7. _____	_____	_____	_____	_____	____
8. _____	_____	_____	_____	_____	____

Additional Accessories:

Type	Use	SN	Date Purchased	Main/ Expansion Unit	Slot
1. _____	_____	_____	_____	_____	____
2. _____	_____	_____	_____	_____	____
3. _____	_____	_____	_____	_____	____

Comments: _____

_____

_____

SOURCE: University of South Alabama Medical Center, Mobile, Alabama. Reprinted with permission.

FIGURE 18–10. Word Processor–Generated Form Labels

Edward, Pat	7344	Data Entry	7982
Jean	7345	Terry, Clint	7983
Richard, Rose	7679	Jim	7984
Darlene	7979	Susan	7985
Sangeeta	7980	Lisa	7986
Gloria	7981		

SOURCE: University of South Alabama Medical Center, Mobile, Alabama. Reprinted with permission.

FIGURE 18–11. Word Processor–Generated Procedure

Scheduling of Personal Computer and Training Room

NOTE: The PC and the training room will be scheduled in the same manner, using the wall calendar to the right of this memo. If the training room is scheduled for a particular day and time, then that means the PC will be unavailable during that period.

Guidelines

1. To schedule yourself for use of the PC; write the time, PC, and your name or department in the top-most available slot for the day desired on the calendar (i.e. 8:00am–9:00am, PC, Richard Swansburg). To schedule the training room; confirm availability of the room with the Health Systems Department, and indicate that it is reserved by writing the time, ROOM, and your name or department where desired (i.e. 8:00am–5:00pm, ROOM, Data Processing).

2. Schedule use of the room or PC at least a day ahead of time, but try not to schedule more than a week in advance.

3. Limit your PC sessions to 2 hours. If the PC is available, then this time limit may be extended.

4. Do not schedule the PC for more than 5 working days in a row. This may be negotiated according to need.

5. Please notify the Information Center of cancellation of reserved time at least 30 minutes prior to that time. If you are 15 minutes late for your reserved time and someone else wishes to use the PC, then your time will be forfeited.

SOURCE: University of South Alabama Medical Center, Mobile, Alabama. Reprinted with permission.

FIGURE 18–12. List of Documents Stored as Compressed Electronic Files

---

```
The IBM Personal Computer DOS
Version 3.20 (C)Copyright International Business Machines Corp 1981, 1986
            (C) Copyright Microsoft Corp 1981, 1986


DisplayWrite 3 DOS Command Task
Type EXIT to Return to task Selection
<D> Type Command: dir/w

   Volume in drive D has no label
   Directory of D:\

CHARGES  TXT    SCHEDULE TXT    CAUSES  TXT    PPSEX    TXT    HIST   TXT
PROGRESS TXT    FORM     TXT    PTCLSCH TXT    RESPONSE TXT    DAY1   TXT
RESPDAYS TXT    TERMMOVE TXT    STUSCH  TXT    STUSCHSH TXT    ROUNDS TXT
MISCLST  TXT    RECOMEND TXT    ORIENT  TXT    RJS      UPR
        19 File(s)        483328 bytes free

DisplayWrite 3 DOS Command Task
Type EXIT to Return to Task Selection
<D> Type Command:
```

SOURCE: University of South Alabama Medical Center, Mobile, AL. Reprinted with permission.

FIGURE 18–13. Data Fields and Types

Num	Field Name	Type	Width	Dec
1	NAME	Character	24	
2	STR__ADDR	Character	24	
3	CITY	Character	14	
4	STATE	Character	2	
5	ZIP__CODE	Numeric	9	0
6	PHONE	Numeric	10	0
7	SEX	Character	1	
8	EMP__TYPE	Character	5	
9	LICENSED	Character	1	
10	LICENSE__NO	Character	14	
11	LIC__REN__NO	Character	14	
12	LIC__DATE	Date	6	
13	EXP__DATE	Date	6	
14	LIA__INS	Character	1	
15	INS__AMOUNT	Numeric	8	0
16	PRIM__AREA	Character	24	
17	UNIT__ASSG	Character	24	
18	PRIM__SHIFT	Character	5	

MODIFY STRUCTURE: >A:\NUPER   Field: 1/18
Enter the field name.
Field names begin with a letter and may contain letters, digits and underscores.

SOURCE: University of South Alabama Medical Center, Mobile, Alabama. Reprinted with permission.

(allowing only numbers in a date format). See Figure 18–13 for an example of data fields and Figure 18–14 for an example of actual data entry.

Once a data base is created, procedures can be established to:

1. Add information.
2. Update information.
3. Display information.
4. Delete information.
5. Generate printed reports.

A menu can also be created to allow easy access to and execution of the procedures; see Figure 18–15 for an example. Most data base tools have application generators which will lead the user through a series of steps to define a data base and its procedures and menus.

The greatest advantage to electronic data base management is the ease in maintaining information and the timely retrieval of this information in report format, as illustrated in Figure 18–16.

Today some software companies have actually integrated all three types of programs into one package. This allows a person to perform word processing, number crunching, and data base management all with the same information. Once a person begins using one of these programs, he or she will begin to develop ideas for other ways to use the program. The big problems a person faces are starting and ensuring that a particular company's software will accomplish the work and function on the microcomputer available.

Computer Graphics

Computers can be used to produce graphics in the form of printed exhibits that can be used for illus-

FIGURE 18–14.   Data Entry

Num	Field Name	Entry
1	NAME	Swansburg, Richard
2	STR_ADDR	31 Country Lane
3	CITY	Mobile
4	STATE	AL
5	ZIP_CODE	36608
6	PHONE	2053432361
7	SEX	M
8	EMP_TYPE	RN
9	LICENSED	Y
10	LICENSE_NO.	02861
11	LIC_REN_NO	1-35855
12	LIC_DATE	123188
13	EXP_DATE	123190
14	LIA_INS	Y
15	INS_AMOUNT	1000000
16	PRIM_AREA	Medicine
17	UNIT_ASSG	MICU
18	PRIM_SHFT	7-3

EDIT: >A:\NUPER   Rec: 1/18

SOURCE: University of South Alabama Medical Center, Mobile, Alabama. Reprinted with permission.

FIGURE 18–15.   Menu of Procedures

Nursing Personnel   **10:21:31 PM**
Master Menu

1. Add Nursing Personnel Record
2. Update Nursing Personnel Record
3. Display Nursing Personnel Record
4. Delete Nursing Personnel Record
5. Report Generation Menu
6. Exit

Key selection number and press enter: 6

SOURCE: University of South Alabama Medical Center, Mobile, Alabama. Reprinted with permission.

tration and teaching. Depending on the printer, graphics can be generated in black and white or color. Graphics can be used as handouts or they can be directed from an individual monitor to larger screens for viewing by large numbers of people. Computer-produced graphics can be converted to overhead transparencies, videotapes, slides, and other teaching aids.

FIGURE 18–16.   A Computer-Generated Report

Registered Nurses
with Licenses Expiring December 1986

Name	License No.	Unit	Shift
Abbott, Patricia M.	1-42345	5S	11–7
Daniels, Mark J.	1-55476	ED	3–11
Meyers, Mary Beth	1-23111	NBN	7–3
Munroe, Jane H.	1-65432	6	7–3
Parker, Harold T.	1-34567	SICU	11–7
Swansburg, Richard J.	1-35855	MICU	11–7
Zieman, Margaret A.	1-43298	3	3–11

Total: 7

SOURCE: University of South Alabama Medical Center, Mobile, Alabama. Reprinted with permission.

FIGURE 18–17.   Computer Graphics

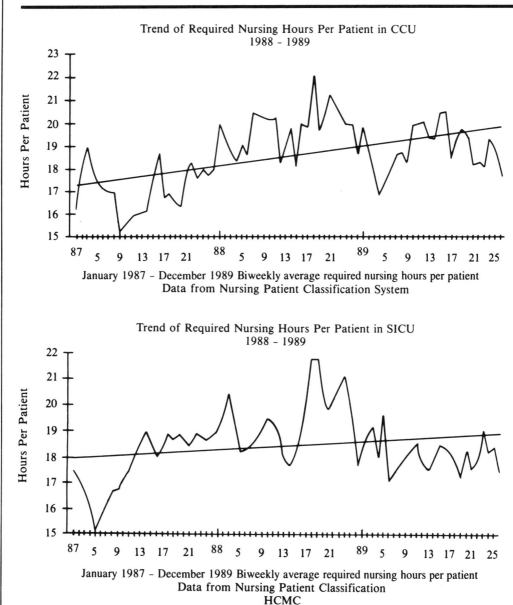

Trend of Required Nursing Hours Per Patient in CCU
1988 - 1989

January 1987 – December 1989 Biweekly average required nursing hours per patient
Data from Nursing Patient Classification System

Trend of Required Nursing Hours Per Patient in SICU
1988 - 1989

January 1987 – December 1989 Biweekly average required nursing hours per patient
Data from Nursing Patient Classification
HCMC

Marks lists the following advantages of computer graphics:

1. They can illustrate the whole picture concisely.
2. They can display trends.
3. They can summarize analysis for planning.
4. They can show relationships between factors.
5. They can provide control information for decision making by quickly providing facts.[11] (See Figure 18–17).

To generate graphics one needs a data base, a computer, and graphics software. The latter is available for microcomputers. A good program should be able to handle line graphs, overlays, pie charts, linear regression analysis, bar graphs, and other graphics.

USING NMISs

Nursing management information systems are software packages developed specifically for nursing services divisions. These software packages have multiple programs or modules which are used to perform various nursing management functions. Most NMISs have modules for patient classification, staffing, scheduling, personnel records, and report generation. Other modules may be included, such as budget development, resource allocation and cost control, diagnostic-related group (DRG) analysis, quality control monitoring, staff development records, modeling and simulation for decision making, strategic planning, short-term demands for forecasting and work planning, and program evaluation.

NMIS modules for patient classification, staffing, scheduling, personnel records, and report generation are often closely interrelated. Patients are classified according to established acuity criteria. The patient classification information is input into the staffing module, and staffing levels are calculated according to various workload formulas. Also, actual staffing is input and a comparison of census, patient acuity, needed staffing, and actual staffing can be made. Schedules are then prepared using the information from the staffing and personnel records modules.

DRG analysis and quality control monitoring are done to associate patient acuity, quality of care, and DRG. This is helpful for establishing future guidelines and care needs for patients according to their DRGs. Budget development is also supported by the census, patient acuity, and needed staffing patterns. This information is invaluable to support requests for additional full-time or part-time help. Finally, the report generation module allows all of the stored information to be retrieved and output in a timely and presentable manner.

Clinical Uses

NMISs and computers can be used to make patient care more effective and economical. Clinical nurses use them for patient care management. Clinical components include patient history, nursing care plans, direct and remote physiological monitoring, physician's order entry and results reporting, nursing progress notes and charting, and discharge planning. This can all be done in the nurses' station or, with the most advanced systems, from individual rooms.

Clinical nurses can use the NMIS to replace manual systems of data recording. This may reduce costs while permitting improved quality of care as well as quality of work life. Those who work in remote locations have access to the clinical components of the NMIS to increase effectiveness and quality of care. All clinical nurses can collect and input clinical data and use the computer to analyze it to formulate treatment plans. They can use quantitative decision analysis to support clinical judgments. Automated consultation can be applied to screen for adverse drug reactions, interactions, and preparation of correct dosages. Computers can be programmed to reject orders that could cause problems in these and other areas, thus preventing medication errors.[12]

Curtin reminds nurses to provide "high touch" in this inhuman "high-tech" world. Technology, computers, and information systems provide the knowledge to save lives or prolong them. Nurses can return control over their lives to patients and families who have lost freedom of action or become unable to understand. Nurses can keep control of cybernetics through the exercise of human compassion.[13]

"High-tech" includes the new scientific knowledge of microelectronics, computers, information, sensors, processors, displays, and education. It has as object the solution of society's total problems, not just those of health care, including nursing.[14]

The Patient Care Profile

Hinson and others describe the use of a total clinical nursing system that includes one computerized form for treatment, Kardex, nursing care plan, and nursing notes, as illustrated in Figures 18–18 and 18–19.

The PCP can be updated by the nurse and/or the unit secretary. It becomes a part of the patient's medical record. Clinical nurses can use it to individualize patient care while nurse managers use it as a source of nursing cost data. It is practical and efficient.

FIGURE 18–18.   Patient Care Profile

```
                            PATIENT CARE PROFILE
    PIEDMONT HOSPITAL          5/16/84   11:45AM           PAGE 1   SHIFT: 1
```

ACTIVITIES OF DAILY LIVING	TRN–09 000187023 2555555 TRN

ACTIVITIES OF DAILY LIVING
   VITAL SIGNS   RT
   OOB   W/ASSIST ꟿ Ⱶ
   BATH   W/ASSIST ꟿ Ⱶ
   FLUIDS   FORCE
   TRANSPORT BY   W/C ꟿ Ⱶ

ALL   REGULAR
CRANBERRY JUICE AT BEDSIDE
NPO AFTER MIDNIGHT

PRC: HARD OF HEARING

TRN–09   000187023   2555555   TRN
   TESTPAT JACK   SEX:M
   ADM: 5/15/84   SRV:URO   SMK:N
   DOB:10/06/21 62 COND:G   LEVEL:1
   HT :5/11   F/I   WT:180/000 P/O
   10000 INTERNIST OTHER
   ALG:PENICILLIN
   DX :NEPHROLITHIASIS

NURSING GOALS
   GL :PT. WILL RECEIVE PRE-OP TEACHING AS
       PER PROTOCOL
   GL :PT. WILL UNDERSTAND WHAT TO EXPECT
       PRE-OP AND IMMEDIATELY POST-OP

ACTIVE ORDERS
   CBC W DIFF (PLATEL 5/16 7:30AM
   SMA 18 BIOCHEM PRO 5/16 7:30AM
   PYELOGRAM INTRAVEN 5/16 AM
   1:MAY HAVE LIQUIDS ON THE DAY OF EXAM
     UNLESS UPPER G.I. SERIES, GALLBLADDER
     SERIES OR SONOGRAM IS ORDERED

NURSING INTERVENTIONS
   1:REVIEW INFORMATION IN PRE-OP BOOKLET
     W PT. INCLUDING PRE-OP PROGRAMS ON
     CHANNEL 13.
   2:REVIEW EXERCISES & EXPECTED
     LIMITATIONS POST-OP WITH PT. (TCDB,
     LOG ROLL, ETC)
   3:EXPLAIN WHAT PT. SHOULD EXPECT PRE-OP
     (PREPS, MEDS, DRESSING, ETC)
   4:REVIEW SEQUENCE OF EVENTS ON DAY OF
     SURGERY (PRE-OP MEDS, STRETCHER TO
     OR, TIME IN RR, RETURN TO ROOM)

TREATMENTS
   1:ANESTHESIA TO SEE PT.
   2:SHAVE AND PREP:MID NIPPLE TO MID
     BACK AND FROM MID AXILLA TO HIP ON
     RIGHT SIDE
   3:PRE OP ON CALL.   DATE:5/17
   4:STRAIN ALL URINE. Ⓓ Y/E/N: ꟿ Ⱶ
   5:INTAKE & OUTPUT Q SHIFT. Ⓓ Y/E/N: ꟿ Ⱶ

DATE: **NURSING NOTES**   **SIGNATURE**

8am Clear yellow urine. No evidence of stones or Ⓡ flank pain. Pt. prepared
for IVP this a.m. Dr. Jones visited —————   *Jane Doe RN*

10³⁰/ᴀ Returned from x-ray. Demerol 100mg. IM RUD for Ⓡ flank pain. *Sally Smith RN*

11³⁰/ₐₘ Pain subsided. Pt. verbalized understanding of information in pre-op
booklet and able to give return demonstration of TCDB ————— *Jane Doe RN*

1³⁰/ₚₘ Urine remains clear yellow. No evidence of stones or Ⓡ flank pain— *Jane Doe RN*

INT	SIGNATURE	INT	SIGNATURE	INT	SIGNATURE
JD	*Jane Doe RN*	MJ	*Mary Jones NA*	SS	*Sally Smith RN*

SOURCE: I. Hinson, N. Silva and P. Clapp, "An Automated Kardex and Care Plan," *Nursing Management*, July 1984, 36.

FIGURE 18–19. Patient Care Plan

Piedmont Hospital	5/16/89 11:41AM	Page 1

```
                              TRN-09              000187023  2555555    TRN
                                TESTPAT JACK                        SEX:M
                              ADM:  5/15/89       SRV:URO      SMK:N
                              DOB:10/06/21 62     COND:G    LEVEL:1
                              HT  : 5/11  F/I      WT :180/000    P/0
                              10000 Internist other
                              ALG :Penicillin
                              DX  :Nephrolithiasis
```

Knowledge Deficit Pre-op
Comfort Alteration Physical
Urinary Elimination Alt Incontinence

Discharge goal	:Pt. verbalizes understanding of significant S&S to report to MD after discharge	Active
Discharge goal	:Pt. verbalizes understanding of type pain to report to MD after discharge	Active
Goal	:Pt. will receive pre-op teaching as per protocol	Active
Goal	:Pt. will understand what to expect pre-op and immediately post-op	Active
Goal	:Pt. will have increased physical comfort	Active
Intervention	1:Review information in pre-op booklet w pt. including pre-op programs on Channel 13.	5/16/84 JD
Intervention	2:Review exercises & expected limitations post-op with pt. (TCDB, log roll, etc.)	Active
Intervention	3:Explain what pt. should expect pre-op (preps, meds, dressing, etc.)	5/16/84 JD
Intervention	4:Review sequence of events on day of surgery (pre-op meds, stretcher to OR, time in RR, return to room)	Active
Intervention	5:Explain what to expect immediately post-op (IV, tubes, dressings, etc.)	Active
Intervention	6:Change dressing PRN	
Intervention	7:Teach pt. to request pain med before pain becomes acute	5/16/84 SS
Intervention	8:Encourage rest (quiet room, limit visitors)	Active
Intervention	9:Change position gradually.D/E/N: __	
Intervention	10:Assist pt. to dangle, D/E:	
Intervention	11:Assist pt. to ambulate progressively D/E/:	
Intervention	12:Teach pt. S&S to report to doctor after D/C (cloudy urine, itching, burning, etc.)	Active

SOURCE: I. Hinson, N. Silva, C. P. Clapp, "An Automated Kardex and Care Plan," *Nursing Management,* July 1984, 40.

The PCP system includes:

1. A Patient Care Profile: activities of daily living, identification data, active orders, treatments, nursing goals, nursing interventions, and nursing notes.
2. Use of nursing diagnoses.
3. Provision of space for handwritten nursing notes.
4. Provision for each nurse to have PCPs of assigned patients on a clipboard.
5. A copy of the PCP for nursing assistant assignments to provide information and make notes and reports.
6. Updating with each shift when a new PCP is printed.
7. A Master Reference Care Plan file from which to select "inappropriate defining characteristics, nursing diagnosis, discharge goals, day-to-day goals, and interventions."
8. A Team Leader worksheet listing patients, diagnoses, and active orders.
9. Patient classifications and staffing requirements.
10. Costing out of nursing care per patient.
11. Completed orders on demand.

In the development of this PCP a vendor was to develop a software package for the HIS. A task force worked with the vendor to develop the care program which was pilot tested. Training of the staff included tutoring.

This system resulted in better documentation and information. It promoted accountability of nurses. The number of forms was reduced. It required top management commitment.[15]

Almost all NMISs have been developed by various management, accounting, and software firms to operate on microcomputers or PCs. These developers sell the hardware, software, documentation, training, and maintenance for their NMISs. Prices will vary according to the hardware bought, how complex and extensive the software is, whether on-site training is wanted, and how much continued support is desired. Nurse administrators can expect a complete system to cost $50,000 to $250,0000.

Implementation of an NMIS

Implementation of an NMIS requires preparation of a management plan, as does the implementation of any other program. The first step is to form a task force or committee to assess the present system and what is wanted by nurse managers and clinical nurses. This assessment should lead to a strategic plan, as acquiring an NMIS requires expenditure of a large amount of human, material, and financial resources. It will include provision for continuous updates, a characteristic of a service economy in the information age.

Assessment. The study team that makes the assessment should include data processors, nurse managers, clinical nurses, and human resource personnel. They can use many references and techniques to gather assessment data. These will include liaison with the data processing department, visits to businesses, industries, and other nursing departments, professional consultants, in-house resources, and the use of phone banks, conferences, and seminars.[16]

Nursing management information systems have to be programmed for individual organizations. There are many models available. Research indicates that nurses should be involved in implementing computer systems or the objectives of such programs will not be realized. A survey of nurses in one hospital had 238 replies. Results indicated nurses in their mid-30s and younger adapted most easily, while those over 50 were more intimidated. Other findings included:

1. Almost two thirds or 65.1 percent of respondents supported the relevance of computers to the enhancement of nursing care and to productivity and effectiveness of nurses.
2. A total of 79.5 percent indicated being able to use computers would give them personal satisfaction.
3. Nearly all—98.7 percent—would attend inservice education on computers.
4. A large majority of 70 percent did not believe a math background was needed for computer competence.
5. A very large majority of 87 percent believed computers were relatively error-free.
6. Nurses want to be able to use computers effectively.[17]

The assessment team will learn capital investment policies and procedures of the institution, as procurement of hardware will fall within the realm of the capital budget. Thus time schedules and budget procedures are important. The team will look at the management style of the division, as the NMIS will reflect centralization or decentralization of control. If there is a desire to increase decentralization and participatory management, development of the NMIS can be used to facilitate these processes.

Availability of space for hardware, personnel, and supplies will be determined. Determination of external environmental influences will be assessed. Does the HIS or higher corporate entity affect NMIS development? In one hospital the mainframe computer was physically located and controlled by the University Computer Services Center, thus placing many restrictions on the HIS and NMIS. The assessment team will analyze types of systems available including hardware and software.

Once a thorough assessment is completed the formal findings are presented to top management and interested others for analysis and approval. The assessment team can be converted to a planning team or a new one can be formed. There should be some uniformity. This is achieved in many organizations by having a nursing systems coordinator whose full-time job is development of the NMIS.

Planning. The second major step in implementing an NMIS is development of the specific management plan. The plan will include objectives, resources needed, communication strategy, a phase-in schedule, a budget that includes operating costs, identification of savings, benefits, and possible revenues, and an evaluation plan. The management plan should be concrete and in writing.

To support the NMIS objectives the team will identify the system requirements needed. They can obtain and evaluate sample requests for proposals (RFPs) from vendors. Criteria for a specific system are recommended.

Security is an important aspect of the NMIS plan. Computers access information about patients and personnel. Each user has an access code that allows them to gain entry to information needed to do their jobs. Provision must be made for confidentiality of records.

A second aspect of security is the protection of software copyright. In this information age we transact intangible property as opposed to tangible property—information business versus manufacturing business. It is difficult to retain control of the

property of computer information. McKenzie-Sanders indicates that the safeguards of software will be protected by law or programs will be given away as a promotion, thus eliminating the need for safeguards.[18]

The NMIS plan should provide for computer downtime. How will critical functions be managed when the computer is down? Procedures and forms will need to be developed to capture and manipulate information during periods of downtime. Also, this information will have to be input into the computer when it becomes available again.

The completed plan is presented to top management for approval. They will coordinate it with the policies and procedures required for approval of capital expenditures, which usually includes action by the board of trustees. With final approval the NMIS is selected and purchased, sometimes through a bidding system that keeps the cost down. Careful planning of the system avoids waste. The NMIS will be expensive.

Implementation. The nursing system coordinator will coordinate implementation of the NMIS, with the involvement of nurse users, throughout the total project. This process will build user trust and confidence. This person will work with the implementation team which includes the key users. The team should keep track of nurses' attitudes toward implementation of computer systems.

Nursing educators can work with the nursing systems coordinator to develop a curriculum for educating nurses in computer use. The organization provides a comfortable setting for nurses to make the best use of computers.[19]

Several writers suggest using the principles of planned change to implement the NMIS. The nursing systems coordinator will be the change agent. Peers will influence others to learn. Audiovisuals, computer terminals, and a system-specific manual are used for training. A pilot test is used on a unit or department. Refer to the chapter on "Implementing Planned Change."[20]

Vendors frequently provide training in use of hardware and software. In addition, there are self-directed training programs.

Evaluation. A predetermined evaluation plan that includes Gantt charts or a similar controlling process is best for keeping the plan on target. Questionnaires, surveys, interviews, observations, and quality circles can all be used to evaluate user acceptance and achievement of objectives. Feedback from these will be used to modify the NMIS.

Nursing Management

Top managers in nursing should not be like those in business and industry who have resisted becoming involved in the use of computers. Computers can be the source of improved nursing decisions about production, administration, and marketing. They can be used to improve delivery of nursing products and services. They support good management. Nurse managers should develop their computer knowledge and skills. Computers can reduce the rate of hiring of additional personnel and improve labor productivity.

Computers have great research capability because of the capacity for capturing large quantities of information in the data bank. This includes:

1. Patient classification systems that measure nursing workloads including volume of patients, differential needs of patients, the nursing care each patient requires, and the amount of nursing time needed for completion of each procedure.

2. Staffing of nursing units and scheduling of unit personnel. The NMIS reduces management time and is precise and practical.

3. Cost accounting and financial management nursing costs can be determined per DRG and patient, hourly and by shift. The system can be used to unbundle the hospital bill and charge for nursing services.

4. Quality assurance audits to process information that analyzes and reports outcome measurements of established nursing standards.

5. Personnel management that profiles demographic information, employment status, educational and license information, certification, and continuing education. (See Figure 18–20.)

6. Research including the application of statistical manipulation of data.

Senior managers are not yet comfortable with using computers to make decisions personally. A three-phase process is used to involve managers in developing the information system at Southwestern Ohio Steel. The three phases are depicted in Figure 18–21.[21]

In applying this process to nursing decisions, nurse managers would come to agreement on the critical success factors in phase one. These would be the factors critical to the success of key nurse executives, key nurse managers, and the nursing organization.

In phase two the nursing decision scenarios would focus on understanding how the systems defined in phase one would deliver the needed information to support key decisions. The development of prototypes reduce monetary and business risks and allow managers to reshape them.

HOSPITAL INFORMATION SYSTEMS

Hospital information systems are large, complex computer systems designed to help communicate and manage the information needs of a hospital. An HIS will have applications for admissions, medical records, accounting, business office, nursing, laboratory, radiology, pharmacy, central supply, nutrition/dietary services, personnel, and payroll. Numerous other applications can exist for any department and for practically any purpose; see Figure 18–22.

Admissions applications include patient scheduling, pre-admissions, admissions, discharges, transfers, and census procedures. Some medical records applications include master patient index maintenance, DRG/diagnosis/procedure coding, physician incompletion of medical records, and medical record locator procedures. Business and accounting procedures include patient insurance verification, billing, billing follow-up, billing inquiry, accounts payable, accounts receivable, and cash processing.

Nursing applications are many. Some applications include order entry, results reporting, nursing care plans, patient classification, staffing, scheduling, nurse's notes, discharge planning, and patient assessments.[22] Other applications included nursing histories, medication profiles, nursing education, nursing research, patient education, quality monitoring, and nursing worksheets or checklists.[23] Still other nursing applications exist.

FIGURE 18–20. *A,* Personnel Management System

```
Jun 2, 1989                    Univ of So. Alabama Med Ctr—NINplus                      1:43 PM
ID: PMED010A/881118                  A. Demographic Information              User ID:      JYE
```

Name: Employee ID:
Home Unit: PICU   Job Title: WC   Status: Full Time

_____ _ ADDRESS _____
1550 Main St

City: Mobile   St: AL 36617-   _____ GENERAL _____
                                                             Telephone : (   )   -
                                                             Soc. Sec. :   - -
_____ TRAVEL INFO _____   Birth Date: / /
Drivers License Number: Maiden:
Drivers License Status: Special Sort Code: 1863
Distance From Hospital: 0.0 Miles
Travel Time To Hospital: 0 Hrs   0 Mins
Means of Transportation:

Comments: WC POSITION

```
CMNDS: A(dd C(hg R(em B(rowse F(ind N(xt P(rv <F1>=Help S(el Q(uit M(ore [ ]
Record Status: AVAILABLE
```

Applications in other areas such as the laboratory, radiology, pharmacy, and central supply may be so voluminous and complex that they have their own subsystems. These subsystems can stand alone and run independently of the HIS, but are usually interfaced to the HIS for information transfer.

Hospital information systems are developed specifically for large mainframe computers and minicomputers. Often several computers are networked together to handle the information needs of large hospitals.

Selection, development, and installation of an HIS can easily take two to five years. The initial cost can be millions of dollars for the hardware and software. Continued yearly maintenance is required and can cost hundreds of thousands or even millions of dollars.

An HIS is an information tool for interdepartmental and intradepartmental use within a hospital. Applications can be developed that benefit multiple departments or only one. When nurse administrators are interested in developing a particular application, they need to weigh the advantages and disadvantages of mainframe versus microcomputer implementation. Also, they should expect development and implementation time and cost to vary depending on the complexity of the application.

AREAS OF FINANCIAL CONCERN

Budgeting

Budgeting has been addressed in a previous chapter. It is an ideal application for the computer. The

FIGURE 18–20. *B*, Personnel Management System (*continued*)

```
Jun 2, 1989                    Univ of So. Alabama Med Ctr—NINplus                    1:42 PM
ID: PMED010A/881118                  B. Job Information                   User ID:    JYE
```

Name: Employee ID:
Home Unit: PICU   Job Title: WC   Status: Full Time

─────────── JOB INFO ───────────   ─────── TERMINATION INFO ───────
  Job Title: WC   Term. Date: / /
  Job — Grade: Status: Full Time   Reason:
  Hours per Week: 0.0   Pay Status: FT–Perm   Len. of Service   Yr   Mo
  Hire Date: 11/19/64   Time on Job: 24 Yr 7 Mo   Rehire Consideration:

══════════════ TRANSFER HISTORY ══════════════
      No   From   To   Date   Reason

```
CMNDS: A(dd C(hg R(em B(rowse F(ind N(xt P(rv <F1>=Help S(el Q(uit M(ore [ ]
Record Status: AVAILABLE
```

(continued)

Charges and Supplies

budget is entered into the computer at the beginning of the fiscal year and expenses are entered on an ongoing basis. At periodic intervals a report is produced. This report will show the budget for that period, the expenses for the period, and the expenses for the year to date. This allows ongoing comparisons of how well the budget is being managed.

The basis for being able to keep track of charges and supplies is a good inventory system and an effective means for charge capturing. The inventory system maintains control over the purchasing, receiving, storage, and distribution of supplies. Effective charge capturing ensures that supplies are charged to either the patient or the department.

For inventory, nurse managers need to have input into the kinds and quantities of supplies needed. They also need to determine the kinds and quantities of supplies to be stocked in the department for patient care and administrative needs. Inventory can be determined from patient needs, quality control, and previous charging patterns.

Effective charge capturing can be made simple by use of the computer. Charges can often be generated through order management. The acknowledgement that a test was completed, a procedure performed, or a medication given can produce supply and professional charges. For example, acknowledging that a proctoscopy has been performed on a patient could automatically generate

FIGURE **18–20.** *C,* Personnel Management System (*continued*)

```
Jun 2, 1989                    Univ of So. Alabama Med Ctr—NINplus              1:44 PM
ID: PMED010A/881118              C. Special Skills & Certificates        User ID:    JYE
```

```
  Name:                                                    Employee ID:
  Home Unit: PICU     Job Title: WC                        Status: Full Time


  ═══════════════════════════ SPECIAL SKILLS ═══════════════════════════
      Special Skill No  . . . . . . .
      Skill Type  . . . . . . . . . . . .
      Experience  . . . . . . . . . . .
      Skill Level  . . . . . . . . . . . .
      Date Last Used  . . . . . . . .
      Date Earned  . . . . . . . . . .


  ═══════════════════════════ CERTIFICATES ═══════════════════════════
       No.       Certificate            Organization            Date Recvd
```

```
CMNDS: A(dd C(hg R(em B(rowse F(ind N(xt P(rv <F1>=Help S(el Q(uit M(ore [ ]
Record Status: AVAILABLE
```

charges for the proctoscope, the examining room, and nursing and physician time.

Charging and revenue reports can be quite beneficial to nurse managers. These reports should be generated weekly or monthly. They identify the kinds of supplies used, procedures performed, and quantities of each. They also identify revenue and loss of revenue.

Patient Classification and Staffing

Since the mid-1970s patient classification systems have been the primary means of identifying nursing staff requirements. The components of these systems are assessments of patient needs, conversion of patient needs into nurse staffing, comparison of calculated staffing with actual staffing, and comparison of staffing with quality of care.[24]

Patient classification systems categorize patients according to the amount of nursing care they require. Nursing care requirements are determined by objective nursing time indicators. Each nursing time indicator has a number of points associated with it. The more nursing time involved, the greater the number of points. The sum of these points determines the category or type to which a patient is assigned. There are typically between four to eight patient types within a classification system. The lowest type identifies a patient who requires minimal nursing care; the highest type patient requires maximal care.

Once all patients are typed, established formulas convert patient type information into recom-

Figure 18–20. *D, Personnel Management System (continued)*

```
Jun 2, 1989                    Univ of So. Alabama Med Ctr—NINplus                    1:45 PM
  ID: PMED010A/881118              D. Recruitment/LOA Information              User ID:    JYE
```

Name: Employee ID:
Home Unit: PICU   Job Title: WC   Status: Full Time

——————————— EDUCATION IN PROGRESS ——————————   ———— PREVIOUS EMPLOYER ————
                                                               Employer No.:
  School: Previous Job:
  Address: Prev. Employer:
  Course: City:
  Degree Program: State:
  Expected Finish: / /   Time On Prev. Job: Yrs,   Mnths

================================ LEAVE OF ABSENCE ================================
        No   LOA Type   LOA Start   LOA Return

```
CMNDS: A(dd C(hg R(em B(rowse F(ind N(xt P(rv <F1>=Help S(el Q(uit M(ore [ ]
Record Status: AVAILABLE
```

(continued)

mended staffing information. This information is used to influence actual staffing. It is also used to support the budget and evaluate quality of nursing care.

More and more nursing departments are using patient classification to do variable billing. In this procedure nursing charges are actually separated from the room charges. Patients are billed for nursing care based upon their classification, not their room accommodation.

Most patient classification systems are marketed and sold as nursing management information systems. The more common systems are implemented on microcomputers, but they are also implemented on mainframes and in combination between the mainframe and microcomputer.

Jobs and the Future

Nurse managers need to be computer literate. All nurses need to know how to interact with a computer; typing will become a necessary technical skill. Computer literacy is beginning to be included in nursing school curriculums.

This means that teaching jobs will change and new positions will open for instructors with computer backgrounds. This will also be true in the work environment. Special positions are already opening in hospitals. Nurses are considered the personnel of choice to fill computer user liaison positions.

These liaison personnel are often referred to as user coordinators. User coordinators promote and

FIGURE 18–20.   *E,* Personnel Management System (*continued*)

Jun 2, 1989   Univ of So. Alabama Med Ctr—NINplus   1:46 PM
ID: PMED010A/881118   P. Continuing Ed.—Optional   User ID: JYE

Name: Employee ID:
Home Unit: PICU   Job Title: WC   Status: Full Time

================ OPTIONAL CONTIN. ED. ================

Program Rec No . . . . .
Program Name . . . . . .
Internal Program . . ?
Start Date . . . .
End Date . . . .
Involvement . . . .
Sponsor . . . .
CEUs / Cont. Hrs . . . .
Hospital Cost . . . . . . $
Employee Cost . . . . $

CMNDS: A(dd C(hg R(em B(rowse F(ind N(xt P(rv <F1>=Help S(el Q(uit M(ore [ ]
Record Status: AVAILABLE

SOURCE: University of South Alabama Medical Center, Mobile, Alabama. Reprinted with permission. System by MDAX.

improve communication between the data processing or information systems department and the other hospital departments. They assist and provide input into the systems analysis and design of new computer applications. They help with computer information and training. Finally, they are an invaluable resource for helping the end user with computer-related problems; see Appendix 18–2 for a sample job description.

In the future one can expect that all nursing jobs will be affected by the computer, and many more new positions will be developed for nurses in the computer area.

Among the jobs generated by computer and information technologies are training, education, technical support, coaching, information analyst, macro design, fourth generation language programmer, librarian, product specialist, using computer manager, and systems development auditing.[25] It has even been suggested that computers will lead to an electronic cottage industry.[26]

With entry into the information age nurse managers should do career planning for themselves and their clinical nurses. New careers in NMIS may be one of the answers to nurse burnout.

TRENDS FOR THE FUTURE

There is little doubt that computers will continue to grow smaller with yet greater capacities. In all like-

FIGURE 18–21.   A Three-Phase Process for Managerial Involvement

Phase One: Linking information systems to the management needs of the business. Key technique: Critical Success Factors Process

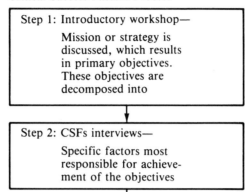

Step 1: Introductory workshop—

Mission or strategy is discussed, which results in primary objectives. These objectives are decomposed into

Step 2: CSFs interviews—

Specific factors most responsible for achievement of the objectives

Step 3: Focusing workshop

Phase Two: Developing systems priorities and gaining confidence in recommended systems. Key technique: Decision Scenarios

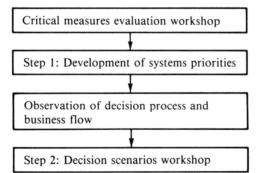

Critical measures evaluation workshop

Step 1: Development of systems priorities

Observation of decision process and business flow

Step 2: Decision scenarios workshop

Phase Three: Rapid development of low-risk, managerially useful systems. Key technique: Prototype Development, Implementation, Use, and Refinement

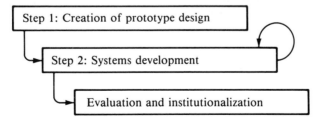

Step 1: Creation of prototype design

Step 2: Systems development

Evaluation and institutionalization

SOURCE: J. F. Rockart and A. D. Cresceuzi, "Engaging Top Management in Information Technology," *Sloan Management Review,* Summer 1984, 6. Reprinted with permission.

FIGURE 18–22. List of Departmental Menus in the USAMC HIS

USAMC MASTER MENU 1   06/05/89   1442
    SELECT ITEM WITH LIGHT PEN OR TYPE OPTION HERE>   <AND PRESS ENTER

---

01) Accounting Department Master	18) Coronary Care Unit Mstr Menu
02) Ancillary Departments Master Menu 1	19) Diag. Radiology Master Menu
03) Ancillary Departments Master Menu 2	20) E.D. Nursing Master Menu
04) Ancillary Departments Super. Master	21) Electronic Mail Master Menu
05) Administration Dept Master	22) Environ. Services Mstr Menu
06) Admitting Department Master	23) External Collect. Agency Menu
07) Burn Center Master Menu	24) Financial Counselor Menu
08) Business Services Cashier/Applic.	25) H.S.F. Master Menu
09) Business Services Cash Super. Menu	26) Internal Audit Master Menu
10) Business Services Clerk Master Menu	27) L&D, or, EAU/RR Master Menu
11) Business Services Follow-up Menu	28) Maintenance Master Menu
12) Business Services Inquiry Mstr Menu	29) Materials Mgmt Master Menu
13) Business Services Master Menu	30) Materials Mgmt Sec. Menu
14) Business Services Supervisor Menu	31) Medical Record Master Menu1
15) Cancer Center Master Menu	32) Medical Record Master Menu2
16) Clinical Laboratory Master Menu	33) Medical Record Master Menu3
17) Collection Manager Menu	34) Mailbox Menu

Mailbox Message Waiting   PM-PROG MENU

AA-SOLIS	BB-SCRNS	CC-PRINTS	DD-DYN2	PF-FWD	00-SIGN OFF

MASTFNCT

A ▉   Aa   —   11

USAMC MASTER MENU 2   06/05/89   1444
    SELECT ITEM WITH LIGHT PEN OR TYPE OPTION HERE>   <AND PRESS ENTER

---

01) Nursing Administration Master Menu	10) Physician Master Menu
02) Nursing Station Master Menu	11) Purchasing Master Menu
03) Nursing Service Technician Menu	12) Quality Assurance Master Menu
04) Nutritional SVC / Dietary Master	13) Receiving Master Menu
05) Operations Master Menu	14) Respiratory Therapy Master Menu
06) Patient Transport Master Menu	15) Social Service Dept. Master
07) Pharmacy Department Master Menu	16) Supply Processing Super. Mstr Menu
08) Physical Therapy Master Menu	17) Supply Processing Technician Menu
09) Physician Maintenance Master Menu	18) Visitor Control/Switchbd Mstr

---

MASTFNDT		PB-BWD		PF-FWD		00-SIGN OFF

A ▉   Aa   —   11

SOURCE: University of South Alabama Medical Center, Mobile, Alabama. Reprinted with permission.

lihood microcomputers will replace minicomputers and maybe even mainframes. Other areas in which we can expect change include robotics, voice communication, optical disks, and expert systems and artificial intelligence.

Robotics

Robots will assist nurses in performing numerous tasks. The most practical use of robotics is in electronic carts, which are used to store and transport drugs, linens, and other supplies. These carts can be remote-controlled and can actually follow predefined routes along the floor. Another example is robotic arms which can be used to do heavy lifting. Possible future applications include procedures humans are unable to perform such as delicate microscopic eye, brain, or spinal surgeries or procedures where direct contact is contraindicated due to health hazards, such as a patient with no immune system or exposure to toxic chemicals or radioactive elements.

Voice Communication and Optical Disks

Voice communication will allow nurses to talk to their computers. Keyboards and bar code readers will not be needed to enter or retrieve information. The computer will be requested to retrieve information or to record it by voice command. Optical disks will revolutionize information storage with their ability to store many times the information in the same space. Microcomputers today use removable floppy diskettes for limited information storage and nonremovable hard disks for volume information storage. New optical laser disks will be removable and the same size as floppy diskettes, but will store up to fifty times as much information as a hard disk.

Conversant computers are widely used in industry. They tell airline baggage handlers which conveyor to put bags on and bank customers their account balances. Conversant computers can identify product deficiencies during manufacturing. They can maintain supply inventories, recording the voice print and processing a spoken reply. They are used to move cameras on spacecraft and to turn on lights and roll up windows of cars. With use of conversant computers, productivity on assembly lines has increased by 25 to 40 percent. Complete

units are available at a cost of about $40,000. Such machines are about 85 percent accurate at present.

Speaker-dependent machines use voice prints so they must be programmed with the user's voice. Speaker-independent machines can understand any speaker. All IBM PCs and Apple Macintoshes have standard built-in speakers but little software is available. Users have not responded well to computer-synthesized voices.[27]

Software today has become much more user-friendly. Almost all software today has help screens and is menu-driven. This means users only have to select what they want to do from a list of items on the screen, and if a problem is encountered help is only a keystroke away. Some computer languages are almost English-like today. What used to take weeks and months to program can now be done in days or weeks. Users are becoming more involved in designing applications on mainframes and handling most things themselves on microcomputers.

Continued or expanded user involvement is a trend of the future. This will occur as users become more knowledgeable about computer hardware and software. Software will continue to become easier for users to manipulate, and software vendors will provide greater support. The best examples are already evident in laboratory, pharmacy, central supply, and nursing management systems, where very little help is involved from data processing personnel.

Expert Systems and Artificial Intelligence

Other future trends in software are expert systems and artificial intelligence. Expert systems are possible today. Nurse administrators have access to a huge quantity of information that is capable of assisting them in making everyday decisions. With expert systems, the nurse manager identifies the management situation, the criteria defining the problem, and objectives for handling the situation. The expert system evaluates the information and provides a listing of alternative ways to manage the situation. The nurse manager then evaluates the alternatives and makes decisions.

Expert systems encode the relevant knowledge and experience of experts to make it available to less knowledgeable and experienced persons. An example would be to take the total knowledge and experience of clinical nurse specialists in neuroscience nursing, encode it in a computer program, and make it available to clinical nurses working in the neuroscience area. They would consult it to solve nursing care problems.

Expert systems encode specialized knowledge including rules and product descriptions to solve difficult problems by supporting human reasoning. They use symbolic reasoning and perform above the level of competence of nonexpert humans. They use heuristic techniques rather than algorithms to provide good answers, but they do not always reach the optimum ones. Heuristic programs use rules of thumb to search through alternative solutions to problems.[28]

Expert systems are software products combining sophisticated representational and computing techniques with expert knowledge. Eventually they will support nursing decision making. While they are not widely used, their use will increase as regional computer systems are established with extensive nursing and medical data bases to link clinical nurse specialists.

An example of a nursing expert system is MANAGER. It is being applied to planning and control of the nursing staff at a regional hospital in Toulouse, France. MANAGER uses three categories of managerial activities as a decision taxonomy: strategic planning, management control, and operational control. This expert system "provides decision makers with an ordered set of plausible solutions." Twelve decision rules are used to control possible nurse transfers among departments. This is one activity of the expert system MANAGER applied to nursing management.[29]

Expert support systems (ESSs) are a further development of expert systems. They are software programs using specialized symbolic reasoning that will help nurses solve difficult problems. ESSs pair humans with expert systems.[30]

With artificial intelligence the machine is actually capable of "thinking" and acting on its own. The difference between artificial intelligence and an expert system is the fact that the machine with artificial intelligence would proceed to make the decision for handling the situation. As an example, in nurse staffing, with an expert system the nurse manager would describe the situation and the machine would supply alternatives for handling the staff. With artificial intelligence the machine could continuously monitor the patients' needs and manage staffing without human intervention. Some individuals do not believe artificial intelligence is possible and at best it appears to be some years away.

Artificial intelligence attempts to develop ideas into computer operations duplicating human intelligence. Such systems use quantitative and qualitative data. Artificial intelligence is being used in robotics, the understanding of natural language, and expert systems.[31]

The industry is now capable of building computerized information systems to appeal to the right and left sides of the brain simultaneously. People share many judgments or assumptions and few symbolic numbers (symbols representing numbers and having a widely perceived meaning) and beliefs. They store facts and use them with a conceptual framework to connect them and then identify them with a particular problem. The conceptual framework is called a schema, cognitive map, or a conceptual model.

Conceptual models are compared with external physical representations by individuals such as artists or engineers. They change perceived differences in one or both. People compare their conceptual models by sending them to others. Each influences the other.

Managers create conceptual models to solve organizational problems by identifying root causes. Market forces determine prices and quality of service. The Advocate Conceptualization/Communication/Creativity Support System (CSS) can be used as a technological tool to manage communications and satisfy stakeholders. The CSS concept will accelerate the corporate change to a systems world view. It will provide the linking corporate language. Ultimately health-care managers will use CSS systems.[32]

Nurse administrators can expect almost anything from computers, but should not expect everything. They should not be concerned that somebody else is using state-of-the-art equipment or software, because if it really is state of the art and beneficial, they will soon be using it themselves.

SUMMARY

The intent of this chapter is to provide an overview of nursing and computers. The computer is a necessary information-handling tool, and most people feel the impact of it on their daily lives. In fact, the computer is now a necessity to manage the complex financial structure of today's health care.

Large mainframe computers are used to support and run highly complex hospital information systems. These HISs have tremendous capabilities for manipulation and storage of information. Almost any nursing application can be implemented through an HIS. With the introduction of the microcomputer, nursing management information systems have developed. These NMISs assist nursing in doing patient classification, analyzing staffing needs and trends, billing patients for nursing care, and developing the nursing budget.

Other general-purpose microcomputer software is also available to assist nursing in doing word processing, number crunching, and record keeping.

Financial areas where nurses need to be particularly adept are in budgeting, tracking of charges and supplies, and patient classification. The budget is the prime tool for managing nursing revenue and expenses. Keeping up with charges and supplies can be simplified with computers; this is often a neglected area where much revenue is lost. Classification of patients is the way in which nurse staffing needs and patterns are determined.

In the future more and more will be accomplished through computers. All nurses will have to be able to interact with these machines. Nursing schools are already incorporating the use of the computer into the nursing curriculum. New positions are being developed for nurses in computer education and support.

The computer has come of age. These machines are tools that already assist nurse managers in performing numerous tasks. They are excellent for the management of all types of information.

NOTES

1. C. R. Carpenter, "Computer Use in Nursing Management," *Journal of Nursing Administration,* Nov. 1983, 17–20.
2. R. D. Zielstorff, "Cost Effectiveness in Computerization in Nursing Practice and Administration," *Journal of Nursing Administration,* Feb. 1985, 22–26.
3. D. E. Gagnon, "Use of Automation in Improving Nursing Efficiency and Operations," *World Hospitals,* 1983, 23–25.
4. R. F. Stein, "An Exploratory Study in the Development and Use of Automated Nursing Reports," *Nursing Research,* Jan.-Feb. 1969, 14–21.
5. B. Moores and I. Wood, "Nursing Allocation Using a Time-Shared Computer," *Nursing Times,* Aug. 18, 1977, 109–112.
6. E. B. Borner, "What Every Manager Should Know About Computers," *Supervisory Management,* May 1984, 16–23.
7. L. J. McCarthy, "Taking Charge of Computerization," *Nursing Management,* July 1985, 35–36, 38, 40.
8. K. Bellinger and J. Laden, "Nurse Use of General Purpose Microcomputer Software," *Nursing Outlook,* Jan.-Feb. 1985, 22–25.
9. S. A. Finker, "Microcomputers in Nursing Administration: A Software Overview," *Journal of Nursing Administration,* Apr. 1985, 18–23.
10. B. Middleton, "Getting Up to Speed on Spreadsheet Software," *Supervisory Management,* Apr. 1986, 12–14.
11. F. E. Marks, "Computer Graphics for Nursing Managers," *Nursing Management,* July 1984, 19–20, 22–23, 25–26.
12. H. W. Gottinger, "Computers in Hospital Care: A Qualitative Assessment," *Human Systems Management,* Fall 1984, 324–345.
13. L. Curtin, "Nursing: High Touch in a High-Tech World," *Nursing Management,* July 1984, 7–8.
14. P. McKenzie-Sanders, "The Central Focus of the Information Age," *Business Quarterly,* Winter 1983, 87–91.
15. I. Hinson, N. Silva, and P. Clapp, "An Automated Kardex and Care Plan," *Nursing Management,* July 1984, 35–36, 38–40, 42–43.
16. L. J. McCarthy, op. cit.
17. S. Krampf and S. Robinson, "Managing Nurses' Attitudes Toward Computers," *Nursing Management,* July 1984, 29, 32–34.
18. P. McKenzie-Sanders, op. cit.
19. S. Krampf and S. Robinson, op. cit.
20. P. R. Bagby, "Orienting Nurses to Computers," *Nursing Management,* July 1985, 30–33; L. J. McCarthy, op. cit.
21. J. F. Rockart and A. D. Crescenzi, "Engaging Top Management in Information Technology," *Sloan Management Review,* Summer 1984, 3–16.
22. "What Nurses Think of Computers," *Nursing Life,* May-June 1985, 28–30.
23. R. D. Zielstorff, Ed., *Computers in Nursing* (Rockville: Aspen Systems Corporation, 1980); G. Clark, "Computers and the Nurse," *The Australian Nurses Journal,* Apr. 1984, 45–47; K. J. Sofaly, "The Nurse and Electronic Data Processing," *Medical Instrumentation,* May-June 1981, 169–170.
24. D. E. Gagnon, op. cit.
25. T. Guimaraes, "Human Resources Needs to Support and Manager User Computing Activities in Large Organizations," *Human Resource Planning,* Feb. 1986, 69–80.
26. P. McKenzie-Sanders, op. cit.
27. N. Madlin, "Conversant Computers," *Management Review,* Apr. 1986, 59–60.
28. F. L. Luconi, T. W. Malone, and M. S. Scott Morton, "Expert Systems: The Next Challenge for Managers," *Sloan Management Review,* Summer 1986, 3–14.
29. C. J. Ernst, "A Relational Expert System for Nursing Management Control," *Human Systems Management,* Fall 1984, 286–293.
30. F. L. Luconi, T. W. Malone, and M. S. Scott Morton, op. cit.
31. Ibid.
32. L. C. Charalambides, "Systematic Organizational Communications," *Human Systems Management,* Apr. 1985, 309–321.

REFERENCES

Adams, R. and P. Duchene, "Computerization of Patient Acuity and Nursing Care Planning," *Journal of Nursing Administration,* Apr. 1985, 11–17.

American Hospital Association, *Strategies: Nursing Management Information Systems* (Chicago: American Hospital Association, 1985), 1–8.

Chang, B. L., "Adoption of Innovations," *Computers in Nursing,* Nov./Dec. 1984, 229–235.

Gilliam, R., "The Use of Computers in Nursing," *International Nursing Review,* Oct. 1968, 308–328.

Graham, N., *The Mind Tool, Computers and Their Impact Upon Society* (4th. ed. St. Paul, MN: West Publishing Company, 1976), 27–28.

Grazman, T. E., "Managing Unit Human Resources: A Microcomputer Model," *Nursing Management,* July 1983, 16, 19–22.

Happ, B., "Should Computers Be Used in the Nursing Care of Patients?," *Nursing Management,* July 1983, 31–34.

Henney, C. R. and R. N. Bosworth, "A Computer-Based System for the Automatic Production of Nursing Workload Data," *Nursing Times,* July 10, 1980, 1212–1217.

Jecmen, C. and N. M. Stuerke, "Computerization Helps Solve Staff Scheduling Problems," *Nursing Economics,* Nov.-Dec. 1983, 209–211.

Jelinek, R. C., T. K. Zinn, and J. R. Brya, "Tell the Computer How Sick the Patients Are and It Will Tell You How Many Nurses They Need," *Modern Hospital,* Dec. 1973, 81–85.

Maknidakis, S. and Wheelright, S. C. *The Handbook of Forecasting: A Manager's Guide* (2d. ed. New York: John Wiley & Sons, 1987).

Minetti, R. C. "Computerized Nurse Staffing," *Hospitals,* July 16, 1983, 90, 92.

Nyberg, J. and N. Wolff, "DRG Panic," *Journal of Nursing Administration,* Apr. 1984, 17–21.

Quinn, S. J., "Computerizing Services in the Nursing Department," *Nursing Management,* July 1984, 16–18.

Romano, C. A., "Computer Technology and Emerging Roles," *Computers in Nursing,* May/June 1984, 229–235.

Willis, R. E. *A Guide to Forecasting for Planners and Managers* (Englewood Cliffs, N.J.: Prentice Hall, 1987).

APPENDIX 18–1.   Glossary of Commonly Used Computer Terms

ABEND: abnormal end of task.

Algorithm: a prescribed set of rules for the solution of a problem in a finite number of steps.

Artificial Intelligence: the capability of a machine that can proceed or perform functions that are normally concerned with human intelligence such as learning, adapting, reasoning, self-correction, automatic improvement.

Bar Code Reader: an optical scanning unit that can read documents encoded in a special bar code. A laser scanner.

Batch Processing: a system approach to processing where similar input items are grouped for processing during the same machine run.

Binary: (1) the number system based on the number 2; and (2) pertaining to a choice or condition where there are two possibilities.

Bit: the smallest unit of data, a binary digit of 0 or 1.

Buffer: intermediate storage, used in input/output operations to temporarily hold information.

Bug: a mistake or error in a computer program.

Byte: a set of eight adjoining bits thought of as a unit.

Central Processing Unit (CPU): the part of the computer that contains the circuits that calculate and perform logic decisions based on a set of instructions.

Compact Disk: a type of disk storage that uses magnetic optical recording and lasers.

CRT (Cathode Ray Tube): cathode ray terminal. The typewriter keyboard or input station.

Data: representation of information in a form suitable for processing.

Database: an electronic storage structure similar to a file.

Disk Storage: a storage device that uses magnetic recording on flat rotating disks.

DOS: disk operating system.

Downtime: the elapsed time when a computer is not operating, may be scheduled for maintenance or unscheduled because of machine or program problems.

Expert Systems: systems that rely on large amounts of information to provide assistance in decision making.

SOURCE: Reprinted from *The Nurse Manager's Guide to Financial Management* by R. C. Swansburg, P. W. Swansburg, and R. J. Swansburg, pp. 330–332, with permission of Aspen Publishers, Inc., © 1988.

APPENDIX 18–1. Glossary of Commonly Used Computer Terms (*continued*)

Field: a unit of information within a record.

File: an electronic storage structure for related records.

Forecasting: describing the possible future, anticipating the impact of present decisions or actions on future activities of nursing. Forecasting uses simple techniques such as graphs and hand calculators, and complicated mathematical models that can be developed using desk top computer software packages.

Hard Copy: printed computer output; reports, listings, documents.

Hardware: the physical computer equipment.

Hospital Information System (HIS): a system designed to facilitate the day-to-day needs of a hospital; a system that stores and manipulates information for interhospital communication and decision support.

Input/Output (I/O): the transfer of data between an external source and internal storage.

Interface: the point at which independent systems or computers interact.

Keyfield: a field within a record that makes that record unique with respect to other records in a file.

Kilobyte: 1,024 bytes or characters.

Laser Scanner: a type of device that utilizes a laser to recognize and receive input.

Mainframe Computer: a large computer capable of being used and interacted with by hundreds of users seemingly simultaneously.

Management Information System (MIS): a system designed to manipulate information to assist in management decision making.

Microcomputer: a small desktop computer built around a microprocessor.

Minicomputer: a medium-size computer smaller than a mainframe but larger than a microcomputer.

Modeling: development of mathematical equations that can be used to fit and balance relationships between or among variables. Forecasting uses models. Managers decide which variables to include and the form of models. In management there are budget models, inventory models, production process models, cash-flow models, models for work-force planning, models of distribution systems, linear programming resource allocation models, and many others.

Modem: a device that converts computer signals into signals for transmission over a telephone line, or vice versa.

Number Crunching: a process of taking huge quantities of numbers and performing mathematical functions on them.

Nursing Management Information System (NMIS): a type of information system geared towards assisting nurse managers in performing their management functions.

On-Line-Processing: a form of input processing where information is input and updated at that time.

Operating System: an organized collection of techniques and procedures combined into programs that direct a computer's operation.

Optical Disk: same as a compact disk.

Printer: a terminal that produces hard copy or printed output.

Program: a set of computer instructions directing the computer to perform some operation.

Random Access: a storage technique whereby a record can be addressed and accessed directly at its location in the file.

Record: a group of related fields of information treated as a unit.

Robotics: machines that work automatically and perform physical movements.

Scenario Projection: use of a scenario or set of planning assumptions to describe and plan for the possible future state of the environment at a point in time and considering the economic, political, social, technological, and natural effects. Scenario projections use trends and trend analysis.

Sequential Access: a storage technique whereby a record can only be addressed and accessed after all those before it have been.

Simulation Forecasting: risk analysis, a procedure that mimics possible or probable business conditions to describe the possible future of each. Simulations stress model structure.

Software: a program or set of programs written to tell the computer hardware how to do something.

Spreadsheet: a specialized type of software for manipulation of numbers.

Table: a collection of data in a form suitable for ready reference.

Trend: systematic pattern of change (increase or decrease) over time based on history or a particular theory. *Example:* an increase in the acuity level of patients over a one-year period.

Trends Extrapolation Forecasting: describing the possible future by projecting the systematic pattern of change (increase or decrease) using the prevailing tendencies of a time series.

(continued)

APPENDIX 18–1. Glossary of Commonly Used Computer Terms (*continued*)

Trend Impact Analysis: analysis of the impact or consequences of the pattern of change (increase or decrease) over time.
Example: How will the increased acuity level of patients over a one-year period affect operational costs, use of resources, cash flow, etc?

Trend Line: a straight line fitted to a graph plotting trends in a time series. It shows the pattern of change (increase or decrease) over time.

User-Friendly (software): easier to use because of menus and help facilities.

Voice Communication: interaction with a computer by voice recognition.

Word Processing: the manipulation of words within documents by a computer.

Word Processor: a specialized type of software for manipulation of printed material.

APPENDIX 18–2. Health Systems Coordinator Job Description

Job Summary

Under the supervision of the Information Systems Manager, interacts between all hospital client departments and Information Systems in the provision of computer support, and the analysis, design, implementation and maintenance of the Hospital Information System (HIS) environment.

Performance Requirements

Responsibilities. The understanding of system structure and informational flow in all hospital departments. Assisting in the coordination activities for providing computer support. Assisting in the development and maintenance of the HIS environment. Assisting in assessing and meeting the ongoing education and information needs of HIS clients. Acts as clearinghouse for all client problems and requests for support relating to information processing. Updating of own knowledge and skills pertinent to job performance.

Physical and Mental Demands. Excellent physical and mental health required. Must be able to make acute sensory perceptions. Must be capable of utilizing appropriate logic, and also able to implement and perform effective problem solving techniques. Stands, sits, and walks during time at work. Operates computer terminals/printers, microcomputers, and related equipment.

Qualifications

Education, Training, and Experience. BSN graduate from an accredited nursing program. Current license as a Registered Nurse in the State of Alabama. A minimum of three years previous clinical experience. Sound knowledge of basic nursing practice and of ancillary departmental functions.

Masters level education from an accredited business administration or computer and information sciences program. Current job performance in a health care information processing environment. A minimum of three years previous information processing experience. Sound knowledge of information processing fundamentals, to include: hardware and software structure, operation, and maintenance; information architecture, storage, and management; and analysis, design, and integration of information systems.

Must have skill in managing resources, and should be excellent problem solver.

Professional Growth. Is expected to pursue programs of education, that will update and maintain professional skills related to the management of health care computer and information support activities.

APPENDIX 18–2. Health Systems Coordinator Job Description (*continued*)

Work Performed

Authority.   Delegated by the Information Systems Manager commensurate with responsibility assigned.

Duties

1. Pursues ongoing education in health care and information processing operations.
2. Performs examinations and interpretations of existing information systems (manual and automated).
3. Assists in the analysis, design, implementation and maintenance of the Hospital Information System and its operating environment.
4. Designs menu and procedure flows, CRT screens, printer formats and forms.
5. Performs liaison, computer support and problem reporting activities between health care client departments and Information Systems personnel.
6. Evaluates and recommends computer hardware and software needs of health care client departments.
7. Develops and writes client procedures, and computer education and reference manuals.
8. Develops and performs client education and training related to computer support and the HIS.

General

Supervised by: Hospital Information Systems Manager

Workers supervised:
Assistant Health Systems Coordinator
Operations Specialist
Job Scheduler
Data Entry Operators
Co-op student assistants

SOURCE: The University of South Alabama Medical Center, Mobile, Alabama. Reprinted with permission.

Supervision

LOUVENIA WARD, M.S.N., R.N.
Assistant Professor of Nursing
Auburn University at Montgomery
Montgomery, Alabama

NATURE AND PURPOSE OF SUPERVISION

Historical Overview

Supervision is the vehicle through which the objectives of an organization are attained. The ultimate objective, of course, is the provision of quality service to meet the needs of patients. Patients and their families are viewed as the most important people within the confines of the hospital. Essentially, they are why the hospital exists.

The term "supervision" stimulates allusions of authority or regimentation to most individuals. Often, it is less than positively viewed. It can be viewed as a directing vehicle of nursing service management.

Supervision is the process by which employees are given the needed resources to accomplish their jobs. Satisfactory patient care depends on people who are enthusiastic, satisfied, and capable. An effective supervisor knows and applies the management principles and practices that stimulate people to be motivated to greater excellence of performance and to greater productivity. Every organization has a mission, philosophy, and objectives. In nursing the objectives pertain to delivering healthcare services to patients using such resources as people who in turn use supplies and equipment. The process of managing these people to accomplish these objectives, the managing of group effort, is supervision.

Two distinct views of supervision may be sketched in as follows:

1. Traditional supervision involves planning work, making decisions, issuing detailed directions and instructions to subordinates, and inspecting results. This type of supervision is restrictive, closely allied with "snoopervision," and stymies initiative and productivity.

2. Modern supervision also involves planning and organizing work, directing and instructing subordinates, and inspecting results, but it goes further. It is based on the philosophy of human dignity and individual worth and the fact that every person is different from every other person. Modern supervision is person-centered. It assumes respect for the individual, recognizes individual differences, and places a high value on the growth potential of each worker.[1]

Supervision is the art of applying the science of behavior technology. Improved or at least satisfactory nursing care of patients is the ultimate purpose of supervision in nursing. The more immediate purpose focuses on the worker—her needs, skills, and ability to do the job. Supervision is concerned with what each worker needs to know to perform his job and with assisting that person to acquire the necessary skills to do the job and develop to his fullest capacity.

Dynamic leadership that utilizes motivational theory will perform supervision that inspires nurses to perform satisfactory nursing care and thus achieve the objectives of the organization.

For all practical purposes just about everyone has a supervisor. Charge nurses are supervised by a head nurse or patient care coordinator, the head nurse supervises the team leader or the primary nurse. The team leader or primary nurse supervises the team member of other nursing care workers. Principles of management are implemented so that work is accomplished by the nursing staff.

One of the primary goals of supervision is to help employees acquire the ability to perform the tasks that they were assigned. Essentially this goal, over the years, has remained unchanged. The supervisor was traditionally considered a role model for clinical practice and indeed had great influence on the professional and clinical growth and development of the staff nurse. The supervisor's influence historically has been an instructive and nurturing one which included monitoring basic skills required in the performance of assigned tasks. The supervisor's role was viewed primarily with respect and was considered to be a desirable professional career option.

The manner in which supervision was practiced was strongly influenced by the style of supervision to which each nurse had been exposed. The main activity was usually the collection of reports or factual information about the patients on the supervisor's assigned units and the relaying of this information to the next shift's supervisor. These reports facilitated discussion, by the supervisors, of many facets of patient care: medical diagnosis, type of surgical operation, vital signs, any unusual occurrences, and so forth. The necessity of these formalities or rituals was questionable, especially since this information was accessible to most staff and other supervisors. However, this type of exchange functioned primarily to facilitate interactions between the staff and the head nurse. Gathering of information was a dominant role at this time, along with minimal discussion or exchange of information relative to the operational management responsibilities of personnel.

The supervisors' management functions extended to include handling complaints regarding nursing care from patients, families, and other hospital departments; reading incident reports; and occasionally taking off orders and answering call lights when the units were extremely busy. There was very little, if any, direct contact with patients. Interactions with families occurred generally when a complaint was voiced or the staff was unable to reach the physician regarding specifics of a patient's care and status.

Additionally the supervisor's duties included making rounds; making decisions about staffing; paperwork related to staff leaves, terminations, and time off; and dealing with issues regarding time cards and payroll.

Supervision Today

The supervisor today must possess the expertise to critically assess the quality of nursing care and outcomes and the knowledge to determine when changes are necessary. Supervisors must be able to manage human resources more efficiently. Directing, facilitating, and evaluating the productivity of large groups of individuals poses a definite challenge to today's supervisors. They must be proficient in skill development, setting priorities, effective communication techniques, task assignments, continuing knowledge acquisition, and motivation on a daily basis.

Trends Affecting Supervision

Nurse managers today are faced with a rapidly growing and changing world that is continually influenced and molded by a variety of factors, including the increasing complexity of medical technology and the increasing fragmentation of the clinical work force into separate health service disciplines.

Cost containment requires that nurse administrators, who manage from 40 to 60 percent of the labor costs in hospitals, function effectively both as professional managers of resources and the environment and as knowledgeable facilitators of the clinical practice of nursing for the provision of effective nursing care. Other outside pressures include increasing consumer awareness and involvement, collective bargaining, and the increasing impact of regulatory agencies. Additional pressures arise from within the nursing profession itself. Issues such as entry-level qualifications, scope of practice, and mandatory continuing education as a prerequisite for relicensure are debated frequently in professional and legislative forums. These elements combine to offer a formidable challenge to today's nurse managers.

Hospitals of today are seen as places of high-technology services where both diagnosis and treatment are streamlined. Procedures that traditionally required invasive and painful interventions, requiring long recovery, are now reduced to mere minutes for noninvasive procedures with a minimal hospital stay.

The alternative to costly health care is to provide care where revenue ceilings are applied to keep costs lower and where costs are curtailed.

Noticeably, consumers are making decisions regarding the kind and amount of service that is desired. Consumers are increasingly comparison shopping for these services, with escalating competition among health-care providers. Nurses, under the guidance of the nurse manager, will need to economize in different ways because the nature of care that is purchased will be directly affected by its availability and cost. Closely aligned to this are the critical ethical issues which will become a significant force in deciding not only the nature of the service provided but the amount of services provided or even permitted. The advent of the prospective reimbursement system for all health-care services has turned the health-care delivery system upside down. Prospective reimbursement has provided the impetus for improved documentation of services provided. All sources of payment for services, both private and public, are concerned about costs and the need to contain them.

These changes in reimbursement procedures have clearly affected the range and style of supervisory practice, primarily by focusing on the need to have a definite plan of care, not just in the nurse's head, but documented. This focus on client care documentation requires a commitment to utilize resources of all kinds in an appropriate and prudent manner.

The nurse manager's ability to maximize available human resources effectively is a relevant issue in determining the outcome of service and care rendered. Failure to recognize the developmental needs of the nursing staff, their contributions, and their psychosocial and economic needs will result in the quality of work being poor and productivity being low.[2]

PRINCIPLES AND FUNCTIONS OF SUPERVISION

Because supervision has been associated with authoritarian behavior, the term "supervisor" appears to be on the wane. More common now are titles like clinical nursing coordinator or nursing practice coordinator. These titles describe jobs that provide an extension of top management, that represent the nurse administrator. Depending on the size of the organization, a supervisor is appointed to cover a geographic area or an area of specialized care. Thus there may be a director or coordinator of medical nursing, pediatric nursing, and so on. Each director or coordinator is an extension of the nurse administrator and is the individual who sees that work is done in her area of responsibility. This area of responsibility is governed by numbers of personnel, numbers of types of patients, kinds of services, and other defining factors.

There are usually an evening supervisor and a night supervisor, each representing the nurse administrator during a tour of duty. Nurse administrators are taking a closer look at these jobs and are performing job analysis. They often find that the job of the supervisor does not require the knowledge and skills of professional nursing. Consequently, non-nurse unit managers have emerged. Charge or head nurses assume the responsibility for their units 24 hours a day. Some nurse managers have replaced the night supervisor with a non-nurse unit manager. The trend is to have only the number of nurse supervisors to accomplish the goals of the department or division of nursing, the number being determined by span of control.

In large organizations and even in small ones, the evening or night supervisor may be titled a director and represent the hospital's chief executive officer.

The following principles of supervision apply to nursing:

1. Supervision is defined by the organizational structure, which will show the lines of authority, including the position to which the supervisor is responsible and those for whom she or he is responsible.

2. Supervision requires a basis of scientific management knowledge, skills in human relations, and the ability to apply principles of management and leadership.

3. The functions of supervision are clearly defined and organized and are accomplished through operating instructions or policy, job descriptions, and job standards.

4. Supervision is a cooperative and democratic process between the supervisor and the workers.

5. Supervision employs management processes, including writing down the mission, philosophy, objectives, and specific plans for accomplishing the objectives for the area of supervisory responsibility. The objectives support those of the division of nursing and the organization and encourage subordinates to develop personal goals that give further support to accomplishment of the mission.

6. Supervision provides an environment that promotes effective communication, stimulates creativity, and furnishes the needed paraphernalia with which nurses perform their primary duties.

7. Supervision has as its ultimate goal the giving of safe, effective, and efficient nursing care that will be satisfactory to clients, workers, and managers. It

develops the potential of both supervisor and supervisee.[3]

Roles

The role of the nurse manager includes participation in planning, priority setting, and policy development; ensuring that nursing practice conforms to law; and acting as an advocate for staff and patients. A synthesis of managerial skills and clinical background contributes significantly to the effective operation of assigned nursing units and representation of the voices of staff and patients. The successful nurse manager must maintain a balance between patient care management, resource management, and fiscal management.

Patient Care Management. The supervisor is involved in supporting the nursing service administrator's planning, implementation, and evaluation of nursing care systems. These outcomes must be accomplished in collaboration among disciplines and achieved at cost-effective levels.[4]

Supervisory responsibilities include:

1. Defining and maintaining standards of practice.
2. Assessing the quality of care rendered by the nursing service.
3. Initiating the development of policies and procedures that govern the nursing service, in collaboration with appropriate other services.
4. Verifying nurses' credentials.
5. Ensuring sound nursing practice.[5]

Resource Management. Supervisors assist in the selection, training, and retention of qualified nursing staff. They assist the nursing staff to use material resources economically.

Fiscal Management. The nurse manager is actively involved in assisting with planning, developing, and implementing fiscal operations for the department. Additionally the nurse manager:

1. Assists in reviewing overall planning objectives for the fiscal year and developing departmental goals compatible with institutional goals.
2. Assists in receiving relevant statistical information to develop the nursing budget.
3. Justifies unit budget projections.[6]

Supervision and the ability to supervise effectively cannot be taken for granted. It is not limited to the person carrying the title of supervisor; everyone responsible for the performance of others must practice supervision. It is necessary even with the most uncomplicated activity; it is vital with the more complex operations involved in professional nursing care. Failure to supervise properly can produce glaring deficiencies in the provision of nursing services. Lack of on-the-scene supervision can result in subordinates making critical decisions about patients without benefit of mature judgment and experience or performing duties for which they are neither qualified nor authorized. The end products are mishaps, accidents, failure of therapy, or even malpractice. At the very least, failure to supervise produces indifferent patient care.

The higher their level of preparation in clinical decision making, the less professional nurses need immediate supervision. It decreases their autonomy: professional nurses want supervisors as mentors and role models.

The Supervisor as a Role Model

Role models are people who act as models for others to emulate. Their behavior is the kind wanted of other nurse practitioners. This means that supervisors should study their own role behaviors and should set the standards for their own conduct. What qualities are wanted of employees? Must they be of good moral character? If so, is the supervisor expected to set the standard of behavior expected of others? This is a loaded question and the answer is obvious. As leaders the supervisors should behave in a moral manner to show them that they believe in honesty, integrity, ethics, and the goal of assisting all people to achieve a high quality of life.

If employees are expected to be industrious, should the supervisor exhibit this trait? If employees are expected to be excellent practitioners, should the supervisor demonstrate excellence of practice? If employees are expected to keep their knowledge and skills current, should the supervisor serve as a model in pursuing continuing education, in reading, and in keeping up to date? If employees are expected to participate as citizens, should the supervisor be involved in community activities? If

the leader is expected to be democratic in managing others, to have employees make decisions and be creative at the practicing level, to spark the motivating forces within individuals to make them set and achieve personal and organizational goals, and to cause them to reach to achieve their highest potentials, what, then, is to be the behavior of a supervisor as role model? Other good qualities could be mentioned, and the conclusion would still be that effective supervision demands hard work from supervisors to qualify themselves as role models for the nursing profession.

Limits of Supervision

The role of the supervisor appears all-encompassing, yet there are limits to what realistically the nurse manager can do effectively. Ignoring these limitations will cause much frustration and overwhelming burn-out. Identification of the boundaries of supervisory practice is essential to successful management.

Nurse managers cannot be all things to all people all the time! Nurses traditionally have felt that they were ultimately responsible for everything. They must take care of everything themselves—not depend on anybody else. This is difficult to accomplish in the manager's role. The supervisor delegates functions to staff to carry out without intrusion. Supervisors should expect staff to possess professional judgment and the capacity to make appropriate clinical decisions and carry them out.

Poor administration will have a profoundly negative impact on the supervisors' ability to perform their responsibilities and to accomplish the goals and objectives of the institution. Supervisors cannot make up for inadequate administrative leadership, nor can the supervisor cover for inefficient, disorganized, or unstable administrators.

Staff workers have a continuous need for self-esteem and recognition. Nurse managers must recognize and encourage this by utilizing skills such as coaching, correcting errors, motivating, providing feedback, delegating, listening, and planning.

There is a risk that the nurse manager may exploit workers' dependency for personal gain, because there always exists tension between independence and dependence in the staff's work. This behavior can be alleviated by understanding why it is occurring and seeking special guidance.

DEVELOPMENT OF NURSE MANAGERS

The dynamic nature of hospital operation mandates that the nurse manager possess the ability to ensure that the care provided patients is of high quality. This mandate requires a serious reorientation of the nurse manager and her new work world. Unlike the past, it is essential that today's nurse managers stay abreast of the operation of the hospital in its totality as well as being responsive and active in planning, implementing, and evaluating the various problems and situations confronting them at their management level.

Management training, particularly near the time of promotion, can make supervisors aware that they are part of the management of the organization. Much has been written on this topic, yet many organizations still let employees make the transition from clinical nurse to supervisor with little or no training, particularly in management skills. Specific sessions should be devoted to their new role as a member of management and the expectations from the organization should be clearly communicated. Without this training supervisors may feel their status has changed very little and that supervising is an extension of the work they have been doing previously.

Results of a survey conducted during a conference of supervisors and directors of nursing services echoed the fact that the complexity and size of a nursing service corresponds to equally large and complex educational and training problems. The participants were asked to list problems they encountered in their work. Their responses included:

1. How to delegate appropriate responsibility.
2. How to act as an effective mediator among the nursing staff.
3. How to choose which problems to solve first.
4. How to develop more effective relations with administration.
5. How to prepare and present budgets.
6. How to improve relations and communications with the medical staff.

7. How to establish adequate controls for drugs, supplies, and equipment.
8. How to determine staffing patterns.
9. How to interest patients in their own care.
10. How to deal with problem behavior of employees.
11. How to balance effectively the needs of patients and the capabilities of nursing personnel.

These responses reflect the need for development of management skills in the areas of interpersonal and interdepartmental relations, nursing care of patients, and employee motivation and control.[7]

Educational programs have been limited and often situated in major urban centers. These programs frequently called for full-time study, which presents a severe hardship to individuals who already are earning salaries that reflect several years of seniority. Furthermore, the university-based and continuing education programs that do exist tend to ignore the differing levels of competence in potential entrants. Thus the burden of relating the learning experience to the hospital setting rests with the learner.

Aydelotte's survey showed a major change in the pattern for education in nursing administration between 1977 and 1982. Her survey indicated that of the nursing service administrators with top administrative status, 51.6 percent had formal degrees in 1977 and only 27.5 percent had master's degree preparation. These figures had increased by 1982 to 99.6 percent with baccalaureate and 61.6 percent with master's degrees.[8]

The 1975–76 National League for Nursing survey showed very significant statistics relative to the field of nursing management. Although there was a marked increase in the number of students enrolled in advanced clinical practice, from 24 percent in 1966 to 69 percent in 1975–76, the enrollment of students in an administrative major declined from 11.3 percent in 1966 to 3.8 percent in 1975–76. This survey also showed a surprising increase of 28 percent, from 2,694 to 3,437 between 1975 and 1976, in the number of graduates from master's programs.

In response to the need for preparing new nurse managers, an outcome-oriented patient care management program was conducted by the American Hospital Association in several regions during 1977, cosponsored by the American Society for Nursing Service Administrators. This program elicited many learning needs from the nurse managers who participated. Identified as among the most prominent learning needs in the area of management skills were:

- How to identify, formulate, and write objectives.
- How to prepare and monitor a budget.
- How to classify patients.
- How to improve documentation of nursing care.
- How to be assertive.
- How to contain costs and implement a cost-awareness program.
- How to handle employee grievances.
- How to implement primary nursing.
- How to introduce and implement change.

Among the most prominent learning needs identified in the area of management knowledge were:

- Management by objectives.
- Primary nursing.
- Synthesis of nursing and managerial roles.
- Fiscal management.
- Personnel management.
- Cost-containment approaches.
- Planning change and the change process.
- Job satisfaction and enrichment.
- Communication, counseling, conflict management, and motivation.
- Labor relations.
- Participatory management.
- Managerial accountability.
- Staffing and scheduling innovations.
- Managing small, rural hospitals.
- Decentralization.[9]

The 1982 survey indicated the percentage of time allocated to each function in the normal work week (see Table 19–1). Swansburg surveyed Alabama's acute care hospitals in 1984 to determine management competencies needed of head nurses (see Appendix 1–1).

Selecting appropriate people to promote to managerial ranks is a concern for most administrators. Demonstrated ability on a technical level does not ensure effective managerial performance. Nurse managers may become dissatisfied if their expectations are unrealistic. A frustrated and ineffective manager has a definite negative impact on the whole organization. The entire climate of a department—cooperation, employee satisfaction, turnover, conflict—are influenced greatly by the nurse manager.

Program development for nurse managers must be an ongoing process. To be effective such programs must not only validly measure management potential, they must be feasible and practical in terms of the existing organizational structure.

KEY PRODUCTIVITY ISSUES IN SUPERVISION

Leadership Style

The term "leadership" implies interaction with people. One of the toughest and most important aspects of a nurse manager's job is interacting effectively with staff. To function effectively the nurse manager acquires fundamental principles that make leadership a learned process rather than a series of duties described and listed in a policy manual. Leadership can only be defined by the behavior manifested by enactment of the nurse manager's role.

Leadership style is the way in which a leader goes about accomplishing her personal and organizational goals. There are, of course, numerous ways of classifying leadership styles, most of which rely on some continuum of behavior patterns. Nurse managers need more than one style of management to succeed; it is therefore essential to recognize the styles and the situations in which each may be most effective.

Likert proposed four styles of leadership that he categorized as management systems. These styles included consultative, participatory, exploitive-authoritative and benevolent-authoritative.[10] Participatory management involves a purposeful inclusion of employees in solving problems. Group decision making and communication are the norm. The management behaviors that characterize a healthy participatory approach include:

1. Identifying appropriate opportunities for participation.
2. Asking interested employees to participate.
3. Clearly communicating the task at hand.
4. Openly sharing known facts, constraints, and expectations.
5. Developing teamwork and a sense of purpose.

TABLE 19–1. Percentage of Allocation of Time to Function and Estimate of Percentage of Time in Normal Workweek

Function or Activity	Number and Percentage Allocating % of Time				Number and Percentage of Nursing Service Administrators Estimating % of Normal Workweek											
	Not Allocated		Allocated		1–2%		3–5%		6–10%		10–20%		Over 20%		Over	
	Number	%	Number	%	Number	%	Number	%	Number	%	Number	%	Number	%	Number	%
Administration	0	0	227	100	—	—	—	—	—	—	—	—	—	—	159	—
Giving direct patient care	193	85.0	34	15.0	18	8.0	8	3.5	5	2.2	3	1.3	—	—	—	—
Formal teaching	119	52.4	108	47.6	48	21.1	39	17.2	16	7.1	4	1.8	1	0.4	—	—
Community related	44	19.4	183	80.6	68	29.9	83	36.6	27	11.9	5	2.2	—	—	—	—
Professional organizational	21	9.3	206	90.7	70	30.8	91	40.1	37	16.3	8	3.5	—	—	—	—
Research	129	56.3	98	43.2	50	22.0	37	16.3	11	4.9	—	—	—	—	—	—
Outside consultation	126	55.5	101	44.5	55	24.2	35	15.5	10	4.4	1	0.4	—	—	—	—
Union-related activities	171	75.3	56	24.7	17	7.5	26	11.5	8	3.5	5	2.2	—	—	—	—
Other	169	74.4	58	25.6	12	5.3	19	8.4	10	4.4	9	4.0	8	3.5	—	—

Note: Data are based on 27 cases.

Source: Myrtle K. Aydelotte, "Report of the 1982 Survey of Nursing Service Administrators," Chicago: American Hospital Association, 1982, 26. Reprinted with permission.

449

6. Soliciting and valuing different points of view.
7. Acquiring appropriate resources for the team effort.
8. Communicating the status of action plans.
9. Teaching the process skills needed to participate effectively.
10. Providing individual coaching and encouragement to team members.
11. Facilitating the process of achieving group consensus.
12. Demonstrating the behaviors of successful teamwork.
13. Actively listening to individuals and appropriately responding.
14. Giving both positive and negative feedback (direct, specific, timely, and descriptive) with the intent to help the person develop.
15. Providing recognition for participation and task completion.[11]

The exploitive-authoritative nurse manager does almost everything in a top-down, dictatorial manner. The benevolent-authoritative nurse manager seeks input from staff occasionally in a very condescending fashion. In the consultative style managers make the assumption that the staff are responsible, concerned, and knowledgeable. Decision making begins to filter into the levels of the organization below the nurse manager. The consultative manager focuses on commitment instead of controls.

Far better performance, in terms of improved patient care, is elicited by consulting staff about methods of procedures or problems and allowing them to participate in finding the best solutions. Nursing staff have ideas of real value and can contribute much when the supervisor consults with them, individually or in groups, concerning the feasibility and workability of an idea or solution to a problem before making a decision.

Consultation with staff regarding decisions requires an open mind and a genuine intention to consult, not just a desire to create the impression. The supervisor must seriously and willingly consider the worker's opinion and suggestions. This does not lessen or weaken the formal authority of the supervisor; the right to make the decision rests with him. But sharing information through discussion of alternate solutions with subordinates before the decision is made gives them an opportunity to participate and make worthwhile contributions.

Consultation of this nature often provides the supervisor with alternative solutions to problems that she may not have considered.

The supervisor should use consultation only on matters where the staff has knowledge on which to draw. For example, one would consult with the clerk on the best way to simplify the routine paperwork, but not on a matter involving the management of direct patient care. The problem must be consistent with the subordinate's ability and within the scope of one's experience; otherwise, consultation will make an employee feel inadequate and frustrated.

Participation in decision making through the use of consultation cannot be used with all employees and in all situations. There will be occasions when the supervisor will need to use firmness and decisiveness in issuing instructions and giving directions.

There is no best way in which to influence people; the style one uses will be greatly influenced by the maturity of the group. This maturity of both the supervisor and the staff also influences the style of leadership that works best. Supervision is a dynamic process and application of any one leadership style requires regular assessment. The new staff member who initially needs reassurance and direction grows in the job until emotional support is needed less and greater independence and autonomy is more important. Therefore, it is necessary for the supervisor to concentrate on which style is used in response to the development level of a particular staff member, so that the supervisor's expectations are consistent with the predicted outcome.

The nurse manager should routinely evaluate leadership style. This self-evaluation enables the nurse manager to accentuate the positive aspects of her style and take steps to minimize the negative aspects. Leadership is discussed in more detail in a separate chapter.

Communication

Major personal characteristics which influence effective supervision include the amount and kind of professional experiences a manager has had and his ability to communicate to those with whom he works. Supervision involves a set of actions that influence members of a group to move toward common goal setting and attainment. There is literally no way communication skills can be separated from management abilities, because the most usual mode of exercising leadership is through the interactive process, which uses communicating as a primary vehicle.

The importance of effective communication to supervision was succinctly stated by La Roux:

> You can have expert knowledge; but if you cannot communicate your ideas clearly, forcefully and fluently, you will have little influence. You can have expert skill; but if you cannot demonstrate your skills to others and move them to action, you will have little power.[12]

Griver cited three areas of communication that can mean success or failure in eliminating conflict among staff, selling your ideas to staff, and reducing cost. Examine yourself in terms of each:

1. Do you commit the error of omission? Do you omit vital information in your written and oral communications?

2. Do you use operational definitions? Do you use specific, precise words to say what you mean—or express yourself in vague, general terms?

3. Do you use problem-solving "dollarization" (computing the dollar impact of the problem) and completed staff work?[13]

Over 80 percent of a supervisor's time is spent in oral and written communication with others. Favorable employee attitudes go hand in hand with good communication. When employees receive the information they want through channels they prefer, communications will be good. What do you want to know from your supervisors? Who do you want to tell you? How do you prefer to receive communication? Most people want to receive information from their supervisors but learn it through the grapevine instead. What is the implication? Have supervisors give their staff information and hold them responsible. Have a program of selection, training, and evaluation of supervisors that has a communication goal. When people receive the information they want, they have a better understanding of how an organization works. There are fewer grievances. Each supervisor should meet with her group a short time each week; 15 minutes will usually suffice. Report news and then have a question-and-answer session. Inspire employees to want the system, since forcing them does not improve communication. Do not propagandize or preach. Avoid labor relations matters, since this is a problem of union and management. Be informative without lecturing. Be frank in acknowledging mistakes. Good communications involve supervisors with their staff. Communication as a supervising or directing function is more fully developed in another chapter.

Motivation

Maintaining staff motivation is a very delicate balancing act for the supervisor. It is indeed a challenge to find a balance within a group so that each person is able to achieve her or his best performance. Obviously, some staff are easier to motivate than others; some need little external stimulation of motivation at all. Those with initiative only need guidance toward the opportunities and resources needed to accomplish their task to be stimulated and satisfied by the work and their achievements.

The staff member who lacks motivation or who is resistant to it is difficult but not impossible to reckon with. Such individuals may cause particular problems if they complain frequently and unnecessarily and influence other staff in the work unit.

Many studies on motivation have provided us with some valuable information on what is important to workers. Motivation is based on the need to have work that is meaningful and to take responsibility for the outcome of that work. Jobs that are fulfilling allow independence, require a variety of skills but also provide feedback. Job satisfaction is usually higher when the job provides the right level of challenge for the person involved.

Unfortunately, this combination of job characteristics does not frequently occur. Supervisors frequently focus on the patient care record and other forms to the exclusion of interpersonal interactions.

A reflection of motivation is productivity. If staff workers feel a sense of ownership of their services they will, undoubtedly, show greater levels of motivation. One way to assist in motivating and rewarding the productive worker is tangible rewards, usually money. Though it is the easiest reward to give, money may too frequently be offered at the expense of other rewards that do more to promote professional growth.

Motivation often can be stimulated through the work environment or by the staff member himself. When staff members are goal-directed, they will act in certain ways to achieve satisfaction in their work. Professionally prepared staff may tend to develop a stronger sense of autonomy and as a result are more apt to be self-motivated. Of course, this should be encouraged. The supervisor has the facilitating role of furthering their sense of satisfaction in the job through feedback which makes motivation work.

Longest has isolated some common elements that increase job satisfaction and motivation. These include achievement, responsibility, interpersonal relationships, and recognition, with salary near the end of an eight-point list.[14] Motivation is more fully developed in a separate chapter.

Delegation

One of the most important facets of a nurse manager's job is that of delegating authority to others. This consists of guiding and supervising the efforts of others toward the attainment of specific goals. In the process of organizing and directing activities, nurse managers are called upon to make decisions that affect the behavior of others, and they must possess knowledge and skills commensurate with this responsibility.

Delegation of authority can result in an organization that is effective in accomplishing group objectives with conservation of time and materials and the greatest return in job satisfaction. Nurse managers have increasingly become aware of the need for guidance in selecting the methods of delegation and for specific tools to prepare them for the task of guiding others.

To be effective, the nurse manager must be ensured of the authority, privilege, and power to carry out the directives within an organization. Effective delegation depends upon the willingness of management to release decision-making powers to members within the system. Delegation never relieves the nurse manager of the basic inherent responsibilities in the position held. The ultimate responsibility includes selecting the best staff member available for the task and providing equipment, resources, and information for the performance of the job. Delegation is not merely telling someone to do a task and expecting it to be done automatically. Delegation means to make use of strengths and abilities of the staff with support and power to make needed decisions and complete the assigned task.

Delegation goes beyond making out work assignments. The experienced nurse manager delegates projects rather than specific tasks. This is an indication of the maturity of both the supervisor and staff to whom tasks are delegated.

Some nurse managers do find it difficult to delegate work. It could be that they do not know to whom to delegate a particular task and what if any, needs to be delegated.

Delegation is likely to work more smoothly in a decentralized organizational structure. A "decentralization of authority and decision making is a fundamental phase of delegation."[15] This may be so; however, a supervisor often has little influence on the organizational structure. The nurse manager must work with the structure in place.

According to Steinmetz, delegation is the act of parceling out selected work that may be in the supervisory or upper-management domain to be done by a staff member.[16] The delegated person is given full responsibility to carry out the assignment to its conclusion.

Ultimately, effective delegation of work should provide the supervisor with time to carry out activities that cannot be delegated. Delegation has clearly failed when the work assigned is not done or is carried out incorrectly, leaving the supervisor to redo the task that was delegated.

Communication is the key link in successful delegation, as in most supervisory activities. Failure to keep staff up to date about changes in plans and let them know what is expected to happen or what is going on now is a violation of the basic spirit of delegation.

SUMMARY

Supervision is the directing function of nursing management, the art of applying the science of behavior technology. It also involves planning, organizing, and evaluating work. Modern nursing supervision is person-centered.

Supervision is affected by increasing and increasingly expensive technology. Supervisors are required to manage the cost of much of this technology.

Supervision is defined by the organizational structure and its lines of authority. It requires a knowledge of scientific management. The functions of supervision should be clearly defined and organized through written policy, job descriptions and job standards. The ultimate goal of supervision is productivity—of safe, effective, efficient, and satisfactory care of patients.

Supervision facilitates patient care management through effective management of personnel and material resources.

The supervisor serves as a role model to clinical nurses. Supervisors need to be developed into effective nurse managers through education and training. They can learn much of the theory from formal graduate programs. Nurse administrators will provide the practice and experience. Education of top nurse administrators continues to increase, with 61.6 percent of members of the American Organization of Nurse Executives having master's degrees in 1982.

Leadership style, communication and motivation are major components of the directing function of management and of the work of the nurse supervisor.

NOTES

1. *USAF Hospital Nursing Service*, AF pamphlet 160-2 (Washington, DC: Department of the Air Force P5-1, 1970).

2. A. C. Bennett, "Effective Management Centers on Human Values," *Hospitals*, July 16, 1976, 50, 73.

3. American Hospital Association, *Role, Function and Qualification of the Nursing Service Administrator in a Health Care Institution* (Chicago: AHA, 1978), 1.

4. Ibid., 4.

5. Ibid., 5.

6. Ibid., 2.

7. Hospital Research and Educational Trust, *Training and Continuing Education: A Handbook of Health Care Institutions* (Chicago: HRET, 1970).

8. M. K. Aydelotte, *Report of the 1982 Survey of Nursing Service Administrators* (Chicago: American Society of Nursing Service Administrators, 1983), 10–12.

9. J. Manez, "The Untraditional Nurse Manager: Agent of Change and Changing Agent," *Hospitals*, Jan. 1, 1978, 65.

10. R. Likert, *New Patterns of Management* (New York: McGraw-Hill, 1961).

11. Hamlin and J. Garrison, "Choosing Between Directive and Participative Management," *Supervisory Management*, Jan. 1986, 15.

12. "Communication and Influence in Nursing," in A. J. Huntsman, and J. L. Binger, *Communicating Effectively* (Wakefield, MA: Nursing Resources, 1981), 11.

13. Griver, J. A., "Communication Skills for Getting Ahead," *AORN Journal*, Aug. 1979 242–249.

14. B. Longest, "Job Satisfaction for Registered Nurses in the Hospital Setting," *Journal of Nursing Administration*, May-June 1974, 46–52.

15. J. Rokich, B. Longest, and K. Darr, *Managing Health Service Organization*, 2d ed. (Philadelphia: Saunders, 1985), 152.

16. L. Steinmetz, *The Art and Skill of Delegation* (Reading, MA: Addison-Wesley Publishing Co., 1976), 4–16.

The Nurse Manager of Staff Development

20

SHARON FARLEY, Ph.D., R.N.
Associate Professor
School of Nursing
Auburn University at Montgomery
Montgomery, Alabama

INTRODUCTION

Staff development must be based on a philosophy of adult education and utilize knowledge of teaching-learning principles and concepts of adult education. Adult learners are people who have a "formal education, a career or employment commitment, identified areas of interest, and family and financial responsibilities."[1] Nurses are adult learners who practice in an environment of rapid change which creates a need for them to update their knowledge and skills or prepare themselves for a different area of expertise.

Nurse managers frequently perform the staff development role. This may be as director of nursing in a smaller hospital, as a head nurse, or from another management position. It may be as a nurse manager teaching a clinical nurse how to present staff development programs.

PHILOSOPHY OF ADULT EDUCATION

Staff development programs must be designed to motivate adult learners to consider the learning

454

process as a natural part of living. People are born into society devoid of knowledge. From the day they are born to the day they die, they live in a society whose institutions are constantly changing. They are capable of learning during this entire life span. Cross believes that "lifelong learning means self-directed growth. It means acquiring new skills and powers—the only true wealth which you can never lose. It means investment in yourself. Lifelong learning means the joy of discovering how something really works, the delight of becoming aware of some new beauty in the world, the fun of creating something, alone or with other people."[2]

Lifelong learning is needed in nursing because of the rapid changes in the health-care delivery system and the changing roles of nursing in that system. Knowledge learned in basic nursing education programs quickly becomes obsolete. Nursing is influenced by public policy, technology, and societal and economic changes.

Nurses' use of technology, which is complex and constantly changing, is a major force in the need for lifelong learning. Nurses will learn to use computers, which are performing some tasks which were once a nursing responsibility. They will learn to work in specialty units and care for critically ill patients with artificial hearts, heart transplants, and other types of advanced surgical techniques. Staff development programs must respond to the needs of nurses practicing under these increased demands.

Educators and nurse managers planning staff development programs should consider that nurses also have lifelong learning needs related to the processes of physical, cultural, political, and spiritual maturation. One of the weaknesses of staff development programs has been their narrow emphasis on the major field of study. Continuing education that focuses on education of the whole person will develop free, creative, and responsible nursing personnel.

Staff development programs to educate the whole person are aimed at building competencies for performing various roles required in human life such as friend, citizen, individual (self), family member, worker, and leisure time user.[3] For example, nurses are adult citizens of the communities in which they live. Educational systems should show them how to participate in social institutions and how to assume their responsibilities, rights, and privileges. They must learn to be people who strive to attain high standards in the institutions in which they actively participate.

CHARACTERISTICS OF THE ADULT LEARNER

Internal Motivation

Malcolm Knowles is generally credited with defining characteristics specific to adult learners. One characteristic is that adult learners are motivated to seek educational experiences by internal motivators such as self-esteem or desiring a better quality of life.[4] Boshier interviewed 453 adult education participants and found that their leading motivators were to become better citizens, to participate in group activity, to relieve boredom, and to live in a more satisfying way.[5] Nurses are likely to perceive a need to learn when they encounter a situation which they cannot handle in their professional practice. Nurses who are pressured into educational experiences often do not learn as well as those who attend because of an identified need. For instance, nurses with associate degrees or diplomas who are pushed by employers to seek a baccalaureate degree are a challenge to educators because they often enter courses with hostility and anxiety which blocks their ability to learn. Educators and managers working with these adult students can recognize the causes and create an educational and work environment that ameliorates them. The readiness of adults to learn is affected by their changing social or life roles rather than by academic pressure. Developmental tasks such as growing older, losing a job, death of a spouse, or divorce will trigger a readiness to learn. Figure 20–1 gives examples of several life roles, developmental tasks associated with those roles, and staff development programs that will assist adults in coping with those roles and tasks.

Self-Direction

Adults are self-directed and want to be perceived as responsible for their own learning. Because of the nature of their jobs, nurses are accustomed to making decisions about their own lives as well as decisions about the health care given to others. When they are placed in situations where their views are not respected or where they feel others are imposing their will, they often experience resentment and

FIGURE 20–1.　Development of Competency for Social Roles

Social Role	Developmental Task	Staff Development
Worker	Finding a job.	Career planning; interviewing skills; how to change jobs; assertiveness training.
	Keeping a job.	Politics of organizations; dealing with change; interpersonal skills; decision-making skills.
	Moving ahead in a job.	Supervision and management skills; executive development, advanced job skills.
	Preparation for retirement.	Financial planning, vocational planning; leisure time planning
Spouse	Living with a spouse.	Marital conflict management.
	Managing a home.	Financial planning; home repair; crisis management; managing job and family.
	Coping with death of a spouse or divorce.	Adjusting to loneliness; establishing new relationships.
Being a self	Maintaining health.	Stress reduction; exercise programs; accident prevention.
	Enjoyment of leisure.	Time management; developing friendships; buying recreational equipment; leisure activites for the elderly.

resistance. They are not likely to remain in a learning situation that threatens their self-esteem or dignity. The nurse manager should employ human relations skills that support the individual nurse's independence and at the same time offer support to that individual's learning needs.

Life Experience

Another characteristic of adults is that they come to the educational activity with a large volume of experience gleaned from their social roles such as parent, worker, citizen, or spouse. Therefore, they are a rich source for one another's learning. When teaching adults, educators should use techniques such as simulation, group discussion, problem-solving projects, and field experiences which make use of the experiences of the learner. Another result of adults' experience is that they have a definite mind-set and they tend to be more closed to new concepts. Their likes and dislikes are more fixed and their attitudes are more difficult to change. Nurse

managers should expose adult learners to experiences that will open their minds to new ideas. One way of doing this is by indicating how the process can be reciprocal, each learning from the other.

Problem-Centered Orientation to Learning

A fourth characteristic of adult learners is that they have a problem-centered orientation to learning. Often coming into learning because of a life problem they want to solve through education, they want immediacy of application. Adults are not patient with information they cannot use in their lives or in their work. Staff development programs should be organized around problem areas rather than subject matter. A computer source titled "Computer Use for Nursing Practice in the Hospital" will be more relevant for nurses than the general course titled "Beginning Computer Skills." Figure 20–2 describes implications of adult learner characteristics for staff development programs.

Figure 20–2.   Implications of Adult Learner Characteristics for Staff Development Programs

Characteristics	Implications
Internal motivation	Students participate in diagnosis of learning needs.
	Opportunities are provided for students to identify gaps in their knowledge related to their occupational and social roles.
Self-direction	Students participate in planning the staff development program.
	Students and teachers share responsibility for developing objectives, designing the course, and identifying resources. Students participate in evaluating progress toward their own goals.
Role of experience as a learning resource	Less use is made of transmittal techniques such as lectures and reading assignments; more of experiential approaches such as case methods, role plays, and discussion.
	Students are encouraged to share experiences and knowledge with class members through group projects and teaching-learning teams.
Problem-centered orientation to learning	Opportunity given for practical application of learning to career or life experiences.
	Staff development programs are organized around problem areas rather than a subject area.
	Programs are flexible enough to accommodate individual student concerns and needs.

THE STAFF DEVELOPMENT PROCESS

Staff development may be defined as "a management program to aid staff in developing skills and knowledge which adds to their professional goals and at the same time increases their value as employees."[6] Staff development is a comprehensive program which includes orientation, in-service education, continuing education programs, and job-related counseling. Orientation introduces employees to new situations and includes content related to philosophies, goals, policies, procedures, personnel benefits, role expectations, and physical facilities. Employees need orientation each time their roles change.

In-service education provides learning experiences in the work setting for the purpose of refining and developing new skills and knowledge related to job performance. These learning experiences are usually narrow in scope and brief because they are aimed at only one competency or knowledge area. For example, a learning experience might be developed to introduce nursing staff in cardiac care to a new, more sophisticated monitor.

Continuing education programs are planned and organized learning experiences which focus on competencies and knowledge employees can use in a variety of settings instead of just a particular agency. Continuing education offerings often give employees new approaches to health-care delivery. Examples of continuing education activities are workshops, conferences, self-learning modules, and seminars.

Staff development also includes job-related counseling, which involves promoting professional growth of employees by helping them give their best job performance. It also involves counseling about promotion possibilities and assistance in obtaining formal training.

Philosophy of the Staff Development Program

The organization needs a statement of beliefs about how it will accomplish its staff development program. The staff development philosophy should relate to the mission and philosophy of the organization of which it is a part. The statement of philosophy should be written by a representative group, not an individual, and be accepted by both staff and administrators.

In writing a philosophy for staff development for health care professionals, beliefs about the following areas need to be addressed:

1. How learning takes place.
2. Teaching methods.
3. Responsibility of employees for their own learning.
4. Organization's responsibility for providing staff development.
5. Clients' rights to health care.

Organization of Staff Development

A staff development program can function under many organizational models and is dependent upon the philosophy of the agency. In a centralized model, there is an agency-wide staff development department, and the educational staff may consist of either nurses or educators who are not nurses. In this model all departments collaborate in determining and planning job needs of their staff. The centralized model facilitates scheduling and use of equipment and may prevent duplication of efforts. The main criticism of this model is separation from nursing staff and perpetuation of an us-against-them attitude.

In a decentralized model, the nursing department has its own organized in-service or staff development department. The nursing staff development department may then adopt a centralized or decentralized model. The strength of a decentralized model is that the specific needs identified by an area can be addressed. The major areas of concern in decentralization are the use and scheduling of classrooms, duplication of efforts, and the cost of providing multiple small programs. A system which attempts to utilize the strengths of both centralization and decentralization is not feasible.

Staff Development Personnel

Nursing service administrators are responsible for staff development in order to promote quality client care. Among their responsibilities are the following:

1. Providing financial and human resources.
2. Establishing policies for staff development.
3. Providing released time and/or finances for staff to attend continuing education offerings.
4. Motivating employees to assume responsibility for their own professional development.
5. Providing mechanisms to identify staff growth needs.
6. Evaluating the effects of staff participation in continuing education offerings on quality of client care.

The staff development coordinator must be both an administrator and a teacher who is able to communicate and establish trust, has knowledge and skills in adult education, has knowledge of training resources and subject matter, and understands the program planning process. As an administrator, the coordinator should understand organizational theory and have skills in budgeting, personnel management, and group process. As a teacher, the coordinator should have educational skills in diagnosing learning needs, developing learning objectives and lesson plans, and selecting and using appropriate teaching techniques.

The professional development staff are selected by the coordinator to work in the planning, implementation, and evaluation of staff development programs. The size of the staff depends on the size of the agency. In small agencies the coordinator may be the only staff member.

Support staff adequate in number and qualifications are essential for staff development. Secretaries need word processing, filing, and public relations skills. Large staff development departments may include staff with computer and audiovisual skills.

Advisory Committees

An advisory committee can be useful for identifying needs and resources and for planning programs. Members of the committee should represent all fields of practice in the agency. Other members may include people with needed expertise. Committee members may increase participation because they can communicate the purpose of staff development programs directly to the people they represent.

Budgets for Staff Development

The amount of budget allocation for staff development depends on staff size, expected number of new employees, and existing resources.[7] The staff development coordinator is responsible for developing and implementing the development budget with input from staff. The agency administration will demonstrate a commitment to staff development by allocating adequate funds for salaries, staff time for training, periodicals, books, audiovisuals, and outside education resources.

ANDRAGOGICAL APPROACH TO PROGRAM DESIGN

The characteristics of adult learners require an *andragogical* approach to curricular development and teaching in staff development programs. Andragogy is the art and science of helping adults learn, in contrast to pedagogy, the teaching of children. This approach assumes that the learners themselves are the facilitators who create a climate that motivates their own achievement.[8]

Mutual Diagnosis of Needs

Effective staff development programs begin with a needs assessment of the learners. A common mistake of staff development planners is to assume they know what adults need to learn. Usually, this assumption leads to an unsuccessful educational program. For adults to be interested and motivated they must enter educational programs because of perceived needs they have identified. Adult learners have a perception of the level of competency they want to achieve and the knowledge they need to help them perform better in their personal lives or work settings. If adult learners' perceptions of their needs differ from those of the planners, they will not participate in the educational offerings. A training program is a waste of money if it does not increase the efficiency and effectiveness of workers.[9] Therefore educational needs assessment is the first step in adult education programming.

Educational Needs Defined

A felt need is a need perceived by the learner, based perhaps on exposure to new situations, increased acuity among patients, or exposure to new information through reading. An ascribed need is a need someone else, such as a head nurse or supervisor, identifies for the learner; such needs are related to factors like performance appraisals or audits.

Needs Assessment Methods

Staff development planners must decide on a method of assessment that will meet their purposes. Following are a list of factors to be considered before designing a needs assessment survey:

1. Target population.
2. Development time.
3. Cost.
4. Financial and human resources.
5. Analysis time.
6. Anonymity.
7. Objectivity.

The needs survey should address content, design of learning activities, and learners' background.[10] Content relates to the specific topics of interest to the learners. Design of learning activities covers such areas as when individuals can attend courses and what kind of learning options (such as workshops or modules) would best facilitate their learning.

When considering a method, it is important to address the needs of the organization as well as those of the learner. Organizational needs are influenced by factors such as the standards of the Joint Commission for Accreditation of Healthcare Organizations, the American Nurses Association Standards for Continuing Education, consumer needs, standards of practice, and the philosophy and objectives of the institution. If staff developers ignore these needs they may lose the support of the sponsoring organization.

Questionnaire/Survey. A questionnaire is perhaps the most frequently used method for assessing needs. Questions on the survey tool may be either forced choice, which allows selection of one of several categories of context needs, or open-ended, which allows more freedom to respond. An example of the latter is a question such as, "If I could learn more about stress management, I would like to learn . . ." The survey tool should be designed with a combination of these two types of questions.

A pilot test of the survey should be done to ensure that it is clear and that the data gathered are complete and relevant. Individuals completing the pilot survey should be asked to comment on whether they understand the questions, how long it took them to complete the questions, and whether other areas should be added. Their responses should then be analyzed by a group and necessary changes made in the questionnaire.

The advantages of the questionnaire are that they are usually easy and convenient to administer and the results are easily computed. Disadvantages include the cost of data collection and analysis. Also, if a mailed questionnaire yields a low return, the data may not result in a representative sample. Figure 20–3 is one example of a broad scale questionnaire.

Observation.   Observation, when used with other methods, is an effective way to assess needs. A head nurse or clinical specialist can observe personnel and perhaps identify learning needs. The effectiveness of this technique is increased if a standardized observation guide is used.

A disadvantage of this method is that observations are subjective and can produce incomplete data. For instance, a nurse observed to be charting incorrectly may do so because of lack of time, not faulty knowledge of the procedure.

Interview.   Interviews of a sample representing the target population is a method that can gather valuable information about needs. Interviews can clarify ambiguous data gathered through surveys. Respondents often feel more comfortable expressing feelings verbally than in writing. A disadvantage is that data collected are difficult to sort, measure, and report.

Open Group Meetings.   Learning needs can be assessed in group discussions if a resource person is available with questions to focus the group on the topic. The resource person should be skilled in group process technique so that all group members can be aided in expressing their learning needs clearly. This method can be time-consuming and of limited value if group members are hesitant about speaking out.

Analysis of Professional Literature.   A systematic review of the previous 6 months to a year of pertinent journals is an excellent means to identify trends and compare national information with the leader's own setting. This method is inexpensive and can be present- or future-oriented. On the negative side, a review of literature is time-consuming because it involves analyzing and synthesizing many articles to find trends. Also, a time lag is involved in publication.

Competency Model.   A competency model is a valuable means for discovering needs of an individual. In building a competency model, a series of statements are developed which identify expected performance or behavior. After the competencies are refined to small units which reflect only single behaviors, individuals can then compare their performance to each behavior. Staff developers can help individuals identify gaps between their level of competency and the desired level. Individuals can then participate in learning activities to close the gaps.

Employee Performance Appraisals.   The performance appraisal can be an effective method for identifying needs if done in a positive way. Appraisals should avoid confrontation, be meaningful instead of demeaning, and be a worthwhile activity that develops staff. People should be encouraged to state their own hopes and aspirations and identify their learning needs. Both the superior and the staff person must have a clear picture of duties and demands of the job and current abilities and level of performance. They should then identify gaps between the desired and actual levels of performance. Staff development programs are then designed to improve performance or prepare the employee for a new position.

Mutual Planning

Once needs are identified and prioritized, appropriate learning experiences must be designed. Adult learners should be able to help plan the educational offerings. Professional nurses are more committed to an activity when they have been involved in the decision-making process. They see themselves as

FIGURE 20–3. Broad Scale Questionnaire

How can Staff Development help meet your needs over the next year? Please answer the following questions. This is an anonymous survey.

Check most appropriate.

1. I am:

___ a. R.N.

___ b. L.P.N.

___ c. NA

___ d. W.C.

2. I work in the following type of nursing area:

___ a. Medical

___ b. Surgical

___ c. Orthopedic/Neuro

___ d. Obstetrical

___ e. Pediatric

___ f. Neonatal

___ g. Emergency room

___ h. Operating room

___ i. Other (specify) _____

3. I have worked in my nursing area for:

___ a. less than 3 months

___ b. 4 to 11 months

___ c. 1 to 3 years

___ d. 4 to 6 years

___ e. over 6 years

4. What is the best time of day for you to attend in-service programs?

___ a. mornings

___ b. afternoons

___ c. evenings

5. What is the best day for you to attend in-service programs?

___ a. Monday

___ b. Tuesday

___ c. Wednesday

___ d. Thursday

___ e. Friday

___ f. Saturday

Circle the most appropriate response, according to your interest, for the following in-service education programs.

4 = I am highly interested.
3 = I am interested.
2 = I am somewhat interested.
1 = I have no opinion or don't know.
0 = I have no interest.

6. 43210   Respiratory care

7. 43210   Wound management

8. 43210   Stress management

9. 43210   Nursing and the law

10. 43210   Communication skills

11. 43210   Nursing process

12. 43210   Use of computers in nursing

13. 43210   Death and dying

14. 43210   Body image

15. 43210   Cost care

16. What other topics would you like included in in-service education programs? _____

_____

_____

self-directed and they will resist a staff development program they think is imposed on them by the establishment. A committee that represents all sub-groups is one mechanism for mutual planning. The nursing service administrator or the education co-ordinator is responsible for appointing the planning committee.

Translating Learning Needs into Objectives

The planning committee should be involved in setting objectives for the learning experience. The staff development director will have to assist the committee in developing objectives, because this is often the most difficult part of the planning process.

Objectives define the type of behavior the learner is to exhibit as a result of the educational experience. Objectives are important because they provide a basis for planning learning activities, selecting methods and materials, and defining and organizing content. Also, objectives provide the guidelines for evaluation. In order for objectives to serve as a workable tool, certain guidelines should be followed:

1. Objectives should be centered on the learner, not the teacher. For example, "the student will list the signs and symptoms of shock"—not "the instructor will present the signs and symptoms of shock."

2. Each objective should have a single subject. Consider an objective such as "state six signs and symptoms of shock and the nursing actions to be taken." The learner may know the six symptoms but not the nursing action. When an objective has more than one subject it may be difficult to evaluate whether the outcome has been achieved.

3. Each objective should include an action verb that describes the behavior to be exhibited such as define, list, explain, or describe. Vague terms such as appreciate, understand, know, or comprehend should be avoided because they are difficult to measure.

Learning outcomes or objectives may be organized into three domains: cognitive, affective, and psychomotor. The cognitive domain includes knowledge, understanding, and thinking skills. An example of a behavioral objective written for the cognitive domain is: "Students will be able to list four positive effects of regular preparation for class on learning outcomes." The affective domain includes those objectives which emphasize feelings, such as interest, appreciation and attitudes. "Students will accept the need for regular class preparation" is an example of an objective written for the affective domain. The psychomotor domain deals with motor skills such as doing, practicing, or demonstrating. An example of a psychomotor objective is: "Students will demonstrate skill in inserting an endotracheal tube." Commonly used words for behavioral objectives are listed in Figure 20–4. A list such as this can be helpful to planning committee members who are unfamiliar with written objectives.

Identifying Content

As with identifying needs and writing objectives, it is also important that staff be involved in identifying content. The staff planning committee can be the vehicle for determining content with the continuing education staff serving as the facilitator. The education staff will assist the committee in defining the target population and refining content so that it achieves the objectives and fits into the time frame. A subject expert should be included on the committee as well as the instructor if the instructor has been identified.

If learning objectives are stated clearly, the content will flow from the objective. For example, the staff development committee identified a need for head nurses to gain additional leadership skills. They then wrote objectives and identified content to meet those objectives. Figure 20–5 gives examples of three of those objectives and the relevant content.

Teaching Methods

To maximize learning, adults should be active learners instead of passive learners. Learning is a shared activity in which both the teacher and the student have responsibilities. This means that the teacher should avoid lecturing and instead stimulate the students to think, discuss, try, and view. If students are active participants, learning is more apt to take place. Following are examples of two methods for facilitating active learning.

FIGURE 20–4. Commonly Used Words for Behavioral Objectives

Cognitive Domain

defines	builds	respects
memorizes	expresses	relates
lists	measures	identifies
selects	plans	matches
states	recalls	

Affective Domain

realizes	exhibits	examines
prefers	participates	studies
conforms	explores	cooperates
helps	joins	enables
complies	is loyal to	shares

Psychomotor Domain

demonstrates	follows directions
imitates	observes
finds	recognizes
sorts	

Self-Instructional Materials. Self-instructional materials such as self-directed modules are one means by which staff can be active participants in the learning process. Self-instructional modules are collections of information, facts, and concepts presented in a step-by-step format. The modules have a set of directions and usually include built-in reinforcements and evaluations of learning. Computer-assisted instruction also utilizes this step-by-step format.

An advantage of self-instructional modules is that the resource is available when a staff member identifies a need—formal classes do not need to be scheduled. Likewise, teaching is not dependent on the availability of a teacher. Third, the method is flexible because staff members can choose the amount and types of learning experiences to meet their needs.

Learning modules are effective only if they are used by staff. Following are some strategies for enhancing module use:

1. Identify characteristics of the user such as previous experience with module learning and other learning styles.
2. Involve staff in developing the modules and in determining the most appropriate areas for module use.
3. Orient staff to the modular format and the self-directed process.
4. Have a facilitator available for learners who desire contact with teachers or colearners.

FIGURE 20–5. Learning Objectives Related to Content

Objective	Content
1. Define the leadership process as related to nursing.	Definition of leadership: formal informal
2. Describe four leadership styles.	Leadership styles: authoritarian democratic permissive laissez-faire
3. Define four bases of power for leaders.	Power bases: reward power legitimate power expert power referent power

FIGURE 20–6. Learning Contract

Learning Objectives	Learning Methods	Standard for Evaluation
The student will demonstrate competencies in interpersonal skills in nursing practices.		
1. With other students	Participate in role playing activities; interact informally with other students; participate in group exercises.	Feedback from instructors and other students indicate that the student facilitates interactions by listening, clarifying, conveying warmth, informing, reflecting, and summarizing.
2. With clients	Interpersonal interactions through assignments including histories, physicals, and clinical interactions. ■ Completes interpersonal assessment (IPA) with two clients. ■ Audio-tape two interactions with clients. ■ Interviews one client in presence of a staff member who is a registered nurse.	IPAs identify patterns in communication as well as facilitators and blocks to communication. Feedback from instructor and staff nurse that student demonstrates skills of attending, clarifying, and informing; recognizes verbal as well as nonverbal communication. During discussion, shows own feelings as appropriate; recognizes client worth and autonomy; evaluates interactions; appropriately terminates the therapeutic relationship; maintains confidentiality of information.

5. Incorporate the module learner program into a career ladder or recognition program.[11]

Learning Contracts. Use of learning contracts is another method of active learning. After learning needs are diagnosed, each learner then writes learning objectives for each need that describes an improvement in performance or a terminal behavior to be achieved. Then, with the instructor's help, the learner identifies how each objective will be accomplished and what resources will be needed. Next the learners indicate how they will demonstrate learning of the specified information skills or concepts. Finally, the learner decides the evaluation criteria or evidence of accomplishment. While the contract is being completed, the instructor or nurse manager acts as a consultant and a facilitator. When the contract is completed the learner gives the instructor materials such as papers, oral presentations, or rating scales to demonstrate successful fulfillment of the contract. The instructor can decide to accept the data as fulfilling the contract or ask for additional evidence.[12] An example of a learning contract is displayed in Figure 20–6.

Creating a Climate for Learning

Presenters of staff development programs must create a climate that will enable adults to have a meaningful learning experience. The physical environment should be made comfortable through proper heating, ventilation, lighting, and access to refreshments and restrooms. Inadequate lighting, noise, uncomfortable temperature, or humidity dis-

FIGURE 20–7. Strategies to Create a Climate for Learning

Climate	Instructional State
Mutual respect	Provide individual name cards.
	Greet each participant by name.
	Learn about each participant's educational background and experience.
	Solicit participants' contributions.
Collaborativeness	Design get-acquainted exercises so participants can share their skills and knowledge.
	Encourage students to work and share with others who have similar needs.
	Encourage cooperative activities such as role playing and shared projects; refrain from encouraging competitiveness.
Mutual trust	Teachers are open in sharing personal information and disclosing their own feelings when appropriate.
	Encourage participants to make independent decisions.
	Allow participants to borrow personal equipment or books.
Supportiveness	Respect each participant's feelings and ideas.

tract from learning. If possible, the color of the room should be bright and cheerful because bright colors promote an optimistic, enthusiastic mood.

The chairs should be comfortable. Learners should not be treated as children, with seating in rows facing the teacher. This arrangement says the teacher imparts knowledge and students take it in. Instead, seating should be in groups or in circles so that learners and the teacher can interact as equals.

Of even more importance than physical climate is the development of a psychosocial and cultural climate that facilitates learning. Figure 20–7 summarizes strategies that can be used to facilitate a climate for learning.

Knowles describes seven characteristics of climate he believes are conducive of learning:

A climate of mutual respect.

A climate of collaboration.

A climate of mutual trust.

A climate of supportiveness.

A climate of openness and authenticity.

A climate of pleasure.

A climate of humanness.[13]

Climate of Mutual Respect. A climate of mutual respect is fostered when instructors take the time to

learn more about learners and their backgrounds. Participants should have name cards and the teacher should greet them by name. Time can be spent learning about participants' educational backgrounds and experience, their current work situation, and their goals in attending the staff development program. Sharing of personal data helps people feel respected as individuals and whole persons, not like just another staff nurse in the emergency room or head nurse on a unit.

Climate of Collaboration. Because adults are rich resources for each other's learning, a climate of collaboration is important. Get-acquainted exercises which allow people to share personal information help participants identify others who share common interests. Participants can communicate their skills and experience to the group to provide a wider range of human resources and encourage sharing of knowledge. An added advantage of these sharing exercises is that self-esteem may be enhanced when individuals realize they have unique skills which others may benefit from. Other techniques to foster collaboration are shared projects, in-class group work, and role plays. Refer to the section on team building for further discussion.

Climate of Mutual Trust. A climate of mutual trust is important to facilitate learning. Students usually have difficulty seeing teachers as trustworthy because teachers are in a position of power. They decide the grades and who passes or fails. Teachers can set the tone for mutual trust by demonstrating that they trust the students. They can do this by allowing the students to make independent decisions or by loaning them equipment or books. Students also are more trusting of teachers they can relate to as whole persons who have interests outside their professions. Teachers as well as learners should share information about their interests and hobbies and perhaps tell an amusing anecdote about themselves. Humor can be used to dissipate tension, and students respond positively to educators who have an appropriate sense of humor.

Climate of Supportiveness.   A climate of supportiveness is one in which learners do not feel threatened. They are able to experiment, practice, and even fail without being unduly criticized. Educators should emphasize learners' strengths instead of their weaknesses.

Climate of Openness and Authenticity.   In a climate of openness all participants are encouraged to make their views known and have them heard by the rest of the group without fear of reprisal, humiliation, or embarrassment. Sometimes adults have to learn how to debate and disagree without anger and resentment. Teachers can demonstrate this behavior by being open and allowing the group to disagree with their ideas. An open environment allows risk-taking behavior and acceptance of new ideas and change.

Climate of Pleasure.   Learning that is fun and pleasurable will motivate staff to be involved in staff development programs. Many adults are conditioned to believe education is dull because of their previous experiences. It may be a challenge for program developers to make learning an adventure. Field trips, guest lectures, and class debates are examples of teaching methods that are exciting diversions that can stimulate learning.

Climate of Humanness.   Knowles sums up his feelings about climate by saying that teachers should provide a climate of "humanness." He believes "learning is a very human activity. The more people feel that they are being treated as human beings, the more they are likely to learn."[14] Knowles believes that paying attention to the physical comforts by providing breaks, refreshments, comfortable chairs, and good lighting, as well as demonstrating caring and respect will help create this climate of humanness.

TEACHING-LEARNING PROCESS FOR ADULT EDUCATION

Staff development programs are often not successful when presenters do not know the educational process and how to use it. Learning involves a change in behavior. Behavior is based on ethical and moral beliefs, cultural backgrounds, and life experiences. Adults resist behavioral changes that are imposed upon them, especially if they do not recognize a need for learning. Presenters of staff development programs must understand characteristics of learning and laws of learning in order to motivate adult learners and facilitate the desired change in behavior.

Learning Is Purposeful

Learning is purposeful; each person learning something new does so in a unique style. One person may actively participate in class learning exercises while another passively depends on the teacher to give information, each responding in accordance with the requirements seen in the situation. Each adult learner has purposes and goals, some unique, others shared; some short term, others for a career or a lifetime. Some want to learn to meet employer demands, some to upgrade work skills, and others to relieve the tedium of everyday living. Learning results when activities further learners' purposes and instruction is related to their goals. A teacher, recognizing that learning is purposeful, would ask attendees to discuss their personal reasons for learning the material. In a continuing education class in ethical practice, for instance, adult learners might say they are learning the material to make ethical decisions related to their jobs.

Learning Is an Individual Process

Learning is an individual process in which a person learns what is experienced. A person's knowledge is a result of experiences. It is affected by previous experience and by individual needs. Although people can learn by rote to recite, they can make such learning a part of their life only if they understand it well enough to apply it correctly in real situations, which they can do if their learning experiences have been extensive and meaningful. If an experience challenges learners, requiring involvement with feelings, thoughts, memories, and physical activity, it is more effective than an experience in which all the learner has to do is commit something to memory. New learning is influenced by what the learner already knows.[15] An adult learner who drove a tractor as a child may easily learn to drive an automobile because of previous knowledge of the principles of steering, braking, and accelerating.

Clearly, learning a skill requires actual experience in performing that skill. Application is important for the older adult learner whose cognitive ability for short-term memory may be decreasing. Young people seem to perform best on tasks requiring quick insight, short-term memorization, and complex interactions. On the other hand as people age, they accumulate knowledge and experience in the use and application of it.[16] Age differences in memory seem to disappear when the material is learned well and opportunities are given for application of skills in practice. Nurses learn how to operate a computer by experiencing using the keyboard and entering data, not by memorizing the procedure book. Nurse managers learn about methods of conflict resolution by relating those methods to personal experiences.

Learning Is Multifaced

Learning is multifaced and occurs from verbal, conceptual, perceptual, motor, problem-solving, and emotional experiences. These elements of learning may occur at the same time and in obvious combinations. For example, in learning to apply the principles of ethical decision making, a class may try to resolve a real ethical dilemma. Each person may approach the task from a different cultural or ethical perspective and this perspective may change as the result of experience. While solving the dilemma, the class also engages in verbal learning and sensory perception.

Learning is also multifaced in that people learn more than one thing at a time. Nurses learning to develop a quality assurance procedure may also be learning cooperation and group dynamics. With guidance from a competent instructor, they may be

learning ethical behavior and professional accountability. This incidental learning may have great impact on the total development of the individual.

Learning Is an Active Process

Learning is an active process in which a person reacts physically or emotionally. Self-motivated participation intensifies motivation, flexibility, and rate of learning.[17] Adults with a history of poor school performance will not be eager to return to a learning situation where they will have another opportunity to fail. On the other hand, people with successful educational experiences in childhood will have a positive attitude toward instruction and their ability to perform and will be motivated to achieve. Those with a positive stance toward learning will seek challenges and new opportunities for growth through learning.[18] If educators want to understand why some adults fail to participate in staff development programs they must begin with an understanding of attitudes toward self and education.[19]

Because learning is an active process, it is not facilitated by a one-way model of education where the teacher imparts knowledge or skill while the student passively absorbs the information. Hale proposes that education is a cooperative rather than an "operative" art, the latter being "one in which the creation of a product or performance is essentially controlled by the person using the art."[20] To facilitate learning, teachers should create an open, nonauthoritarian atmosphere where students can react and respond both emotionally and intellectually. For example, when instructors teach students about burnout among registered nurses, they might describe bureaucratic behaviors that will elicit a strong emotional response from participants. Instructors can encourage students to argue back and forth over the validity of the behaviors described. If the learning process is a process of changing behaviors, clearly the process must be an active one.

LAWS OF LEARNING

Early in this century one of the pioneers in educational psychology, Edward L. Thorndike, postulated several laws of learning which seemed generally applicable to the learning process. Although in the years since, other psychologists have found that learning is a more complex process than some of these laws suggest, they still provide insight into the learning process. The laws that follow are not necessarily as Thorndike stated them. During the years they have been restated and supplemented. In essence, however, they may be attributed to him. The first three are the basic laws as originally identified: the law of readiness, the law of exercise, and the still generally accepted law of effect. Three laws were added later as a result of experimental studies: the law of primacy, the law of intensity, and the law of recency.

Law of Readiness

People learn best when they are ready to learn and do not learn much if they see no reason for learning. When there is no motivation to learn, there is no learning. Motivation enhances learning and achievement because people work longer, harder, and with more vigor and intensity when they have strong purposes, clear objectives, and readiness for learning.[21] Increased time spent in learning activities increases achievement.[22] Motivated students are easier to teach because they are cooperative, open to learning, and process information more readily than unmotivated students. Also, eager students spawn enthusiastic teachers who are willing to give their best effort.

Teachers do not have to wait for readiness to develop naturally; there are things that teachers can do to foster it such as exposing adults to effective role models, engaging them in career planning, and helping them diagnose gaps in their knowledge.[23] However, under certain circumstances, the teacher can do little to motivate a person to learn. Personal problems, poor health, or outside responsibilities or interests may overshadow a person's desire to learn.

Law of Exercise

The law of exercise states that those things most often repeated are best remembered. It is the basis of practice and drill. The mind can rarely retain, evaluate, and apply new concepts or practices after a single exposure. People do not learn to give an injection in one class; they learn by applying what they have been told. Every time they practice, the learning is reinforced. The teacher must provide opportunities for adult learners to practice or re-

peat, and must see that this process is directed toward a goal. Repetition can be of many types, including recall, review, restatement, and physical application.

Law of Effect

A third law is the law of effect. This law is based on the emotional reaction of the learner. It states that learning is strengthened when accompanied by a pleasant or satisfying feeling. An experience that produces emotions of joy, curiosity, optimism, affection, and confidence puts people in a positive mood for learning. However, experiences that lead to emotions of apathy, boredom, defeat, frustration, or anger increase stress and decrease learning. If an instructor attempts to teach the entire computer instruction manual to nurses during the first class, they are likely to feel inferior, frustrated, and dissatisfied and drop out.

Teachers can evoke pleasant student emotions by demonstrating a willingness to answer questions and offer explanations, being interested in students, giving positive feedback, and displaying confidence in themselves and in the students. Conversely, teachers can evoke unpleasant emotions by threats, being sarcastic, giving only negative feedback, or acting in a superior manner. Adults who leave a learning situation feeling positive and motivated about what they have learned are more likely to have a future interest in what they have learned and to return to future staff development programs.

Law of Primacy

A fourth law of learning is the law of primacy. Primacy, the state of being first, often creates a strong, unshakable impression. If a nursing student learns to give an injection incorrectly, the teacher will have a difficult task in unteaching the bad habits and reteaching the good ones. Unteaching is more difficult than teaching. Adults in a staff development program have a history of formal and informal learning experiences. If they are secure with their level of knowledge and skills they may resist new information and change in procedures. This resistance to new learning can be decreased if learners are involved in planning and goal setting for a staff development program and if the need for changes in procedure is communicated to them.

Law of Intensity

The law of intensity states that a vivid, dramatic, or exciting learning experience teaches more than a routine or boring experience. Friedrich Nietzsche said that against boredom, even the gods themselves struggle in vain. Learning appears to be an area where people are vulnerable to the powerful emotion of boredom. Boredom decreases learning because it disrupts and diminishes a person's ability to maintain effort and attention, and it leads to irritability, fatigue, strain, distractibility, and carelessness.[24]

Teachers can decrease boredom and create stimulating learning experiences by providing variety in personal presentation style, methods of instruction, and learning materials and by providing realism. Students can learn more about cardiopulmonary resuscitation and find the lesson more exciting if they can watch someone resuscitate a patient rather than listening to a lecture on the subject. The teacher can use a variety of methods and teaching aids to bring excitement into the classroom. Mockups, color slides, movies, filmstrips, posters, photographs, and other audiovisual aids can add vividness to classroom instruction. Demonstrations, skits, and panels do much to intensify learning experiences. The work situation is an ideal place to learn to apply the knowledge and skills related to the practice of nursing.

Law of Recency

The sixth law of learning is the law of recency. Other things being equal, what was most recently learned is best remembered. Conversely, the farther a learner is removed in time from a new understanding, the more difficult it is to remember. It is easy, for example, to recall an address used during the day, but may be impossible to recall an unfamiliar one used the previous week. If a nursing student is to give an injection but has not performed the procedure for three months, the instructor will need to brief the student before the injection is given to the patient. As people age they may have difficulty with short-term memory, unless new information is related to previously learned material and applied in practice. Recognizing the law of recency, the teacher should plan a summary for a lesson or an effective conclusion for a lecture which restates or reemphasizes important matters, to make sure the adult learner remembers them.

All the laws of learning are not apparent in every learning situation. These laws manifest themselves singly or in groups; it is not important to determine which law operates in what situation. However, understanding the laws of learning aids a teacher in dealing intelligently with motivation, participation, and individual differences, the three major factors that affect learning.

Motivation is the force that causes a person to move toward a goal; the participation factors mean that students learn best when they are active; the individual difference factor indicates that students learn differently based on differences in intelligence, cultural background, experience, interests, desire to learn, and countless other psychosocial, emotional, and physical factors.

ROLE OF THE TEACHER IN ADULT EDUCATION

Nurse managers who use the principles of adult education, are facilitators more than teachers. Their role is primarily to design procedures that facilitate the acquisition of knowledge, attitudes, and skills by the learners. The facilitator links learners with content resources such as peers, knowledgeable people in the community, and media and material resources. Carl Rogers believes that educators are facilitators and sharply attacks the concept of teacher as used in pedagogical theory:

> Teaching in my estimation is a vastly overrated function. Having made such a statement, I scurry to the dictionary to see if I truly mean what I say. "Teaching means to instruct." Personally I am not much interested in instructing another in what he should know or think. "To impart knowledge or skill." My reaction is, why not be more efficient, using a book or programmed learning? "To make to know." Here my hackles rise. I have no wish to make anyone know something. "To show, guide, direct." As I see it, too many people have been shown, guided, directed. So, I come to the conclusion that I do mean what I said. Teaching is for me, a relatively unimportant and vastly overvalued activity.[25]

The "critical moment" in performing the role of facilitator is the personal relationship between the educator and the learner. This relationship is dependent on the facilitator possessing certain attitudinal characteristics, such as the ability to be open, flexible, and spontaneous. This means facilitators are willing to answer questions and offer explanations. They expose their feelings, they state their opinions, and they respect the opinions of others. They display confidence in themselves and in the students. When educators tell students that they are partners in facilitating learning they create an atmosphere that stimulates exchange of ideas.

The andragogical approach demands that teachers feel at ease in situations in which they do not have complete control. They share with the students the tasks of goal setting, designing learning experiences, deciding on content, and evaluation. They must give up dominant roles and instead assume roles of facilitators, experts, peers, and resource persons.

ROLE OF THE LEARNER IN ADULT EDUCATION

Students as well as teachers have to assume new roles as active participants who share responsibility for their own learning. At first these new roles will be uncomfortable for adults whose past educational experiences have taught them to be passive recipients of courses designed by others.

Nurse managers as teachers in staff development programs must be aware that learners vary in their degree of responsibility. They must be willing to help them become active participants. Learners' confidence increases when they learn how to design their own learning experiences and see their efforts leading to effective and exciting educational experiences.

EVALUATION PROCEDURES

Evaluation is essential to provide staff with information to improve programs or to determine if training programs should be continued or dropped. Each course, seminar, class, or workshop should be evaluated when it is completed to see if the program met the needs it was designed to meet. Evaluation includes both learner and program evaluation.

Learner Evaluation

Adult learners must have a sense of progress toward their goals and should be involved in evaluating their learning. Teachers should involve learners in developing mutually acceptable criteria and methods for measuring progress toward the learning objectives. If objectives are written in behavioral terms the standard for evaluation is included in each objective. It can then be observed whether the knowledge, skill, attitude, or practice is accomplished.

When measuring learning a before-and-after approach should be used so that learning can be related to the training program. If possible, learning should be measured objectively, as by a written test. Also, if practical, a control group should be compared with the experimental group that receives the training.

There are several types of techniques that can be used to evaluate learning:

1. Observation of skills or behavior is often useful. Observation guides need to be developed and observers need to be told specifically what they should be scrutinizing. Validity may be a problem if learners perform in a particular way because they are being observed, or if the perception of the observer is incorrect.

2. Paper-and-pencil methods such as true/false, multiple choice, or fill-in-the-blank tests are frequently used. Pretesting and post-testing should be done so comparison can be made. For some students tests produce anxiety which may contribute to poor test results.

3. Inobtrusive measures when used with other evaluation data can be valuable. Examples of inobtrusive measures are chart reviews, audits, wear of textbook pages, or numbers of staff using self-directed learning modules.

Program Evaluation

The content, process, and method of a program offering should be evaluated. A survey or questionnaire is often used to elicit information that indi-

FIGURE 20–8.   Evaluation Questionnaire

Purpose.   To provide feedback to program planners so presentations can be improved

Complete the following anonymously.

Evaluation of the Burn Therapy course: August 12. Circle the number representing your feelings about each statement.

	Strongly Disagree	Disagree	Agree	Strongly Agree	No Opinion
1. The content presented is applicable to my work.	1	2	3	4	5
2. The objectives of the program were clear to me.	1	2	3	4	5
3. The content presented reflected the objectives.	1	2	3	4	5
4. The content presented was what I expected.	1	2	3	4	5
5. The content was valuable to me.	1	2	3	4	5
6. The instructor's presentation was clear and informative.	1	2	3	4	5
7. The instructor made good use of audiovisuals.	1	2	3	4	5
8. The level of presentation was too theoretical.	1	2	3	4	5
9. The level of presentation was not practical.	1	2	3	4	5

Please respond to the following questions.

10. What were the most positive aspects of this presentation?

11. What did you like best about the presentation?

12. Please make any other comment or suggestion.

13. Suggestions for future presentations.

---

cates participants' reaction to the program. Information that can be obtained by a survey includes:

1. What the participants liked or disliked about the program.
2. Whether the faculty or speakers were prepared.
3. Whether objectives were met.
4. How well the offering was organized.
5. Whether the facilities were adequate.
6. Suggestions for improvements.
7. Suggestions for future offerings.

Problems arise if the questionnaires are too long or unwieldy for the participants or for the person who must tabulate them. Guides for preparing question-naires include:

1. Determine what you want to find out and avoid any unnecessary questions.
2. Design the form so that most reactions can be tabulated by a computer.
3. Make the form anonymous.
4. Give participants opportunity for additional comments.
5. Pilot-test the questionnaire on a simple target audience.

Figure 20–8 is an example of an evaluation questionnaire.

Use of Evaluation Data

Evaluation data can point out needed changes in the program or can indicate future educational needs. Evaluation can demonstrate if a program is worth-while and if it justified the expenditure of time and energy. Funding sources, board members, and ad-ministrative superiors require evaluation data for decisions about support of the staff development programs.

Evaluation data can be used as a public relations marketing tool to enhance the image of the pro-gram. Favorable participant comments can be pub-lished.

Evaluation studies can be published in journals so others can learn from the data if they are plan-ning similar programs. Comparison data can be beneficial for future program planning.

SUMMARY

The purposes of staff development include the improvement of care given to clients and the im-provement of participants' quality of life. Nurse managers who present successful staff development programs understand and apply the laws of learn-ing and principles of adult education. Staff mem-bers as adult learners are self-directing and want to be involved in diagnosing their learning needs, developing objectives, and evaluating their own learning. They have a wide variety of experiences on which to build new learning and they are looking for experiential types of teaching techniques that

allow them to share their knowledge. They want educational programs which are problem-centered and which they can apply in their work or life roles. Nurse managers as teachers in staff development programs are facilitators of learning. This role is enhanced if the educator possesses certain at-tributes such as openness, flexibility, and sponta-neity.

NOTES

1. C. E. Smith, "Planning, Implementing, and Evaluating," *Nurse Educator*, Nov.-Dec. 1978, 31–36.
2. K. Cross, *Adults as Learners* (San Francisco: Jossey-Bass, 1982), 16.
3. M. Knowles, *The Adult Learner: A Neglected Species*, 2d ed. (Houston: Gulf Publishing, 1978).
4. Ibid.
5. R. Boshier, "Motivational Orientations of Adult Education Participants: A Factor Analytic Exploration of Howle's Ty-pology," *Adult Educational Journal*, Feb. 1971, 3–26.
6. G. Morrow-Winn, "Elements of Staff Development," *Journal of the American Health Care Association*, Sept. 1981, 19–26.
7. Ibid.
8. M. Knowles, *Andragogy in Action* (San Francisco: Jossey-Bass, 1984).
9. M. Moore and P. Dutton, "Training Needs Analyses," *Academy of Management Review*, July 1978, 532–545.
10. P. Yoder Wise, "Needs Assessment as a Marketing Strategy," *Journal of Continuing Education in Nursing*, Sept./Oct. 1981, 5–9.
11. E. Zebelman, K. Davis, and E. Larsen, "Helping Staff Nurses Use Learning Modules," *Nursing and Health Care*, April 1983, 198–199.
12. M. Knowles, *Andragogy in Action*, op. cit.
13. Ibid.
14. Ibid.
15. Ibid.
16. K. Cross, op. cit.
17. R. Wlodkowski, *Enhancing Adult Motivation to Learn* (San Francisco: Jossey-Bass, 1972), 33.
18. R. B. Lovell, *Adult Learning* (New York: John Wiley & Sons, 1980).
19. K. Cross, op. cit.
20. C. O. Howle, *The Design of Education* (San Francisco: Jossey-Bass, 1972), 33.
21. J. M. Keller, "Motivational Design of Instruction," in C. M. Riegeluth, Ed., *Instructional Design Theories and Models: An Overview of Their Current Status* (Hillsdale, NJ: Erlbaum, 1983).
22. T. Levin and R. Long, *Effective Instruction* (Alexandria, VA: Association for Supervision and Curriculum Development, 1981).
23. M. Knowles, *The Modern Practice of Adult Education: From Pedagogy to Andragogy*, 2d ed. (Chicago: Follet, 1980).
24. R. Wlodkowski, op. cit.
25. As cited in M. Knowles, *The Adult Learner*, op. cit.

Conflict Management

21

INTRODUCTION

Any organization in which people interact has a potential for conflict. Health-care institutions include many interacting groups: staff with staff, staff with patients, staff with families and visitors, staff with physicians, and so on. These interactions frequently lead to conflicts.

Conflict relates to human feelings including feelings of neglect, of being viewed as taken for granted, of being treated like a servant, of not being appreciated, of being ignored, and of being overloaded. It relates to a lack of self-esteem and not being treated as worthy. The individual's feelings build into anger to the point of rage. This results in overt behaviors like brooding, arguing, or fighting. The individual can let feelings and behavior get in the way of work. Productivity declines, sometimes purposefully, and mistakes are made.

CAUSES OF CONFLICT

Defiant Behavior

Defiant behavior can create conflict. It produces guilt feelings in the person to whom it is directed. The nurse manager should take the position that the person expressing defiance is responsible for the conflict. Defiance is a threat to rational dialogue; it violates the acceptable protocols for adult interaction.

The defiant person challenges the authority of the nurse manager through obstinate and intransigent behavior. This behavior may be both verbal or nonverbal.

Murphy describes three versions of the defier. The first of these is the Competitive Bomber who simply refuses to work. Such people mutter statements that translate into "go to the devil." They scowl and will even walk away from the nurse manager or off the job.[1] Competitive defiers can be aggressive underminers who plan deliberate assaults. They comment about unfair and terrible working conditions, manipulation, and lousy schedules. These behaviors are done to provoke managerial response. If they do not elicit a response, they sulk and pout to win the pity of peers or even higher management.

The second defier is the Martyred Accommodator, who uses malicious obedience. They work and cooperate but do so mockingly and contemptuously. They complain and criticize to enlist the support of others.

A third category of defier is the Avoider. These defiers avoid commitment and participation. They do not respond to the nurse manager. When conditions change they avoid participating.[2]

Stress

Conflict leads to stress, fear, anxiety, and disruption in professional relationships. These conditions can, in turn, increase the potential for conflict. Stressors include "having too little responsibility, lack of participation in decision making, lack of managerial support, having to keep up with increasing standards of performance, and coping with rapid technological change."[3] Stress costs in 1973 were estimated at 1 to 3 percent of the gross national product. If anything, they have risen since then.

Burnout is a result of stress. Nurse managers burn out maintaining a support system for the care givers. Clinical nurses burn out from trying to give high-quality nursing care.

Confrontation, disagreements, and anger are evidence of stress and conflict. Stress and conflict are caused by poorly expressed relationships among people, including unfulfilled expectations.

Stress in patients leads to iatrogenic ailments, complications, and delayed recovery. It may be created by depression and anxiety. Stressed staff cannot cope with stressed patients, and this leads to inefficiency, job dissatisfaction, and insensitive care. Ultimately the staff are provoked into conflict. They too can develop iatrogenic ailments, just like their patients. Families of patients can add to stress if they are not managed appropriately. Increased stress for patients and staff decreases effective use of time. Such problems increase patient care costs, as they increase the length of the illness and decrease nursing efficiency and effectiveness. The next time, the patients may go somewhere else for care, whether at

their own initiative or on the recommendations of physicians, relatives, friends, or acquaintances.[4]

Space

When nurses have to work in crowded spaces they must interact constantly with other staff members, visitors, and physicians. This is particularly true of crowded critical care units. Such conditions cause stress that leads to burnout and turnover.

Physician Authority

Physicians are trained to be in authority over nurses. Today's nurses want to be more independent, to have professional responsibility and accountability for patient care. They spend more time with patients than physicians do and often have valid proposals for altering therapeutic measures. Physicians sometimes ignore their suggestions, indicating they do not want feedback. Nurses become angry as their self-worth diminishes. Communication fails, particularly two-way communication.[5]

Beliefs, Values, and Goals

Incompatible perceptions or activities create conflict. This is particularly evident when nurses hold beliefs, values, and goals different from those of nurse managers, physicians, patients, visitors, families, administrators, and so on. Nurses' values may boil over into conflicts related to ethical issues involving "do not resuscitate" orders, callous statements that belittle human worth, abortion, abuse, AIDS, and other problems. Personal goals frequently conflict with organizational goals, particularly with regard to staffing, scheduling, and the climate within which nurses work.

Nurses who have to violate their personal standards will lash out at the system. This is demeaning to them and causes loss of self-esteem and emotional stress. They must know that they are valued; that their beliefs, values, and personal goals are respected. Like other people, nurses act to protect their personal or public images when confronted or invaded. They respond in terms of other people's expectations of them, as they want approval. They will defend their rights and their professional judgments. The ego is easily bruised and becomes a big problem in conflict. Defense becomes more heated when one or both parties to conflict are uninformed or manipulated. When nurses are not recognized or respected they feel helpless, and they feel hopeless when they are unable to control the situation.[6]

Other Causes[7]

Change creates conflict that in turn impedes change. People who are not prepared for change will fight it or fail to support it. They are threatened.

Organizational climates and leadership style can create conflict if different managers set conflicting rules. Disciplinary problems can result from inadequate orientation and training and poor communication.

Off-the-job problems affect work performance, leading to disciplinary problems and conflict. These include marital discord, drug use, alcoholism, mental stress, and financial problems.

Age can create stress and conflict. As employees age, they resent increased scrutiny of their work. Clinical nurses cannot always keep up with physical demands of work as they grow older. They become fearful of being able to compete with younger nurses and build up resentment that can lead to conflict.

Nurse managers are professional managers and directors of clinical nursing practice. They must cope with forces internal and external to the nursing organization. Pressures include cost containment, effectiveness of patient care, collective bargaining, consumer awareness and involvement, regulatory agencies, entry-level qualifications, scope of practice, and mandated continuing education.

Computers are replacing many activities of middle managers in business and industry. Centrally controlled departments are being replaced with ad hoc forces, project teams, and small, autonomous business units. This results in downsizing within the organization, with decentralization and fewer levels of management, thus increasing pressures to increase output without increasing the number of managers. Managers face increased accountability and more demanding performance evaluations. The remaining managers become anxious, insecure, and doubtful about the future, resulting in malaise and conflict. As hospitals implement nursing management information systems, this situation can affect nurse managers.

People who have been discriminated against, such as racial minorities, may have "chips on their shoulders" and resent real or imagined slights. They may respond with confrontation, defensiveness, anger, and other conflict-producing behaviors. Persistent racial prejudice and discrimination are also an important source of workplace conflict.

CONFLICT MANAGEMENT

Discipline

In using discipline to manage or prevent conflict, the nurse manager must know and understand the organization's rules and regulations. If they are not clear, the nurse manager should seek help to clarify them. Discipline is the last resort in correcting undesirable employee behavior. Rules and regulations must be reasonable and work-related. Rules that are unreasonable or reflect personal biases invite infractions.

The following rules will help in managing discipline:

1. Discipline should be progressive.
2. The punishment should fit the offense, be reasonable, and increase in severity for violation of the *same* rule.
3. Assistance should be offered to resolve on-the-job problems.
4. Tact should be used in administering discipline.
5. The best approach for each employee should be determined. Managers should be consistent and should not show favoritism.
6. The individual should be confronted and not the group. Disciplining a group for a member's violation of rules and regulations makes them angry and defensive, increasing conflict.
7. Discipline should be clear and specific.
8. It should be objective, sticking to facts.
9. It should be firm, sticking to the decision.
10. Discipline produces varied reactions. If emotions are running too high, a second meeting should be scheduled.
11. The nurse manager performing the discipline should consult with her supervisor. One should expect to be overruled sometimes. Knowing the boundaries of authority and the supervisor will avoid most overrules.
12. A nurse manager should build respect, trust, and confidence in his ability to handle discipline.[8]

Considering Life Stages

Most organizations will include nurses at all life stages. Conflict can be managed by supporting individual nurses in achieving goals that pertain to their life stage. Three developmental stages are:

1. The young adult stage. This is the stage during which the nurse is establishing a career. People at this stage pursue knowledge, skills, and upward mobility. Conflict may be prevented or managed by facilitating career advancement.

2. The middle age, during which the nurse becomes reconciled with his achievement of life's goals. This nurse helps to develop careers of younger nurses.

3. After age 55, adults integrate their own ego ideals with their accomplishments. At this stage the nurse is thinking in terms of completing her work and retiring.[9]

Communication

Communication is an art essential to maintaining a therapeutic environment. It is necessary to accomplishing work and resolving social and emotional issues. Supervisors prevent conflict with effective communication and should make it a way of life. To promote communication that prevents conflict:

1. Teach nursing staff effective communication and their role in it.
2. Provide factual information to everyone—be inclusive, not exclusive.
3. Consider all aspects of a situation—emotions, environmental considerations, verbal and nonverbal messages.
4. Develop basic skills of:
   4.1 Reality orientation, by direct involvement and acceptance of responsibility in resolving conflict.
   4.2 Physical and emotional composure.
   4.3 Having positive expectations that generate positive responses.
   4.4 Active listening.
   4.5 Giving and receiving information.[10]

Active Listening. Active or assertive listening is essential to managing conflict. To be sure the per-

ceptions of nurse managers are correct, they can paraphrase what the angry or defiant employee is saying. Paraphrasing clarifies the message for both. It can help to cool off the situation as it gives the employee time and opportunity to hear the supervisor's perception of the emotions expressed.

Active or assertive listening is sometimes called stress listening. Powell suggests these techniques for stress listening:

1. Do not share anger; it adds to the problem. Remain calm and matter-of-fact.
2. Respond constructively in both verbal and nonverbal language. Be cheerful but sober. Maintain eye contact. Prevent interruptions. Bring the problem into the open. Make the employee comfortable. Act serious. Always be courteous and respectful.
3. Ask questions and listen to the answers. Determine the reasons for the anger.
4. Separate fact from opinion, including your own.
5. Do not respond hastily. Plan a response.
6. Consider the employee's perspective first.
7. Help the employee find the solution. Ask questions and listen to responses. Do not be paternalistic.[11]

Solving problems of angry confrontation requires stress listening. The nurse manager guides the process to a joint solution.

Quality Circles

Quality circles have been used to reduce stress by increasing employee motivation. They have been used with participatory management, membership in standing committees, leadership development programs, exercise classes, career ladders, job enrichment, and nursing grand rounds. These programs reduced turnover from 37.6 percent in 1980 to 20 percent in 1982 at one hospital.[12]

Assertiveness Training

Assertive nurses, including managers, will stand up for their rights while recognizing those of others. They are straightforward, being free to be themselves. Assertive nurses know they are responsible only for their own thoughts, feelings, and actions. They can help others deal with their anger and thus prevent conflict. They know their strengths and limitations. Rather than attack or defend assertive nurses, the nurse manager should assess, collaborate, and support, remaining neutral and nonthreatening. They can then accept challenges.

Assertiveness can be taught through staff development programs. In these programs nurses are taught to make learned, thoughtful responses. They learn to accept responsibility rather than blame others. They learn when to say "no," even to the boss. They learn to hold people to a standard. When they are dissatisfied they do something to increase their satisfaction. Most of these assertive behaviors can be learned with case studies, role playing, and group discussion.

When they finish their training, assertive nurses will reinforce their expectation that others will do their job by positive comments. Praise and consideration promote wellness and positive individual behavior, which are linked to effective management and communication. Nurse managers learn that direct communication of support to the staff increases their job satisfaction.

Assertive nurses focus on data and issues when offering constructive criticism to the boss or constructive feedback to the staff. This encourages dialogue and produces solutions to problems rather than conflict. They ask for assistance or for delay when it is needed.

People usually respond positively to assertion and negatively to aggression. Some people respond negatively to assertion.[13]

Assessing the Dimensions of the Conflict

Greenhalgh[14] has developed a system for assessing the dimensions of a conflict. His view is that conflict may be considered to be managed when it does not interfere with ongoing functional relationships. Participants in a conflict have to be persuaded to rethink their views. A third party must understand the situation empathetically from the participants' viewpoints. The conflict may be the result of a deeply rooted antagonistic relationship.

Greenhalgh's Conflict Diagnostic Model has seven dimensions, each with a continuum from "difficult to resolve" to "easy to resolve." Once the dimensions of the conflict have been assessed, those viewpoints that fall in the difficult-to-resolve domain should be shifted to the easy-to-resolve domain (see Table 21–1).

The Issue in Question. It has already been stated that values, beliefs, and goals are difficult issues to bring to a reasonable compromise. Principles fall into the same category, since they involve integrity and ethical imperatives. The third party must persuade the conflicting parties to acknowledge each other's legitimate point of view. How can principles be maintained but the organization and employees be saved?

The Size of the Stakes. The size of the stakes can make conflict hard to manage. If change threatens somebody's job or income, the stakes are high. The third party must try to keep egos from being hurt, postponing action if necessary. What will the parties settle for? Precedents create potential for future conflicts: "If I give in now, what will I have to give up in the future?"

Interdependence of the Parties. People must view resources in terms of interdependence. If one group sees no benefits from the distribution of resources, they will be antagonistic. A positive-sum interdependence of mutual gain is needed.

Continuity of Interaction. Long-term relationships reduce conflict. Managers should opt for continuous, not episodic, interaction.

Structure of the Parties. Strong leaders who unify constituents to accept and implement agreements reduce conflict. When informal coalitions occur, involve their representatives to find and implement agreements.

Involvement of Third Parties. Conflicts are difficult to resolve when participants are highly emotional resorting to distorting nonrational arguments, unreasonable stances, impaired communication, or personal attacks. Such conflicts can be solved with a prestigious, powerful, trusted, and neutral third party. The third party can be an outside consultant, mediator, or arbitrator. The inside manager who acts as judge or arbitrator polarizes; inviting a third party makes it public. Third parties have to be involved when the nurse manager, as party to a conflict, cannot resolve it.

TABLE 21–1. Conflict Diagnostic Model

Dimension	Viewpoint Continuum	
	Difficult to Resolve	Easy to Resolve
Issue in Question	Matter of Principle	Divisible issue
Size of stakes	Large	Small
Interdependence of the parties	Zero sum	Positive sum
Continuity of interaction	Single transaction	Long-term relationship
Structure of the parties	Amorphous or fractionalized, with weak leadership	Cohesive, with strong leadership
Involvement of third parties	No neutral third party available	Trusted, powerful, prestigious, and neutral
Perceived progress of the conflict	Unbalanced: One party feeling the more harmed	Parties having done equal harm to each other

Perceived Progress of the Conflict. Parties should be convinced that the score is equal and enough suffering has occured.

TECHNIQUES OR SKILLS FOR MANAGING CONFLICT

Aims

When involved in managing conflict, the nurse manager must aim for broadening of understanding about problems. Help the parties to see the big picture rather than the limited perspectives of each party. Aim to increase the possible number of alternatives in resolving the conflict. If possible, encourage conflicting parties to voice several possibilities acceptable to each. Then work on a compromise. This stimulates their interaction and involvement, another aim of conflict management. Other aims include better decisions and commitment to decisions that have been made.

Strategies[15]

Avoidance. Avoidance is a strategy that allows conflicting parties to cool down. The nurse manager involved in a conflict can sidestep the issue by saying, "Let's both take time to think about this and set a date for a future talk." This approach allows both parties to cool down and gather information. Avoidance can be used when the issue is not critical or when the potential damage of immediate confrontation outweighs the benefits. In the latter case a third party may have to be involved. Certainly the nurse manager as third party can tell the parties to a conflict, "I want you both to go on with your work while I take time to determine the facts and analyze them." Then set a not-too-distant date for the future meeting.

Accommodation. The nurse manager who is party to a conflict can accommodate the other party by yielding and placing the other's needs first. This is a particularly good strategy when the issue is more important to the other person. It maintains cooperation and harmony and develops subordinates by allowing them to make decisions.

Competition. A nurse manager as supervisor can exert position power at a subordinate's expense. This enforces the rule of discipline. It is an assertive position that does not foster commitment to conflict resolution on the part of the subordinate.

Compromise. Taking a middle ground may resolve a conflict. It should be a temporary strategy when time is needed to work out a permanent satisfactory position. A compromise that leaves both parties dissatisfied is not a good one.

Collaboration. When both parties collaborate to resolve conflict, they will both be satisfied. This is especially true of important issues. There should be integration of insights. This takes time and energy. A consensual solution wins full commitment.

One of the areas in which collaboration could resolve conflict is that of physician-nurse relationships. In one study undertaken "to examine the personal organizational and managerial factors that contribute to nurse-physician collaboration on patient care units," the findings were:

1. There was a weak inverse relationship between collaboration and length of employment (personal factor).
2. There was no significant relationship between collaboration and education (personal factor).
3. Although turnover was low due to system's rewards, productivity was low also (organizational factor).
4. There was low physician involvement in hospital's affairs (organizational factor).
5. There was a significant positive relation between primary nursing and collaboration (organizational factor).
6. There was greater collaboration on critical care units (organizational factor).
7. Collaboration and trust were increased by open communication, managed conflict, and meetings (managerial factor).
8. Collaboration increased with control of organizational stress (managerial factor).
9. Orientation, in-service education, and discussion with all groups produced positive collaboration (managerial factor).
10. Positive collaboration was related to standardization of work and skills, supervision, mutual adjustment, and group methods including rounds (managerial factor).[16]

One could conclude that collaboration leads to satisfaction among nurses. Collaboration can be better achieved through managerial factors and organizational factors than through personal factors.

Specific Skills

The following is a list of skills to use in managing conflict. Many are preventive.

1. Establish clear rules or guidelines and make them known to all.
2. Create a supportive climate with a variety of options. This makes people feel comfortable to make suggestions. It energizes them, promoting creative thinking and leading to better solutions. It strengthens relationships.
3. Tell people they are appreciated. Praise and confirmation of worth are important to everyone for job satisfaction.
4. Stress peaceful resolution rather than confrontation. Build a bridge of understanding.
5. Confront when necessary to preserve peace. Do so by educating people about their behavior. Tell them the behavior you perceive, what is wrong with it, and how it needs to be corrected.
6. Play a role that does not create stress or conflict. Do not play an ambiguous and fluctuating role that creates confusion among employees.
7. Judge timing that is best for all. Do not postpone indefinitely.
8. Keep the focus on issues and off personalities.
9. Keep communication two-way. Tune into the message, to correct interpretation, and to the feeling level of the employee. Reassure people by listening to them unload and dump. What is the real problem?
10. Emphasize shared interests.
11. Separate issues and confront those that are important to both parties.
12. Examine all solutions and accept the one most acceptable to both parties.
13. Avoid overriding your better judgment, becoming defensive, reprimanding the individual, cutting off further expression of feelings, and monopolizing the conversation. These responses increase frustration and are ineffective management techniques.
14. If conflict is evident at the decision-making or implementation stages, work to reach an agreement. Commit to a course of action serving some interests of all parties. Seek agreement rather than power.
15. Understand barriers to cooperation or resolution and focus on the dynamics of conflict to resolve it.

16. Distinguish between defiant behavior and normal on-the-job mistakes. Defiance is usually an individual behavior. Determine who the defier is and prepare for the confrontation emotionally and intellectually. Deal with one defiant person at a time. Establish authority and competence. Interview privately; teach, evaluate, resolve, guide, and deal with the defier. Do this immediately and follow up in two days. Discuss behavior and consequences including possible termination, keeping calm and steady. Assume adults have a sense of courtesy and cooperation. When challenged, respond on the spot and stand your ground. Then move to a private area or remove yourself from the scene.

17. Be a sponge to a charge by an angry person.

18. Determine who owns the problem. Take responsibility for it as if you own it and say thanks.

19. Determine needs that are being ignored or frustrated and need recognition and nurturing.

20. Help distinguish demands from dreams.

21. Build trust by listening, clarifying, and allowing the challenges to unwind completely. Give feedback to make sure you understand. Let people know you care and that you trust them. Indicate recognition of other viewpoints and willingness to work to improve the relationship. Be factual. Ask for feedback. Work out a common bridge of "must" items. If a staff nurse or other employee has a valid point, recognize it, apologize if need be, and be genuine.

22. Renegotiate problem-solving procedure to forestall further anger, distrust, and defensiveness.[17]

RESULTS OF CONFLICT MANAGEMENT

If attention is given to the role of the nurse manager in creating a climate for productive work by nurses, many of the causes of conflict will be eliminated. Knowledge of and skill in managing conflict when it occurs is an active role of nurse managers.

Zemke indicates that stress and work pressure in themselves are stimulating. They make managers more positive, more upbeat, and more concerned about their employees. In his survey he found that downsizing motivates good performance, improves output, and eliminates nonproductive jobs that can cause morale problems and conflict. With changes in the reimbursement system for hospitals, nurse managers will be confronted with stress, work pressure, and downsizing.[18]

Nurse managers cannot be bypassed in resolving conflicts. A study of conflicts between management and unions in the Engineering and Water Supply Department of Australia resulted in initiation of participatory management activities. To avoid alienation of managers, they and the workforce were involved in a democratic relationship. A pilot study was done in which a committee was formed to focus on safety and potential losses. Minutes went to everyone. As a result there was a 20 percent drop in the accident rate compared with the previous 5-year average. There was also more effective identification of training needs and more effective communication. A conclusion is that when managers and employees work together, communicate with each other, and all receive the same information, much conflict disappears or is resolved.[19]

Conflict can be a positive source of energy and creativity; it can be constructive when properly managed. Otherwise conflict can become dysfunctional and destructive, draining energy and reducing both personal and organizational effectiveness.

Conflict can destroy initiative or creativity and cause hostile and disruptive behavior, loss of team spirit, and loss of the desire to work toward common goals, resulting in deadlocks and stalemates. Managed conflicts do not escalate.[20]

SUMMARY

The interrelationships among nurses and other personnel, patients, and families offer many potentials for conflict. For this reason nurse managers should know how to manage conflict.

Causes of conflict include defiant behavior, stress, crowded space, physician authority, and incompatibility of values and goals.

Conflict can be prevented or managed by discipline, consideration of people's life stages, communication including active listening, use of quality circles, provision of assertiveness training for nurse managers, and assessment of the dimensions of the conflict.

Aims of conflict management include broadening understanding about problems, increasing alternative resolutions, and achieving a workable consensus on decisions and genuine commitment to decisions made. Specific strategies include avoidance, accommodation, competition, compromise, and collaboration. In addition nurse managers can learn and use specific skills to prevent and manage conflict.

Conflict management keeps conflict from escalating, makes work productive, and can make conflict a positive or constructive force.

NOTES

1. E. C. Murphy, "Managing Defiance," *Nursing Management*, May 1984, 67–69.
2. Ibid.
3. D. R. Faulconer and V. B. Goldman, "Managerial Stress," *Nursing Administration Quarterly*, Winter 1983, 32.
4. E. C. Murphy, "Communication and Wellness: Managing Patient/Staff Relationships," *Nursing Management*, Oct. 1984, 64–68.
5. G. S. Wlody, "Communicating in the ICU: Do You Read Me Loud and Clear?," *Nursing Management*, Sept. 1984, 24–27.
6. M. B. Silber, "Managing Confrontations: Once More into the Breach," *Nursing Management*, Apr. 1984, 54, 56–58.
7. E. C. Murphy, "Practical Management Course," *Nursing Management*, Mar. 1987, 76–77; American Hospital Association, *Role, Functions, and Qualifiactions of the Nursing Service Administrator in a Health-Care Institution* (Chicago: AHA, 1978); R. Zemke, "The Case of the Missing Managerial Malaise," *Training*, Nov. 1985, 30–33; M. A. Palich, "What Supervisors Should Know About Discipline," *Supervisory Management*, Oct. 1983, 21–24; and L. Greenhalgh, "SMR Forum: Managing Conflict," *Sloan Management Review*, Summer 1986, 45–51.
8. M. A. Palich, op. cit.
9. E. C. Murphy, "Practical Management Course," op. cit.
10. E. C. Murphy, "Communication and Wellness," op. cit.
11. J. T. Powell, "Stress Listening: Coping with Angry Confrontations," *Personnel Journal*, May 1986, 27–29.
12. D. R. Faulconer and V. B. Goldman, op. cit.
13. C. C. Clark, "Assertiveness Issues for Nursing Administrators and Managers," *Journal of Nursing Administration*, July 1979, 20–24.
14. L. Greenhalgh, op. cit.
15. H. K. Baker and P. I. Morgan, "Building a Professional Image: Handling Conflict," *Supervisory Management*, Feb. 1986, 24–29.
16. A. C. Alt-White, M. Charns, and R. Strayer, "Personal Organizational and Managerial Factors Related to Nurse-Physician Collaboration," *Nursing Administration Quarterly*, Fall 1983, 8–18.
17. H. K. Baker and P. I. Morgan, op. cit.; E. C. Murphy, "Practical Management Course," op. cit.; R. Lamkin, "Communicating Effectively," *B&E Review*, July 1984, 16; H. K. Baker and P. I. Morgan, "Building a Professional Image: Using 'Feeling Level' Communication," *Supervisory Management*, Jan. 1986, 20–25; E. C. Murphy, "Managing Defiance," op. cit.; L. Greenhalgh, op. cit.; and M. B. Silber, op. cit.
18. R. Zemke, op. cit.
19. D. Filmer, "Improving Communications in Large Organizations," *Work and People*, Feb. 1985, 12–14.
20. H. K. Baker and P. I. Morgan, "Building a Professional Image: Handling Conflict," op. cit.

REFERENCES

Levenstein, A., "Negotiation versus Confrontation," *Nursing Management*, January 1984, 52–53.

Swansburg, R. C., and P. W. Swansburg, *Strategic Career Planning and Development for Nurses* (Rockville, MD: Aspen, 1984).

Templeton, J., "For Corporate Vigor, Plan a Fight Today," *Sales Management, The Marketing Magazine*, June 15, 1969, 32–36.

Controlling or Evaluating

INTRODUCTION

The final element of management discussed by Fayol was control. He defined control as:

> verifying whether everything occurs in conformity with the plan adopted, the instructions issued, and principles established. It has for its object to point out weaknesses and error in order to rectify them and prevent recurrence.[1]

Controlling or evaluating was defined by Urwick as "seeing that everything is being carried out in accordance with the plan which has been adopted, the orders which have been given, and the principles which have been laid down."[2] Urwick referred to three principles:

1. The principle of uniformity ensures that controls are related to the organizational structure.
2. The principle of comparison ensures that controls are stated in terms of the standards of performance required, including past performance. In this sense controlling means setting a mark and examining and explaining the results in terms of the mark.
3. The principle of exception provides summaries that identify exceptions to the standards.[3]

It is important that controlling be done on a factual basis. When issues arise people should be made to meet with each other and settle them through direct contact. To stimulate cooperation, they need to participate from the beginning. Nurse managers can teach people to cooperate across departmental lines and to let reason and common sense prevail.[4] Management authors, including nurses, have described the controlling process as follows:

1. Establish standards for all elements of management in terms of expected and measurable outcomes. These are the yardsticks by which achievement of objectives are measured.
2. Apply the standards by collecting data and mea-

suring the activities of nursing management, comparing standards with actual care.

3. Make any improvements deemed necessary from the feedback.
4. Keep the process continuous for all areas including:
   4.1 Management of the nursing division and each subunit.
   4.2 Performance of personnel.
   4.3 Nursing process/product.[5]

This may be expressed as a formula:

$$Ss + Sa + F + C \longrightarrow I$$

Standards set plus Standards applied plus Feedback plus Correction will yield Improvement.

CONTROLLING AS A FUNCTION OF NURSING MANAGEMENT

Dovovan is one of the few nursing authorities who has written of controlling as a major function of nursing management. Other authors have expended considerable space devoted to quality assurance and performance evaluation. Dovovan stated that control is "the sum of the findings of the means in use to determine whether the goal is being achieved."[6] Control includes coordination of numerous activities, decision making related to planning and organizing activities, and information from directing and evaluating each worker's performance. Control is also viewed as being concerned with records, reports, organizational progress toward aims, and effective use of resources. Kron and Gray indicated that control uses evaluation and regulation, whereas other authors have suggested that controlling is identical to evaluation.[7] Koontz and Weihrich defined controlling as "the measurement and correction of the performance in order to make sure that enterprise objectives and the plans devised to attain them are accomplished."[8]

Systems Theory

Feedback and adjustment comprise the control element of nursing management. Output is described or defined in terms of the patient in the patient care model and is measured by quality assurance indicators. In case management these indicators are predicted and met on a timed basis. Discharge planning will take note of them. When the outcomes or indicators fall short the information is fed back to the clinical nurses who make adjustments in the case management plan and the process controlled by the critical path. Both the patient and the nurse are system inputs, while throughput consists of nursing actions related to patient outcomes and managerial actions related to setting goals for nurses' behavior. Quality assurance is the process by which the nursing product or process is measured and action prescribed to correct deficiencies.

Similarly, systems theory can be applied to performance evaluation of the registered nurse as output. Input is still the patient and the nurse, with throughput the managerial actions related to goals for nurses' behavior. A performance results contract between the clinical nurse and nurse manager spells out agreed-upon performance goals or results. When they are not being met the nurse manager discusses the deficiency with the clinical nurse and they agree upon corrective actions. In an open system the process is continuous.

Management's job is not complete with satisfaction of nursing values; the management values of efficiency and economy must also be addressed. An effective control system has standards, measuring tools, and a surveillance process culminating in corrective action. A quality control program for measuring patient care will have these same components.[9]

Controlling is the second physical act of administration, the first physical act being directing. It is the fourth and final element of the Administrative Composite Process (ACP), planning and organizing being the conceptual acts. All functions of management—planning, organizing, directing, and controlling—occur simultaneously. Inputs include resources other than the clinical nurse,[10] such as supplies, equipment, and plant: all of the direct and indirect cost elements used in achieving the outputs. Nurse managers will use staffing reports, budget status reports, and other information to control the functioning system. These reports are both monitoring devices and feedback to the clinical nurses and care managers.

Controls as Management Tools

In the process of measuring the degree to which predetermined goals are achieved and applying necessary corrective actions to improve performance, policies and procedures are used as standards. Also, observations, questions, patient charts, patients, and health-care team members serve as sources of data. Corrective actions can be corroborative, disciplinary, or educational.[11] In the process of feedback, a positive experience will stimulate motivation and contribute to the growth of employees.[12]

Controls are management tools for improving performance. Among the controls are rules which are needed to let people know what is expected of them and how functions can be coordinated. Communication as information is essential to control. Self-control is essential to managerial control as it is the highest form of control. Self-control includes being up to date in knowledge, giving clear orders, being flexible, understanding reasons for behavior, helping others improve, increasing skills of problem solving, staying calm under pressure, and planning ahead. People should be told the facts in language that they understand and words that have the intended meaning. Effective nursing managers set limits and make them known to their employees. Then when the line is crossed the appropriate disciplinary action should be taken. The latter is achieved by corrective action that is consistently applied after checking the facts.[13]

Controls can be separated into two elements, mechanical and sociological. There are three stages of control, the first two being the mechanical elements: (1) a predetermined definition of standards for a level of performance, and (2) measurement of current performance against the standards. The third, taking corrective action if it is indicated, is the sociological element.[14] Nurse managers will avoid the unintended consequence of control, noncompliance. Since control can be perceived as a threat from unwanted power and authority, it can trigger defense mechanisms such as aggression, repression, and others. Lemin advocated the following of McGregor's approaches to control: (1) time, (2) a high degree of mutual trust, (3) a high degree of mutual support, (4) open and authentic communications, (5) clear understanding of objectives, (6) respect for differences, (7) utilization of member resources, and (8) a supportive environment. These approaches will lead to conflict resolution, changed beliefs and attitudes, genuine innovation, genuine commitment, strengthened management, and prevention of unintended consequences of control.[15]

Ten characteristics of a good control system are:

1. Controls must reflect the nature of the activity.
2. Controls should report errors promptly.
3. Controls should be forward-looking.
4. Controls should point out exceptions at critical points.
5. Controls should be objective.
6. Controls should be flexible.
7. Controls should reflect the organizational pattern.
8. Controls should be economical.
9. Controls should be understandable.
10. Controls should indicate corrective action.[16]

Nurse managers will remain cognitive that the best way of ensuring the quality of nursing service provided in the patient units is to establish philosophy, standards of care, and objectives. At least two of these activities, philosophy and objectives, involve planning, further evidence that the major functions of management take place simultaneously.[17] Controlling mechanisms also include accreditation procedures, consultants, evaluation devices, rounds, reports, inspections, and nursing audits.[18]

Nurses activate the processes of control. This function involves the use of power and should be used by nurse managers to promote openness, honesty, trust, competence, and even confrontation. It involves value systems, ethical decision-making, self-control, professional self-regulation, and control by an aggregate of professionals. It is emerging as a system of quality control programs. The dimensions of quality assurance programs are quality of care including accessibility and beliefs and attitudes of patients about health care, structure of health care, processes of care, professional competence, outcomes of care, and self-regulation. Audits and budgets are the major techniques of control.[19]

Control functions can be differentiated among levels of managers. For example, the head nurse manager of a unit is concerned with short-range operational activities including daily and weekly schedules, assignments, and effective use of resources. This nurse manager also keeps records of absences and incidents and prepares personnel appraisals: control activities subject to quick changes.

Two methods of measurement are used to assess achievement of nursing goals: task analysis and quality control. In task analysis, the head nurse inspects the motions, actions, and procedures laid out in written guides, schedules, rules, records, and budgets. It is a study of the process of giving nursing care. It measures physical support only; relatively few tools have been developed to do task analysis in nursing. In quality control the head nurse is concerned with measurement of the quality and effects of nursing care. Mechanisms or models for doing this have been developed by the American Nurses Association (ANA), the Joint Commission on Accreditation of Healthcare Organizations (JCAHO), and others. Many quality assurance techniques are referred to as audits.[20]

STANDARDS

A prime element of the management of nursing services is a system for evaluation of the total effort. This includes a system for evaluation of the management process as well as the practice of nursing and all nursing care services. Evaluation requires standards that can be used as the yardsticks for gauging the quality and quantity of services. The key source for these standards, which are available for both management and practice, is the ANA, whose publications include *Standards for Organized Nursing Services and Responsibilities of Nurse Administrators Across All Settings* and *Standards of Nursing Practice.* Several functional yardsticks can be developed using these source documents. They can be of assistance in developing the objectives of the division of nursing and of each ward, unit, and clinic. Objectives are developed into operational or management plans, and systematic and periodic review of accomplishments of these objectives will be part of the evaluation system. In addition, a management evaluation system can be developed with a similar format. Further evaluation can be effected through development of criteria for nursing rounds by the nurse executive and other nurse managers. Performance standards can be used for individual performance, and criteria can be developed for collective evaluation of patient care. The latter may include the standards for use during nursing rounds as well as criteria for the quality assurance program.

Performance evaluation and quality assurance are dealt with in succeeding chapters. Standards are established criteria of performance, planning goals, strategic plans, physical or quantitative measurements of products, units of service, person-hours, speed, cost, capital, revenue, program, and intangible standards.[21] They have also been defined as "an acknowledged measure of comparison for quantitative or qualitative value, criterion, or norm," and as "a standard rule or test on which a judgement or decision can be based." Nurse managers develop, in collaboration with clinical nurses, the "clinical nursing criteria against which to measure patient outcomes and the nursing process."[22] These standards are stated as patient outcomes and as nursing care processes.

Koontz and Weihrich identified eight categories of standards:

1. Physical standards using patient acuity ratings to establish nursing hours per patient day.
2. Cost standards, of which the cost-per-patient day for supplies would be an example.
3. Capital standards, of which a new program of monetary investment, such as a patient teaching staff, would be a part.
4. Revenue standards, including the revenue per hour of nursing care received by patients.
5. Program standards, such as those designed to develop a new nursing service for changing peoples' behavior regarding exercise, eating, or other health activity.
6. Intangible standards, which could include staff development costs in nursing.
7. Goals are frequently used as standards in nursing management. Intangible standards are being replaced by goals, including those for qualitative measurements.
8. Strategic plans, as control points for strategic control. As nurse managers increase their involvement in strategic planning they will need to perform strategic control.[23]

Figure 22–1 shows an example of an evaluation plan for nursing services.

CONTROLLING TECHNIQUES

Although evaluation operational plans are controlling techniques, other specific controlling techniques can be developed including planned nursing

FIGURE 22–1.   Operational Plan

Mission Statement to Which Objective Applies.   The division of nursing has a stated philosophy and has objectives. Personnel of each department or unit within the division will have their own philosophy and will set up their own objectives. The objectives will be continuously evaluated and a written statement as to progress will be sent to the chair's office each August and February

Philosophy Statement to Which Objective Applies.   We believe that a continuous evaluation of the activities of the division of nursing is necessary to assess how effectively the needs of the patients are being met and to take action to improve nursing service when indicated. Research must be performed, and the results must be analyzed, adapted, and implemented to modify nursing procedures and practices for the attainment of more effective patient care.

Objective 6.   The patient benefits from close nursing supervision to all nonprofessional personnel who give patient care, and the patient benefits from continuous evaluation of the nursing care given and of performances of all nursing service personnel based on professional standards.

Plans for Achieving Objective	Action and Accountability	Target Dates	Accomplishments
1. Plan and execute a system of continuous evaluation and appraisal of nursing services	1. Make complete rounds throughout the hospital at least once a day from nursing office. Establish a system of formal nursing rounds by chair, assistants, and clinical nursing coordinators monthly.	Apr. 23, 1989	Doing.
	2. Do a monthly nursing audit. Have committee chair brief the chair of the division of nursing afterward.	Dec. 1, 1989	Criteria for 45 conditions completed; 10 more under development. Committee combined with other disciplines. Criteria applied to four conditions with retrieval by medical records personnel and corrective actions taken.
	3. Develop standards for patient care. Use ANA Standards of Nursing Practice for evaluating patient care. Obtain copies for all charge nurses.	Jan. 1, 1989	Obtained. Being developed into checklist by committee of staff nurses. Will cross-check with job performance standards.
	4. Develop standards for personnel performance.	Dec. 31, 1989	Completed for clinical nurses I, II and III, charge nurse, in-service education coordinator, clinical coordinator, chair and assistants, operating room supervisor and staff nurses, public health nurse, and rehabilitation nurse.
	5. Set up a system whereby supervisors attend: a. Change-of-shift reports.	Jul. 1, 1989	Receiving reports and need to plan for their use. Will discuss with supervisors.

Figure 22–1. Operational Plan (*continued*)

Plans for Achieving Objective	Action and Accountability	Target Dates	Accomplishments
	b. Unit conferences.		
	c. Unit in-service programs.		
	6. Review and use ANA *Standards for Organized Nursing Services and Responsibilities of Nurse Administrators Across All Settings* to develop an evaluation and inspection checklist.	Dec. 1, 1989	
2. Study organization	1. Reorganize as needed. Have organizational chart printed.	Jul. 1, 1989	Done as hospital policy.
	2. Write policy on unit policies and procedures.	Jul. 1, 1989	Done as nursing operating instruction 160-2-4.
3. Establish a counseling program for all nursing personnel.	1. Program counseling sessions for all head nurses. Have them do the same for those they supervise.	Jan. 1, 1989	All done once by Jan. 1, 1989.
	2. Use the job performance standards.		

rounds by nurse managers from all levels, checklists from ANA *Standards for Organized Nursing Service and Responsibilities of Nurse Administrators Across All Settings,* ANA *Standards of Nursing Practice,* JCAHO *Accreditation Manual for Hospitals,* and other published standards of third-party payers such as Medicare and Medicaid.

Nursing Rounds

An effective controlling technique for nursing managers is planned nursing rounds. They can be placed on a schedule and can include all nursing personnel. Rounds cover such issues as patient care, nursing practice, and unit management. To be effective, the results should be discussed with appropriate nursing personnel in a follow-up conference. Part of the evaluation process takes place as a result of the communication occurring during the rounds. Figure 22–2 shows a protocol for planned monthly nursing rounds.

Nursing Operating Instructions

Nursing operating instructions or policies become standards for evaluation as well as controlling techniques; see Figure 22–3.

The ANA *Standards for Organized Nursing Services and Responsibilities of Nurse Administrators Across All Settings* can be developed into a check list for evaluating the management processes of nursing services. See Exhibit 22–4 for an *excerpt* from these standards.

The ANA *Standards of Nursing Practice* can be implemented in several ways. One way is to convert these into a checklist and evaluate their use, as in Figure 22–5. The entire set of standards can be developed into a checklist along these lines.

Written protocols should be developed to implement a program for the evaluation process. Another way these protocols may be implemented is by using them to develop the evaluation standards, as in Figure 22–6.

FIGURE 22–2. Protocol for Planned Monthly Nursing Rounds

1. The chair, assistant chair, and other appropriate nursing personnel will make nursing rounds monthly.
2. Time is 10:00 to 11:00 A.M. unless otherwise indicated.
3. Schedule:

Ward	Day
1F	1st Tuesday
2A	1st Wednesday
2B	1st Thursday
2F	2nd Tuesday
ICU	2nd Wednesday
4A	2nd Thursday
3A	2nd Friday
3-OB	3rd Tuesday 10:30 to 11:30 A.M.
3F	3rd Wednesday
4B	3rd Thursday 11:00 A.M. to 12:00 noon
5A, CCU	4th Tuesday
5B	4th Wednesday

4. All unit nursing personnel are welcome to attend these rounds with their head nurse. Patient care needs come first. The following areas will be covered as rounds are made to each patient's bedside:
   a. Nursing histories.
   b. Nursing care plans.
   c. Nursing notes.
   d. Nurses' signatures on necessary documents.
5. Other management areas of note will be discussed after bedside rounds:
   a. Equipment and supplies.
   b. Staffing and assignments.
   c. Narcotic registers.

Gantt Charts

Early in this century, Henry L. Gantt developed the Gantt chart as a means of controlling production. It depicted a series of events essential to the completion of a project or program. It is usually used for production activities.

Figure 22–7 shows a modified Gantt chart that could be applied to a major nursing administration program or project. The five major activities that the nurse administrator has identified are segments of a total program or project. It could be applied to a project such as implementing a modality of primary nursing. These are possible nursing actions for such a project:

1. Gathering of data.
2. Analysis of data.
3. Development of a plan.
4. Implementation of the plan.
5. Evaluation, feedback, and modification.

Figure 22–7 is only an example. Application of this controlling process by nurse managers would be specific to the project or program, the time elements for the various activities varying with each. Also, these five major activities could be modified by using subcategories of activities with estimated completion times. The nurse manager's goal is to com-

FIGURE 22–3. Operating Instructions

1. Special care units will maintain policies and procedures relative to their mission. These procedures will be reviewed, updated, and signed at least annually.
   a. Intensive care unit.
   b. Critical care unit.
   c. Newborn/intensive care unit nursery.
   d. Renal dialysis.
2. Special care units will maintain a list of equipment needed to achieve their mission.
3. Supplies and equipment
   a. Blount resuscitator will have percent-adaptor to increase oxygen concentration.
   b. Ambu resuscitator will have tail on to increase oxygen concentration.
   c. Humidification will not be used with oxygen with Ambu resuscitator.
   d. Trays from Central Sterile Supply will be returned as soon as used so that instruments will not be lost or misplaced.

FIGURE 22–4. Checklist: Standards for Organized Nursing Services and Responsibilities of Nurse Administrators Across All Settings, Standard I

Standard I: Organized Nursing Services have a philosophy and structure that ensures the delivery of effective nursing care.

Criterion	Yes	No
1. The philosophy and structure are compatible with established professional standards, *Nursing: A Social Policy Statement* and *Code for Nurses with Interpretative Statements,* standards of regulatory agencies, and the mission of the organization within which nursing services are provided.		
2. The philosophy of organized nursing services provides to individual nurses the authority and accountability for the clinical management of nursing practice.		
3. The philosophy provides for a structure that facilitates participative management.		
4. A written organizational plan specifies lines of authority, accountability, and responsibility for all nursing personnel.		
5. The philosophy supports the representation and participation of nurses in professional organizations and community and governmental activities related to health care.		

SOURCE: Reprinted with permission from *Standards for Organized Nursing Services and Responsibilities of Nurse Administrators Across All Settings,* © 1988, American Nurses' Association, Kansas City, MO, p. 3.

FIGURE 22–5. Evaluation of Implementation of ANA Standards of Nursing Practice

---

Section: wd 3C
Date: Oct. 15, 1989
Evaluator: F. Jules, R.N.

Standard I: Assessment Factors

	Yes	No	Example
1. Collection of data about the status of the patient was systematic and continuous. The data were accessible, communicated, and recorded.			
a. Health status data collected included:			
Growth and development			
Biophysical status			
Emotional status			
Cultural, religious, socioeconomic background			
Performance of activities of daily living			
Patterns of coping			
Interaction patterns			
Patient's perception of and satisfaction with his health status			
Patient's health goals			
Environment (physical, social, emotional)			
Available and accessible human and material resources			

SOURCE: Reprinted with permission from *Standards of Nursing Practice,* © 1973, American Nurses' Association, Kansas City, MO, p. 3.

FIGURE 22–6. Standards for Evaluation of the Controlling (Evaluating) Function of Nursing Administration of a Division, Service, or Unit

1. An evaluation plan exists and is used for each nursing department, service, or unit.
2. Each evaluation plan is specific to the needs and activities of the individual department, service, or unit.
3. Evaluation findings are given in immediate feedback to subordinate nursing personnel.
4. Standards are accurate, suitable, and objective.
5. Standards are flexible and work when changes are made in plans and when unforeseen events and failures occur.
6. Standards mirror the organizational pattern of the nursing division, service, or unit.
7. Standards are economical to apply and do not produce unexpected results or effects.
8. Nursing personnel know and understand the standards.
9. Application of the standards results in correction of deficiencies.

plete each activity or phase *on or before* the projected date.

Milestones and Critical Control Points

Master evaluation plans should have critical control points. Critical control points are specific points in the production of goods or services at which the nurse administrator judges whether the objectives are being met, qualitatively and quantitatively.

They tell whether the plan is progressing satisfactorily. They pinpoint successes and failures and the causes. Critical control points tell managers whether they are on target with regard to time, budget, and other resources. Milestones are segments or phases of specific activities of a project or program that are projected to occur within a time frame.

Figure 22–8 represents a modified Gantt chart with networks of milestones and critical control points. The critical path is $1 \rightarrow 2 \rightarrow 3 \rightarrow 4 \rightarrow 5 \rightarrow 6 \rightarrow 7 \rightarrow 8 \rightarrow 9 \rightarrow 17 \rightarrow 18$. Line 5 represents evaluation of all other nursing actions.

This is a simplified illustration of control techniques. Case management also uses critical paths with milestones and control points. Any major nursing program could have dozens or even hundreds of milestones and critical control points. This system may also be known by the name PERT (program evaluation and review technique).

Application of the milestone technique involves establishing a network of controllable pieces in planning and controlling a project or program. Each piece of the project or program is also allocated a prorated portion of the total budget. A nurse manager could use this technique to evaluate the actual amount of estimated budget expenditure at the end of each step of activity (monthly) of the project or program. These will be the critical control points as each would culminate in the achievement of a milestone. Each event may represent a budgeting allocation, a time event or span, or a continuum of several or all of these. Bar graphs are frequently used to depict milestone budgeting. Budgeting is a major controlling technique in any of its forms.[24]

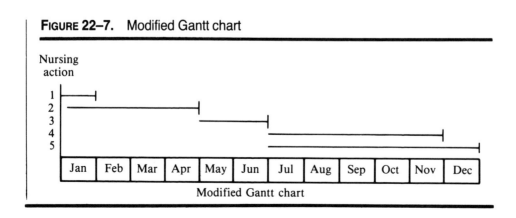

FIGURE 22–7. Modified Gantt chart

Nursing action

| | Jan | Feb | Mar | Apr | May | Jun | Jul | Aug | Sep | Oct | Nov | Dec |

Modified Gantt chart

FIGURE 22–8. Milestones and Critical Control Points

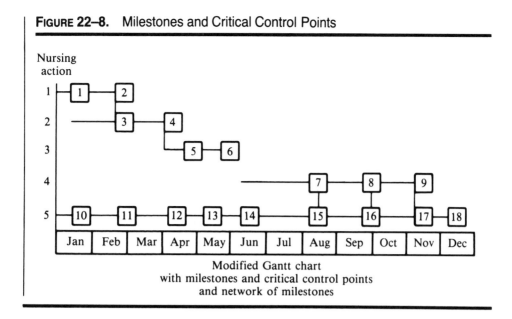

Modified Gantt chart
with milestones and critical control points
and network of milestones

Program Evaluation and Review Technique (PERT)

The program evaluation and review technique (PERT) was developed by the Special Projects Office of the U.S. Navy and applied to the planning and control of the Polaris weapon system in 1958. It worked then; it still works; and it has been widely applied as a controlling process in business and industry.

PERT uses a network of activities. Each activity is represented as a step on a chart. A time measurement and an estimated budget should be worked out including:

1. The finished product or service desired.
2. The total time and budget needed to complete the project or program.
3. The starting and completion dates.
4. The sequence of steps or activities that will be required to accomplish the project or program.
5. The estimated time and cost of each step or activity.
6. Three paths for steps 5 and 6:
   a. the optimistic time.
   b. the most likely time.
   c. the pessimistic time.
7. Calculation of the "critical path," the sequence of the events that would take the longest time to complete the project or program by the planned completion date. The reason this is the critical path is because it will leave the least slack time.[25]

Why should nurse managers use the PERT system for controlling? It forces planning and shows how pieces fit together. It does this for all nursing line managers involved. It establishes a system for periodic evaluation and control at critical points in the program. It reveals problems and is forward-looking. PERT is generally used for complicated and extensive projects or programs.

Many records are used to control expenses and otherwise conserve the budget. These include personnel staffing reports, overtime reports, monthly financial reports, expense and revenue reports, and others. All these reports should be available to nurse managers to help them monitor, evaluate, and adjust the use of people and money as part of the controlling process.[26]

MASTER CONTROL PLAN

A master controlling or evaluating plan can be used by nurse managers to fulfill this important management function. It can be a general plan for all with each manager adding specific items for their management area. A sample basic master control plan is depicted in Exhibit 22–9.

FIGURE 22–9. Master Controlling Plan

Objective 1.   Inspect for and identify the presence of written, current, and practical statements of mission, philosophy, and objectives for the division of nursing and each of its component units. They should reflect the purposes of the health-care organization and give direction to the nursing care program.

Actions
 1. The written statements of mission, philosophy, and objectives were current (reviewed or revised within past year).
 2. They existed for the division of nursing and for each department, ward, unit, and clinic.
 3. They were written by appropriate nursing personnel, representative of people who will accomplish them.
 4. The philosophy reflected the meaning of clinical practice.
 5. The philosophy was developed in collaboration with consumers, employees, and other health-care workers.
 6. The objectives were specified, written in behavioral terms, and achievable.
 7. They guided the process of implementing the philosophy.
 8. They were used for orientation of newly assigned personnel and were otherwise widely distributed and interpreted.
 9 They supported the mission, philosophy, and objectives of the institution.
 10. Nursing personnel knew the rights of individuals and served as advocates for these rights.

Objective 2.   Inspect for and identify the presence of written operational or management plans for accomplishment of the objectives of the division of nursing and each of its component units.

Actions
 1. The written operational or management plans were current (entries within past 30 days).
 2. They existed for the division of nursing and for each department, ward, unit, and clinic.
 3. They included specific actions to be taken to achieve objective, target dates, and names of personnel assigned responsibility for each action.
 4. They were used to evaluate progress; accomplishments were listed.

Objective 3.   Inspect for and identify the presence of an organizational plan for the division of nursing and each of its component units.

Actions
 1. The organizational plan was current; it agreed with actual organization when checked.
 2. It existed for the division of nursing and for each department, ward, unit, and clinic.
 3. It showed the relationships between component parts, spelling out the major functions of each, and it showed relationships with other services.
 4. The organizational plan supported the mission assigned to personnel.
 5. All nursing functions were managed by the nurse administrator.

Objective 4.   Inspect for and identify the presence of adequate policies and procedures for guidance of personnel of the division of nursing and each of its component units.

Actions
 1. Policies and procedures of the division of nursing and of each department, ward, unit, and clinic were current (reviewed within past year).
 2. Policies and procedures did not duplicate those of higher echelons.
 3. Policies and procedures were not obsolete, restrictive, or inappropriate in context.
 4. Content of location of policies and procedures was known by people who needed this information.

FIGURE 22–9. Master Controlling Plan (*continued*)

5. Policies and procedures for special care units included:
   a. Function and authority of unit director.
   b. Admission and discharge criteria.
   c. Criteria for performance of special procedures, including cardiopulmonary resuscitation, tracheostomy, ordering of medications, admistration of parenteral fluids and other medication, and the obtaining of blood and other laboratory specimens.
   d. The use, location, and maintenance of equipment and supplies.
   e. Respiratory care.
   f. Infection control.
   g. Priorities for orders for laboratory tests.
   h. Standing orders, if any.
   i. Regulations for visitors and traffic control.
6. The nursing annex to the disaster plan was current and included:
   a. Recall procedures.
   b. Assignment procedures.
   c. Training plan.

Objective 5.　Inspect for and identify the presence of job descriptions and job standards for all personnel throughout the division of nursing.

Actions
1. Job descriptions and job standards existed and were current throughout the division of nursing (reviewed within past year).
2. Nursing personnel participated in formulating them.
3. Nursing personnel were classified according to competence and salaries were commensurate with qualifications and positions of comparable responsibility within the agency and the community.
4. Job descriptions were used for purposes of counseling and helping employees to be productive.
5. They were used for orientation of newly assigned personnel.
6. They described the functions, qualifications, and authority of each position identified in the organizational plan.
7. They were readily available and known to each employee.
8. There was a designated nurse leader for the division of nursing who was a registered nurse with educational and experiential qualifications in nursing practice and the administration of nursing services.

Objective 6.　Inspect for and identify the presence of a master staffing plan for the division of nursing and each of its component units.

Actions
1. A master staffing plan existed and was current for the division of nursing and each department, ward, unit, or clinic. It showed authorized versus assigned personnel and was reviewed at least monthly.
2. Adequate personnel policies existed to give guidance to nursing personnel in the planning of time schedules and to allow for mobility so that personnel could be matched to jobs.
3. Avenues of communication existed to give input from nursing personnel to the nurse administrator regarding staffing problems.
4. An active plan existed for sponsoring newly assigned personnel and for identifying their special training and experience and their desired assignments.

Objective 7.　Inspect for and identify the presence of a planned counseling program for all personnel of the division of nursing.

(continued)

Figure 22–9. Master Controlling Plan (*continued*)

Actions

1. The nurse executive had a planned program for counseling with managers, including charge nurses.
2. Counseling occurred at least every 6 months on a scheduled basis.
3. Charge nurses counseled with individual staff members on a scheduled basis at least once every 6 months.
4. The counseling process included discussion of progress toward personal objectives and revisions resulted from the sessions. Job standards were reviewed and special educational and experience goals were discussed and acted on.
5. Records of counseling sessions were available and were reviewed.
6. A career progression plan was operational.

Objective 8. Inspect for and identify the presence of a system of evaluation of nursing activities in the division of nursing and each of its component units.

Actions

1. A system for evaluation of the division of nursing and each of its departments, wards, units, and clinics was in operation.
2. Change-of-shift reports and ward conferences were being periodically evaluated (at least once every 6 months).
3. Management plans indicated current evaluation of accomplishment of objectives (within past 30 days).
4. Management personnel, including the nurse executive, made planned ward rounds at least monthly and checked all aspects of department, ward, unit, or clinic management, including:
   a. Narcotic registers.
   b. Nursing histories.
   c. Nursing care plans.
   d. Nursing notes.
   e. Drug levels and security.
   f. Supplies and equipment.
   g. Assignment procedures.
   h. Patient records.
5. The quality assurance program was in effect, and at least one problem per month had been evaluated since June 1, 1989.
6. There was provision for inclusion of other health-care disciplines and consumers in evaluating the nursing care programs.
7. Results of evaluation were used to assess planning for change.

Objective 9. Inspect for and identify the representation of division of nursing personnel on institution-wide and departmental boards, committees, and councils.

Actions

1. The division of nursing was represented on institution-wide boards, committees, and councils whose activities affected nursing personnel directly.
   a. Social actions.
   b. Personnel boards such as awards and benefits.
2. Nursing service committees had specific objectives.
3. Membership was current and representative of all appropriate segments of the nursing staff.
4. Minutes of meetings reflected progress toward objectives and follow-up of problems.

Objective 10. Inspect for and identify the existence of a working public relations program that serves as a means of communication between personnel of the division of nursing and the community they serve.

Actions

1. Evaluation programs existed to tell consumers of the nursing services available to them and to receive feedback from consumers on the types of services they needed.

FIGURE 22–9. Master Controlling Plan (*continued*)

---

2. There was a planned program to publicize nursing activities and recognize contributions and accomplishments of nursing personnel.

Objective 11. Inspect for and identify the existence of a planned program for training and continuing education for all division of nursing personnel.

Actions

1. Written statements of mission, philosophy, and objectives existed and were current (reviewed within past year).
2. An operational or management plan for the accomplishment of objectives was current (entries made within past 30 days).
3. The plan listed activities, set priorities and target dates, assigned responsibility, and provided for continuous evaluation.
4. The plan provided for identification of training and continuing education needs, including input from participants, translation of needs into objectives, and the accomplishment of objectives.
5. An orientation program existed and included philosophy and objectives of organization and nursing service, personnel policies, job descriptions, work environment, clinical practice policies and procedures, and operational policies and procedures.
6. Supplemental classes were taught to meet on-the-job training needs.
7. Training programs were documented.
8. The program supported career advancement.

Objective 12. Inspect for and identify the existence of procedures and policies for providing needed primary nursing care to patients.

Actions

1. Collection of data on each patient was sufficient to permit identificaiton and assessment of the patient's needs and to institute an individual plan of care. Included were admission data and patient's nursing history.
2. The nursing care plans included the nursing diagnoses, prescriptions for care, and patients' teaching needs.
3. The plan was used to provide care to the patient, and there was an ongoing reassessment of the patient's needs with appropriate changes made in the plan of care.
4. There was evidence that nursing actions required by physicians' orders, plans of nursing care, and hospital policies were accomplished appropriately. Observations of patient's progress and response to actions were made and recorded.
5. There was evidence of interpretation and implementation of the ANA *Standards of Nursing Practice*.
6. Nursing administration had a plan for reviewing the requirements for giving credentials to individuals and health-care organizations and for participating in their implementaiton.
7. Guidelines existed for assignment of personnel based on level of competence.
8. There were policies to use unit managers and ward clerks to perform clerical, managerial, and indirect service roles.
9. Nursing administration provided resources to accomplish primary nursing care to patient: facilities, equipment, supplies, and personnel.

SUMMARY

Controlling or evaluating is an ongoing function of nursing management occurring during planning, organizing, and directing activities. Through this process standards are established and then applied, followed by feedback that leads to improvements. The process is kept continuous.

Each nurse manager should have a master plan of control that incorporates all standards related to these actions. This plan can be applied to obtain immediate feedback and meet the objectives of control established for the unit, department, or division. The plan will verify results, provide instructions, and apply principles of uniformity, comparison, and exception.

Controls include policies, rules, procedures, self-control or self-regulation, discipline, rounds, reports, audits, evaluation devices, task analysis, and quality control. They should reflect the nature of the activity and be forward-looking, objective, flexible, economical, and understandable. They should lead to continuous action.

Standards are the yardsticks for evaluation and include ANA *Standards for Organized Nursing Services and Responsibilities of Nurse Administrators Across All Settings* and *Standards of Nursing Practice.* Other standards include management plans, goals, programs, costs, revenues, and capital. Physical standards use Gantt charts, critical control points, milestones, and PERT. Each nurse manager should have a master evaluation plan.

NOTES

1. H. Fayol, trans., *General and Industrial Management* by C. Storrs (London: Sir Isaac Pitman & Sons, 1949), 107.
2. L. Urwick, *The Elements of Administration* (New York: Harper & Row, 1944), 105.
3. Ibid., 107–110.
4. Ibid., 113–117.
5. H. Koontz and H. Weihrich, *Management* (New York: Mc-Graw-Hill, 1988), 490–492; R. M. Fulmer and S. G. Franklin, *Supervision: Principles of Professional Management* (2d. ed. New York: Macmillan, 1982), 214–216. R. M. Hodgetts and D. F. Kuratko, *Management* (2d. ed. New York: Harcourt Brace Jovanovich, 1988), 376; H. S. Rowland and B. L. Rowland, *Nursing Administration Handbook* (Germantown, MD: Aspen, 1980), 20; P. F. Drucker, *Management: Tasks, Responsibilities, Practices* (New York: Harper & Row, 1973), 495–505; and T. Kron and A. Gray, *The Management of Patient Care: Putting Leadership Skills to Work,* 6th ed. (Philadelphia: W. B. Saunders, 1987), 179–180.
6. H. M. Donovan, *Nursing Service Administration: Managing the Enterprise* (Saint Louis: C. V. Mosby, 1975), 155.
7. T. Kron and A. Gray, op. cit., 100.
8. H. Koontz and H. Weihrich, op. cit., 490.
9. B. J. Stevens, *The Nurse as Executive,* 2d ed. (Wakefield, MA: Nursing Resources, 1980), 284.
10. C. Arndt and L. M. D. Huckabay, *Nursing Administration: Theory for Practice with a Systems Approach,* 2d ed. (Saint Louis: C. V. Mosby, 1980), 22–46.
11. P. Franck and M. Price, *Nursing Management,* 2d ed. (New York: Springer Publishing, 1980), 135.
12. M. L. Holle and M. E. Blatchly, *Introduction to Leadership and Management in Nursing* (Monterey, CA: Wadsworth Health Services Division, 1982), 178–185.
13. A. Levenstein in *The Nurse as Manager,* M. J. F. Smith, Ed. (Chicago: S-N Publications, 1981), 17–33.
14. B. Lemin, *First Line Nursing Management* (New York: Springer, 1977), 47–51.
15. Ibid.
16. R. M. Fulmer and S. G. Franklin, op. cit., 216–217.
17. I. G. Ramey, "Setting Standards and Evaluating Care," in S. Stone et al., Eds., *Management for Nurses* (Saint Louis: C. V. Mosby, 1976), 79.
18. H. M. Donovan, op. cit., 160–169.
19. M. Beyers and C. Phillips, *Nursing Management for Patient Care,* 2d ed. (Boston: Little, Brown, 1979), 109–141.
20. L. M. Douglass, *The Effective Nurse: Leader and Manager* (3d. ed. Saint Louis: C. V. Mosby, 1988), 180–184.
21. H. Koontz and H. Weihrich, op. cit., 490, 492–494.
22. J. M. Ganong and W. L. Ganong, *Nursing Management,* 2d ed. (Rockville, MD: Aspen, 1980), 191.
23. H. Koontz and H. Weihrich, op. cit., 492–494.
24. H. Koontz and H. Weihrich, op. cit., 520–521; R. M. Fulmer and S. G. Franklin, op. cit., 221–227; M. Beyers and C. Phillips, op. cit., 134–135; and H. S. Rowland, op. cit., 495–505.
25. H. Koontz and H. Weihrich, op. cit., 521–525.
26. J. M. Ganong and W. L. Ganong, op. cit., 257.

REFERENCE

Swansburg, R. C., *Management of Patient Care Services,* (Saint Louis: C. V. Mosby, 1976).

Quality Assurance

23

OVERVIEW

As discussed in the preceding chapter, a master evaluation or controlling plan is needed to evaluate the whole program of any nursing department, service, or unit. One of the major elements of such a plan will be a quality assurance program. As the costs of hospital and all aspects of health care keep increasing, quality assurance programs are essential to ensuring that the quality of care is maintained, and indeed, that quality care is delivered. The assumption is that nursing must be accountable to its clients for the care rendered by its practitioners.

Quality assurance programs began in hospitals in the 1960s with voluntary implementation of nursing audits. The term has emerged in the health-care industry as a synonym for evaluation or as a major evaluation activity. Quality assurance has been defined as "estimation of the degree of excellence in patient health outcomes and in activity and other resource outcomes."[1]

Part of evaluation involves determination of management effectiveness of how well objectives, outcomes, or results have been achieved. Another part involves efficiency, the cost of achieving objectives. Quality assurance not only involves evaluation, it involves its use to secure improvement.

COMPONENTS OF A QUALITY ASSURANCE PROGRAM

A quality assurance program and plan is composed of the following components:

1. Clear and concise written statements of purpose, philosophy, and objectives.
2. Standards or indicators for measuring the quality of care.
3. Policies and procedures for using such standards for gathering data. These policies define the organizational structure for the quality assurance program.

497

4. Analysis and reporting of the data gathered, with isolation of problems.
5. Use of the results to prioritize problems.
6. Monitoring of clinical and managerial performance and ongoing feedback to ensure problems stay solved.
7. Evaluation of the quality assurance system.

Statements of Purpose, Philosophy, and Objectives

The first element of a planned quality assurance (QA) program will be development of clear and concise statements of purpose, philosophy, and objectives. A group developing a tool to evaluate QA programs indicated that only 50 percent of studies done during a 7-year period in a 700-bed medical center stated their individual purposes.[2] Every program needs objectives and every study a purpose; see Figure 23–1 for an example of mission and purpose statements.

Standards for Measuring the Quality of Care

Standards define nursing care outcomes as well as nursing activities and structural resources needed.

FIGURE 23–1. Mission and Purpose Statements

Mission. The mission of the Quality Assurance Plan of the University of South Alabama Medical Center is directly reflective of the mission of the University of South Alabama Medical Center. As stated in the policy, "Functional Plan of Organization of the University of South Alabama Medical Center" (from Mission Statements), the Department of Quality Assurance "ensures that the quality of patient care at the University of South Alabama Medical Center is optimal through a unified program for patient care evaluation activities."

Purpose. The purpose of the Quality Assurance Plan of the University of South Alabama Medical Center is to ensure that all patients receive the optimal quality of care.

SOURCE: Courtesy of the University of South Alabama Medical Center, Mobile, Alabama.

They are used for planning nursing care as well as for evaluating it. Outcomes include positive and negative indexes.

Various organizations issue indexes. The Health Care Financing Administration (HCFA) discloses projected and actual hospital mortality rates by diagnostic-related group (DRG) annually. HCFA is preparing to disclose physical quality indexes. The Joint Commission on Accreditation of Healthcare Organizations (JCAHO) will issue clinical and organizational performance measures and outcomes by 1991. Indicators will include severity of illness or risk adjustment mechanisms. Providers doing an excellent job as well as those doing a poor job will be identified.

Other organizations collecting data for quality measurement are the American Hospital Association, Voluntary Hospitals of America, National Committee for Quality Healthcare, and the National Association of Health Data Organizations. They will gather, analyze, and publish data on quality of health care for consumers, employers, and the government. These standards will include performance standards for providers. The objectives are to achieve improvement in the health status of patients, to reduce unnecessary utilization of health-care services, and to meet specifications of patients and purchasers. The standards will address social, psychological, financial, clinical, and management concerns.[3]

Outcomes or indexes serve as an estimate or judge of the value, rank, or degree of excellence; see Figure 23–2.

Policies and Procedures

The third element of a quality assurance program is to develop policies and procedures for using standards or indicators for gathering data to measure the quality of care. They will define the organizational structure for the QA program and will prescribe the tools for gathering data.

ORGANIZATIONAL STRUCTURE

The organizational structure of a quality assurance program is defined by organizational policy covering all departments and the medical staff. If the organization is large enough there will be a QA

FIGURE 23–2. Standards of Nursing Care for Sixth Floor

The following standards are directed toward nursing care that is provided for all patients regardless of social, economic, or religious status.

Standard 1. When admitted to the sixth floor, the patient and family will be oriented to hospital and room by a nursing employee, who will explain hospital policies including visiting hours, smoking, etc., in an unhurried, warm manner.

Standard 2. A registered nurse will interview the patient, or family responsible for the patient, to obtain a complete health history. This information will be written on the admission data profile and will become a part of the medical record, accessible to all medical personnel.

Standard 3. An R.N. will make an assessment of the patient with regard to the reason for admission and chief complaint. The individualized nursing care plan will be developed from this assessment.

Standard 4. The nursing staff will evaluate and revise the nursing care plan as necessary. The care plan will be discussed with other patient care disciplines by means of report, patient care conferences, etc.

Standard 5. Patient care will include the following on a daily basis:

1. A.M. care
   a. Daily bath—self, given, or with assistance.
   b. Mouth care—self, given, or with assistance.
   c. Hair grooming—self, given, or with assistance.
   d. Skin care—special attention to be given to areas of potential breakdown.
   e. Change linens on the bed; clean linens for bath.

2. P.M. care
   a. Skin care.
   b. Mouth care.
   c. Freshen patient's linens and straighten room.
3. Hygiene
   a. Handwashing before and after meals.
   b. Handwashing after use of bedpan and/or urinal.
4. Activity
   a. As ordered—proper positioning in bed or chair.
   b. Active or passive physical therapy.
5. Assessment of nutritional needs and diet instruction.
6. Assistance with meeting needs of bowel and bladder elimination.
7. Ensurance of necessary rest and sleep.
8. Administration of medication and treatments according to correct procedures.
9. Ensure a safe environment.

Standard 6. The nursing staff will give the patient and family support by:

1. Attentive listening.
2. Reassurance.
3. Observance of unusual behavior.
4. Therapeutic intervention.
5. Assistance with spiritual needs.

Standard 7. A registered nurse will provide the patient and/or family with appropriate patient teaching and discharge planning which include:

1. Explanation of all procedures and nursing measures utilized.
2. Teaching of self-care.
3. Discussion and presentation of discharge plan with other patient care disciplines.

SOURCE: Courtesy of the University of South Alabama Medical Center, Mobile, Alabama.

department. Otherwise there will be a full-time or part-time person assigned to oversee the program. QA programs are tailored to the institution and to accomplishment of program objectives. The QA policy should contain an organizational and functional scheme, as in Figure 23–3.

QA committees frequently function at the level of both the organization and the nursing department. Both levels should have representation from clinical nurse caregivers since the entire process concerns the quality of patient care.

Committees will usually be defined by policy

FIGURE 23–3. Sample Quality Assurance Policies, Procedures, and Information Flowchart

UNIVERSITY OF SOUTH ALABAMA MEDICAL CENTER
DEPARTMENT OF QUALITY ASSURANCE
POLICIES AND PROCEDURES

Policies. The policies of the Department of Quality Assurance are in effect the policies of the University of South Alabama Medical Center.

Additional policies within the department are:

I. All information and data obtained in the department through monitoring activities shall remain confidential except to the extent that it is used for quality assurance and credentialing purposes.

II. Any information obtained through monitoring activities which could indicate that a patient (or patients) are at risk of harm will be reported immediately to administration and to the attending physician or the chair of the admitting service department.

III. Each person in the department is expected to keep abreast of JCAHO requirements concerning quality assurance to the extent that the person is involved in quality assurance activities.

IV. It is the responsibility of the personnel in the Department of Quality Assurance to keep up to date on current literature, methods, and procedures for performing quality assurance activities.

V. All personnel in the Department of Quality Assurance are also expected to keep up to date on the University of South Alabama Medical Center's policies.

VI. Each employee in the Quality Assurance Department is expected to render responsible service to the department and to the University of South Alabama Medical Center.

VII. All new personnel in the Department of Quality Assurance are expected to become familiar with the policies and procedures of the University of South Alabama Medical Center and the Department of Quality Assurance.

VIII. Each employee in the Department of Quality Assurance is expected to provide in-service training pertaining to quality assurance activities as necessary.

IX. All data presented to the Quality Assurance Committee shall be reviewed by the quality assurance director or quality assurance coordinator, the assistant administrator for the Quality Assurance Department, and the chair of the Quality Assurance Committee prior to the committee's meeting.

X. The quality assurance plan for the University of South Alabama Medical Center will be reviewed and revised as necessary but at least annually.

Procedures

1. *Core Criteria.* Core criteria for the nine clinical departments which admit patients will be captured on a monthly basis. These criteria, along with an analysis of the data, will be sent to the departments for discussion at the monthly departmental meetings. The core criteria include:

Volume indicators—

Number of admissions (retrieved from Medical Records monthly report).

Number of discharges (retrieved from Medical Records monthly report).

Number of in-house surgical procedures (when indicated—retrieved from Medical Records report).

Number of ambulatory surgical procedures (when indicated—retrieved from Medical Records report).

FIGURE 23–3. Sample Quality Assurance Policies, Procedures, and Information Flowchart (*continued*)

Quality/appropriateness indicators—

Number of incident reports (reported from Risk Management).

Number of patient complaints (retrieved from patient questionnaires, nursing QA reports, ancillary QA reports).

Number of readmits within 30 days (highlight readmits within 15 days—captured from data processing report).

Number of patients leaving against medical advice (captured from data processing report).

Number of delinquent medical records (end of month—captured from data processing report).

Percent nosocomial infections (reported from infection control monthly report).

Gross death rate (percent—from medical records department monthly report).

Number of complications (this parameter *must* be captured by medical staff).

Number of potential problems referred from other medical staff committees (captured from review of minutes from medical staff departmental meetings, hospital committee meetings, and other quality assurance reporting mechanisms).

Number of unexpected returns to operating room (OR) (captured from OR monthly quality assurance monitoring report).

Number of delinquent operative reports (captured from medical records department monthly quality assurance monitoring report).

Number of preop/postop diagnoses that differ (captured from OR monthly quality assurance monitoring report).

Charts lacking history and physical 24 hours after admission (percent of those reviewed for service—captured from quality assurance monitor reviewing percentage of admissions for each service).

Blood wastage (percent of total wastage—captured from monthly transfusion service quality assurance monitoring report—all transfusions reviewed).

DRG Status (percent reimbursement—calculated for all patients on all services, based on dollar-per-dollar reimbursement per DRG [excludes monies received for education]).

Any unexpected indicators (any indicators discovered through quality assurance activities that do not fall into above criteria).

2. *Monitoring activities.* Monitoring performed by quality assurance personnel will include:

History and Physicals—One day a week, 25 percent of each service's admissions will be monitored to see whether valid histories and physicals are on the medical record and are signed by a licensed physican within 24 hours of admission. The history should be current (taken on admission) and the physical should include all major systems and examination on admission.

Preliminary anatomic diagnosis and final anatomic diagnosis.

Compliance with hospital bylaws.

Patient response.

Blood product loss.

Blood appropriateness.

(continued)

FIGURE 23–3.   Sample Quality Assurance Policies, Procedures, and Information Flowchart (*continued*)

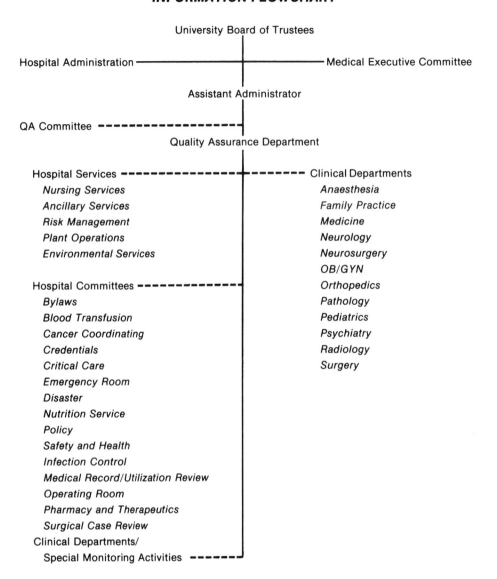

QUALITY ASSURANCE PLAN
INFORMATION FLOWCHART

University Board of Trustees

Hospital Administration ——————————— Medical Executive Committee

Assistant Administrator

QA Committee ----------------------

Quality Assurance Department

Hospital Services ---------------------- Clinical Departments

Nursing Services   *Anaesthesia*
Ancillary Services   *Family Practice*
Risk Management   *Medicine*
Plant Operations   *Neurology*
Environmental Services   *Neurosurgery*
                                    OB/GYN
Hospital Committees -------------   *Orthopedics*
Bylaws   *Pathology*
Blood Transfusion   *Pediatrics*
Cancer Coordinating   *Psychiatry*
Credentials   *Radiology*
Critical Care   *Surgery*
Emergency Room
Disaster
Nutrition Service
Policy
Safety and Health
Infection Control
Medical Record/Utilization Review
Operating Room
Pharmacy and Therapeutics
Surgical Case Review
Clinical Departments/
   Special Monitoring Activities -------

Explanation of Information Flowchart

University Board of Trustees.   The ultimate responsibility for ensuring that patients at the University of South Alabama Medical Center receive optimal patient care lies with the University of South Alabama Board of Trustees. The authority and accountability for achieving this goal are delegated to the University of South Alabama Medical Center's administration and the Medical Executive Committee. Policies for implementation of this authority include:

FIGURE 23–3. Sample Quality Assurance Policies, Procedures, and Information Flowchart (*continued*)

1. The Board of Trustees exercises overview responsibility for the effectiveness and efficiency for achieving quality patient care at the University of South Alabama Medical Center.
2. The Board of Trustees authorizes the administration of the University of South Alabama Medical Center to establish a Department of Quality Assurance which will serve to centralize and implement a quality assurance plan for the Medical Center. In addition, the president of the medical staff is authorized to appoint a multidisciplinary committee to oversee quality assurance activities at the Medical Center. The chair shall be a physician member of the committee.
3. The Board of Trustees authorizes the Medical Executive Committee to exercise overview responsibility for the effectiveness and efficiency of the quality assurance plan. This function will be accomplished through a tracking plan designed to channel quality assurance information to the Executive Committee on a scheduled basis. The Medical Committee shall be expected to act on any unresolved problems tracked to the committee.

The Quality Assurance Department. The Quality Assurance Department has the responsibility of establishing, implementing, and revising the quality assurance plan (hereafter referred to as the plan) for the University of South Alabama Medical Center. The plan is subject to review and approval by hospital administration, the Medical Executive Committee, and the Quality Assurance Committee. The plan shall be revised at least annually and shall encompass all aspects of quality assurance activities for the University of South Alabama Medical Center.

The Quality Assurance Committee. The Quality Assurance Committee (hereafter referred to as the committee) shall be a multidisciplinary committee appointed by the president of the medical staff. The committee shall meet monthly and shall receive reports of monitoring activities from all hospital departments and hospital committees. The functions of the committee shall include but are not limited to:

1. Reviewing monitoring reports presented at monthly committee meetings.
2. Discussing, recommending, and acting on problems identified through monitoring activities.
3. Reviewing and approving criteria for each department's monitoring activities (includes existing and new criteria).
4. Referring identified problems to Executive Committee for actions as necessary.
5. Reviewing reports from hospital committees.
6. Discussing, recommending, and acting on problems identified through hospital committee reports.
7. Referring problems identified through hospital committee reports to the Executive Committee for action as necessary.
8. Reviewing and approving at least annually the quality assurance plan.

Clinical Departments. The clinical departments of the University of South Alabama Medical Center include:

Anesthesia	Orthopedics
Family Practice	Pathology
Medicine	Pediatrics
Neurology	Psychiatry
Neurosurgery	Radiology
OB/GYN	Surgery

These departments shall develop valid criteria to assess the quality of patient care given by the medical staff of the department. The nine departments which admit patients shall receive the core criteria (developed and approved by the Quality Assurance Committee) from the Quality Assurance Department on a monthly basis. The departments which do not admit patients (anesthesia, pathology, radiology) shall also receive information from the Quality Assurance Department and shall develop criteria to assess the quality of care delivered by their physicians.

(continued)

FIGURE 23–3.   Sample Quality Assurance Policies, Procedures, and Information Flowchart (*continued*)

The results of these monitoring activities shall be reflected in the minutes of monthly departmental meetings. In addition, the minutes shall reflect recommendations, actions, and follow-up on problems identified through monitoring activities. These minutes shall be reviewed by the Medical Executive Committee. This committee shall act on any unresolved problems.

Hospital Services.   Hospital services, including the Nursing Department, Ancillary Services, Risk Management, Plant Operations, and Environmental Services, will routinely monitor important aspects of care rendered through their departments and will present a report on a scheduled basis to the Quality Assurance Committee.

Hospital Committees.   All hospital committees will report results of their activities on a scheduled basis to the Quality Assurance Committee.

Clinical Departments—Special Monitoring Activities.   Special monitoring activities requested by clinical departments will be reported to the Quality Assurance Committee on a regular basis and with approval of the chair of the clinical department involved.

SOURCE: University of South Alabama Medical Center, Mobile, Alabama. Reprinted with permission.

---

that includes the purpose, membership, and functions designed to support the QA program. Clinical nurses will have hours assigned to accomplish their QA committee function.

TOOLS FOR COLLECTING QA DATA

Standards are not evaluation instruments. Tools or instruments should be selected to collect evidence that indicates standards are being met. There are various standardized instruments available. If the QA committee decide to develop new tools they will need to determine reliability and at least content validity.

There are three basic forms of nursing audits: structure audits, process audits, and outcome audits.

Structure Audits

Structure audits focus on the setting in which care takes place. They include physical facilities, equipment, caregivers, organization, policies, procedures, and medical records. Standards or indicators will be measured by a checklist that focuses on these categories.

Structure can include such content as staff knowledge and expertise, in addition to policies and procedures. Content related to specific nursing care to meet established standards will be included in nursing process audits.

Process Audits

Process audits implement criteria for measuring nursing care to determine if nursing standards of practice are being met. They are task oriented. Process audits were first used by Maria Phaneuf in 1964 and were based upon the seven functions of nursing established by Lesnick and Anderson. The Phaneuf audit is retrospective, being applied to measure the quality of nursing care received by the patient after a cycle of care has been completed and the patient is discharged. The seven subsections of the Phaneuf audit are:

1. Application and execution of physicians' legal orders.
2. Observation of symptoms and reactions.
3. Supervision of the patient.
4. Supervision of those participating in care (except the physician).
5. Reporting and recording.
6. Application and execution of nursing procedures and techniques.

7. Promotion of physical and emotional health by direction and teaching.

The Phaneuf model uses a Likert scoring system. It does not evaluate care not recorded.[4]

The Quality Patient Care Scale (Qual PacS) is a process audit that measures the quality of nursing care concurrently. Its six subsections are:

1. Psychosocial—individual.
2. Psychosocial—group.
3. Physical.
4. General.
5. Communication.
6. Professional implications.

The nurse is evaluated by direct observation in a nurse-patient interaction. A 15 percent sample of nurses on a unit is considered adequate. Both of these process audits use the performance of the first-level staff nurse as a standard for safe, adequate, therapeutic, and supportive care.[5]

The Qual PacS audit was developed from the Slater Nursing Competencies Rating Scale. The Slater model references five staff nurses from best to poorest, contains eighty-four questions, and takes 2½ to 3 hours to administer per nurse-patient interaction. Qual PacS reduced the questionnaire to sixty-eight items.[6]

Other open system audits include Commission on Administrative Service in Hospital (CASH) Scale and the Medicus Corporation Nurses Audit. They also measure or monitor action, assessment, and clinical skills.

A nursing process audit tool has been developed to evaluate independent nursing functions based on the nursing process. Each step of the nursing process can be evaluated independently or the process can be evaluated as a whole. The audit can be used concurrently or retrospectively. While it is one component of the QA program of a mental health nursing service, nurse managers could use it as a model for other nursing services.

In this model the medical record is randomly selected and audited in the presence of the primary nurse or a meeting is scheduled with her or him for feedback. Scores are developed for:

1. Assessments (thirteen categories).
2. Planning (reassessment, identified needs, nursing diagnosis, expected outcomes, and nursing actions).
3. Implementation (chart progress point, date, days, dates not met).
4. Evaluation (documentation reflects progress toward achieving expected outcomes).
5. Discharge summary (current health status and discharge planning summary).

Feedback from measurement information is expected to result in a change in nursing care with documentation of corrective actions. This tool uses rational standards of practice, collects data for research, can be used for staff development, and improves patient care.[7]

Outcome Audits

Outcome audits are also either concurrent or retrospective. They evaluate nursing performance in terms of established patient outcome criteria. The National Center for Health Services developed an outcome audit based on Orem's description of nine categories of self-care requirements:

1. Air.
2. Water/fluid intake.
3. Food.
4. Elimination.
5. Rest/activity/sleep.
6. Social interaction and productive work.
7. Protection from hazards.
8. Normality.
9. Health deviation.

These categories are evaluated in terms of:

1. Evidence that the requirement is met.
2. Evidence that the patient has the necessary knowledge to meet the requirement.
3. Evidence that the patient has the necessary skill and performance abilities to meet the requirement.
4. Evidence that the patient has the necessary motivation to meet the requirement.[8]

Outcome criteria are set for selected topics. They can evaluate specific aspects of nursing care for particular groups such as cancer patients, perioperative patients, intensive care patients, and others. Patients are grouped for efficiency: DRGs, like treatments, like needs, geography, life stages, illness stages, and like standards. A determination is made as to whether the outcomes are met. If not, deficiencies are corrected and followed up.

The Nurse Executive.   The nurse executive plays an active role in outcome audits. This includes guidance in the development of protocols by nursing peer panels. The nurse executive teaches methods of developing nursing measurement criteria, including those related to cost management. The nurse executive ensures that the QA program is a total system and participates in that system through monitoring it and thereby evaluating institutional effectiveness.

Nursing Peer Groups.   Nursing peer groups write criteria and compare them to the actual results. They identify the causes of problems and recommend or take action to improve or solve these problems. They make reports to the chief nurse executive as well as the QA committee. They collaborate with other groups and disciplines. Practicing nurses in local situations will write pertinent criteria. They can work with other institutions locally and can use national models for reference;[9] see Figure 23–4.

Triad Models

Some nursing quality assurance models employ a triad of structure, process, and outcome. Measurement criteria are referenced by code to specific structural, process, or outcome standards. A modular approach has been used in which patient conditions were related to five areas: patient rights, developmental stage of patient, social groups, therapy-associated needs, and medical diagnoses. Standards for each patient group were developed and used to construct the evaluation instrument.

The modular design for QA provides discrete components that can be used independently or in different combinations. This design has three modules:

1. Patient care standards.
2. Outcome, process, structure trail.
3. The standard with derived measurement criteria.[10]

Outcome indicators also include mortality rates and infection rates.

FIGURE 23–4. Guidelines for Developing Sets of Outcome Criteria Statements

1. Screening criteria are a crucial factor that, if not met, may indicate a significant deficiency in nursing care.
2. The purpose of screening criteria is to survey a large number of cases and quickly determine acceptable levels of patient outcomes.
3. The outcome stated in the criteria must be possible to achieve.
4. Criteria should be statements of specific outcomes representing optimal achievement.
5. Criteria should be written as specifically as possible, including the time when they are to be measured and the measurement to be used to determine if the criteria have been met.
6. In establishing criteria, one should select the most critical time for the measurement of the identified outcome for a particular patient population.
7. Criteria must be appraisable. However, the ease of measurement should not be used as the sole basis for accepting or rejecting potential criteria. If criteria are important, some assessment can usually be obtained.
8. Criteria should be stated to yield a dichotomous distinction (yes-no).
9. Criteria should be phrased in positive terms (presence of) rather than negative terms (absence of), when applicable.
10. Criteria should be pertinent to the particular patient population under consideration. For example, for the ambulatory patient receiving photocoagulation of the eye, skin care is not a priority. Hence, criteria would not be written for skin care.
11. Criteria should be free from bias. Each patient to whom criteria are applied should be equally likely to be able to meet the criteria. For example, the skin condition of an aged patient and a youth might require different criteria.
12. A set of criteria applicable to a specific patient population may include criteria for outcomes of care for members of the family or significant others.

Establishing criteria is a "pencil and eraser" operation. Criteria will change as values and scientific knowledge change and as health-care practices change. Thus criteria should be revised at regular intervals.

Source: Reprinted with permission from *ANA Guidelines for Review of Nursing Care at the Local Level,* © 1977, American Nurses' Association, Kansas City, MO. 21-22.

PROBLEM IDENTIFICATION

Analysis and reporting of the data gathered from the evaluation process leads to problem identification and isolation. Evidence comes from primary sources such as the patient and personnel and from secondary sources including the patient's chart and family. Evidence is gathered through rounds, observations, and records. There should be active patient and family participation. QA addresses current problems. Nurse managers look for patterns or trends of deviation from normal. They also identify deficiencies relating to other departments that affect nursing care.

PROBLEM RESOLUTION

Once problems have been defined and isolated, plans are made to solve them on a priority basis. Those that are critical are addressed first and plans are immediately made and implemented to resolve them. Those involving the safety and welfare of the patient take first priority. Other factors used in determining priority will include severity, frequency, benefit, cost-effectiveness, elimination, reduction, association with professional liability, and impact on accreditation. The first consideration is always based on the impact on patient care.[11]

Solutions and corrective action for problems will be assigned to appropriate nursing departments, services, and units. The need is to resolve problems, not just evaluate them.

MONITORING AND FEEDBACK

The QA process is a cyclic one that requires monitoring of clinical and managerial performance and feedback to ensure that problems stay solved. Follow-up can be expensive and difficult. Its breadth should determine what should be covered. Problems of a multidisciplinary nature such as those involving occupational therapy, physical therapy, speech pathology, and nursing can be one consideration.

The cyclic process will continue to set standards of care, take measurements according to those standards, evaluate data from multiple sources, recommend improvements, and above all, ensure that improvements are carried out.

SYSTEM EVALUATION

Although nurses defend their right to define and regulate the quality of care, they often do not pursue QA activities. In a study of nurse managers, staff development nurses, and clinical nurses in ten metropolitan hospitals it was found that most nurses believed QA involved all levels of nursing personnel but not as part of their daily work. Twenty-five percent viewed it as an accreditation requirement. Peer review and patient care audits ranked low against direct patient care activities. Less than 50 percent of respondents wanted to participate in these activities.[12]

Nurses with formal QA experience were more likely to want to write standards for their specialty, to participate in peer review, and to want to be on QA committees. They were more interested in QA associated with direct patient care.[13]

Many QA programs are developed without thorough assessment of the needs of those to be served or of the resources available. Many programs are continued without evaluation and evidence of their positive contributions to health care. These include hospice and cardiac rehabilitation programs.[14]

Several models for QA program evaluation have been developed. These include the James model and the Renzulli key features model.

The James Model

The James model of evaluating the nursing department QA programs is a triad or structure-process-outcome model. It describes and measures effort, performance, adequacy of performance, efficiency, analysis of the process, and unforeseen objectives. Data comes from patient records, incident reports, reports form third-party payers, staff interviews and observations, profile analysis from previous audits, marketing reports, patient surveys, product sampling and testing, and direct observation. QA programs can be total evaluation programs that evaluate the nursing department or division as a whole. A goal attainment model establishes objectives and management plans. When objectives are measured, further actions are taken based upon the results.[15]

The Renzulli Key Features Model

The Renzulli key features model can be used to evaluate health-care delivery programs. Evaluation is done by teams for specific areas such as (1) needs assessment to determine the need for change, (2) program design, (3) program implementation, and (4) program and/or process evaluation.

The Renzulli key features model has four key elements:

1. Investigation of all direct and indirect *factors* bearing on a participating program's effectiveness.
2. Consultation of prime interest groups to identify the *key features,* those major factors or variables that make the programs successful.
3. Examination of objectives to identify the *prime interest groups* among all people involved with the program.
4. Use of formative and summation evaluation, including the best use of time in the overall functioning of the evaluation system.[16]

There are four steps in using the Renzulli key features model for total nursing department evaluation:

1. Front-end analysis—The major concerns of each prime interest group are identified from written materials, developing and administering questionnaires, conducting interviews, and making observations of the program in action.

2. Synthesis of input information and instrument development—A model is developed listing prime interest groups and key features. Possible sources of data are noted and a determination is made of instruments for data gathering. The key features must accurately express the concerns of prime interest groups. There must be appropriate relationships between key features and instruments used to gather data. The evaluation must be concerned with economy and parsimony in gathering data.

3. Data collection and analysis—Important aspects of data collection and analysis include selection and training of collectors, timing, and a plan for data analysis including consultation.

4. Preparing the evaluation report—There should be interim and final reports following the same predetermined format organized around each prime interest group and key feature. These reports should include sources of data, methods, instrument description, technique used for data analysis, positive and negative results, and a summary of highlights of major findings.[17]

Maciorowski, Larson, and Keane developed and tested another tool to evaluate QA studies. It evaluated four aspects of the nursing process: problem identification, methods, analysis, and follow-up.[18] Their questionnaire is reproduced as Figure 23–5.

The nurse manager should view QA as part of the total evaluating function of nursing management rather than as a distinct entity. A model for evaluation of all nursing services, including clinical practice, management, teaching, and research should be selected in consultation with representative nurses working in these areas. It should be a model that produces results in a timely and economical manner.

MANAGEMENT PROCESSES INVOLVED IN QUALITY ASSURANCE

Quality assurance is important to accountability of nurses who want to control their practice areas. Many groups are seeking evidence that outcomes of nursing care are of good quality and represent a cost-effective use of resources. Accountability for nursing practice is still diffused by the employment environment and this fact must be corrected by nurse managers.

Involvement of Practicing Nurses

Practicing nurses can be stimulated to increase their positive attitudes about QA by direct behavioral experience. Nurse managers should find out reasons these nurses view QA unfavorably. They will correct and change this viewpoint by various strategies that include:

FIGURE 23–5. Assessment of Quality Assurance Studies

Directions: Read the report of the study in its entirety. Respond "yes" to items below when you can find a specific statement to support your answer. Otherwise, respond "no."

Study title _____ Type: Retrospective _____ Concurrent _____

Year _____ Dept. _____ Total # pts. studied _____

	% Yes	No
1. Problem statement		
a. Reason for study is stated	_____	_____
b. Reason is based on an identified problem	_____	_____
c. Study is related to nursing practice (vs. activities of medical pharmacy or others)	_____	_____
d. Reason is described as a nursing problem or diagnosis	_____	_____
e. Evidence that costs/risks of problem were considered (*i.e.,* risks of problem identified are greater than costs of the study)	_____	_____
2. Methods		
a. Subject selection criteria are stated	_____	_____
b. Rationale for sample size is described	_____	_____
c. Individuals collecting data are identified	_____	_____
d. A description of how study tools and/or methods were developed is included	_____	_____
e. Tools or forms used are included	_____	_____
3. Findings/plan of action		
a. Findings are summarized	_____	_____
b. Findings are reported in relation to total population at risk (*e.g.,* # of UTI over # of catheterized patients)	_____	_____
c. A plan of action supported by study results is formulated	_____	_____
d. Action plan aims at solving the problem defined	_____	_____
e. Outcomes of action plan are measurable	_____	_____
4. Follow up		
a. Person(s) or group(s) responsible for implementation of action plan are named	_____	_____
b. There is a specified time frame for implementation of action plan	_____	_____
c. Mechanisms for follow-up are described	_____	_____
d. There is evidence that follow-up occurred (*e.g.,* dates of action, names of people contacted)	_____	_____
e. There is evidence that the stated problem is either resolved or further action is planned	_____	_____
Total Score (add "yes" answers)	_____	

SOURCE: L. F. Maciorowski, E. Larson, and A. Keane, "Quality Assurance: Evaluate Thyself," *Journal of Nursing Administration*, June 1985, 38–42. Reprinted with permission.

1. Having practicing nurses choose QA topics.
2. Providing release time for practicing nurses to participate in QA activities, including attendance at committee meetings and time for QA audits.
3. Providing rewards such as performance results achievement records that can lead to pay raises, promotions, educational opportunities, or special assignments.
4. Targeting QA to patient care outcomes, the very essence of nursing practice.
5. Involving clinical nurses in management through such techniques as quality circles, employee involvement programs, participatory management, decentralization, "adhocracy," and quality of work life.

Resources

QA programs are labor-intensive, requiring efficient and effective use of resources that include personnel, physical plant, supplies, equipment, policies, and procedures. Nurse managers should be selective in determining areas to be evaluated, considering time and difficulty as well as safety and urgency. They should sample the standards rather than dogmatically evaluating every one. This will require placing priority on standards and even making a decision whether to eliminate some that are not critical.

Efficiency

Efficiency is related to two questions: Was the care accomplished in a way that conserved resources? Did it meet practice standards?[19] The computer is a labor-saving device for developing and conducting a QA program. Nurse managers will use it and teach other practicing nurses to use it. It can be used to track the QA process.

Standards will be kept up to date and accessible to all units. A loose-leaf notebook or the computer memory are efficient for easy access. Standards should be cross-indexed.

Charts can be labelled so as to be easily retrieved for nursing QA evaluation. They can be coded by nursing diagnosis or nursing care standards.[20]

Other elements of efficiency and effectiveness include:

1. Identification of the impact of nursing care on the health of the patient—results or outcomes measured in terms of the patient's health status. Do the notes meet such a standard?
2. A QA program should be practical enough to be used in all clinical nursing settings.
3. Samples should be random and are effective when done on a schedule but unannounced.
4. Nursing personnel should serve on QA committees long enough to be proficient.
5. When more than one person is administering criteria, each should grade.
6. Higher patient acuity combined with shorter lengths of stay should be noted as they require greater nursing efficiency and effectiveness.
7. Interdisciplinary QA programs should be effective and efficient so nurses will not do the work of other disciplines. Nursing is interdependent with other groups and organizations, ethically and operationally.
8. Planning is necessary to enhance resilience and a sense of responsibility. Planning helps nurse managers move into an uncertain future by blueprinting where they want to go as well as how and whether they will reach their goal. Planning can be used to develop scenarios for managing the future, changing the culture of nursing organizations, developing interpersonal skills, and making a creative response to risk taking.[21]
9. Each nurse should be held responsible for self-improvement and for delivering a high standard of patient care.

Consumer Involvement

Consumers will be involved in all aspects of a QA program including discharge planning. They know what they want and are demanding quality with economy. Nurses can teach patients to do pricing of health care that includes calling providers of all health services and establishing prices. Then consumers can negotiate with providers to accept their insurance as payment in full. Consumers can be taught to negotiate discounts for making prompt payments and billing their insurers themselves.

Training and Communication

Training and communication are important elements of a total QA program. Training includes interpersonal skills, stress management, and conflict management. Learning is a cyclic or continuous process. Nurse managers who play educator roles develop self-awareness by applying learning principles to their own behaviors. Patient education requires an interdisciplinary team approach.

Communication of QA findings including problems, resolution of problems, and results must be clear. Both physicians and employees need to be kept up to date. Quality must be provided and communicated to be successful. This means that providers as well as consumers will know the status of the quality of care being rendered.

Quality in the marketplace is defined by employers, employee benefit consultants, physicians, and consumers—not by providers (even though physicians are providers, as are hospitals, nurses, and other caregivers). The reason physicians determine quality is they have control over all orders for diagnosis and treatment procedures. Only one-half of consumers, employers, and employee benefit consultants ever differentiate between high- and low-quality hospitals. Two-thirds of physicians do.[22]

Good employee relations and consumer relations programs are necessary for success in the marketplace and their good quality must be communicated. Consumers want quality factors in this order:

1. Warmth, caring, concern.
2. Expert medical staff who are concerned, thorough, and successful.
3. Up-to-date technology/equipment.
4. Specialization/scope of services available.
5. Outcome.[23]

Nurses sometimes tend to emphasize technology and specialization rather than warmth, caring, and concern.

RESEARCH AND QUALITY ASSURANCE

Nursing quality assurance programs can be combined with research programs. Nursing research is being done in clinical settings to improve patient care. Research can be sold to nurse managers because it provides prestige, advanced knowledge for nursing professionals, and a data base for clinical nursing practice.[24]

Nursing research can be used to evaluate management issues such as staffing, cost management, and staffing retention. It produces new knowledge of the relationship between process and outcome. Combining quality assurance with research makes efficient use of personnel and other resources to link research with a mandatory process; to increase the probability that research will relate to patient care; and to increase sharing of successful quality assurance programs with others outside the institution.[25]

Researchers describe and discuss while QA personnel implement and monitor change. Researchers use sophisticated tests of association, correlations, and statistical significance while QA studies summarize findings as percentages and proportions. Integration requires interpersonal skills to manage territoriality.[26]

Hermon relates quality assurance and research. She defines QA as "an ongoing component of all health-care systems, providing the health-care provider with an ongoing mechanism to assess level of care against a well-defined and measurable 'standard of care.' " QA is complemented by nursing research.[27]

RISK MANAGEMENT

Risk management has an altogether different connotation today than it did in the 1960s. It was then touted by business and industry as the venture approach to new business, to taking a chance on the unknown. The risk manager was an entrepreneur who purposefully formed small new companies to develop new products that would create new sales and more profit dollars. This manager was responsible for the success or failure of the new venture of patent protection, technical know-how and marketing methods.[28] While venture management is alive and well in U.S. business and industry, risk management has evolved into a defense against the spiraling costs of institutional liability premiums generated by successful and costly malpractice suits.

Goal of Risk Management

The goal of risk management is to have a program that will identify and correct deficient patterns of care, thereby preventing malpractice suits. Some liability insurers require that a risk management program be in place before insuring. Some states require a risk management program for licensure.[29] In its high-visibility context, a risk management program is designed to reduce system and personnel failures.

Since the 1960s, emphasis on civil and consumer rights has generated increased legal challenges to all health-care providers, including nurses. The possibility that accidents or negative outcomes will occur in health care is a reality. The consumer knows this and frequently agrees to the possibility in writing. However, when a negative outcome occurs, the same consumers expect compensation for the loss. According to the National Association of Insurance Commissioners Closed Claims Study, 85 percent of all loss dollars paid by insurance companies are for claims origination in the hospital setting.[30]

Health care, including nursing, is big business and costly. The consumer views hospitals, physicians, and nurses as being in business to make money. Injuries and deaths occur in health-care institutions and at the hands of professional personnel. Many can be prevented, a fact recognized by the general public that results in increased malpractice litigation even when care meets established standards of practice.

The objectives of a hospital risk management program are:

1. Protection of hospital assets and earning power from large awards that will cause financial instability. This frequently includes liability insurance for employees while they are working for the institution.
2. Injury control or elimination.
3. An effective and economical program.[31]

Activities

Risk management activities include internal audits of hospital procedures and educational activities, effective claims management by investigating and managing claims, an effective patient representative program, and effective insurance management.[32]

The risk management process consists of:

1. Identification of pure risks.
2. Analysis of risks for possible loss frequency and security.

3. Development of risk control and risk financing techniques.
4. Implementation techniques.
5. Maintenance of program for effectiveness and modification as needed.[33]

Audits

Audits of hospital procedures are a quality assurance technique and part of the evaluating function of nursing management. From initiatives of the risk management program, personnel must be educated in the process. This will include knowledge of the reasons for the program, its goals, and their roles in the risk management program and frequent feedback concerning their own status and that of the organization with regard to the risk management program. Audits and incident reports are usual sources of identification of pure risks.

The educational program should be coordinated through the staff development or education department. Specific classes can be given by the risk manager, who may act as a consultant for risk management content of other classes. Classes should be given over shifts and often enough to allow all employees to attend. They should be related to job factors for various classes of employees. Professional hands-on personnel will have different interests than technical and support personnel.

Claims Management

Claims management includes analysis of risks for possible loss frequency and severity—the assessment of potential claims based on data analysis. It also includes development of risk control and risk-financing techniques as well as implementation techniques. To accomplish this the risk manager uses written and verbal reports to investigate potentially compensable events and losses and their causes, thereby determining liability and settlement value. Recommendations are made to administrators that include write-offs of specific charges or entire bills. Also, many claims can be settled out of court for small sums.

It is important that the risk manager be able to determine where the institution and personnel are *not* at fault. Some claims should go to litigation with jury trials.

The Patient Representative. Many large health-care institutions employ patient representatives. These individuals may be nurses or other professionally educated individuals with strong interpersonal skills. They see that patients and families are attended to and satisfied with all aspects of their care and treatment.

Among the services provided by patient representatives are orientation of patients and their families to hospital policies, procedure and to services provided; resolution of complaints, making phone calls, mailing letters, notarizing documents, making transportation arrangements, and daily follow-up survey samples of patients following discharge. Patient representatives can be assisted by volunteers.[34]

Insurance Management by Risk Manager. Effective insurance management is accomplished by the risk manager who maintains the program for effectiveness and modifies it as necessary. This includes review of areas of risk on a scheduled basis and design of preventive measures. It includes identification of hazards that cannot be eliminated because the positive therapeutic outcomes far outweigh the possible negative ones.

The risk manager uses carefully planned public relations, makes private explanations, apologizes when necessary, and collects, prepares, and presents evidence.[35] The risk manager's job is further described in Figure 23–6.

INCIDENT REPORTING

Incident reporting is an effective technique of a good risk management program. The tool itself should be constructed to collect complete and accurate information. This will include the name, address, age, and condition of the individual involved; exact location, time, and date of the incident; description of the occurrence; physician's examination data; bedrail status; reason for hospitalization; witnesses; and extent of out-of-bed privileges.

Use of Incident Reports

Incident reports are used to collect and analyze future data for the purpose of determining risk control strategies. They are prepared for any unusual occurrence involving people or property, whether or not injury or damage occurs.

FIGURE 23–6. Risk Manager Competencies

1. Keep an up-to-date manual, including policies, lines of authority, safety roles, disaster plans, safety training, procedures, incident and claims reporting, procedures, and schedule and description of retention/insurance program.
2. Update programs with changes in properties, operation or activities.
3. Review plans for new construction, alterations, and equipment installation.
4. Review contracts to avoid unnecessary assumptions of liability and transfer to others where possible.
5. Keep up-to-date property appraisal.
6. Maintain records of insurance policy renewal dates.
7. Review and monitor all premium and other billings and approve payments.
8. Negotiate insurance converage, premiums, and services.
9. Prepare specifications for competitive bids on property and liability insurance.
10. Review and make recommendations for coverage, services, and costs.
11. Maintain records and verify compliance for independent physicians, vendors, contractors, and subcontractors.
12. Maintain records of losses, claims, and all risk management expenses.
13. Supervise claim-reporting procedures.
14. Assist in adjusting losses.
15. Cooperate with director of safety and risk management committee to minimize all future losses involving employees, patients, visitors, other third parties, property, and earnings.
16. Keep risk management skills updated.
17. Prepare annual report covering status, changes, new problems and solutions, summary of existing insurance and retention aspects of the program, summary of losses, costs, major claims, and future goals and objectives.
18. Prepare annual budget.

The incident report is discoverable by the plaintiff's attorney. For this reason it should be prepared in a timely manner to ensure accuracy and objectivity of reporting. It must be complete and factual. The incident report is corrected as any other medical record and should not be altered or rewritten. It

FIGURE 23–7.   DOs and DON'Ts of Incident Reporting

DOs	DON'Ts
■ For any event involving patient mishap or serious expression of dissatisfaction with care.	■ Place blame on anyone.
■ For any event involving visitor mishap or property.	■ Place on the patient's chart.
■ Be complete.	■ Make entry about an incident report on the patient's chart.
■ Follow established policy and procedure.	■ Alter or rewrite.
■ Be prompt.	■ Report hearsay or opinion.
■ Act to reduce fear by the nursing staff.	■ Be afraid to consult, ask questions, or complete incident reports. They can be part of your best defence and protection.
■ Correct as any medical record.	■ Prescribe in the M.D.'s domain.
■ Include names and identities of witnesses; record their statements on separate pages.	■ Be cold and impersonal to patients, families, or visitors.
■ Report equipment malfunctions including control numbers. Remove them from service for testing.	
■ Keep the report confidential.	
■ Report to nurse manager.	
■ Confer with risk manager.	
■ Work to provide nursing care to meet established standards.	
■ Attend all staff development programs.	
■ Confirm all telephone orders in writing.	

should contain no comments criticizing or blaming others. To keep the incident report from being discoverable it must be sent from preparer to attorney to assure confidentiality. Nurse managers frequently insist on reviewing them. They can obtain accurate information from the patient's chart and from conversations with the preparer. The incident report should be prepared in a single copy and should never be placed on the patient's chart.

Attorneys can prepare abstracts of data from collective incident reports. Thus they identify the number of occurrences of particular incidents. The information will be used by the risk manager to do his or her job, including trend analysis to establish patterns and education and training of personnel.[36] See Figure 23–7.

While it may be institutional policy to send the incident report to the risk manager, an alternative method of notification is better. The preparer can call the risk manager and the nurse manager and give them verbal information to investigate and evaluate deviations from the standard of care and for making corrections. To accomplish this managers will have to establish a climate of trust that supports incident reporting by nurses. The JCAHO requires incident reporting.

According to Poteet, the majority of successful suits against nurses fall into nine risk categories. These are:

1. Administration of medication.
2. Assisting in the surgical suite.
3. Falls.
4. Burns.
5. Electric shocks.
6. Injuries due to faulty equipment.
7. Nosocomial infection.

8. Mistaken identity.
9. Misinterpretation of signs and symptoms.[37]

These would be included in a planned staff development program as would fire safety, disaster procedures, work hazards, radiological and laser safety, sanitation and infection control. Specific staff development programs would focus on malpractice and legal liability, including standards of care, informed consent, documentation, professional competence, and relevant laws. Other programs would focus on these fundamental concepts in nursing care:

1. Sensitivity to patients.
2. Identification of patients.
3. Environment.
4. Mental competence of patients.
5. Moving and lifting.
6. Transport of patients.[38]

ACCIDENT REPORTING

Incidents involving employees are frequently referred to as accidents. Follow the same principles as for incident reporting. These will usually be covered by institutional policy and procedure. Perceptions vary too much to require personnel to discriminate between incident and accident. An accident is an incident and many incidents are accidents.

INFECTION CONTROL

A major area for quality control and risk management is infection control. Infections acquired in hospitals are termed *nosocomial* infections. Many hospitals will have full-time infection control nurses. They investigate all reported nosocomial infections. A source of data is the medical laboratory. It is good policy to have all laboratory reports positive for infectious diseases routed to the infection control nurse. They will be investigated and procedures implemented to prevent their spread and future development.

Staff development is a major function of infection control. Standards followed are those of the Center for Disease Control.

DISCHARGE PLANNING

Schuman, Ostfeld, and Willard studied discharge planning in an acute care hospital. The need for this function was recognized in 1944, and 32 years later studies indicated that it was still being poorly done. The research team indicated that the head nurse supervises the function of discharge planning by nurses and supports their communication with physicians.[39] The competency required of the head nurse is to supervise staff nurses, who need to provide discharge planning that makes each patient aware of necessary precautions related to diagnosis and therapy, their medical regimens including times to take medication, dietary restrictions, and where to go for help. The fact is that patients suffer decreased functional capacity after discharge. Discharge planning decreases hospital readmission rates by fostering compliance with therapy. Instruction increases the importance of therapy in the eyes of the patient. The authors suggested that "nurses tend to be the most qualified personnel to delineate a patient's nursing needs following discharge and tend also to be aware of his need for ancillary services."[40]

SUMMARY

Quality assurance programs make certain that patient care is delivered that meets established standards. QA programs have as their objective the determination of whether the actual service provided matches predetermined criteria of excellence. Quality assurance also involves continuous action to improve deficiencies.

QA is a management process that provides a sound basis for decision making and problem solving. Management of care by competent clinical nurses and nurse managers ensures the quality of that care.

NOTES

1. M. J. Zimmer, "A Model for Evaluating Nursing Care," in *Management for Nurses: A Multidisciplinary Approach*, M. S. Berger, D. Elhart, S. C. Firsich, S. B. Jordan, and S. Stone, Eds. (St. Louis, MO: C. V. Mosby, 1980), 47–52.
2. L. F. Maciorowski, E. Larson, and A. Keane, "Quality Assurance: Evaluate Thyself," *The Journal of Nursing Administration*, June 1985, 38–42.

3. L. Edmunds, "A Computer Assisted Quality Assurance Model," *Journal of Nursing Administration*, Mar. 1983, 36–43; A. DeLotto, "Examining Quality of Care Becomes Top Industry Priority," *Amherst Quarterly*, Winter 1988, 1–3.

4. B. J. Curtis and L. J. Simpson, "Auditing: A Method for Evaluating Quality of Care," *Journal of Nursing Administration*, Oct. 1985, 14–21; M. A. Wandelt and M. D. Phaneuf, "Tools for Evaluation," *Management for Nurses*, op. cit., 229; H. S. Rowland and B. L. Rowland, *Nursing Administration Handbook*, 2d ed. (Rockville, MD: Aspen, 1985), 468–495.

5. Ibid.

6. Ibid.

7. B. J. Curtis and L. J. Simpson, op. cit.

8. Ibid.

9. H. S. Rowland and B. S. Rowland, op. cit.

10. L. Edmunds, op. cit.

11. H. S. Rowland and B. L. Rowland, Eds., "Quality Assurance," *Hospital Legal Forms, Checklists, and Guidelines* (Rockville, MD: Aspen, 1988), 26:1–26:14.

12. S. R. Edwardson and D. I. Anderson, "Hospital Nurses' Valuation of Quality Assurance," *Journal of Nursing Administration*, July-Aug. 1983, 33–39.

13. Ibid.

14. B. H. Munro, "A Useful Model for Program Evaluation," *Journal of Nursing Administration*, Mar. 1983, 23–26.

15. G. M. Wolff, "Systems Management: Evaluating Nursing Departments as a Whole," *Nursing Management*, Feb. 1986, 40–43.

16. B. H. Munro, op. cit.

17. Ibid.

18. L. F. Maciorowski, E. Larson, and A. Keane, op. cit.

19. H. S. Rowland and B. L. Rowland, *Nursing Administration Handbook*, op. cit.

20. L. Edmunds, op. cit.

21. R. Allio, "Forecasting: The Myth of Control," interview with Donald Michal, *Planning Review*, May 1986, 6–11.

22. D. C. Coddington and K. D. Moore, "Quality of Care As A Business Strategy," *Healthcare Forum Journal*, Mar./Apr. 1987, 29–32.

23. Ibid.

24. E. Larson, "Combining Nursing Quality Assurance and Research Programs," *Journal of Nursing Administration*, Nov. 1983, 32–34.

25. Ibid.

26. Ibid.

27. S. A. Hermon, "QA at St. Joseph's—Every Nurse's Responsibility, Every Nurse's Obligation," *Nursing Directions* (St. Joseph's Hospital Centers), July 1987, 1–3.

28. R. Levy, "The Go-Go World of the Risk Manager," *Dun's Review*, Nov. 1967.

29. G. W. Poteet, "Risk Management and Nursing," *Nursing Clinics of North America*, Sept. 1983, 457–465.

30. Ibid.

31. A. P. Sielicki, "Current Philosophy of Risk Management," *Topics in Health Care Financing*, Spring 1983, 3.

32. H. S. Rowland and B. L. Rowland, Eds., *Hospital Legal Forms, Checklists and Guidelines*, op. cit., 28:1–28:58.

33. A. P. Sielicki, op. cit.

34. "QAs Pave the Way: The Quest for Quality," *Hospital Profiles*. Alabama Hospital Association, December 1987/January 1988, 1, 4–5.

35. D. Joseph and S. K. Jones, "Incident Reporting: The Cornerstone of Risk Management," *Nursing Management*, Dec. 1984, 22–23.

36. G. W. Poteet, op. cit.; H. S. Rowland and B. L. Rowland, op. cit.; and K. H. Henry, ed., *Nursing Administration and Law Manual.* (Rockville, MD: Aspen, 1985), 9:1–9:39.

37. Ibid.

38. Ibid.

39. J. E. Schuman, A. M. Ostfeld, and H. N. Willard, "Discharge Planning in an Acute Hospital," *Archives of Physical Medicine and Rehabilitation*, July 1976, 343–347.

40. Ibid.

REFERENCES

Blake, P., "Incident Investigation: A Complete Guide," *Nursing Management*, Nov. 1987, 36–41.

Breland, D., "Medical Care Crisis Feared in State," *Mobile Register*, Sept. 25, 1985, B1, B6.

Buros, O. K., *Mental Measurements Yearbooks* (Highland Park, NJ: Gryphon Press, 1938, 1940, 1949, 1953, 1959, 1965, 1972, 1978).

Chun, K. T., S. Cobb, and J. R. P. French, Jr., *Measures for Psychological Assessment: A Guide to 3,000 Original Sources and Their Applications* (Ann Arbor: Institute for Social Research, University of Michigan, 1975).

Deep, W. M., "Dilemma of a Malpractice Insurer's Appointed Defense Attorney," *PLN* (Insurance Corporation of America), Sept. 1985, 2–5.

Kinloch, K., "For Nurses Only: Should Nursing Administrators Use Incident Reports as a Risk Management Tool?," *The Canadian Nurse*, Nov. 1982, 16–17.

"Malpractice Crisis Threatens Health of Medical Profession," *The Alexian Way*, Summer 1985, 3–9.

Purgatorio-Howard, K., "Improving a Quality Assurance Program," *Nursing Management*, Apr. 1986, 38–40, 42.

"QAs Pave the Way: The Quest for Quality," *Hospital Profiles* (Alabama Hospital Association), Dec. 1987/Jan. 1988, 1, 4–5.

Renzulli, J. S., "Key Features: A Practical Model for Program Evaluation," *Curriculum Trends*, Feb. 1972, 1–6.

Renzulli, J. S., *A Guidebook for Evaluating Programs for the Gifted and Talented* (Ventura, CA: Office of the Ventura County Superintendent of Schools, 1975).

Smeltzer, C. H., B. Geltman, and K. Rajki, "Nursing Quality Assurance: A Process, Not a Tool," *The Journal of Nursing Administration*, Jan. 1983, 5–9.

Spicer, J. G., and G. M. Lewis, "Using Theory to Promote Change," *Nursing Administration Quarterly*, Winter 1981, 53–57.

Ward, M. J., and C. E. Lindeman, Eds., *Instruments for Measuring Nursing Practice and Other Health Care Variables*, 2 vols., DHEW Publication HRA78-53 (Hyattsville, MD: U.S. Department of Health, Education, and Welfare, 1979).

The JCAHO publishes the *Quality Review Bulletin*, which is available from: Cashier, Joint Commission, 875 North Michigan Avenue, 22nd Floor, Chicago, IL 60611. Subscriptions are $70 ($80 outside the continental United States).

Performance Appraisal

24

INTRODUCTION

Performance appraisal is a control process in which employees' performances are evaluated against standards. The literature on performance appraisal is voluminous, indicating its value to management. Considerable research has been done on various aspects of the performance appraisal process.

Neither employees nor managers like performance appraisal. Some employees view performance appraisal as being more valued by top management than by themselves and their supervisors. Some managers do not like to do performance appraisals because it makes them feel guilty. "Did I do justice by the employee?" As writers of performance appraisals, managers are concerned that they may "cast something in stone" that is inaccurate, may be criticized on written grammar and spelling, say something illegal about the ratee, or may not be able to be substantiated.[1] Other managers are afraid of employees' reactions to ratings. Also, performance appraisal requires careful planning, information gathering, and an extensive formal interview, a time-consuming process. Managers perform activities of short duration, attend ad hoc meetings, perform non-routine behavior and focus on current information, all short-term activities in comparison with ongoing performance appraisal.[2] The process is usually not interactive, moves slowly, is passive, is isolated, and is not people-oriented.[3]

Measurement of performance is imprecise. Often the focus is upon the format, not the people. In some organizations the human resources department sends the rating forms to the departments shortly before the end of the fiscal year. They have to be completed immediately and are done with little or no training and preparation of either rater or ratee. The result is distrust by employees and dread by managers.

A survey of Fortune 1300 companies (1000 industrial and 300 nonindustrial) indicated that 29 percent of hourly workers are not evaluated by a formal appraisal system. Thirty-nine percent of respondents indicated that, where used, performance appraisal systems are "extremely effective" or "very effective." They are underappreciated.[4]

Performance appraisal systems require top management commitment. They can be tied to the planning cycle by relating them to personnel budgets or including them as a management plan.

PURPOSES OF PERFORMANCE APPRAISAL

Performance appraisal is a nurse manager's most valuable tool in controlling human resources and productivity. The performance appraisal process can be used effectively to govern employee behavior in order to produce goods and services in high volume and of high quality. Nurse managers can also use the performance appraisal process to govern corporate direction in selection, training, career planning, and rewarding of personnel. The Fortune 1300 survey indicated that 80 percent used appraisal systems to justify merit increases, provide feedback, and identify candidates for promotion, all considered short-range goals. They were linked to long-range goals of performance potential for succession planning and career planning, but could be much more useful in strategic planning. Fifty-eight percent used performance appraisal to identify strengths and weaknesses, while 39 percent used it for career planning. Eighty-nine percent used it for general guidelines for salary increases, while only 1 percent used it for forced distribution for bonuses. Forced distribution sets a limit on the number of high-level ratings.[5]

In addition to being used for promotions, termination, selections, and compensations, performance monitoring has been found to make employees effective. It is a managerial tool that can facilitate performance levels that achieve the company's mission and objectives.[6]

Appraisal systems are needed to meet legal requirements including those for standardized forms and procedures, clear and relevant job analysis, and trained raters. When they do not, disciplinary actions including termination do not stand up in court.[7]

Motivation

A goal of performance appraisal is to stimulate motivation of the employee to perform the tasks and accomplish the mission of the organization. Promotions, assignments, selection for education, and increased pay are among the goals of the employee that stimulate this motivation. If performance appraisal is to improve performance, the science of behavioral technology should be employed. This science has as its basis the premise that consequences will influence behavior. People will work more willingly if supervisors or managers exercise concern for their feelings and needs. A basic question here is, what rewards will the employee work for?

Analyzing Problems Using Behavioral Technology. The usual answer to identified problems is to give the employees more training. Consider an example involving the writing of nursing notes. A nurse executive made scheduled ward rounds on a monthly basis. One of the announced activities that she would perform was to evaluate the quality of nursing notes in relation to the nursing care plan. Since this facility was using the problem-oriented system, the nursing notes were to describe progress in relation to each nursing problem and the prescribed nursing approaches. Time after time there were omissions in the recording system. The standard approach to the problem was to give more in-service education to the personnel making the nursing notes. Finally, the nurse executive sat down with key managers to analyze the problem. These were the questions they asked themselves:

What were the consequences of proper recordings?

Financial: Salary had not been affected by writing satisfactory nursing notes. They were a requirement of the job description and the job standards.

Supervision: Few comments by supervisors had related to satisfactory recordings.

What were the consequences of improper recordings?

Financial: Salary had not been affected by writing unsatisfactory nursing notes. Salary increases had been approved regardless of the quality of the nursing notes.

Supervision: There had been criticism by nurse managers of omissions and improper recordings by clinical nurses.

In further discussion it was decided that more in-service education classes were not going to solve the problem. The approach would be a positive one. Personnel who consistently wrote especially good nursing notes would be rewarded. An attempt would be made to give their salary increases early. Also, supervisors would overtly recognize and comment on the satisfactory nursing notes while refraining from criticism of omissions and unsatisfactory ones. In-service education would be used only for personnel who did not know the techniques of writing problem-oriented nursing notes.

This approach is also illustrated by the experience of Ms. Bins, a nurse executive who received daily written reports on selected patients. Much of this information was useless to her, since few comment related to the nursing problems of patients or the prescribed nursing care. Progress was not usually indicated. The reports were composed mostly of trivia. She decided to reinforce the behavior she desired and ignore the undesirable behavior. Consequently she wrote positive comments on the reports that contained a nursing diagnosis and prescription and described progress and returned these reports to the charge nurses. Within weeks progress was pronounced; nurses were writing reports that gave the nurse executive excellent knowledge of the patients' conditions as well as of the workload and performances of nursing personnel.

Designing Learning Systems Using Behavioral Technology. Where safety is involved, it is not enough to teach people skills that prevent injuries to themselves and to patients. Supervisors should be taught to reinforce the correct behavior. Such behavior should be reinforced directly after the act. Verbal reinforcers are often as effective as monetary ones. They are particularly effective if followed by monetary rewards. When managers become skilled in the principles of behavioral technology, they know the amount of reinforcement needed by individual employees. The act should be identified with the reinforcement if the latter is to be effective. Reinforcement should be genuine so that the employee will recognize the correlation between the desired behavior and the reward.[8]

Salary Problems. Performance evaluation is used to determine and provide equitable salary treatment. Jobs within groups of professionals such as engineers, physicians, chemists, physicists, and nurses have the same basic characteristics. There are differences in the complexity of jobs. One could say that the job of a nurse assigned to a special care unit is more complex than that of one assigned to an intermediate care unit. This could be true to the extent that the depth of complexity exists. Contrast this with the complexity of managing the care of an active intermediate care unit of twenty to forty-five patients. The *breadth* of complexity of the nursing care of many patients with differing problems who are treated by many physicians directing medical care plans and many nonprofessional workers appears to be equivalent to the *depth* of complexity of intensive nursing care. In fact, some nurses want to be assigned to special care units, not because of the dynamics of the situation, but because their sphere of operations is encapsulated. Is one entitled to more salary than another? The job analysts say "yes" if special training is required, if complicated specialized equipment is being used, and if the nurse is required to make more independent and critical judgements.

Certainly the jobs of all professionals can be evaluated by using the yardsticks of conventional performance appraisal techniques. However, arguments abound regarding the relationship between performance appraisals and salaries and promotion. Some writers say keep performance appraisals well away from times of salary increases and promotions.[9] In a survey of 875 companies, 32 percent experimented with some form of performance-based pay.[10]

Kirkpatrick recommends separating appraisals for merit salary increases from appraisals for performance improvement. Those used for merit salary increases look backward at past performance, look at total performance, compare one individual to others doing same job, are subjective, and are done in an emotional climate. Appraisals done for performance improvement look ahead, are concerned with detailed performance, are compared with what is expected in standards, goals, and objectives, and are conducted in a calm climate.[11]

For performance reviews related to salary administration, nurse managers would explain to subordinates the basis of decisions. They would be fair and would be totally understood by the managers, who would allow employees to react even to the point of discussing them with higher management. If a high salary increase results, the nurse manager communicates the good news to the employee. Three months should elapse between appraisals for salary administration and those for improved performance.[12]

Expectancy theory states that "the greater a person's expectancy [i.e. subjective probability] that effort expenditure will lead to various rewards, the greater the person's motivation to work hard."[13] Rewards of high value should be obtainable and related to job performance. Employees will repeat rewarded behavior and they will be retained, thus maintaining productivity.

Research indicates that productivity increased on a range of 29 to 63 percent with output-based pay plans versus time-based pay plans. Also, individual incentive plans are better than group incentive plans.[14]

Pay is the most powerful motivator of performance and people will not work without it. Also, other financial incentives such as shift differentials, education pay, and certification pay are positive motivators. Research has shown that productivity actually drops with time-based rewards and hourly wages. Good employees will leave rather than work with poorly performing ones. Rewards should be related to job performance. The results can be seen by correlating rewards across individual performances. There should be substantial differences in the rewards. Kopelman suggests a mixed-consequence system: rewards for good performance; deductions for poor performance. The latter requires coaching, training, counseling, reassigning, or terminating. Important job responsibilities and behaviors deserving of high rewards can be determined from job analysis. They should be related to difficult performance standards or goals.[15]

The Xerox Experience. Prior to 1983, Xerox had a traditional appraisal system tying merit pay increases to performance rating. Employees were dissatisfied with the lack of an equitable rating distribution. Ninety-five percent of employees were at level 3 or 4 of a four-level rating system. Forced distribution was used to control the numbers of employees above or below a specific level. There were no preplanned objectives, the focus being on the summary rating. A task force was used to develop a performance feedback and development process with the following characteristics:

1. Objectives were set between manager and employee.
2. The evaluation was documented and approved by a second-level manager.
3. An appraisal review was held at the end of 6 months, with review and discussion of objectives and progress. The written report was signed by both.
4. A final review was held at 1 year.
5. The process emphasized performance feedback and improvements.
6. A merit increase discussion was held 1 to 2 months later.
7. There was agreement on personal goals related to communications, planning, time management, human relations, and professional goals (specialty and job).
8. There were financial and human resource management objectives.
9. Managers were trained in the process.

Regular surveys of the Xerox system indicated that 81 percent of employees understood their work group objectives better, 84 percent considered appraisal fair, 72 percent understood how merit pay was determined, 70 percent met personal and professional objectives, and 77 percent favored the system.[16]

Other Purposes of Performance Appraisal

An effective appraisal generates understanding and commitment, leading to productivity. Career development and performance appraisal support each other if they share objectives, recognition, concern, and communication. Usually nurse managers take charge of performance appraisal while employees take charge of career development. They can be brought together for mutual benefits.

Talent development can be a mutual goal and benefit of the two programs. Performance input supports future options and paths for future growth and development of employees.[17]

Performance appraisals can also be used to confirm hiring decisions. This is particularly true when new employees have a probationary period before becoming permanent. This is a crucial period as employees can be terminated without the extended termination process. Effective nurse managers will use this period to counsel and coach the employee to effective performance. The performance appraisal will document the process.

DEVELOPING AND USING STANDARDS FOR PERFORMANCE APPRAISAL

Performance Standards

Performance standards are derived from job analysis, job descriptions, and job evaluation and other documents detailing the qualitative and quantitative aspects of jobs. They are established by authority, which may be the agency in which they are used or a professional association such as the American Nurses' Association (ANA). They are measuring sticks for qualitative and quantitative evaluation of the individual's performance. They should be based on appropriate knowledge and practical enough to be attained. Like other documents, they must be kept up to date. Job or performance standards for the nurse manager may be developed using the ANA *Standards for Organized Nursing Services and Responsibilities of Nurse Administrators Across All Settings.*

Performance standards are written for a job and are used to measure the performance of the individual filling the job. Employees should know that these standards are being used and what they are. They may be asked to bring them to their supervisor for scheduled counseling. They may also be asked to list their accomplishments in relation to the standards. This makes performance counseling less of a threat and allows employees to recognize and discuss their accomplishments. They may be guided into recognition of those areas where their performance falls short and to voice goals for improvement in these areas. This method of using performance standards has been found to be effective.

The ANA Congress for Nursing Practice has developed and published standards of practice in several areas: nursing practice, community health nursing practice, geriatric nursing practice, maternal-child health nursing practice, psychiatric-mental health nursing practice, medical-surgical nursing practice, emergency room nursing practice, cardiovascular nursing practice, orthopedic nursing practice, operating room nursing practice and others. The ANA *Standards of Nursing Practice* can be used in the development of performance standards.

Figure 24–1 is an example of performance standards for a clinical nurse.

The nurse manager controls nursing productivity with standards that measure nursing performance. Standards are based on history or past experience and "gut level appraisal by the person in charge."[18] They include establishment of criteria, planning goals, and physical or quantitative measurements of products, units of service, labor-hours, speed, and the like.[19]

A standard has been defined as "an acknowledged measure of comparison for a quantitative or qualitative value, criterion, or norm." A criterion is "a standard rule or test on which a judgement or decision can be based." Nurse managers develop, in collaboration with clinical nurses, the "clinical nursing criteria against which to measure patient outcomes and the nursing process."[20]

Koontz and Weihrich identified eight categories of standards.[21] They are listed in chapter 22, Controlling or Evaluating.

Accuracy and fairness of performance appraisal comes from having an objective, standards-oriented performance appraisal plan. The plan should have objectively defined task standards that can be measured in terms of output and observable behavioral change. These performance standards will relate to both the quantity and quality of work; the who, how, when, where, and what is produced. They will include production standards.[22]

Performance evaluation includes standards for experience, complexities of job, trust level, and understanding of work and mission. Friedman recommends developing job standards based on four to eight core responsibilities. For nurse managers these core responsibilities could be in the major management functions of planning, organizing, directing, and controlling. They could also be related to the roles of clinician, teacher, administrator, consultant, and researcher. Finally, they could relate to self-development. Desired behaviors, outputs, or results under each core responsibility are then developed as performance objectives. Objectives are related to or combined with behaviors as standards for performance evaluation.[23]

FIGURE 24–1.   Performance Standards—Clinical Nurse

Performance Standards

1. Type of work: Nursing care of patients
   Major duty: Performs the primary functions of a professional nurse (50 percent of working hours).
   a. Obtains nursing histories on all newly admitted patients.
   b. Reviews nursing histories of all transfer patients.
   c. Uses nursing histories to make nursing diagnoses determining patients' needs and problems.
   Using this information:
   d. Initiates a nursing care plan for each patient.
   e. Lists goal(s) for each nursing need or problem.
   f. Writes nursing prescription or orders for each patient to meet each need or problem and goal.
   g. Applies the plan of care giving evidence of knowledge of scientific and legal principles.
   h. Executes physicians' orders.
2. Type of work: Management of nursing personnel.
   Major duty: Plans nursing care of patients on a daily basis (14 percent of working hours).
   a. Rates each patient according to number and complexity of needs and goals.
   b. Knows abilities of each team member.
   c. Makes a daily assignment for each team member.
   d. Discusses assignment with each team member at the beginning of each shift.
      1. Listens to taped report with team members.
      2. Sees that team members review physicians' orders and nursing care plans.
      3. Answers questions arising from these activities.
   e. Confers with charge nurse and ward clerk periodically to ascertain whether there are any new orders.
   f. Plans for a team conference at a specific time and place, and tells team members.
   g. Incorporates division and unit philosophy and objectives into team activities.
   h. Assists with assignment of L.P.N. and R.N. students, including them as active team members according to their backgrounds and learning needs.
3. Type of work: Management of nursing personnel.
   Major duty: Supervises team activities (10 percent of working hours).
   a. Makes frequent rounds to assist team members with their care of patients. At the same time, talks to and observes patients to determine:

   1. New needs or problems.
   2. Progress. Confirms these observations with patient if possible.
   b. Conducts 15- to 20-minute team conference using a specific agenda that has been made known to team members at previous day's conference.
      1. Involves all team members.
      2. Solicits comments on new problems or special problems of patients and updates selected nursing care plans as needed.
      3. Assigns roles for next day's team conference.
   c. Writes nursing progress notes and updates remaining nursing care plans.
      1. Assists technicians with writing notes as needed for training. Otherwise reads and countersigns their notes. Writes own notes.
      2. Updates those nursing care plans not done at team conference. Recognizes this is a professional nurse's responsibility.
      3. Reads notes of L.P.N.s and R.N.s.
   d. Communicates nursing service and hospital policies to team members on a daily basis through referral to such information as daily bulletins, minutes of meetings, and changes in regulations.

4. Type of work: Management of equipment and supplies.
   Major duty: Identifies needs; plans and submits requests for new and replacement equipment and supplies to charge nurse (1 percent of working hours).
   a. While working with team members identifies malfunctioning equipment and supply shortages and reports same to charge nurse and ward clerk on a daily basis.
   b. Submits requests for new equipment and supplies to charge nurse on a quarterly basis.

5. Type of work: Training.
   Major duty: Identifies training needs of team members and plans activities to meet needs (5 percent of working hours).
   a. Identifies specific training needs of individual team members through daily observation of their performance and interviews.
   b. Evaluates performance through use of performance standards. Makes these standards known to each team member and holds them responsible for meeting standards.
   c. Plans counseling and guidance of each team member on an individual basis, at least quarterly.

FIGURE 24–1.   Performance Standards—Clinical Nurse (*continued*)

d. Plans and conducts unit in-service education programs at least monthly. Involves team members.

e. Recommends team members for seminars, short courses, college programs, and correspondence courses.

f. Thoroughly orients all new team members. Conducts skill inventory during initial interview and plans on-the-job training for those needed skills in which team member is not proficient.

g. Submits budget requests for training materials and programs to charge nurse annually.

h. Makes reading assignments and allows time for team members to use library resources.

6. Type of work: Planning patient care.

   Major duty: Coordinates nursing resources essential to meeting each patient's total needs and goals (5 percent of working hours).

   a. Consults with patients' physicians daily.

   b. Requests consultations of clinical nurse specialists. This may include clinical nurse specialists in pediatrics, mental health, medical/surgical, radiology, public health, and rehabilitation.

   c. Consults with other personnel as needed, including chaplain, social worker, recreation worker, occupational therapist, physical therapist, pharmacist, and inhalation therapist. Coordinates with physicians and charge nurse as needed.

   d. Supports philosophy of having ward clerks assume non-nursing activities by assisting with their training as needed on a daily basis, to help them become proficient in their duties.

   e. Aggressively pursues having ward clerks do administrative tasks and nursing team members perform the primary functions of nursing. The latter most commonly occurs at patients' bedsides.

7. Type of work: Teaching patients.

   Major duty: Teaches patients to care for themselves after discharge from the hospital (5 percent of working hours).

   a. Plans teaching as a major rehabilitation goal of each newly admitted patient. Includes it as part of nursing assessment and enters it on the nursing care plan.

b. Reviews and updates teaching plans daily.

c. Involves resource people in teaching program.

d. Refers cases to visiting nurse for follow-up.

e. Makes follow-up appointments for assessment of progress toward nursing goals with a clinical nurse.

f. Involves families in teaching as indicated.

8. Type of work: Evaluation of care process.

   Major duty: Conducts audits of nursing care (3 percent of working hours).

   a. Audits nursing records on a daily basis.

   b. Performs bedside audit on a weekly basis.

   c. Audits closed charts of discharged patients on a monthly basis.

   d. Reviews patient questionnaires.

   e. Discusses results of all audits with team members as a group and on an individual basis.

9. Type of work: Personnel administration.

   Major duty: Rates performances of team members (2 percent of working hours).

   a. Writes performance reports.

   b. Discusses reports with individuals to learn their personal goals.

10. Type of work: Self-development.

    Major duty: Pursues a program of continuing education activities (5 percent of working hours).

    a. Sets own goals for self-development, including a reading program and a set of educational goals for short courses, conventions, workshops, college courses, and management courses.

    b. Participates in division and departmental in-service education programs.

    c. Participates in nursing service committee activities.

    d. Participates in research projects.

    e. Participates as a citizen in the community through involvement in professional organizations and service projects.

    f. Assumes responsibility for knowledge of, progress in, and utilization of community resources such as:

       1. Health groups.
       2. Civic groups.
       3. General education groups.
       4. Nursing recruitment.
       5. Others.

Job analysis, job descriptions, and job evaluations are important sources of standards for performance evaluation.

Job Analysis

Edwards and Sproull list "objective performance dimensions, developed by management and employees" as a necessity for effective performance appraisal. They are developed from job analysis. "Performance criteria should be: (1) measurable through observation of behaviors of the job, (2) clearly defined, and (3) job-related." Nurse managers and nursing employees would agree on the meaning and priority of each measurement. These standards need not be quantifiable but must be keyed to observable behavior:[24]

Observable Behavior→ Job Analysis→ Job
Standards

Basing performance appraisal on job analysis makes it more relevant and establishes content validity.[25] Job analysis systematically gathers information about a particular job. It "identifies, specifies, organizes, and displays the duties, tasks, and responsibilities actually performed by the incumbent in a given job."[26]

The job analysis will reveal overlaps among jobs so that they can be modified. It can be used to improve efficiency and proficiency by identifying skills certification, altering staffing levels, reassigning staff, selecting new employees, altering management, establishing training objectives and standards, developing career ladders, and improving job satisfaction.[27]

A procedure for doing job analysis is as follows:

1. Name the job specifically, e.g., nurse manager, oncology.
2. Go to the work place, identify the target nurses working in the job family, and talk to them. Ask these questions:
    2.1 What are the characteristics of a good clinical nurse?
    2.2 What are the characteristics of a poor clinical nurse?
    2.3 How does a good clinical nurse differ from a poor clinical nurse?
    2.4 How does a good clinical nurse perform tasks better than others?
    2.5 Give examples of effective performance by a clinical nurse.
    2.6 Why is this clinical nurse effective?
    2.7 Give examples of ineffective performance of a clinical nurse.
    2.8 Why is this clinical nurse ineffective?
    2.9 Describe a clinical nurse who performs the job better than anyone else. Why?
    2.10 What job skills would you look for if you had to hire someone to do clinical nursing? Why?
    2.11 Describe the prior training or experience needed to effectively perform clinical nursing. Why is this so?
3. Have the job incumbents list all duties, tasks, and responsibilities (DTRs) that they perform. Do for a specific time period.
4. As manager, list all DTRs that the job incumbents perform. Do by observation for specific time period coinciding with incidents. These can be prepared one to each index card.
5. Compare the two lists and aim for consensus between job incumbents and manager.
6. State the duties, tasks, and responsibilities in specific, clear behavioral terms.
7. Determine the four to eight job task categories to be used, such as managerial, direct care, maintenance, and interpersonal.
8. Classify each DTR into the four to eight core job categories.
9. List the DTRs by priority. Use consensus. This will improve efficiency.
10. Evaluate DTRs for specificity, indicating how and when they will be performed.
11. Review with the team, eliminating those with low priority. Rewrite items as needed, making each a unique job skill stated in understandable language.
12. Set standards of performance, including the percentage of time each is to be done.
13. List constraints: education, experience, physical, and emotional.
14. Write a summary of the unique facets of the job.
15. Prepare a job analysis questionnaire and administer it to all personnel with the same job title.[28] See Figure 24–2 for format.

Research has shown no significant differences on job analysis information between effective and ineffective retail store managers. Research has also shown no significant difference between high job

FIGURE 24–2. Job Analysis Questionnaire

Title: Head Nurse

Check here if you ever do the task	<Relative time spent>	<Training emphasis>
in your present job:	<Lo><Avg><Hi>	<Lo><Avg><Hi>
_____ 1. (List DTRs)	123456789	123456789
_____ 2.		

SOURCE: Modified from E. P. Prien, I. L. Goldstein, and W. H. Macey, "Multidomain Job Analysis: Procedures and Applications," *Training and Development Journal,* Aug. 1987, 68–72.

---

performers' perceptions of their jobs' demands and those of low job performers among police officers. Since these research studies are few and inconclusive in relation to the literature on the subject, nursing researchers should do research in these areas. The described method of developing a master inventory of knowledges, skills, and abilities could be used by nurse managers to develop job analyses.[29]

Job analysis leads to a job description of the work expected by the institution, which can be used for performance appraisal.

Job Descriptions

The Job Description as a Contract. A job description is a contract that should include the job's functions and obligations and tell the person to whom the worker is responsible. It is a written report outlining duties, responsibilities, and conditions of the work assignment. It is a description of a job and not of a person who happens to hold that job. "That many executives recognize the importance of obtaining good position descriptions is reflected in a survey made several years ago by the American Management Association. In this study, seventy firms reported a median fee of $20,000 paid to management consultants for preparation of their job descriptions. Most significantly, 95 percent of the respondents reported that the expenditure was 'definitely worth-while.' In two instances the fee paid for this service approached $100,000."[30] Most formats include a job title, statements of basic functions, scope, duties, responsibilities, organizational relationships, limits of authority, and criteria for performance evaluation.

What Are Job Descriptions Used For? There are many organizations that do not have job descriptions. Still others do not use those they have. Poor management practices are usually evident in the output or productivity of employees and in the behavior they exhibit that indicates their attitudes about nursing work. As an example, they may devote a large proportion of their duty hours to non-nursing work and avoid primary practices of nursing related to clinical services to consumers.

Job descriptions are used for many purposes:

1. To establish a rational basis for the salary structure, thus showing why one job pays more than another. For example, job descriptions should show why a charge nurse earns less than a director of nursing.
2. To clarify relationships between jobs to avoid overlaps and gaps in responsibility.
3. To help employees analyze their duties so that they will have a better understanding of their jobs.
4. To help define the organizational structure and support or give evidence for its revision.
5. To reassign and fix functions and responsibilities in the entire agency.
6. To evaluate job performance.
7. To orient new employees to jobs.
8. To assist in hiring and placement of employees.
9. To establish lines of promotion within the department.
10. To identify potential training needs.
11. To critically review the existing nursing practices within the agency.
12. To maintain continuity of all operations in a changing work environment.

13. To improve the work flow.
14. To provide data as to proper channels of communication.
15. To develop job specifications.
16. To serve as a basis for planning staffing levels.

Introduction of a system using job descriptions requires planning and should be built into the operational or management plan for accomplishment of departmental objectives. In fact, job descriptions should relate to specific objectives of management. It takes time to develop good job descriptions and introduce them into a management system. Many changes in the dynamic environment of a health-care agency, such as changes in personnel, departmental or agency objectives, budget, and technology, create the necessity for periodic review and revision of job descriptions. Time should not be wasted preparing job descriptions that will not be put to daily use. They should be available to all personnel so that they will know the dimensions of their jobs, who in the agency can help them in their work, how their performances will be evaluated, and the opportunities for advancement. To make the data more useful, numerical values may be assigned to the important elements of the specific duties, as in Figure 24–1.

To avoid bias, data for job descriptions should be gathered from several sources. Data may be collected from interviewing the job incumbent, having an incumbent keep a log of duties performed during a specific time period, observation, and a questionnaire (job analysis).

The person preparing the job descriptions should determine the uses that will be made of them so that needed information may be included. It is probably best to introduce job descriptions during a time of favorable economic outlook when employees will be less threatened by them. They should be introduced to the staff registered nurses first. Managers may fear increased workloads and grievances. It is important to consult with all employees and allow them to discuss, comment, and recommend changes in the job descriptions for positions they will fill. This makes development of job descriptions a cooperative venture, leading to consensus, effective management, and effective performance appraisal. Language used in the job descriptions should be simple and understandable. They are guides; rigid application will result in negative behavior. As an example, some personnel have re-

fused to perform certain duties that were not included in their job descriptions. Job descriptions should define minimum standards for effective job performance and employment and should not be too detailed. "Performs other duties as directed" is evasive and should not be put into a job description.

A format is needed for quality and thoroughness of job descriptions. Kennedy recommends the following parts:

1. Header: job title, name and location of incumbent, immediate superiors.
2. Principal purpose or summary; overall contribution of incumbent.
3. Principal responsibilities, including percentage of time spent on each.
4. Job skills: knowledge, skills, and education.
5. Dimension or scope: quantifies such areas as the budget, size of reporting organizations, impact on bottom line.
6. Organizational chart.
7. Problem-solving examples.
8. Environment.
9. Key contacts.
10. References guiding incumbent's actions.
11. Supervision given and received.[31]

Job descriptions can be written to comply with some legal, regulatory, and accrediting requirements. The following are examples:

1. Licensing laws of the state, rules of accrediting agencies, and Medicare and Medicaid regulations can be met through job descriptions.
2. They can be used for job rating and classification.
3. They can be used to determine whether jobs are exempt or nonexempt.
4. They can be used in recruitment, selection, evaluation, and retention.[32]

Figure 24–3 presents a job description for a bedside nurse in a U.S. hospital about 1887.

Figure 24–4 is a job description for a generalized clinical nurse in 1989.

Job Evaluation

Job evaluation is a process used to measure exact amounts of base elements found in jobs. Laws require men and women to be paid equally for equal

FIGURE 24–3.   1887 Job Description

In its publication, *Bright Corridor,* Cleveland's Lutheran Hospital published this job description for a bedside nurse in a U.S. hospital in 1887:

In addition to caring for your fifty patients, each bedside nurse will follow these regulations:

1. Daily sweep and mop the floors of your ward; dust the patient's furniture and window sills.
2. Maintain an even temperature in your ward by bringing in a scuttle of coal for the day's business.
3. Light is important to observe the patient's condition. Therefore, each day fill kerosene lamps, clean chimneys, and trim wicks. Wash the windows once a week.
4. The nurse's notes are important in aiding the physician's work. Make your pens carefully; you may whittle nibs to your individual tastes.
5. Each nurse on day duty will report every day at 7:00 A.M. and leave at 8:00 P.M., except on the Sabbath, on which day you will be off from 12:00 noon to 2:00 P.M.

6. Graduate nurses in good standing with the director of nursing will be given an evening off each week for courting purposes, or two a week if you go regularly to church.
7. Each nurse should lay aside from each payday a goodly sum of their earnings for her benefits during her declining years, so that she will not become a burden. For example, if you earn $30 a month you should set aside $15.
8. Any nurse who smokes, uses liquor in any form, gets her hair done at a beauty shop, or frequents dance halls will give the director of nurses good reason to suspect her worth, intentions, and integrity.
9. The nurse who performs her labors, serves her patients and doctors faithfully and without fault for a period of five years will be given an increase by the hospital administration of $.05 a day, providing there are no hospital debts that are outstanding.

FIGURE 24–4.   Position Description

Title: Generalized Clinical Nurse (GCN)

General Description   The GCN is a professional nurse with academic preparation at the B.S.N. level or above, who provides expert nursing care based upon scientific principles; delivers direct patient care and serves as a consultant or technical advisor in the area of health professions; and serves as a role model in the leadership, management, and delivery of quality nursing care by integrating the role components of clinician, administrator, teacher, consultant, and researcher.

Qualifications

A. Educational
   1. Graduation from an accredited school of nursing.
   2. Bachelor of Science in Nursing degree required.
B. Personal and Professional
   1. Current state professional nursing license.
   2. Knowledge of and experience in preventive care (screening and teaching).
   3. Demonstrated knowledge and competence in nursing, communication, and leadership skills.

4. Ability to analyze situations, recognize problems, search for pertinent facts and make appropriate decisions.
5. Ability to coordinate orientation and continuing education of clinic staff utilizing appropriate teaching strategies.
6. Ability to apply principles of change, organizational theory, and decision making.
7. Membership and participation in professional organizations desirable.
8. Recognition of civic responsibilities of nursing.
9. Ability to communicate effectively both in writing and verbally.
10. Evidence of professional manner and conduct.
11. Optimum physical and emotional health.

Organizational Relationships.   The GCN is administratively responsible and accountable to the nurse administrator. He or she is responsible for assessing, teaching, coordinating, providing appropriate care, and making referrals when necessary.

(continued)

FIGURE 24–4. Position Description (*continued*)

Activities

A. Clinician
  1. Give direct patient care in selected patient situations and serve as a behavioral model for excellence in practice.
  2. Assist the nursing personnel in assessing individual patient needs and formulation of a plan of nursing care; write nursing orders, when appropriate, for implementation of nursing plan; and assist the nursing personnel in documenting the effectiveness of the individualized care.
  3. Set, evaluate, and re-evaluate standards of nursing practice; communicate these standards to the nursing personnel; and change standards as necessary.
  4. Evaluate nursing care given to patients within the clinical area (assessing and teaching); when appropriate, make recommendations for improvement of that care.
  5. Function as a change agent; identify the barriers to more comprehensive health-care delivery, modify behavior, and introduce new approaches to patient care.
  6. Collaborate with other health-care providers and make appropriate referrals when necessary.

B. Teacher
  1. Provide an atmosphere conducive to learning.
  2. Teach appropriate prevention measures to clients.
  3. Direct the orientation of new staff and student nurses to ease their role transition and improve their skills, attitudes, and practices.
  4. Consider the needs of the adult learners (nursing personnel) as well as the clinicians' knowledge and expertise when planning continuing education to the clinical practice.
  5. Initiate or assist with the planning, presenting, and evaluating of continuing education programs for clinic staff.
  6. Guide and assist staff and nursing students as they assume the responsibility of patient teaching.

C. Administrator
  1. Function as a change agent and appraise leadership, communication, and change processes in the orga-

nization and assist with direct strategies for change as necessary.
  2. Work collaboratively with hospital personnel and other health-care providers in planning care and making referrals.
  3. Make recommendations relative to improving patient care and staff and student requirements to the appropriate administrative personnel.
  4. Support and interpret the clinical policies and procedures.

D. Self-Development
  1. Assume responsibility for identifying own educational needs and upgrade deficit areas through independent study, seminar attendance, or requesting staff development programs.
  2. Evaluate own nursing practice and instruction of others and the effect these have on the quality of patient care.

E. Consultant
  1. Conduct informal conferences with nursing personnel concerning patient care of specific health problems, the problem patient, or other pertinent problems related to nursing as suggested by the staff.
  2. Assist personnel to develop awareness of community agencies/resources available in planning patient care.
  3. Serve as a resource person to patients and their families.

F. Researcher
  1. Determine research problems related to preventive care, nursing clinics, etc.
  2. Conduct research studies to upgrade independent nursing practice.
  3. Demonstrate knowledge of the current research applicable to the clinical area and apply this knowledge in nursing care when appropriate.
  4. Research clinical nursing problems through the development and testing of relevant theories, evaluation, and implementation of research findings for nursing practice.
  5. Promote interest in reading and reviewing of current publications dealing with the delivery of preventive care to ambulatory patients.

work requiring equal skill, knowledge, effort, and responsibility under similar working conditions. This is an important factor in the fight to achieve pay equity for women and hence for nurses.[33]

Job evaluation rates jobs within a given agency. Although several job evaluation systems exist, the Hay Job Evaluation System is reported to be the best known. It was developed by the Hay Group, a Philadelphia-based consulting firm in 1951 to approve managerial, technical, and professional positions.[34]

The Hay System attempts to measure exact amounts of base elements found in all jobs, including (1) know-how, (2) problem solving, and (3) accountability. Know-how includes practical procedures, specialized techniques, scientific disciplines, managerial know-how, and human relations skills. Problem solving includes the job's thinking environment and thinking challenge. Accountability includes freedom to act, input of the job on the corporation, and the magnitude of the job. Observations of Hay System use indicate that the percentage of specialized know-how decreases with high-level positions, indicating problem solving and accountability to be the real pay-off factors.[35]

Work Classification

Helton reports a system for work classification to improve white-collar work. It includes four categories: specialist, professional, support, and clerical. Professional and specialist jobs involve a significant amount of cognitive effort, are not routine, and are challenging. Criteria used to classify white collar work are (1) work range, (2) work structure, (3) control, and (4) cognitive effort. Applied to nursing the M.S.N. nurse would be a specialist, the B.S.N. nurse a professional, the A.D./diploma/L.P.N. nurse a support person, and aides and clerks would be equivalent to clerical workers. It would be economical to develop or integrate the latter into one job.[36]

The classical approach is to design jobs and then find or fit people to them. Over 80 percent of all employees are reportedly satisfied with their jobs.

A 1974 national survey of white collar workers put "interesting work" first and "good pay" seventh. The behavioral approach uses job enlargement and job enrichment. Job enlargement uses horizontal loading to add tasks of equal difficulty and responsibility to jobs. Job enrichment uses vertical loading to add tasks that increase difficulty and responsibility of jobs. Both have beneficial results, including

increased productivity. In thirty-two experiments involving job redesign, thirty indicated impact; the median increase in productivity was 6.4 percent. Employee satisfaction increased in twenty cases and was tied to more pay for increased work plus less supervision and more autonomy. To make job redesign effective nurse managers need to make accurate diagnosis and real job changes. They need to address technological and personnel system constraints, support autonomy, have a bureaucratic climate, have union cooperation, have top management and supervising management support, have individuals ready, and have contextual satisfaction with pay, supervision, promotion opportunities, and coworkers.[37] Some people indicate autonomy and bureaucracy are incompatible. Bureaucratic activities that support professional nurses' autonomy are desirable.

TRAINING

A lack of training is considered a management and organizational shortcoming in which managers allow employees to give unsatisfactory performance. Allowing unsatisfactory performance to exist indicates substandard management. Nurse managers should be educated to make effective performance appraisals that will maintain employee's productivity. Training will entail coverage of such subjects as motivational environment, appropriate job assignment, proper supervision, establishing job expectancies, appropriate job training, interpersonal relationships, interviewing, coaching, counseling, and performance appraisal methods.

Training raters makes performance appraisal work. The goal of such training is improved productivity. A 2-day training program can give nurse managers a conceptual understanding of performance appraisal as a management system for transmitting, reinforcing, and rewarding the behaviors desired by the organization. Raters need to know how performance appraisals will be used. Research indicates that raters have been found to vary ratings depending upon their uses. Refresher training is recommended after one year. Performance appraisal training can be conducted with other management development programs.[38]

An effective appraisal system will have an objective, reliable method to evaluate whether raters are qualified. Training of raters should focus on specific evaluating errors. Research indicates that rater training decreases accuracy because the raters become more sensitive to typical rating error and change their responses, thus creating new errors. Training programs should be designed to increase awareness of this fact and correct for it. Raters will be trained to capture all components of an individual's contribution to the organization, including qualitative behavior. All behavior does not reduce to quantitatively measurable performance.[39]

Training based on feedback is specific. Training of raters should address behavior observation, documentation of critical performance incidents that support the consensus of an evaluation by a team, sensitivity to employees in legally protected categories, and performance criteria.[40]

FEEDBACK

Feedback has been discussed in the section on management by objectives (MBO), a process used in performance appraisal, particularly among management personnel.

An analysis of sixty-nine articles reporting 126 experiments in which feedback was applied indicated feedback with goal setting and/or behavioral consequences was much more consistently effective than feedback alone. Daily and weekly feedback produced more consistent effects than monthly feedback. Also, feedback accompanied by money or fringe benefits of food and gasoline produced improvements in behavior more often than praise. Graphs were the feedback mechanism producing the highest proportion of consistent effects. The conclusion is that feedback graphically presented at least weekly, plus tangible rewards, yields effective work performance.[41]

Other areas for training raters include techniques to overcome cognitive limitations, keeping a diary being one of them. Training will include providing specific feedback to raters on timeliness, completeness, rating errors (1.5 to 2 hours per error), and quality and consistency of ratings. Training methods include case studies, role plays, behavioral modeling, discussion, and writing exercises that evaluate actual appraisals relating them to job descriptions.[42]

Feedback closes the loops by tying the appraisal process together. It informs the ratee of achievements in comparison to expectations. It will be timely, constructive, and objective and ensure that the ratee knows and can respond. The goal is to have good results continued by eliminating frustrations which lead to lowering of goals and of performance.[43]

Rater feedback from team evaluation consensus (TEC) addresses systematic inconsistencies including unlawful bias. Correction by feedback creates improved accuracy of system, improved morale, increased worth, and increased productivity. TEC, which is discussed in more detail below, identifies inaccurate raters for directed training or elimination as raters.[44]

Feedback can be provided through coaching, counseling, and interviewing.

Coaching

The appraisal rater is a leader and a coach. Coaching for job performance is similar to coaching for athletic performance. As a coach the rater does continuous reinforcement of tasks done well and helps with other tasks. In addition the rater uses knowledge of adult education to train the employees to accomplish assigned work, does two-way communication, and has the necessary resources to do the job.

Coaching can include walking around to observe and listen for examples of work, good or bad. The rater coach praises the good and helps improve the bad with a joint action plan. Coaching makes performance evaluation useful.[45]

Coaching is year-long evaluation and discussion of performance. It eliminates surprises. Progress discussions can be brief, regular, frank, open, factual, and include the employee's viewpoint. In the latter instance the rater does not try to achieve truth but to discuss perceptions. The coach also removes obstacles to satisfactory performance. If the consequences are not working to improve unsatisfactory performance, the coach changes them. The ultimate resort is to transfer or terminate the employee.[46]

Counseling

Counseling can be the most productive function of supervision. Counseling interviews are for the purpose of advising and assisting an individual to grow and develop self-direction, self-discipline, and individual responsibility. The counseling interview is a helping relationship involving direct interaction between the counselor (rater) and the counselee (ratee). In a counseling interview there is a personal face-to-face relationship. One person helps another recognize, accept, examine, and solve a certain problem.

Nursing managers can use the counseling interview to offer support and:

- Help workers develop realistic pictures of themselves, their abilities, their potential, and their deficiencies.
- Explore courses of action.
- Explore sources of assistance.
- Accept incontestable limitations and learn to live with them, whether physical, emotional, or intellectual.
- Make choices and improve capabilities.

Unless they have had special training, most nurse managers are not qualified for in-depth, extensive counseling in areas involving personality structure or analysis of psychological or emotional conditions. They must beware of tampering with the psyche of the worker. They should in these cases know and be able to recommend sources of help.

Although counseling interviews are conducted to promote desirable behavior, the term "counseling" should not be used synonymously with the term "reprimand." Reprimands belong more properly in the progress and informational type of interview. One often hears a supervisor say "I have counseled him on what will happen if he does not improve." This is not counseling; this is informing a worker of the consequences of certain types of behavior or performance.

There are three approaches that can be used for the counseling interview—directive, nondirective, and elective. When using the directive approach, the interviewer knows in advance what will be discussed. This approach gives advice, makes suggestions, and helps the individual make meaningful decisions. The interviewer may even take some action on the decisions made. This approach can be used quite successfully with career counseling.

The nondirective approach starts with the individual being counseled: his or her strengths and weaknesses, potential, and problems. The individual takes responsibility for solving the problems; the counselor aids by listening. This is the ideal approach for personal counseling, but requires skill. The person being counseled says what he or she wants and freely expresses feelings. The interviewer

must hide personal feelings and not express personal ideas. The counselor is a mirror only, reflecting the thoughts, ideas, and emotions of the counselee. This technique gives the individual an opportunity to think through problems out loud. Usually the employee will come up with some kind of answer or course of action. In using the nondirective approach it is most important that there be no interruptions or advice on a course of action.

With the exception of the pre-employment interview it is advisable to keep notes during the interview and write a summary afterward. This should indicate any decisions made during the interview and any follow-up action that should be taken. A comment should be made in terms of how well the interview accomplished its purpose. No notes should be taken during the pre-employment interview, although a summary of the interview and the decision reached should be written up immediately afterwards. Taking notes during the actual interview discourages the applicant and makes it difficult to obtain the information needed.

Career progression depends on present and past duty performance, personal initiative, motivation, professional development, and growth potential. Performance counseling of subordinates is vitally important so they will know where they stand, how well they are doing, and where they can improve. The goal of this counseling is to improve present and future performance, not make a critical examination of the past. The informal day-to-day performance counseling dealing with current activities and immediate performance is important and must be continuous, but it is not enough. Planned, careful performance counseling, scheduled at regular intervals, is needed to encourage self-improvement and further development. During the counseling interview the supervisor and subordinate work together to set targets in response to the job description requirements and also targets for future job progression. These are put into writing and progress is reviewed at the next session.

Performance counseling results from observation and evaluation of performance based on job standards. Anecdotal records may be kept and will yield facts to support written ratings or reports.

When counseling employees on performance problems the rater uses a problem-solving approach. This includes reaching agreement that a problem exists, discussing alternative solutions, agreeing on a solution, and following up on progress.[47]

Interviewing

Interviewing is covered in another chapter. The problem-solving approach is also more effective than "tell-and-see" or "tell-and-listen" appraisal interviews. High ratee participation produces greater rater satisfaction. The problem solving rater has a helpful and constructive attitude; does mutual goal setting with the ratee; focuses on solutions of problems; and acts with the knowledge that harsh criticism does not improve behavior.[48]

PEER RATINGS

Research has shown that an individual's peers, the people she or he works with from day to day, are a more reliable source for identifying the capacity for leadership than are the person's superiors. The armed services have found that peer nominations for leadership are significant predictors of future performance. Democratic procedures, having peers select the person to be promoted, would probably be threatening to many nurse managers. It has been found that peer selection differs little from selections of superiors. Occasionally peers see a member or their group as a leader when superiors do not. Peer rating is valid if the members of the group have sufficient interaction and they are reasonably stable over time. It is also valid if the position is important within the organization. Peer rating does help to identify potential leaders who go unnoticed by superiors. Where several individuals are equally qualified for a position, peer ratings may single out the one with the highest informal leadership status.[49]

Peer rating is the professional model of appraisal used by physicians. It is gaining in interest and use among professional nurses. It is advocated as part of a system to make performance appraisals more objective, the theory being that multiple ratings will give a more objective appraisal. They can be obtained from multiple managers, project leaders, peers, and even patients.[50]

SELF-RATINGS

Self-rating is another method of performance appraisal that is little used. In the Fortune 1300 study, 96 percent of appraisals were done by immediate supervisors.[51] Problems with self-rating are the same as with supervisory rating, indicating the need for training of the self-rater as well as the supervisory rater.[52]

Employee-developed performance appraisals have been found to be tougher than those of supervisors. Employees are the subject matter experts and do wider coverage of their jobs. Proactive, they establish expectations beforehand. Appraisal interviews are done after self-evaluation. They are done with a common agenda and without surprises, so conversations are more productive. Objectives are under the employee's control. The job elements and performance indicators come from both employees and supervisors so they are legally defensible, broad in perspective, and elicit employee commitment.[53]

Self-evaluation can be developed by using small groups. Having a good job description facilitates development of good behavioral-expectation appraisal forms. They become customized for each position. The human resources department can provide a facilitator and other support. Some questions that will facilitate performance indicators are:

■ Think of who has been most effective at this element or task. What behaviors and results can you cite to support your choice?
■ Think of the behaviors or results that made you say to yourself, "It would be good if everyone did that."
■ What are the "tricks of the trade" related to this task or element?
■ Think about times when you perform this task well and other times when you are not as successful. What causes the difference?
■ How is the average performer different from the excellent one?
■ If you were training someone, what would you emphasize?[54]

Self-rating has been found to be threatening as the employee places herself or himself in view of others. It is a participatory management approach that research supports. Employees who view the organization as being open are more favorable to participating in performance appraisals.[55]

Employees can be trained to research their own performance and the work environment. They can make self-assessments against goals and expectations and analyze them. Employees can also be trained to influence management communication skills and to provide information and advice, express their needs, and learn the style of influence to use on the manager. Thus employees become proteges of proactive performers.[56]

OTHER RATING METHODOLOGIES

Other rating methodologies are less common than supervisor ratings, peer ratings, and self-ratings. They include team evaluation consensus (TEC) and behavior-anchored rating scales (BARS).

Team Evaluation Consensus

Team Evaluation Consensus (TEC) uses multiple raters, a method claimed to minimize rater bias and inaccuracies. It uses peers, managers, and immediate supervisors for a total of two to eight raters. Direct comparisons are made with other employees or with performance benchmarks of "outstanding" or "consistently exceeds."[57]

Behavior-Anchored Rating Scales

Behavior-Anchored Rating Scales (BARS) list specific descriptors of good, average, and poor performance for each of several to many job aspects. Extensive analysis is required to develop these descriptions, making them time-consuming and difficult to develop. Returns are slight.[58]

PERFORMANCE EVALUATION PROBLEM AREAS

It is largely assumed that merit rating systems of performance evaluation help to develop subordinates and prepare to attest to their readiness for pay increases, promotions, selected assignments, or penalties. When such systems have been scrutinized, three main problem areas have been found:

1. Subordinates have not been motivated to want to change.
2. Even when people recognize a need for a change, they are unable to do so.
3. Subordinates become resentful and anxious when the merit system is implemented conscientiously.[59]

Contrast the following two situations. The same job standards are applied in each case. In the first situation the subordinate is handed a completed rating form and is told to read and sign it. She does so but immediately appeals to the next highest level of supervision, saying that it is the lowest rating she has received in 15 years of work and she has never been counseled that the quality of her performance has been slipping. Even though the situation is resolved in favor of the subordinate, she is no longer satisfied to work for the supervisor and has to be transferred.

In another situation the job standards are discussed with the subordinate before they are used. The subordinate is asked to identify those performance factors and responsibilities that are really important to the success of the unit. She is asked to write out the goals of her job as she sees them. They are fully discussed between supervisor and subordinate. Progress is discussed at the request of the subordinate and at stated intervals. As a result the subordinate is assisted in planning educational activities that she will accomplish in preparation for the career she desires.

Which situation meets the criterion of an effective performance appraisal?

There are many pitfalls and deficiencies in performance appraisal. Many managers defend it as a system for improving performance. As used, it probably has negative influences, since most people know their shortcomings better than a supervisor. Criticisms by people who have not been adequately trained to manage an appraisal system cause employees to be anxious and frustrated, to feel themselves failures, and, in some cases, to withdraw.

What are the weaknesses? The rater is influenced by the most recent period of performance, an influence that may be positive or negative. Without objective measurements and records, raters tend to focus on the few outstanding activities that are vivid in their minds. Personal feelings influence raters, causing positive or negative halo effects. In many instances the performance is appraised without clear job definitions, job descriptions, and job standards. The employee seldom knows the yardsticks by which performance is being measured. Raters are either lenient or tough, making a great variance in value judgments. Attitudes about whether the employee deserves a pay increase influence the rater. Some managers believe that all employees are average, and they project their beliefs by rating all alike.[60]

Other rating errors include:

■ Leniency/stringency error. The rater tends to assign extreme ratings of either poor or excellent.
■ Similar-to-me error. The rater rates according to how he views himself.
■ Central tendency error. All ratings are at the middle of the scale.
■ First impression error. The rater views early behavior that may be good or bad and rates all subsequent behaviors similarly.

Other problems of performance appraisal include racial bias, focus on longevity, and complacency of managers. In their usual form they are intrinsically confrontational, emotional, judgmental, and complex. A survey of 360 managers in 190 corporations indicated that 69 percent viewed objectives as unclear; 40 percent saw some payoff but 29 percent saw minimal benefits; 45 percent were only partially involved in setting objectives for their own performance; 81 percent indicated regular progress reviews were not conducted; 52 percent said guidelines for collecting performance data were haphazard or nonexistent; a scant 19 percent viewed performance appraisal as properly planned; and only 37 percent viewed meetings as highly productive, while 30 percent saw no worthwhile results.[61]

Performance appraisals are extrinsically affected when format is improper due to lack of manager preparation, confusion about objectives, once-a-year activity, and overreliance on forms. Also, there is the extrinsic area of inappropriate values and attitudes: avoidance of conflict to avoid unpleasantness; lack of respect in failing to take the appraisal seriously; and misuse of power causing the ratee to be beaten down, resentful, and uncommitted.[62]

EFFECTIVE MANAGEMENT OF PERFORMANCE APPRAISAL

How do we overcome these pitfalls or deficiencies? First, we must be aware of them. Second, we can learn the management-by-objectives approach and treat people as people. Employees will know by what yardsticks they will be measured. The appraisal will be a joint project. It will be a helpful situation for rater and ratee. Usually, if the situation is working right, the ratee will push herself or himself.

A complex and lengthy evaluation form has not proved effective in rating personnel. Many managers have reduced their rating system to a limited checklist and a write-up that asks for strengths and weaknesses with specific examples to justify each. Many managers will agree to the following principles for a rating system:

1. It should be a simple and effective plan.
2. The procedures and uses of the plan should be understood and agreed upon by line management.
3. Factors to be rated should be measurable and agreed upon by managers and subordinates.
4. Raters should understand the purpose and nature of the performance review. They should be taught to use the system, observe, write notes including a critical incident file, organize notes and write evaluations that include examples of evidence, edit their reports, and conduct effective review interviews.
5. Raters should understand the meanings of the dimensions rated including their relative weights. Managers are reported to be able to distinguish between only three levels of performance: poor, satisfactory, and outstanding.
6. Criticism should promote warmth and the building of self-esteem with both the rater and the ratee.
7. The process should be organized and used to manage people on a daily basis.
8. Praise or suggestions for improvement should be done at the time of the event.
9. Standards of performance should be set and modified at the time of the event.
10. Performance standards should be valid, reliable, and fair.
11. Managers should be rewarded for good performance evaluation skills.
12. Professionally accepted procedures should be used for job analysis, developing job-related observable performance criteria, and job classifications. This approach ensures fairness as

processes are applied systematically and uniformly throughout the organization.

13. Use a fair employment posture committed to equal opportunity. A conscientious and equitable appraisal system reduces lawsuits and assures fairness and confidence.

14. Measure work output, not habits and traits such as loyalty *unless* they are described by observed behavior examples.

15. Use multiple ratings including those of ratees subordinates.[63]

SUMMARY

Performance appraisal is a major component of the evaluating or controlling function of nursing management. It is disliked by both raters and ratees. If used appropriately and conscientiously the performance appraisal process will govern employee behavior to produce goods and services in high volume and of high quality.

Purposes or uses of performance evaluation are multiple. In nursing it is used to motivate employees to produce high-quality patient care. The results of performance appraisal are often used for promotion, selection, termination, and improving performance.

Performance appraisal is a part of the science of behavior technology and should be viewed as part of that body of knowledge that relates to the management of human behavior. Nurse managers need this knowledge to manage the clinical nurse effectively and efficiently as a human resource.

When used for merit pay increases—a retrospective use—performance appraisal should be separated from that which looks to the future. Output-based pay plans have been more effective than time-based pay plans.

Performance appraisal should be done as a system with:

1. Clearly defined performance standards developed by rater and ratee.
2. Objective application of the performance standards—both rater and ratee measuring the latter's performance against the standards.
3. Planned interval feedback with agreed-upon improvements when indicated.
4. A continuous cycle. Raters and ratees should trust each other.

Job analysis and job description are essential instruments of behavior technology used in performance appraisal. They provide objectivity and discriminate among jobs.

Coaching, counseling, and interviewing are skills of an effective performance appraisal system. In addition to supervisor ratings, performance appraisal can include peer ratings, self-ratings, team evaluation consensus (TEC), and behavior-anchored rating scales (BARS).

Problems with performance appraisal systems include poor preparation of raters and ratees, problems of recency, positive and negative halo effects, lack of use of standards, leniency/stringency errors, similar-to-me errors, central tendency errors, and first impression errors.

A simple, well-planned performance appraisal system can be devised. It will be successful when understood by employees and will require considerable supervisory effort using nursing management theory.

NOTES

1. S. Krantz, "Five Steps to Making Performance Appraisal Writing . . ," *Supervisory Management*, Dec. 1983, 7–10.
2. R. Zemke, "Is Performance Appraisal a Paper Tiger?" *Training*, Dec. 1985, 24–32.
3. S. Krantz, op. cit.
4. C. J. Fombrun and R. L. Land, "Strategic Issues in Performance Appraisal: Theory and Practice," *Personnel*, Nov.-Dec. 1983, 23–31.
5. Ibid.
6. C. E. Schneier, A. Geis, and J. A. Wert, "Performance Appraisals: No Appointment Needed," *Personnel Journal*, Nov. 1987, 80–87.
7. R. Zemke, op. cit.
8. D. M. Brethower and G. A. Rummler, "For Improved Work Performance: Accentuate the Positive," *Personnel*, Sept./Oct. 1966, 40–49.
9. A. Levenstein, "Feedback Improves Performance," *Nursing Management*, February, 1984, 65–66.
10. R. Zemke, op. cit.
11. D. L. Kirkpatrick, "Performance Appraisal: When Two Jobs Are Too Many," *Training*, Mar. 1986, 65, 67–79.
12. Ibid.
13. R. E. Kopelman, "Linking Pay to Performance Is a Proven Management Tool," *Personnel Administrator*, Oct. 1983, 60–68.
14. Ibid.
15. Ibid.
16. N. R. Deets and D. T. Tyler, "How Xerox Improved Its Performance Appraisals," *Personnel Journal*, Apr. 1986, 50–52.

17. B. Jacobson and B. L. Kaye, "Career Development and Performance Appraisal: It Takes Two to Tango," *Personnel,* Jan. 1986, 26–32.
18. R. M. Fulmer and S. G. Franklin, *Supervision: Principles of Professional Management* (2d. ed. New York: Macmillan, 1982), 214–215.
19. H. Koontz and H. Weihrich, *Management,* 9th ed. (New York: McGraw Hill, 1988), 490–494.
20. J. M. Ganong and W. L. Ganong, *Nursing Management,* 2d ed. (Rockville, MD: Aspen Publications, 1980), 191.
21. H. Koontz and H. Weihrich, op. cit., 493–494.
22. B. Blai, "An Appraisal System That Yields Results," *Supervisory Management,* Nov. 1983, 39–42.
23. M. G. Friedman, "10 Steps to Objective Appraisals," *Personnel Journal,* June 1986, 66–71.
24. M. R. Edwards and J. R. Sproull, "Safeguarding Your Employee Rating System," *Business,* Apr.-June, 1985, 17–27.
25. S. Price and J. Graber, "Employee-Made Appraisals," *Management World,* Feb. 1986, 34–36.
26. D. Ignatavicius and J. Griffith, "Job Analysis: The Basis for Effective Appraisal," *The Journal of Nursing Administration,* July-Aug. 1982, 37–41.
27. J. Markowitz, "Managing the Job Analysis Process," *Training and Development Journal,* Aug. 1987, 64–66.
28. D. Ignatavicius and J. Griffith, op. cit.; J. Markowitz, op. cit.; E. P. Prien, I. L. Goldstein, and W. H. Macey, "Multidomain Job Analysis: Procedures and Applications," *Training and Development Journal,* Aug. 1987, 68–72.
29. P. R. Coaly and P. R. Sackett, "Effects of Using High- Versus Low-Performing Job Incumbents as Sources of Job Analysis Information," *Journal of Applied Psychology,* Aug. 1987, 434–437.
30. C. Berenson and H. O. Ruhnke, "Job Descriptions: Guidelines for Personnel Management," *Personnel Journal,* January 1966, 14–19.
31. W. R. Kennedy, "Train Managers to Write Winning Job Descriptions," *Training and Development Journal,* Apr. 1987, 62–64.
32. H. S. Rowland and B. L. Rowland, Eds., *Hospital Legal Forms, Checklists, and Guidelines* (Rockville, MD: Aspen, 1987), 23:28.
33. A. Waintroob, "Comparable Worth Issue: The Employer's Side," *The Hospital Manager,* July-Aug. 1985, 6–7.
34. TNA's Professional Services Committee, "Nurses and the Comparable Worth Concept," *Texas Nursing,* Apr. 1985, 12–16.
35. "How to Establish the Comparable Worth of a Job—Or One Way to Compare Apples and Oranges," *California Nurse,* Mar./Apr. 1982, 10–11; TNA's Professional Services Committee, op. cit.
36. B. R. Helton, "Will the Real Knowledge Worker Please Stand Up?," *Industrial Management,* Jan.-Feb. 1987, 26–29.
37. R. G. Kopelman, "Job Redesign and Productivity: A Review of the Evidence," *National Productivity Review,* Summer 1985, 237–255.
38. D. C. Martin and K. M. Bardol, "Training the Raters: A Key to Effective Performance Appraisal," *Public Personnel Management,* Summer 1986, 101–109.
39. M. R. Edwards and J. R. Sproull, op. cit.
40. Ibid.
41. F. Balcazar, B. L. Hopkin, and Y. Suarez, "A Critical, Objective Review of Performance Feedback," *Journal of Organizational Behavior Management,* Fall 1985/Winter 1985–86, 65–89.
42. D. C. Martin and K. M. Bardal, op. cit.; M. G. Friedman, op. cit.
43. T. A. Ratcliffe and D. J. Logsdon, "The Business Planning Process—A Behavioral Perspective," *Managerial Planning,* Mar./Apr. 1980, 32–38.
44. M. R. Edward and J. R. Sproull, op. cit.
45. C. E. Schneier, A. Geis, and J. A. Wert, op. cit.
46. V. D. Lachman, "Increasing Productivity Through Performance Evaluation," *The Journal of Nursing Administration,* Dec. 1984, 7–14.
47. Ibid.
48. D. C. Martin and C. M. Bardol, op. cit.
49. G. S. Booker and R. W. Miller, "A Closer Look at Peer Ratings," *Personnel,* Jan.-Feb. 1966, 42–47.
50. M. G. Friedman, op. cit.
51. C. J. Fombrun and R. L. Land, op. cit.
52. R. Zemke, op. cit.
53. S. Price and J. Graber, "Employee-Made Appraisals," *Management World,* Feb. 1986, 34–36.
54. Ibid.
55. M. P. Lovrich, "The Dangers of Participative Management: A Test of Unexamined Assumptions Concerning Employee Involvement," *Review of Public Personnel Administration,* Summer 1985, 9–25.
56. B. Jacobson and B. L. Kaye, op. cit.
57. M. R. Edwards and J. R. Sproull, op. cit.
58. R. Zemke, op. cit.; M. R. Edwards and J. R. Sproull, op. cit.
59. W. M. Fox, "Evaluating and Developing Subordinates," *Notes and Quotes,* April 1969, 4.
60. J. C. Coyant, "The Performance Appraisal: A Critique and an Alternative," *Business Horizons,* June 1973, 73–78.
61. R. E. Lefton, "Performance Appraisal: Why They Go Wrong and How to Do Them Right," *National Productivity Review,* Winter 1985, 54–63.
62. Ibid.
63. S. Krantz, op. cit.; D. C. Martin and K. M. Bardol, op. cit.; C. Logan, "Praise: The Powerhouse of Self-Esteem," *Nursing Management,* June 1985, 36, 38; M. G. Friedman, op. cit.; C. E. Schneier, J. A. Geis, and J. A. Wert, op. cit.; M. R. Edwards and J. R. Sproull, op. cit.; E. Y. Breeze, "The Performance Review," *Manage,* February 1968, 6–11.

REFERENCES

American Hospital Association Council on Nursing and the American Organization of Nurse Executives, *Guidelines: Role and Functions of the Hospital Nurse Executive* (Chicago: American Hospital Association, 1985).

Davis, D. S., A. E. Greig, J. Burkholder, and T. Keating, "Evaluating Advance Practice Nurses," *Nursing Management,* Mar. 1984, 44–47.

Fouracre, S., and A. Wright, "New Factors in Job Evaluation," *Personnel Management,* May 1986, 40–43.

Idaszak, J. R., and F. Drasgow, "A Revision of the Job Diagnostic Survey: Elimination of a Measurement Artifact," *Journal of Applied Psychology*, Feb. 1987, 69–74.

Lawler, F. E. III, "What's Wrong with Point Factor Job Evaluation?," *Management Review*, Nov. 1986, 44–48.

Lee, M. A., "How to Use Job Analysis Technique," *Restaurant Management*, Apr. 1987, 84–85.

Meyer, A. L., "A Framework for Assessing Performance Problems," *The Journal of Nursing Administration*, May 1984, 40–43.

Murphy, K. R., B. A. Gannett, B. M. Herr, and J. A. Chen, "Effects of Subsequent Performance on Evaluation of Previous Performance," *Journal of Applied Psychology*, Aug. 1986, 427–431.

Pollock, T., "The Fine Art of Speaking from a Desk," and "How Do You Look to Your Boss?," *Production*, July 1985, 27–29.

Pollock, T., "Are You Getting Better?," *Production*, Aug. 1985, 33.

Reed, P. A., and M. J. Kroll, "A Two-Perspective Approach to Performance Appraisal," *Personnel*, Oct. 1985, 51–57.

Schnake, M. G. and M. P. Dumler, "Affective Response Bias in The Measurement of Perceived Task Characteristics," *Journal of Occupational Psychology*, June 1985, 159–166.

St. John, W. D., "Leveling with Employees," *Personnel Journal*, Aug. 1984, 52–57.

Weingard, M., "Establishing Comparable Worth Through Job Evaluation," *Nursing Outlook*, Mar./Apr. 1984, 110–113.

How to Do a Merit Pay Increase

INTRODUCTION

Merit is a term that is becoming increasingly associated with performance and pay increases, particularly for teachers and university faculties and staffs. Merit means that employees receive what they earn or deserve. Their pay and rewards are based on the degree of competence they demonstrate in performing their jobs. Merit systems can include both rewards and punishments. The general goal of a merit performance and pay system is to reward people on an incremental scale so that the top achievers or performers are paid the highest salary.

A merit pay system must have four components:

1. Individual performance standards.
2. Measurement scales.
3. A budget.
4. An award procedure.

These procedures must meet Standard NR.3 of the Accreditation Manual for Hospitals, which states:

> **NR.3.7** Job descriptions for each position classification of registered nurses and other nursing personnel specify standards of performance and delineate the functions, responsibilities, and specific qualifications of each classification.
>
> **NR.3.7.1** Job descriptions are made available to nursing personnel at the time they are hired and when requested.
>
> **NR.3.7.2** Job descriptions are reviewed periodically and revised as needed to reflect current job requirements.
>
> **NR.3.8** A written evaluation of the performance of registered nurses and other nursing personnel is made at the end of the probationary period and at a defined interval thereafter.
>
> **NR.3.8.1** The evaluation is criteria-based and relates to the standards of performance specified in the individual's job description.
>
> **NR.3.8.1.1** An annual evaluation is recommended.[1]

538

Merit pay increases are an employee incentive program. Employees who have their competencies developed, encouraged, and recognized have better attitudes about their work and their employers. These employees will work to achieve organizational objectives that are supportive of their personal objectives.

Merit pay increases are extrinsic rewards or punishments. The reward can be in the form of promotion, praise, recognition, criticism, social acceptance or rejection, or fringe benefits.[2]

Many of these rewards or punishments are activated with a total merit pay increase system. Extrinsic rewards need to be associated with the intrinsic rewards that come from employee's participation in making decisions about their work and the conditions under which they will perform their work. Professional nurses want control of their nursing practice. They want to participate in management decisions about how they will accomplish this. As a result they will receive intrinsic rewards from having made the organization successful, as they have contributed to that success.

FIGURE 25–1. Policy on Evaluation of Personnel Performance

All nursing service employees will have a criteria-based performance evaluation as follows:

1. Initiated upon employee orientation.
2. At the end of the probationary period (6 months).
3. Annually (to be initiated during the following evaluation period for all employees). The annual performance evaluation will be cosigned by the head nurse or supervisor and employee and filed in the employee's personnel file.
4. Upon termination of employment or transfer from one unit to another. When an employee terminates employment or transfers there shall be an evaluation conference. A completed performance results contract will be cosigned by the employee and head nurse/supervisor, then placed in the personnel file.

Conferences and renegotiation concerning the criteria-based performance evaluation may occur as often as the employee/supervisor deems necessary.

SOURCE: Courtesy of the University of South Alabama Medical Center, Mobile, Alabama.

PERFORMANCE STANDARDS

Individual performance standards are written criteria developed by the supervisor in conference with the individual to be evaluated. They evolve from an established, more generalized set of job performance criteria, the job description. These performance standards are tailored to the individual's abilities and goals as well as the common expectations of themselves and their supervisor. They should be measurable and they should be objectively applied. The supervisor and employee can both observe or know that the standard has been met. These standards can be written in the format of a Performance Results Contract related to the job description. Figure 25–1 represents a division of nursing policy. The procedure for implementation of this policy involves use of a job description (Figure 25–2) and a performance results contract (Figure 25–3).

MEASUREMENT SCALES

The weights assigned to each key results area can be in terms of units or percentages. It is more practical to assign up to 1.0 unit to each key results area and determine the percentage of achievement at the annual or final conference. This allows objectives to be added, modified, or deleted without readjusting the percentage weight. In Figure 25–3 the weights are the numbers assigned to each key results area. The total of these is 100. If the employee achieves 90 then the percentage of achievement for merit pay purposes is 90 percent. This figure is used to allocate budgeted wage and salary increases.

BUDGET

Personnel pay increases are usually projected in the operational budget represented by excerpt in Table 25–1. They can be related to increases in the consumer price index, to the market place, or the financial status of the institution. The last must be a major consideration. The organization personnel department usually prepares a cost analysis by position (Table 25–1). This is the bridge for merit pay increases for the total nursing division.

FIGURE 25–2. Sample Job Description for Clinical Nurse Consultant

Job Summary   Performs the primary functions of facilitator, teacher, and resource person in assessing, planning, organizing, implementing, and evaluating staff development programs for a specified area or clinical group on a 24-hour basis. Performs selected primary clinical functions of a professional nurse.

Performance Requirements   Responsible for: Designing programs which facilitate the attainment of standards of care established by the Joint Commission on Accreditation of Healthcare Organizations and the University of South Alabama Medical Center. Assists nursing staff to acquire the knowledge and skills necessary to fulfill their role expectation in nursing service. Fosters a climate in which nursing staff identify their own learning needs and seek opportunities to meet these needs. Initiates and/or participates in studies and research activities related to staff development and health care.

Physical demands: Excellent physical and mental health required. Must be able to make acute sensory perceptions. Stands, sits, or walks during most of the time at work. Uses good posture and body mechanics in working with patients.

Special Demands: Assumes total responsibility for setting and achieving objectives for a given clinical assignment to assist nursing staff to maintain and improve their competency in the provision of health care. This will include periodic tours or hours of duty with the evening and night personnel. Must use tact and be able to effectively coordinate with personnel of all other departments. Promotes and exercises leadership in affecting appropriate changes. Applies concepts of adult education in planning, implementing, and evaluating learning experiences. Participates in centralized programs within staff development.

Qualifications   Education: Graduate of an accredited school of nursing. Current registered nurse license for state of Alabama. Knowledge in clinical area, in principles of adult education, and in managing people.

Training and experience: Master's degree in nursing, three years clinical experience or bachelor's degree in nursing, three years clinical experience with education training and work toward a master's degree.

Professional growth: Is expected to pursue programs of continuing education including professional meetings, education conferences, and college courses that will update and maintain professional knowledge and skills related to the management of the unit or ward, its people and material resources, and its patients.

Work Performed   Authority: Delegated by the director of nursing for staff development commensurate with responsibilities assigned.

Duties: To provide learning opportunities for a specified group and serve as a resource person for nursing service in general.

1. Collaborate with the nursing service personnel to provide educational programming consistent with expected clinical performance through such means as:
   1.1 Participating in regularly established meetings of the Nursing Council.
   1.2 Establishing meeting times with head nurses and other leadership personnel concerned with specific programming.
   1.3 Contributing to the development of philosophy, objectives, policies, procedures, and position descriptions for the nursing service department.
   1.4 Participating in establishing priorities for staff development activities.
2. Provide leadership in formulating the philosophy and objectives of the nursing service department.
3. Project and implement a budget that will provide the necessary human and physical resources to achieve goals of the program, cost-effectiveness, and cost containment by:
   3.1 Utilizing short- and long-range goals as a basis for budget planning.
   3.2 Involving appropriate people in preparation and review of the budget.
   3.3 Identifying adequate funds needed to plan, conduct, and evaluate the staff development program.
   3.4 Maintaining budget control by comparing actual expenditures with current budget at regular intervals.
   3.5 Evaluating cost-effectiveness and cost containment in the achievement of program goals as a basis for planning the budget for the next fiscal year.
4. Identify learning needs of employees by using, but not being limited to:
   4.1 Position descriptions.
   4.2 Personal observations and those of others.
   4.3 Interviews, questionnaires, surveys, and reports.
   4.4 Minutes of meetings.
   4.5 Policies, procedures, and directives.
   4.6 Current literature.
   4.7 Incident/accident reports.

FIGURE 25-2. Sample Job Description for Clinical Nurse Consultant (*continued*)

4.8 Quality assurance review.

4.9 Employee performance appraisals.

4.10 Achievement results of personnel in relation to expected outcomes of staff development offerings.

4.11 The employee's identification of his or her own learning needs.

4.12 Established standards of care.

4.13 Conferences with supervisory personnel and the director of nursing service.

5. Plan offerings that correlate with the total program or curriculum and lead to the desired behavior. Steps in planning include:

5.1 Establishing priorities for learning.

5.2 Allowing sufficient planning time.

5.3 Setting reasonable and attainable objectives.

5.4 Determining criteria for measurement of expected behavioral change(s).

5.5 Developing course outlines and teaching strategies.

5.6 Identifying appropriate media, teaching methods, and resources.

5.7 Arranging for space, equipment, and teaching aids.

5.8 Informing participants and others concerned about the offerings.

6. Communicate the plan for the program to encourage and foster participation and cooperation through:

6.1 Discussing plans with appropriate individuals and/or groups.

6.2 Utilizing posters, flyers, newsletter copy, and other materials to publicize educational offerings.

7. Implement the established plan to meet learning needs by:

7.1 Establishing an effective teaching/learning climate.

7.2 Exercising flexibility in use of time, space, equipment, and instructional plans.

8. Evaluate results of the total staff development program effort as well as specific learning offerings.

9. Participate with others in counseling personnel about their educational needs.

10. Initiate and/or participate in studies and research activities related to staff development education and evaluate reported studies and research findings for application to staff development programming.

11. Develop and maintain a recording system to document achievement of program goals and objectives and serve as a guide for planning by:

11.1 Determining types of records to be maintained in the categories of total program, single offering, individual, and budget.

11.2 Designing a system in which essential information is recorded and easily retrieved.

11.3 Utilizing records for evaluating accomplishment of goals and objectives for research purposes and future planning.

12. Orient personnel to philosophy, objectives, policies, procedures, role expectations, and physical facilities of the institution through a planned orientation program.

13. Coordinate cardiopulmonary resuscitation certification classes for all nursing personnel.

14. Direct and/or participate in the evaluation of new products.

15. Pursue activities which further the staff development educator's own professional growth and development by:

15.1 Seeking new concepts in professional and other relevant literature and sharing such knowledge and information with colleagues.

15.2 Participating in inter- and intradepartmental meetings within the health-care facility.

15.3 Participating in professional organizations and community projects.

15.4 Attending workshops, seminars, and academic courses.

15.5 Engaging in appropriate independent learning activities or projects.

SOURCE: Courtesy of the University of South Alabama Medical Center, Mobile, Alabama.

AWARD PROCEDURE

Nurse administrators take all performance results contracts for each category of nursing personnel and add up the percent totals for all persons (for the nurse in Figure 25–3 this was 90 percent). The total for Registered Teaching Nurse II (RTN II) positions was 1.911 percent. This number is divided into the total budgeted dollars for RTN II which was

FIGURE 25–3. Sample Performance Results Contract

1. Scope of Responsibility: As clinical nurse consultant, assumes responsibility to improve the quality of health care received by the patient in her defined clinical area of expertise through role modeling, teaching, consultation and research. The consultant assists nursing personnel to achieve their full potential and satisfaction in providing effective, efficient, and individualized care to patients and their families. The clinical nurse consultant is self-directive, determining the priorities of her role through inter- and intradisciplinary collaboration. She evaluates her own practice based on the attainment of individual objectives. She is responsible to the director of nursing for staff development.

2. Key Results Areas

Performance Results	Individual's Performance
2.1 Schedule monthly meetings with head nurses of each unit to discuss needs and to plan for utilization of clinical consultant in meeting those needs.	I would like to see more assertive behavior in this area. Meetings were often put off & not enough consistent followup—head nurses to set a time. 8%
2.2 Present inservice for each area as contracted with head nurses.	Observations and needs should be made by both parties in setting up classes. This area has improved since Jan. in some units. 7%
2.3 Work with department members to evaluate and revise nursing orientation program.	Done. New schedule completed. Meeting held—head nurses of 5th, 6th, 7th, and 8th floors. 10%
2.4 Orient new staff to orientation program.	Worked with (name). 10%
2.5 Co-ordinate nursing orientation program with Staff Development, Personnel Relations and Nursing Service.	Continuous need for smooth co-ordination & double checking on dates. 9%
2.6 Review and revise medication exam as necessary.	Recommendation made to (name). 10%
2.7 Assist in teaching CPR as directed.	Class taught as scheduled. 10%
2.8 Continue to coordinate and present Drug Update.	Aminoglycoside (Antihypertensive agents, Penicillin, March) Series started in Sept. Was delayed in start. Need for assertion in meeting this objective. 9%
2.9 Present classes based on needs survey.	Equipment Fair done. Coordinated with (name). 10%
2.10 Participate in critical care course—present emergency re-insertion of tracheostomy tube.	Content approved by Alabama Board of Nursing. Very poor evaluations from second class with many negative comments written and verbalized. 7%

Complete for Terminal Evaluation Only:

	Excellent	Good	Fair	Poor
Attendance				
Initiative				
Quantity of work				
Quality of work				
Cooperation				

Eligible for rehire _____ Yes _____ No

FIGURE 25–3. Sample Performance Results Contract (*continued*)

3. *Authority Codes*
    A. Does without reporting
    B. Does and Reports
    C. Gets approval before doing
    D. Participates in
    E. Recommends to supervisor
    F. Assists supervisor under direction

Summary

    (Name) has been flexible in coming in for classes on 3–11 and 11–7 shifts. She has completed most of the areas on her performance contract satisfactorily. She is generally well received by new employees and helpful in their orientation to USAMC.

    I would like for (Name) to take more initiative and to be more assertive in identifying needs with the head nurses of the clinical units and in addressing those needs promptly and consistently. She has been active in emergency admission unit and I would like for her to be more active on 6th and 9th floors and the burn unit.

    I would also ask (Name) to address her concerns and questions to me directly.

Director Staff Development
May 8, 1989

SOURCE: Courtesy of the University of South Alabama Medical Center, Mobile, Alabama.

TABLE 25–1. Budget for Four Percent Merit Pay Increase

Position Classification	Hospital Nursing Positions					
	FTE Filled	Total Current Salaries	Cost	FTE Vacant	Total Current Salaries	Cost
Licensed practical nurse	84.50	$1,108,339	$44,334	9.00	$110,021	$ 4,401
RTN I—clinical level I	249.00	4,607,379	184,295	18.00	312,794	12,512
RTN I—clinical level II	14.00	292,921	11,717	1.00	20,255	810
RTN I—clinical level III	1.00	22,755	910	0.00	0	0
RTN I (working supervisor)	45.00	893,820	35,753	0.00	0	0
Registered teaching nurse II	20.00	443,126	17,725	2.00	38,438	1,538
Nursing service supervisor I	11.50	266,910	10,676	2.00	40,228	1,609
	425.00	$7,635,250	$305,410	32.00	$521.736	$20,869
Total cost: Annual			$305,410			$20,869
Monthly			$25,451			$1,739

SOURCE: Courtesy of the University of South Alabama Medical Center, Mobile, Alabama.

$19,263 (the sum of the amounts for filled and vacant positions in Table 25–1.) For each percent, each person in this category will be allocated $10.08. A person who receives a 90 percent merit pay increase will receive 90 × $10.08 = $907.20 (see Table 25–2). This amount is transferred to a personnel action memorandum and processed through payroll. Each employee is told by their supervisor how much merit pay they will receive.

THE PROCESS

Step 1: Employee and supervisor have an appointed conference to establish the key results areas (objectives) that the employee will accomplish over an agreed-upon period of time. These will include organizational objectives of the supervisor and personal objectives of the employee. Each will come to the conference table prepared to present their objectives in an atmosphere of mutual trust and cooperation. At this conference the wording of the key results areas will be negotiated, weights will be assigned to each, time frames will be established, controls or reporting authority will be established,

and the approximate date will be set for the next evaluation conference.

Step 2: A definitive date is established and the next conference is held. At this conference the supervisor and employee discuss progress in accomplishment of key results areas. They modify objectives by negotiation, discard those they agree are no longer relevant, add new ones as needed, and discuss and record progress in accomplishment of each. This conference and all succeeding ones can be scheduled at earlier dates should either supervisor or employee request it.

Step 3: Conferences are scheduled at 1- to 3-month intervals until the probationary period is completed, the annual rating is required, or the employee transfers or terminates. At these times the contract is summarized, signed by both employee and supervisor, and filed in the employee's personnel folder. The weights assigned by negotiated discussion are totalled and a number is assigned. This number is used in allocating the merit pay increase.

As has been discussed earlier merit pay is a difficult procedure to implement as employees may not agree with the outcome. Also, supervisors are hesitant to make decisions that give employees variable pay increases. Some experts suggest that merit performance appraisal be separated from performance appraisal for future performance. The author has found that the two can work together when planned, communicated, and fairly applied.

TABLE 25–2. Calculating merit increase for RTN II positions

Percent	Amount	Percent	Amount
100	$1008	71	$716
99	998	70	706
98	988	69	696
97	978	68	685
96	968	67	675
95	958	66	665
94	948	65	655
93	937	64	645
92	927	63	635
91	917	62	625
90	907	61	615
89	897	60	605
88	887	50	504
87	877	40	403
86	867	30	302
85	857	20	202

SOURCE: Courtesy of the University of South Alabama Medical Center, Mobile, Alabama.

SUMMARY

Merit pay increases are designed to reward employees for past performance based on the degree to which they meet the standards of their jobs. Merit pay increases include use of individual performance standards developed by individual employees and their supervisors. A measurement scale is used to quantify the degree by which the employee meets the agreed upon standards. A budget is established to pay for the merit pay increase based upon award procedures known to employees and supervisors.

NOTES

1. "Nursing Services NR.3," *Accreditation Manual for Hospitals* (Chicago, IL: Joint Commission On Accreditation of Healthcare Organizations, 1989), 136.
2. D. McGregor, *Leadership and Motivation* (Cambridge, MA: MIT Press, 1966), 203–204.

Author Index

545

Subject Index